CD

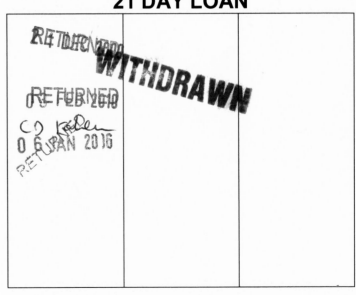

Metastatic Carcinomas
of Unknown Origin

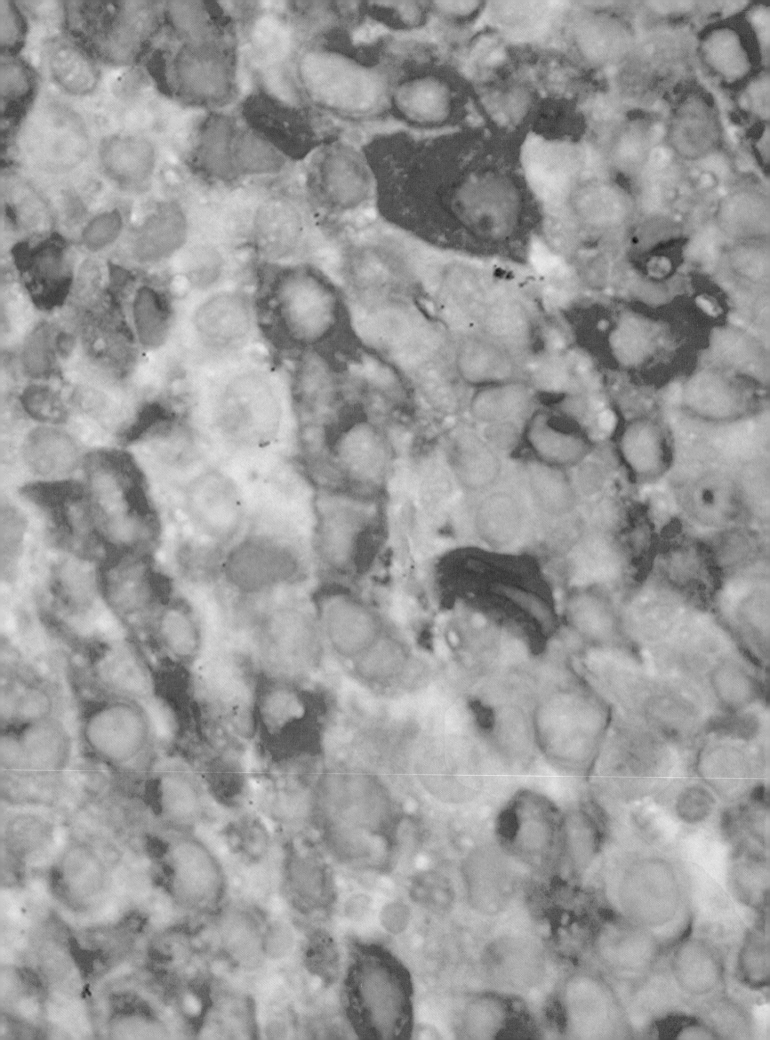

Metastatic Carcinomas of Unknown Origin

EDITOR

Mark R. Wick, MD

Department of Pathology

Division of Surgical Pathology and Cytopathology

University of Virginia Health System

Charlottesville, Virginia

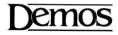 New York

Acquisitions Editor: R. Craig Percy
Book Designer: Steven Pisano
Compositor and Indexer: Egerton Group
Printer: RR Donnelley

Visit our website at www.demosmedpub.com

Library of Congress Cataloging-in-Publication Data

Metastatic carcinomas of unknown origin/editor, Mark R. Wick
   p. ; cm.
   Includes bibliographical references and index.
   ISBN 1-933864-32-X (hardcover: alk. paper) 1. Cancer of unknown primary origin. I. Wick, Mark R., 1952-
   [DNLM: 1. Neoplasms, Unknown Primary. QZ 202 M58728 2008]
   RC268.48.M48 2008
   616.99'4071–dc22   2008007705

Medicine is an ever-changing science undergoing continual development. Research and clinical experience are continually expanding our knowledge, in particular our knowledge of proper treatment and drug therapy. The authors, editors, and publisher have made every effort to ensure that all information in this book is in accordance with the state of knowledge at the time of production of the book.

Nevertheless, this does not imply or express any guarantee or responsibility on the part of the authors, editors, or publisher with respect to any dosage instructions and forms of application stated in the book. Every reader should examine carefully the package inserts accompanying each drug and check with a physician or specialist whether the dosage schedules mentioned therein or the contraindications stated by the manufacturer differ from the statements made in this book. Such examination is particularly important with drugs that are either rarely used or have been newly released on the market. Every dosage schedule or every form of application used is entirely at the reader's own risk and responsibility. The editors and publisher welcome any reader to report to the publisher any discrepancies or inaccuracies noticed.

Made in the United States of America

08 09 10 11 5 4 3 2 1

Contents

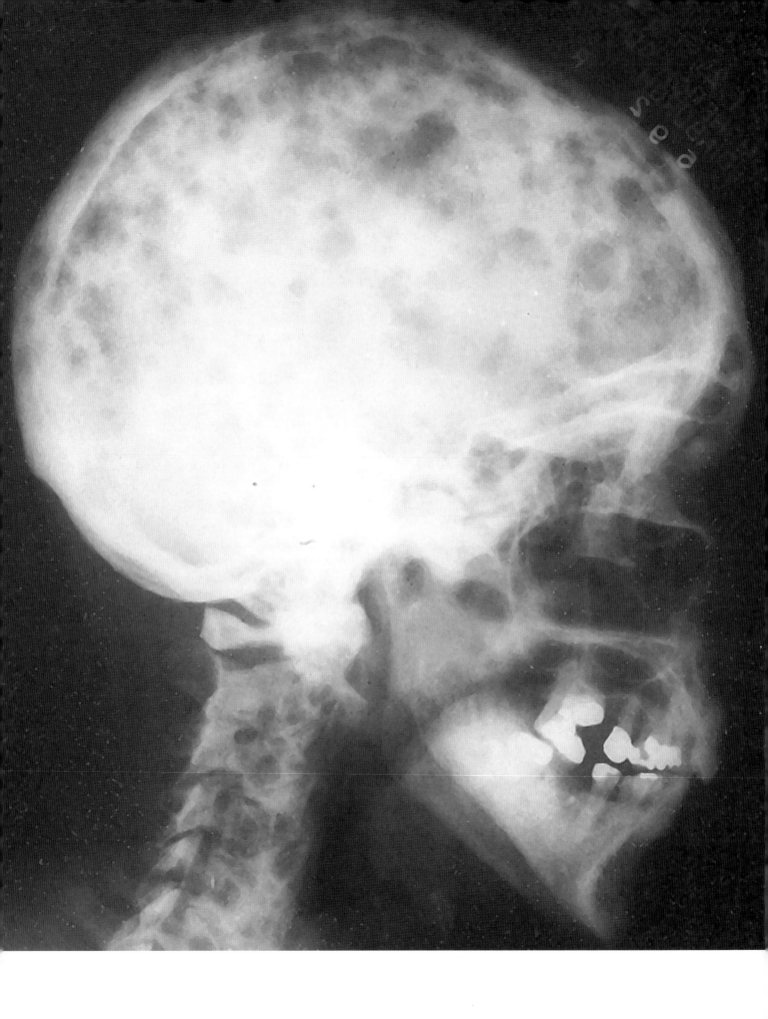

Preface

THE AMERICAN CANCER SOCIETY estimated that more than 30,000 new cases of metastatic carcinoma of unknown origin (MCUO; also known as "carcinoma of unknown primary" [CUP]) would be identified in the United States in 2007. That figure corresponds to approximately 2% of all new cancers seen yearly in this country. One may surmise that the relatively low incidence of MCUO relegates it to only peripheral clinical interest. However, viewed in another manner, the *total* of new cancer cases—of all types—that are seen each year in at least 25 of the U.S. states is *less than* 30,000. Moreover, epithelial malignancies of the thyroid, ovary, endometrium, pancreas, stomach, esophagus, and larynx are individually less common yearly than MCUO, as are new cases of acute leukemia or glioma. Thus, carcinoma of uknown origin poses a larger problem for American—and international—physicians than one might think at first glance.

Because treatment plans for carcinomas are typically predicated largely on the primary sites of those tumors, uncertainty regarding their anatomic derivations is anxiety provoking. Neither the patient nor the physician usually feels empowered or confident after a diagnosis of MCUO has been made. Common questions in that scenario include: "Is the diagnosis correct?"; "Has the clinical or pathologic evaluation been inadequate?"; "What is the optimal treatment approach?"; and "What is the prognosis?"

This monograph was conceived as a framework for approaching these issues, with input from physicians in six countries who have a special interest in, and substantial experience with, MCUOs. The book is divided into five topic areas, covering clinical presentations, methods of pathologic evaluation, techniques for topographic localization, treatment and prognosis of MCUO, and postmortem validation studies pertaining to those subjects. Although our knowledge of this difficult area of oncology (and pathology?) will undoubtedly continue to evolve, the contents of this text are felt to be completely current as of this writing.

I have edited all of the chapter manuscripts personally, and if any mistakes or misstatements are present in them I take the responsibility. The individual authors have been given license to present their topics as they saw fit; as a result, inevitable redundancy of some topic coverage will be seen by the careful reader. I believe this is a positive feature of the book, because it serves to emphasize points that several different contributors—despite different experiences—feel are important.

Finally, because virtually all physicians are expected to educate their peers, associates, and trainees in this day and age, an effort has been made to illustrate the book as thoroughly as possible. A companion CD-ROM contains all of the color versions of the images found in the text. That disk is intended for use in hospital teaching conferences and other medical education activities.

I am indebted to Mr. Joseph Hanson and Mr. Craig Percy of Demos Publishing, who respectively solicited and coordinated this book project. I sincerely hope that readers will find it to be useful in their clinical practices.

Mark R. Wick, MD
Department of Pathology
Division of Surgical Pathology and Cytopathology
University of Virginia Health System
Charlottesville, Virginia

Acknowledgment

The editor is grateful to Jane, Robert, and Morgan, who gave me time that would otherwise have been spent with them so that this book could be completed. The consistently strong support of colleagues at the University of Virginia Medical Center (Charlottesville, Virginia) is also warmly acknowledged.

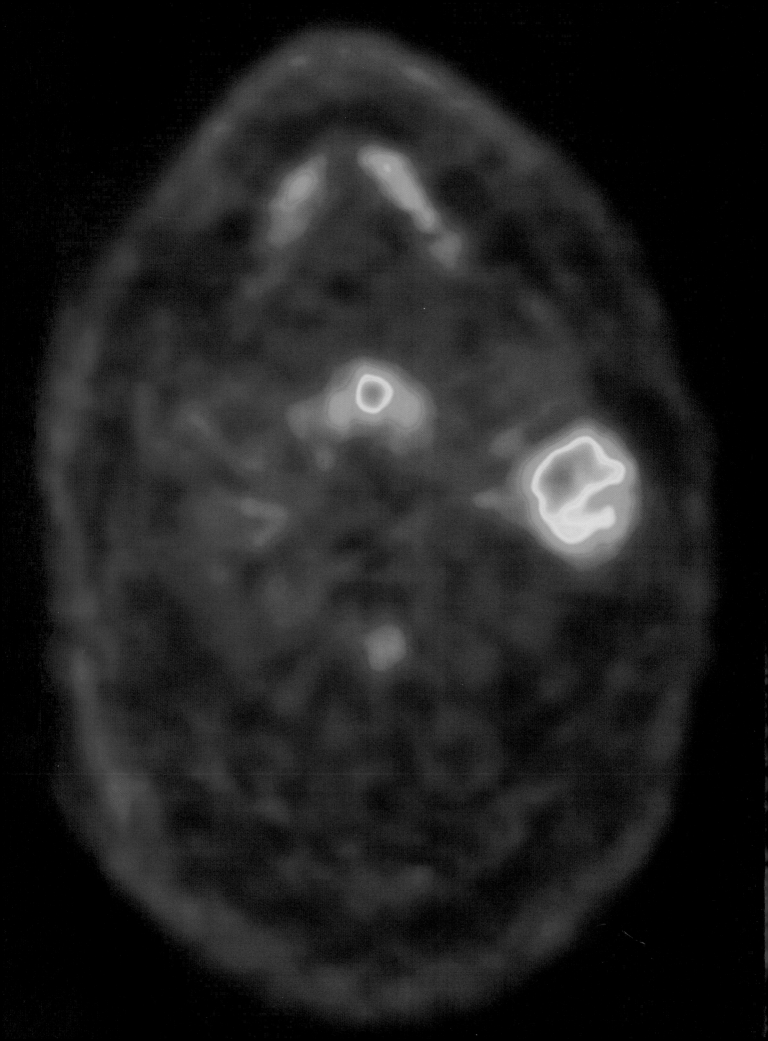

Contributors

Åke Berglund, MD
Department of Oncology
Akademiska Sjukhuset
Uppsala, Sweden

Rohit Bhargava, MD
Department of Pathology
University of Pittsburgh
Magee-Women's Hospital
Pittsburgh, Pennsylvania

Jeffrey E. Carter, MD
Department of Surgery
Wake Forest University
Winston-Salem, North Carolina

Lisa A. Cerilli, MD
Department of Pathology
University of New Mexico
Albuquerque, New Mexico

Katherine Chorneyko, MD
Department of Pathology and
Molecular Medicine
McMaster University
Hamilton, Ontario, Canada

David J. Dabbs, MD
Department of Pathology
University of Pittsburgh
Magee-Womens Hospital
Pittsburgh, Pennsylvania

Marieke T. De Graaf, MD
Departments of Medical Oncology
and Neurology
Erasmus University Medical Center
Rotterdam, The Netherlands

Henry C. Ho, MD
Division of Gastroenterology
University of Virginia Health System
Charlottesville, Virginia

LeRon Jackson, MD
Department of Surgery
Mayo Clinic
Rochester, Minnesota

Michel Kahaleh, MD
Division of Gastroenterology
University of Virginia Health System
Charlottesville, Virginia

Edward A. Levine, MD
Department of Surgery
Wake Forest University
Winston-Salem, North Carolina

Abhijit Mazumder, PhD
Vericlex LLC
Warren, New Jersey

James W. Patterson, MD
Departments of Dermatology
and Pathology
University of Virginia Health System
Charlottesville, Virginia

Nicholas Pavlidis, MD
Department of Medical Oncology
Ioannina University Medical School
Ioannina, Greece

George Pentheroudakis, MD
Department of Medical Oncology
Ioannina University Medical School
Ioannina, Greece

James F. Reibel, MD
Department of Otolaryngology
University of Virginia Health System
Charlottesville, Virginia

Jeffrey S. Ross, MD
Department of Pathology
Albany Medical College
Albany, New York

Pascal Sève, MD, PhD
Department of Internal Medicine
Hotel Dieu
Hospices Civils de Lyon
Lyon, France

Vanessa M. Shami, MD
Division of Gastroenterology
University of Virginia Health System
Charlottesville, Virginia

Perry Shen, MD
Department of Surgery
Wake Forest University
Winston-Salem, North Carolina

Peter A. E. Sillevis Smitt, MD, PhD
Department of Neurology
Erasmus University Medical Center
Rotterdam, The Netherlands

Anders E. Sundin, MD
Department of Radiology
Akademiska Sjukhuset
Uppsala, Sweden

Mark R. Wick, MD
Department of Pathology
Division of Surgical Pathology and Cytopathology
University of Virginia Health System
Charlottesville, Virginia

Metastatic Carcinomas
of Unknown Origin

Clinical Presentations of Metastatic Carcinomas of Unknown Origin

PASCAL SÈVE

■ INTRODUCTION

In a general medical oncology service, metastatic carcinomas from an unknown primary site (CUPs) constitute as many as 3% to 5% of referred patients with solid tumors. However, this incidence varies depending on the definition of CUP, the extent of the investigations that are performed, and the details of the patient population (1, 2). Several terms have been used for CUP, such as "unknown or occult primary tumor," "carcinoma or adenocarcinoma of unknown primary site," "metastases of unknown origin," "metastases from unknown primary tumors," and "tumors of unknown or unidentified origin." CUPs represent clinical problems that necessitate significant interactions between pathologists, oncologists, and primary physicians. Despite recent advances in molecular diagnostics, immunohistochemistry, gene expression profiling, and imaging technology, the diagnosis of patients with CUPs continues to be a real dilemma for practicing oncologists. The goal of this review is to recount the clinical presentations of these enigmatic tumors.

■ DEFINITION

CUPs represent a heterogeneous group of metastatic carcinomas for which no primary site can be detected even after a thorough medical evaluation. The primary lesion, which has escaped detection by radiographic and endoscopic studies, is rarely identified during the subsequent lifetime of the patient. In historical studies, only 15% of CUPs were associated with a definite primary neoplasm (3). A thorough evaluation at autopsy improves these figures somewhat; in 51% to 85% of cases primary lesions are found postmortem in CUP patients. They are usually small tumors that caused no symptoms or signs during life (3–10). The "parent" neoplasm is most often present in the lung (17–23%) or the pancreas (20–37%). The second tier of frequency regarding the primary site concerns lesions of the large bowel (4–10%), the liver (3–11%), the stomach (3–8%), and the kidney (4–6%). The least common locations for the parent neoplasm are the breasts (2%), ovaries (3–4%), and prostate (3–4%). New and sophisticated imaging techniques, such as positron emission tomography (PET) scanning, and improvement of surgical pathological evaluations will likely increase the number of cases in which a primary tumor can be localized during life.

The difficulty in detecting a "parent" tumor for CUP has two possible explanations. One is that the primary tumor has involuted and is not detectable when metastasis becomes evident. Although it is not a common phenomenon, spontaneous tumor regression has been well described in reference to several neoplasms. The second explanation is that the phenotype and genotype of the primary tumor favor metastasis over local growth (11). In that scenario, a small primary tumor might rapidly yield metastatic lesions, the growth of which greatly outstrips that of the parent lesion.

The definition of CUP has varied over time according to the inclusion criteria that were used and the evolution of diagnostic tools. In the early 1970s, some researchers argued that the diagnosis of CUP could be made only if the primary tumor was not found at autopsy (12). In other studies, all patients presenting with metastases whose primary tumors were not found after an initial clinical examination were labeled as having CUP (13, 14). Other authors placed cases in this category at the time the initial diagnosis was made (15) and limited inclusion to particular histological types (10, 15). Today, the diagnosis of CUP requires several elements:

1. Histologically confirmed metastatic carcinoma
2. Negative results of a detailed historical and physical assessment, including pelvic and rectal examination, with regard to finding a likely primary tumor site
3. Negative results of chest radiography, ultrasonography, or computed tomography (CT) of the abdomen and pelvis, vis-à-vis localization of a primary neoplasm
4. Determination of serum prostate-specific antigen (PSA) levels in men and mammography in women that fail to demonstrate an origin of the tumor
5. In certain cases, CT of the thorax and endoscopic evaluations that are negative (Table 1) (16, 17)

In most studies of CUP, cases of lymphoma, metastatic melanoma, and sarcoma have been rightly excluded. Initial light microscopic diagnosis of the biopsy specimen usually identifies one of four main histological types, and cases should be categorized accordingly (18): (*i*) well or moderately differentiated adenocarcinoma; (*ii*) poorly differentiated carcinoma (PDC) or poorly differentiated adenocarcinoma (PDA); (*iii*) squamous cell carcinoma (SCC); and (*iv*) "undifferentiated" carcinoma of small cell, large cell, or spindle cell and pleomorphic types. Approximately 50% of patients with CUP have category 1 tumors, 30% have undifferentiated carcinomas or PDCs, 15% have SCCs, and 5% have undifferentiated neoplasms. With modern pathological characterization, most tumors in the last of these groups can be better defined; they include PDC, neuroendocrine carcinomas, lymphomas, germ cell tumors, melanomas, sarcomas, and embryonal malignancies ("blastomas") (Table 2) (19). Only carcinomas should be included in the CUP category.

One goal of the diagnostic evaluation is to identify CUPs that are in treatable subsets. These include tumors with neuroendocrine features, SCC involving cervical lymph nodes, adenocarcinomas in women that present with metastasis to axillary lymph nodes, peritoneal carcinomatosis in women, blastic bone metastases in men, and midline malignancies, usually in young men, that are probably extragonadal germ cell tumors (18, 19). These patients represent only 15% of individuals with CUP, but their identification is crucial to optimal treatment and outcome.

Table 1 Clinical and laboratory data required to define a patient as having a carcinoma of unknown primary origin

Histologically confirmed metastatic cancer

Detailed medical history

Complete physical examination (including, skin, thyroid, breast, pelvic, and rectal exams)

Full blood count

Biochemistry

Histopathologic review and use of immunohistochemistry

CT of the abdomen and pelvis

Mammography (in certain cases)

CT of the thorax (in certain cases)

Prostate-specific antigen evaluation (in certain cases)

Endoscopic procedures (in certain cases)

Alpha-fetoprotein and gonadotrope chorionic hormone evaluation (in certain cases)

Source: From Refs. 16, 17.

Table 2 Histological classification

Histology	Incidence (%)
Well or moderately differentiated adenocarcinoma	50
Poorly differentiated adenocarcinoma/carcinoma	30
Squamous cell carcinoma	15

Undifferentiated neoplasms
  Unspecified carcinoma
  Neuroendocrine tumors
  Lymphomas
  Germ cell tumors
  Melanomas
  Sarcomas
  Embryonal malignancies
	5

Source: From Ref. 19.

The scenario of an unknown primary can be very unsettling to both the patient and the treating physician. The anxiety provoked by this clinical scenario may be caused by the uncertainty over treatment and an assumption of a grim prognosis, but this disease entity actually represents a group of diseases with potentially widely divergent outcomes. When grouped together, patients with metastases from an unknown primary site reported by registries, have a median survival of three months (2, 20), but it is important to recognize that there are certain patient subgroups that have more responsive tumors and better prognoses. It is essential to conduct a consistent and thorough diagnostic evaluation to determine if a patient falls into one of these favorable subgroups, although one should avoid the use of needless, invasive tests. This approach enables the physician to optimize the treatment regimen for each patient.

■ EPIDEMIOLOGY

Data from epidemiology surveys and large registries indicate that CUPs constitute between 2.3% and 4.2% of all human cancers (Table 3) (1, 21–28). Among overall solid-tumor incidence in the United States, CUPs represented approximately 40,000 of the 950,000 new cases per year (29). The annual age-adjusted incidence is 7 to 12 cases per 100,000 population per year in the United States

(24) and 18 to 19 cases per 100,000 population per year in Australia (21). In the Netherlands, almost 2500 new patients are diagnosed annually, giving an age-standardized incidence rate of 6.7 per 100,000 for male and 5.3 per 100,000 for females (30). CUPs therefore were considered as the seventh to eighth most frequent type of cancer and the fourth most common cause of cancer death in both males and females. However, more recent studies showed a lesser incidence of CUPs (24). For example, according to the National Cancer Institute's 2003 Surveillance, Epidemiology and End Results data, 30,000 (2%) new cases of cancers of "other and unspecified primary sites" were diagnosed in the United States. The estimated incidence continues to decrease each year (25). In 2006, the American Cancer Society estimated that CUPs would represent 27,680 of the 1,399,790 (1.98%) new cancer cases and 45,260 of the 564,830 deaths expected to occur in the United States (31). CUPs are more frequent than esophageal, gastric, and ovarian cancers. According to this estimation, CUPs are the 12 most frequent types of cancer and the fourth most common cause of cancer death in both males and females. In referral centers, the median age at presentation is approximately 60 years, with a marginally higher frequency in males. However, in populations described by registries, patients are 10 years older, and the American Cancer Society estimates a higher frequency in females (14,360 vs. 13,320). In children, CUPs represent less than 1% of diagnosed solid tumors.

■ Table 3 Epidemiology of carcinoma of unknown primary origin			
Geographical Areas (Ref.)	**Source**	**Frequency (%)**	**Period**
USA (24)	SEER	2.3	1973–1987
USA (25)	SEER	2	2003
Australia (21)	New South Wales Registry	4.2	1970–1990
Netherlands (Southeast) (28)	Eindhoven Cancer Registry	4	1984–1992
Finland (26)	IARC	2.5	—
Germany (23)	—	7.8	1968–1984
Russia (Dniepropetrovsk region) (22)	—	3.6	—
Switzerland (Vaud and Neuchatel Canton) (1)	Local Registries	2.3	1984–1993
Japan (27)	IARC	3	—

Abbreviations: SEER, Surveillance Epidemiology and End Results survey; IARC, International Agency for Research on Cancer.

■ CLINICAL PRESENTATIONS

Natural History of CUPs

CUPs represent a unique phenomenon in which a primary tumor is able to metastasize before its site of origin is large enough to be identified. The natural history of patients with CUP differs considerably from that of patients with known primary neoplasms. Early dissemination, unpredictability of metastatic patterns, and overall aggressiveness typify the fundamental characteristics of these tumors. Rapid distant spread is reflected by the clinical absence of symptoms related to a primary tumor.

"Unpredictability of metastatic pattern" in CUP cases refers to differences in the incidence of metastatic sites that they involve, as compared with those of known primary carcinomas (5). For example, ovarian carcinoma presenting as a CUP involves the bones in 30% of cases, whereas if it is a known primary lesion, osseous metastases are seen in only 1% to 10%. Similarly, pancreatic carcinoma presenting as a CUP has a fourfold higher incidence of osseous involvement, whereas prostatic CUP has seven times more hepatic metastasis compared with a known primary neoplasm. Pancreatic CUP metastasizes to the lungs in 78% versus 40% for known pancreatic tumors. The incidence of brain metastasis in gastrointestinal (GI) CUPs is 16% to 19%, but involvement of the central nervous system (CNS) is uncommon in the usual clinical course of known GI cancers.

It seems that CUPs do not undergo "type 1" progression (from a premalignant lesion to a malignant one) but are instead fully malignant from the outset ("type 2" progression). The main difference, however, between CUPs and other type 2 malignancies is that the former lesions do not form a clinically apparent primary mass and commonly do not pursue a predictable pattern of metastasis.

General Statements

The diagnosis of CUP is usually suspected after obtaining the case history and performing a physical examination. Common sites of involvement at presentation are the liver, lungs, bones, and lymph nodes, but other locations certainly may also be affected. Table 4 considers the frequency with which certain anatomic sites are involved. There is considerable variation in tumor distribution, depending on the histological tumor types. More than 50% of CUP patients present with multiple metastasis sites, and approximately 30% of them have involvement of three or more organs (2, 9, 16, 32, 33). Those data differ considerably from findings in patients with known primary tumors, in whom <15% have metastasis in three or more sites.

The characteristic clinical features of CUPs include the following:

1. A short history of local symptoms (e.g., pain, swelling, and cough) that are related to the site(s) of metastasis
2. A brief history of constitutional symptoms (e.g., weight loss, malaise, fatigue, and fever), often related to hepatic metastases
3. Obvious abnormalities on physical examination, such as palpable masses at a single site, or, more frequently, at multiple sites
4. The possible presence of paraneoplastic syndromes (e.g., superficial migratory thrombophlebitis; hypercalcemia; neurologic dysfunction) (see Chapter 2)

Clinicopathologic CUP groups that usually share an unfavorable outcome can be separated from others that represent comparatively favorable subsets.

Unfavorable Subsets of CUP

METASTATIC CUP PRIMARILY AFFECTING THE LIVER. Patients with hepatic metastases represent one of the most common subgroups of CUP, accounting for approximately 25% of all cases. After nodal metastasis, involvement of the liver is the second leading manifestation of secondary carcinoma in general (34). Metastatic lesions in other organs can also be seen at diagnosis in the liver-centered CUP subset, but hepatic disease is the predominant finding. Common clinical presentations of such patients include right upper quadrant abdominal pain, epigastric pain, abdominal swelling, jaundice, and weight loss. In referral patients with suspected CUP and hepatic metastases, tumors of the lung, colon and rectum, and pancreas comprised the majority of eventually discovered primary malignancies. Adenocarcinoma (57%) and poorly differentiated to undifferentiated carcinoma (32%) are the most frequently encountered histological categories in this CUP subset (34). Neuroendocrine carcinomas and squamous carcinomas represent 7% and 3% of cases.

Short survival times in these CUP patients have led many investigators to recommend only limited diagnostic evaluations; expensive and time-consuming radiological or endoscopic studies identify a primary tumor in <10% of cases (34, 35). Debate continues as to the most appropriate diagnostic approach, particularly concerning the use of endoscopic methods. Current recommendations (17) propose that complementary procedures be used, including thoracoabdominal CT scanning, imaging of the pelvis (CT or ultrasound), and mammography in women who have adenocarcinoma or undifferentiated carcinoma. One is well advised to limit the assessment of serum tumor markers to PSA, alpha-fetoprotein (AFP), and human chorionic gonadotrophin beta subunit (β-HCG) when the clinical picture is

Table 4 Sites of metastasis in patients with unknown primary site

Site of Involvement	Abbruzzese et al. (16); n (%)	Culine et al. (33)	Hess et al. (32)	Lortholary et al. (163)	Sève et al. (20)	van de Wouw et al. (2)
Liver	202 (31)	47 (31)	331 (33)	51 (16)	153 (39)	244 (24)
Lung	NS	60 (40)	263 (26)	42 (13)	82 (21)	NS
Pleura	NS	18 (12)	112 (11)	15 (5)	76 (20)	NS
Lymph nodes	244 (37)	87 (58)	418 (42)	176 (57)	155 (40)	114 (11)
Peritoneum	39 (6)	18 (12)	90 (9)	21 (7)	90 (23)	92 (9)
Bone	184 (28)	67 (45)	289 (29)	99 (32)	75 (19)	82 (8)
Brain	50 (8)	7 (5)	64 (06)	24 (8)	32 (8)	18 (2)
Elsewhere	NS	26 (17)	NS	48 (15)	81 (21)	81 (8)
No. of sites						
1	259 (39.4)	44 (29)	408 (41)	109 (35)	168 (43)	NS
2	220 (33.5)	61 (41)	295 (29)	NS	128 (33)	NS
>2	178 (27.1)	45 (30)	297 (30)	NS	93 (24)	266 (26)
Total	657 (100)	150 (100)	1000 (100)	311 (100)	389 (100)	1024 (100)

Abbreviation: NS, not specified.

compatible with a prostatic carcinoma or germ cell tumor (16). Assays of AFP will also facilitate the detection of multicentric or satellitotic hepatocellular carcinoma, which can simulate multiple hepatic metastases (Fig. 1). Colonoscopy has generally not been recommended in liver-centered CUP cases unless there are clinical symptoms or signs relating to the alimentary tract. However, we believe that the latter procedure is indeed useful, because of the emergence of new medical and surgical strategies, including targeted monoclonal antibody therapy, which have improved the prognosis of metastatic colorectal carcinoma. Colonoscopy should be done in cases with a familial history of colorectal cancer, or in patients with an apparently exclusive and possibly resectable hepatic mass, especially if they have a good performance status (PS) (36). Immunohistochemical studies of tumor tissue that reveal a keratin 7–negative and keratin 20–positive adenocarcinoma favor a colorectal or gastric source, and would also justify endoscopic evaluation (37).

The prognosis of the hepatocentric CUP subset is poor, with a median survival of six to nine months in studies performed at cancer centers (CC). However, case examples in this subgroup that concern metastatic neuroendocrine carcinomas (especially well-differentiated ones) appear to have a better response to treatment and a longer survival (34, 38).

METASTATIC CUP PRINCIPALLY AFFECTING THE LUNGS. Patients with pulmonary parenchymal metastases usually present with multiple peripheral nodular lesions, at least some of which are usually pleural based. The lung-centered CUP subgroup accounts for 5% to 10% of all CUP patients. Adenocarcinomas with varying levels of differentiation are the most frequently seen in this cohort. In CC patients referred for lung-centered CUPs, neoplasms of the lungs, breasts, kidneys, and colon represent the most frequently discovered tumor sources (39).

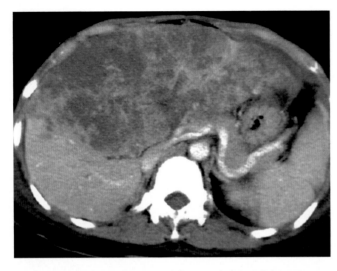

FIGURE 1 Abdomen CT scan. Multicentric hepatocellular carcinoma simulating multiple hepatic metastases. Assay of alpha-fetoprotein will be systematic in case of undifferentiated tumor to avoid ignoring a hepatocarcinoma.

In cases where only a single peripheral lung nodule is present, without evidence of any extrapulmonary tumor (Fig. 2), the usual doctrine is to consider such a lesion as a primary lung cancer and treat it accordingly. Visualization of an endobronchial lesion at broncho-scopy or by direct visualization at thoracotomy provides even stronger evidence for origination of the tumor in the lung.

The prognosis for lung-centered CUPs is poor, especially for most patients with multiple metastases. Young individuals (<40 years of age) with possible germ cell or trophoblastic tumors, however, stand apart as a special subset. For young men, the measurement of serum AFP and HCG, testicular ultrasonography, and thoracoabdominal CT scanning are indicated (17). In young women, HCG levels and pelvic ultrasonography are appropriate.

METASTATIC CUP PRINCIPALLY AFFECTING THE PLEURA. Malignant pleural effusions are common in patients with CUP, but in a small group of individuals they can be the only manifestation of demonstrable metastasis. This cohort accounts for 3% to 12% of all CUP patients. Viewed from another perspective, 6% to 15% of all malignant pleural effusions are related to CUPs (40). Dyspnea is the most common presenting symptom in pleura-centered CUP cases, and it is seen in >50% of them. Others symptoms include weight loss, anorexia, malaise, and chest pain (41). Adenocarci-noma is the main histological tumor type; primary sites in the lungs, breasts, and ovaries should be excluded (39). The differential diagnosis of pleural epithelial mesothelio-ma and metastatic carcinoma—especially of the so-called pseudomesotheliomatous type (42–44)—can be extremely difficult at both the clinical and histopathological levels. The radiological picture of a diffusely thickened pleura or tumor encasing the lung (Fig. 3) favors the interpretation of malignant mesothelioma, but is far from definitive evidence of it. Pathological examination of tumor tissue, including an immunohistochemical panel of well-defined antibodies (45), not only conclusively identifies meso-thelioma but also provides information on a likely anatomic source for metastatic carcinomas in the pleura. A thoracoscopic pleural biopsy is the most advisable for that purpose, resulting in a definite pathological diagnosis

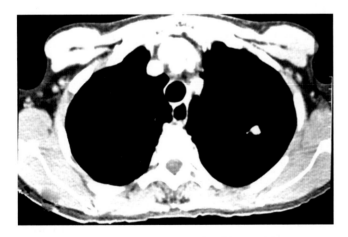

FIGURE 2 Chest CT scan. Single peripheral lung nodule.

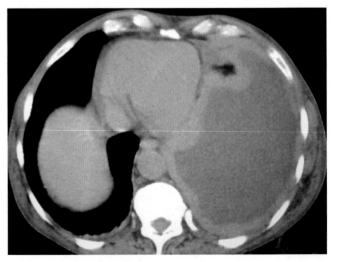

FIGURE 3 Chest CT scan. Malignant mesothelioma with left pleural effusion and diffusely thickened pleura.

in 95% of cases. Diagnostic yields of other procedures are 62% for pleural fluid cytology and 44% for "closed" (cutting-needle) pleural biopsy (41).

The most effective nonpathological investigation in this CUP subgroup for detection of a primary tumor is a CT scan of the thorax (46). Bronchoscopy, although frequently done in this context, is unhelpful in patients who have negative CT scans (46).

In general, the prognosis of this CUP subset is adverse. In a series by Abbruzzese et al. on CUPs, those cases presenting with a malignant pleural effusion did particularly poorly. They had a median survival of approximately six months, and none was alive after 20 months (16). Bonnefoi and Smith reported a median survival of 12 months in a comparable study, and 10% of patients were alive at two years (46).

METASTATIC CUP PRINCIPALLY AFFECTING THE BONES. Almost 20% to 25% of CUP patients present with bone symptoms caused by metastases, and bone scintigraphy is positive in >50% of cases (Fig. 4). Axial and proximal appendicular portions of the skeleton are especially involved (47). Presenting symptoms are dominated by bone pain at the site of the lesion or the general anatomic region in which it is located (48). They may also

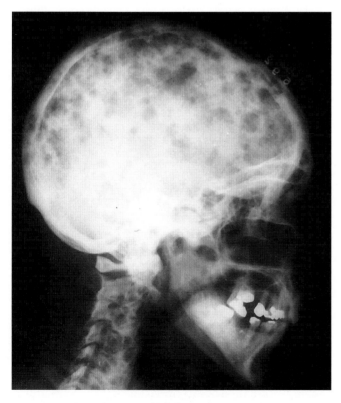

FIGURE 4 Cranial X-ray. Multiple bone metastases are present.

be accompanied by neurological dysfunction, primarily represented by nerve root pain. Hypercalcemia, bone swelling, and pathological fractures are less common.

Histological examination of the intraosseous lesions provides a definitive diagnosis of CUP, excluding hematological malignancies and sarcomas. Adenocarcinoma is again the main CUP tumor type in this context. Site-selective antibodies such as thyroid transcription factor-1 (TTF-1), PSA, estrogen and progesterone receptor proteins (ERP/PRP), and gross cystic disease fluid protein-15 (GCDFP-15) (a marker of breast epithelium) can be helpful in suggesting an anatomic source for the intraosseous tumor. Although "blind" iliac crest biopsy was recommended in the past for evaluation of bone-centered CUPs (49, 50), recent advances in interventional radiology now favor the use of guided percutaneous bone biopsies.

In CUP patients with bone metastases, the lungs, breasts, prostate, and kidneys represent the most common sites for primary malignancies (39, 48). Recent studies have shown an increase in the proportion of patients with lung cancer in that CUP subgroup (48). Although thyroid carcinomas do have a propensity for osseous metastasis, the inaugural involvement of bone is exceedingly rare as a presentation of those tumors. Vandecandelaere et al. compared two series concerning bone metastases in which primary sites were sought. The studies, separated by 30 years, showed that a primary site could not be localized in 38% of cases in the more recent analysis as compared with 27% in the earlier series (48).

Thoracic and abdominal CT scans, mammograms in women, and PSA assays in men are considered useful for determining a possible site of the primary tumor. In contrast, examination of the GI tract and pelvic imaging seldom have been thought to be effective in that regard (51). This opinion is based on the results of retrospective studies (48, 51, 52). A prospective assessment by Rougraff et al., however, showed that CT scans of the thorax could detect lung carcinomas in cases where plain chest radiographs were felt to be normal (53). Routine assays of multiple tumor markers in CUP patients with bone metastases are costly and, in my opinion, unhelpful. Although thyroglobulin is a specific indicator, routine assays for that analyte are not warranted because of the low overall incidence of thyroid cancer involving bones.

METASTATIC CUPS PRINCIPALLY AFFECTING THE BRAIN. Metastatic CUPs in the CNS may be represented by solitary or multifocal lesions. Up to 15% of all patients with brain metastases have no clearly identified site of tumor origin despite extensive evaluations. Approximately 50% have a single intracerebral mass that is detected by CT scans (Fig. 5) or magnetic resonance imaging (MRI),

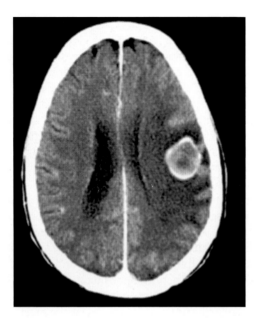

FIGURE 5 Brain CT scan. Solitary metastatic lesion with mass effect.

and the rest have two or more lesions. The most common intracranial locations for CUPs are the frontal and parietal lobes, followed by the temporal and occipital lobes (54).

Headache is the most common presenting symptom in this CUP subset, being present in >50% of cases; it may be the only manifestation of disease. Others problems include motor deficits, seizures, nausea and vomiting, and paresthesias (54).

Histopathologically, intracranial CUPs are most frequently adenocarcinomas, followed by SCCs. Anatomic origins for intracerebral metastases of known primary tumors include the lungs (39–64%), breasts (13–17%), kidney (4–13%), GI tract (3%), and the endometrium or vulva (5–8%). CUP cases account for only 5% (39, 55–57). Prostatic, ovarian, testicular, and bladder cancers rarely involve the brain. In patients for whom brain metastases are the only manifestation of CUP, lung carcinoma is the most frequently discovered primary tumor (54).

The prognosis of CUP cases with brain-centered metastases generally is poor; thus, most treatment is palliative (58). Nevertheless, a subgroup of those patients, with solitary lesions, may benefit from surgical excision and have a better prognosis (59). Nguyen et al. showed that a minority of cases treated with complete resection and radiotherapy lived for five or more years (54).

MALIGNANT ASCITES OF UNKNOWN ORIGIN AND NONPAPILLARY-SEROUS CARCINOMATOUS HISTOLOGY. Some patients with malignant ascites have nonpapillary carcinomas; they are as likely to be men as women. In females who present with disseminated

peritoneal carcinomatosis, the tumor usually originates in the ovary. Occasionally, carcinomas in the breasts, lungs, or GI tract (e.g., stomach or vermiform appendix) can produce this pattern of metastatic spread. The median age of this CUP subset is approximately 67 years. The patients have stage III and IV peritoneal carcinomatosis, according to the scheme advanced by Gilly (60).

Adenocarcinoma is once more the main histological tumor type. In cases with mucin-producing adenocarcinomas, often with signet-ring cell differentiation, a GI (especially gastric and appendiceal) origin should be suspected. As is true of malignant pleural effusions, clinicopathologic differential diagnosis with epithelial mesothelioma can be difficult, especially for nonmucinous neoplasms.

The tumors in these CUP cases are generally not responsive to chemotherapy. The median survival is only 1.5 months (60, 61).

Favorable Subsets of CUP

WOMEN WITH PAPILLARY SEROUS ADENOCARCINOMA OF THE PERITONEUM. As previously mentioned, among all patients with CUP, there are certain subgroups that have relatively favorable outlooks after appropriate therapy. The first of them is represented by patients with peritoneal carcinomatosis and serous papillary carcinomatous histology.

Peritoneal carcinomatosis in women is commonly associated with known primary tumors, usually in the ovaries, GI tract, or breasts. However, in some examples of diffuse peritoneal carcinomatosis, no primary lesion is detectable in any of those sites or elsewhere. These cases frequently show the histological features of ovarian carcinoma; specifically, many of them are classified as papillary serous adenocarcinomas with the formation of psammoma bodies. This clinicopathologic scenario has been called "multifocal extraovarian serous carcinoma," "papillary serous peritoneal carcinoma" (PSPC), "peritoneal mesothelioma," "peritoneal papillary (serous) carcinoma," "primary peritoneal carcinoma," "serous surface papillary carcinoma," "multiple focal extraovarian serous carcinoma," and "small ovarian carcinoma." PSPC belongs to the Mullerian family of neoplasms, including ovarian papillary serous carcinoma (OPSC), endometrial papillary serous carcinoma, and serous papillary carcinoma of the uterine cervix or Fallopian tube. These tumors have generally similar histological and clinical features.

Two theories have been proposed to explain the development of PSPC. The first is that germ cells resting along the gonadal embryonic pathway give rise to eventual malignancies. According to the second paradigm, malignant transformation occurs by oncogenic transformation of the coelomic epithelium in the abdominal serosa and ovarian surfaces (62, 63). Although ovarian carcinomas appear to have a clonal origin (64), at least some PSPCs are multifocal (65–67).

To better define the patient population with the PSPC form of CUP and to develop an organized treatment strategy for it, the Gynecologic Oncology Group defined a concise set of criteria for this diagnostic category:

1. Both ovaries must be either physiologically normal in size or enlarged only by a benign process
2. Tumor bulk in extraovarian sites must be greater than that seen on the surface of either ovary
3. Microscopically, an ovarian tumor component must be nonexistent, confined to the ovarian surface with no evidence of cortical invasion, or involve the ovarian cortical stroma with a tumor diameter of no more than 5 mm, with or without surface growth
4. The histomorphological characteristics of the tumor must be predominantly of the serous type, that is, comparable to those of ovarian serous papillary adenocarcinoma of any grade

The feasibility of these criteria was confirmed in a retrospective review by Chan et al. (68).

The first report of PSPC was by Swerdlow in 1959 (69). Another subsequent communication in 1982 called attention to the poor outlook of women who presented with peritoneal carcinomatosis and had no definable tumor (70). However, Hochster et al. thereafter reported their experience with three such patients, two of whom had long-term remissions with cisplatin-based chemotherapy. They suggested PSPC could be successfully treated with regimens that were effective for ovarian carcinoma (71). Another similar report of five patients soon followed (72). By 2006, as many as 400 patients with PSPC were reported, and it was suggested that approximately 10% of women with "metastatic ovarian cancer" actually had PSPC (62, 68, 73–77). The incidence of PSPC has increased over the last decade (78).

The interpretation of these studies is complicated by variable diagnostic terminology, diverse treatment approaches, and the retrospective nature of the reports. The PSPC form of CUP is more common in women with a family history of ovarian cancer, but preventive oophorectomy, as expected, does not protect them from the disease (79). As is true of ovarian carcinoma, the incidence of PSPC is increased in patients with BRCA1 mutations (80). Isolated cases of PSPC have also been reported in men (81).

Most recent studies confirm that the clinical presentation of PSPC is indistinguishable from that of advanced ovarian carcinoma of International Federation of Gynecology and Obstetrics (FIGO) stage III and IV (82). Affected patients are usually postmenopausal Caucasians who present with abdominal pain (29–63%), abdominal distension (64–78%), GI complaints (7–30%), and weight loss (11%). The most common finding on physical examination is ascites (60–100%), while a pelvic mass is demonstrable in up to 55.6% of patients and an abdominal mass is seen in 25.9 to 100%. Some patients also manifest pleural effusions (6–16%), parenchymal hepatic metastases (11–13%), and extraabdominal lymph node involvement (3–6%) (74, 75, 78, 83, 84).

Radiological findings that suggest the diagnosis of PSPC are diffuse microcalcification of the peritoneum, which is felt to occur in relation to psammoma body formation (Fig. 6). Multicentric peritoneal disease is typical, with omental involvement being particularly prominent (85). The serum CA-125 level is often >1000 U/mL, and, not uncommonly, it is markedly elevated (78, 84, 86).

The diagnosis of PSPC requires that the surgeon identifies grossly normal ovaries or minimal surface involvement of them by tumor. Fromm et al. arbitrarily chose a maximum tumor diameter of 4 mm in the ovaries as exclusionary for the diagnosis of PSPC (62). The histologic image of PSPC features a micropapillary growth pattern with irregularly sized and shaped papillae, areas of stromal invasion, and focally solid epithelial growth. Psammoma bodies are commonly encountered throughout the lesion. The immunophenotype of PSPC is generally analogous to that of serous papillary ovarian carcinoma. Tubulopapillary mesotheliomas are variants of epithelial mesothelioma that may be confused with PSPC. Ber-EP4, MOC-31, and ERP/PRP are useful markers in making that discrimination pathologically (43, 87).

A few small studies have been performed to assess possible differences in biomarker levels in PSPC as compared with OPSC. For example, Kowalski et al.

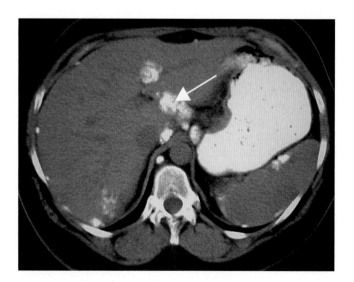

FIGURE 6 Abdomen CT scan. Diffuse microcalcification of the peritoneum suggests the diagnosis of primary serous papillary carcinoma.

evaluated ploidy and overexpression of p53 or HER-2/*neu* in 44 patients with PSPC and in 44 with OPSC (88). Differences were found in HER-2/*neu* overexpression (59% of PSPC cases vs. 36% of OSPCs), but they were not related to prognosis. Chen et al. showed that PSPC and OPSC have comparable immunophenotypes for HER-2/*neu*, p53, *bcl*-2, and nm23-H1 (89).

Outcome studies have shown survival rates in PSPC cases that are better than (90), similar to (62, 68, 75, 76, 82, 91), or worse than those of patients with FIGO stage III or IV OSPC (78, 92–94). A significant survival advantage pertains to those cases in which the post-treatment residual tumor measures ≤1 cm in greatest dimension (95).

Patients with PSPC are treated with surgical debulking and chemotherapy regimens that are similar to those used for ovarian carcinoma. The PSPC–CUP subset is associated with better survival than that seen in other CUP cases (74), especially if optimal cytoreduction is achieved (84, 86, 96).

WOMEN WITH ADENOCARCINOMA INVOLVING ONLY AXILLARY LYMPH NODES. The second possible CUP subgroup with favorable prognosis is that of patients with adenocarcinomatous metastases to axillary lymph nodes. Initially, evaluation of these patients is guided by gender. Men who present in this manner should undergo evaluation for a primary lung cancer. The GI system and thyroid should also be evaluated in attempts to identify a primary neoplasm.

Isolated axillary adenocarcinoma in women most likely represents a manifestation of mammary carcinoma (Fig. 7). Of all women with breast cancer, 0.3% to 1% have involvement of the axillary lymph nodes as the seminal indicator of an occult malignancy (97). This

uncommon situation was first described by Halsted in 1907 (98). He reported three patients suffering from "occult breast cancer" who presented only with axillary metastases. This situation remains a difficult and troublesome one for both patients and physicians, because the inability to localize a primary tumor causes uncertainties regarding diagnosis and treatment. "Occult" breast cancer presenting with axillary lymphadenopathy (OBCAL) requires every effort to be made toward detecting a small breast tumor (99, 100). These CUP lesions are staged as T0/N1 or N2/M0 (stage II or IIIa) in the UICC/AJC classification.

The mean age of women in this CUP subset coincides with that of others who have "ordinary" breast cancer, at 45 to 55 years of age (101, 102). The diameter of the axillary masses is often surprisingly large. Both Haagensen (103) and de Andrade et al. (104) reported a mean size of 4.7 cm; in a series from the Curie Institute, it was 3 cm (105). Seventy percent of patients with OBCAL have N1 disease; only 5% present with disseminated disease (102). Rarely, one may observe axillary node metastases in patients with a history of breast carcinoma on the contralateral side (106). In such cases, it is difficult to define whether the new lesions are metastases from the previous neoplasm or derivatives of a new, occult tumor in the ipsilateral breast. Genotypic studies may be necessary to address this point (107).

The assessment of patients with axillary lymphadenopathy begins with a careful history and physical examination. These may exclude a benign cause, which is most common (108, 109), or a noncarcinomatous tumor such as lymphoma or metastatic melanoma. A fine-needle aspiration (FNA) biopsy or needle-core biopsy can be obtained as the initial diagnostic test. A negative result does not exclude malignancy, and should prompt an excisional biopsy (97).

The pathological evaluation of involved lymph axillary nodes in metastatic carcinoma cases should include immunostains for ERP and PRP. Expression of these receptor proteins is found in >50% of patients, and it provides corroborative evidence for an underlying breast cancer (110); similar comments apply to tumor positivity for GCDFP-15. In our opinion, HER-2/*neu* immunostains should also be included, with an eye on future treatment.

By definition, an occult breast carcinoma is not detectable by mammography; therefore, additional imaging studies must be performed. These include ultrasonography of the breasts, as well as MRI and PET scanning. Breast sonography has been recommended, but, in this particular context, it has shown unacceptable rates of false positivity and false negativity and poor detection of occult carcinomas (111). On the other hand, color Doppler ultrasonography may detect a "tumor flow signal" and prove to be more successful, as shown by Lee et al. (112).

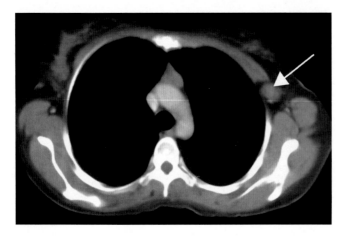

FIGURE 7 Chest CT scan. Left axillary lymphadenopathy due to adenocarcinoma involving only axillary lymph nodes.

Of late, MRI of the breast has been used to identify a primary site in some cases. This technique has a high sensitivity, ranging from 88% to 100% (113). Its specificity is much less, as low as 35% in some reports (106). Suspicious foci in *any* imaging study should be biopsied. Some analyses have specifically shown that MRI can identify primary tumors in most women (75–86%) with OBCAL (114–116). Negative results predict a low likelihood of finding the tumor with a mastectomy.

PET scanning has been used successfully in women with OBCAL; it is particularly attractive as an imaging method in patients with fibrocystic changes and radiodense breasts, or others who have undergone augmentation mammoplasties (106). Moreover, PET is capable of detecting occult regional or distant metastases. Its application is currently limited by high cost and constrained spatial resolution, which precludes detection of breast carcinomas <1 cm in diameter (117).

Survival of patients with OBCAL is generally the same, stage for stage, as that of women with known breast cancer and axillary lymph nodal metastases (106, 109). Five-year actuarial survival rates after treatment range from 36% to 79% (106). Most patients fall into clinical stage II, and their prognosis is determined by the number of metastatically involved nodes. Those with less than four positive nodes have a more favorable outcome. Hormonal receptor status is also important; ERP-positive cases have a better prognosis (102). In spite of this, reliable prognostic analyses have been difficult to perform because of selection biases in retrospective series and small sample sizes.

Patients with OBCAL should be treated as though they had stage II or stage III breast carcinomas. With N1 disease, adjuvant chemotherapy, hormonal therapy, and trastuzumab should be administered. This recommendation is based on improvements in disease-free and overall survival rates for patients who were so treated. Surgical management is more controversial. When the occult breast carcinoma is found by imaging studies, breast-conservation therapy will often be proposed because the tumors are relatively small, but no prospective trial of limited versus total mastectomy has been performed in this context. Patients with negative MRI scans should have axillary lymphadenectomies and could be treated by breast irradiation alone rather than mastectomy. Again, however, long-term clinical trials are needed to further evaluate these options (97, 118). Mere observation of the breast is not a recommended course of action (97, 106, 118). In patients with N2 disease and "fixed" nodes, preoperative neoadjuvant chemotherapy is suggested, using guidelines for stage III breast cancer. In nonresponsive tumors or in very elderly women, radical radiotherapy is the treatment of choice.

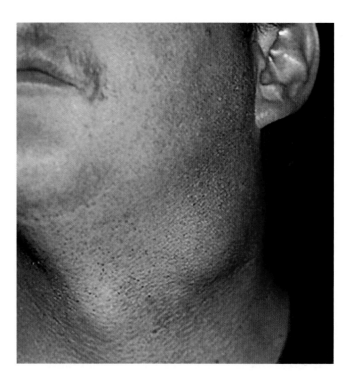

FIGURE 8 Cervical node metastases representing metastatic squamous carcinoma.

METASTATIC SQUAMOUS CARCINOMA PRINCIPALLY INVOLVING CERVICAL LYMPH NODES. Another subset of CUP patients with relatively favorable survival rates is that in which metastatic SCC presents in the cervical lymph nodes and is seemingly limited to them (Fig. 8). This syndrome is not common, comprising 2% to 9% of malignancies in the head and neck (119). In a Danish national study, the annual incidence of cervical node metastases from squamous carcinoma at an unknown primary site (CNS–CUP) was 0.34 cases per 100,000 persons per year, and it remained stable over a 20-year period (120). The number of new cancers in the head and neck cancers concurrently increased, suggesting that the proportion of CNS–CUP cases actually diminished.

The mean age at diagnosis in this CUP subgroup has varied in different series from 55 to 65 years, but a younger median age in some studies may be explained partially by their inclusion of undifferentiated tumors, possibly including metastatic nasopharyngeal carcinoma (the latter malignancy can be seen in children as well as in adults). As is true of other individuals with carcinomas of the head and neck, the majority of CNS–CUP patients are men with a significant history of alcohol and tobacco use. The median interval between the first appearance of symptoms and diagnosis is approximately three months.

The most frequently involved lymph nodal area in CNS–CUP cases is level II, followed by level III; other nodal stations are less commonly affected (119). Unilateral nodal disease is the most common; bilateral lymphadenopathy is seen in only 10% of cases. Median nodal size is 5 cm (range 2–14 cm), and there is an apparent prevalence of N2 cases.

Metastases in the upper and middle neck are generally attributed to cancers of the head and neck, whereas metastases of SCC in the lower neck (i.e., the supra-clavicular area) are often associated with primary tumors below the clavicles, especially represented by lung carcinomas. FNA for cytopathologic diagnosis is recommended before a neck dissection is performed. However, if FNA is unproductive because of negative results or paucicellular specimens, formal lymphadenectomy should be undertaken. Another hypothetical option is that of excisional lymph node biopsy, but an increased risk of distant metastasis has been suggested after this procedure.

The diagnosis of CNS–CUP requires proper physical examination including a thorough evaluation of the head and neck mucosa. This may be accomplished with fiberoptic or rigid endoscopy, with the latter being done under general anesthesia. Biopsies are usually taken from all suspicious sites or obtained blindly from the likely sites of tumor origin. These include the base of the tongue, tonsils, pyriform sinus, and nasopharynx on the lesional side. If the tonsil is not present, a biopsy of the tonsillar fossa should be performed.

Imaging studies of the head and neck include CT scanning and MRI (Fig. 9). The detection rate with CT is approximately 15% to 20%. In cases where there are suggestive findings on clinical examination or imaging, panendoscopy with biopsy is successful in identifying a primary tumor in up to 65% of patients. The most common sites for a definable primary lesion (in 82% of cases) are the tonsil or tonsillar fossa and the base of the tongue. Some patients also present with synchronous primary tumors. In recent years, the incidence of occult primary tumors in the nasopharynx, hypopharynx, and supraglottic larynx has decreased.

In cases with negative radiographic examinations, e.g., CT scanning and MRI, a primary tumor can sometimes be detected by using a functional imaging modality such as PET. Rusthoven et al. did a comprehensive review of the efficacy of fluorodeoxyglucose (FDG)–PET in detecting primary tumors presenting with cervical metastasis of a CUP (121). The overall sensitivity, specificity, and accuracy of the procedure were 88.3%, 74.9%, and 78.8%, respectively. FDG–PET delineated 24.5% of tumors that were undetected by other imaging modalities, and it was also sensitive in detecting previously unrecognized regional or distant metastases. Nonetheless, FDG–PET had a low specificity for tonsillar tumors and a

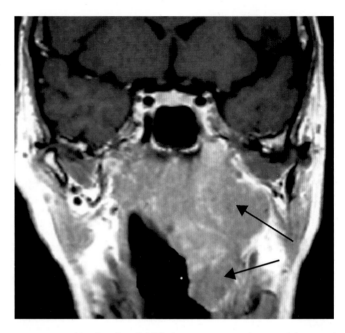

FIGURE 9 Head and neck MRI. A mass occupies the tongue base and hypopharynx, representing squamous carcinoma.

low sensitivity for carcinomas at the base of the tongue. Proof that FDG–PET improves the prognosis of patients with CNS–CUP is not yet available. We therefore consider this technique to be an option in cases in which other conventional imaging studies are negative.

A systematic bilateral tonsillectomy, even in the absence of visible lesions, has been recommended for CNS–CUP (17); up to 25% of occult primary tumors are detected in this manner. This is most true when presenting metastases are seen in the subdigastric lymph nodes, followed by the submandibular and midjugular nodes. In cases involving the supraclavicular nodes, an intrathoracic primary tumor must be considered and checked for with thoracic CT scanning and endoscopic evaluation. Cases showing the presence of undifferentiated carcinoma should be assessed with serologic studies for Epstein–Barr virus (EBV) or detection of EBV-DNA in the tumor tissue by in situ hybridization. These measures help delineate undifferentiated nasopharyngeal carcinomas, particularly in young males from North Africa or Southeast Asia (122).

The five-year survival rates for CNS–CUP range from 35% to 50%, and long-term tumor-free survival has been documented. Nodal status is considered to be the most important prognostic factor. In fact, the prognosis in CNS–CUP cases appears to be equivalent to that observed in patients with known primary tumors and a similar nodal stage. In cases where a neck dissection is done, other prognostic factors come into play, including the number of positive lymph nodes, the histological grade of the tumor, and extranodal extension by carcinoma. Over the last 30 years, probably due to better pretreatment evaluation and more effective therapy, local tumor control has improved in cases of CUP of the head and neck. However, proof that the latter effect translates into improved survival remains elusive.

The treatment of the CNS–CUP subset follows the guidelines for locally advanced squamous carcinomas of the head and neck (120, 123). Surgery alone is an inferior approach and is recommended only in highly selected patients, particularly those with pN1 disease and no extranodal tumor extension. Radiotherapy of the ipsilateral cervical nodes alone is inferior to irradiation to both sides of the neck, together with the mucosa in the entire pharyngeal axis and larynx. Again, although recommended, this intensive irradiation protocol has not been shown definitively to prolong survival. The role of systemic chemotherapy in this setting is undefined, but concurrent chemoradiotherapy seems to be particularly beneficial for patients with N2 or N3 disease.

ISOLATED INGUINAL LYMPH NODE METASTASIS OF SQUAMOUS CARCINOMA.

Isolated inguinal involvement by carcinoma defines an uncommon CUP subset, and the most common histological tumor type seen in this context is undifferentiated (anaplastic) carcinoma (124). Lymphoma and metastatic melanomas of unknown origin should be excluded pathologically in such circumstances. SCC or mixed squamous carcinoma–adenocarcinoma is considered a special entity because of its better prognosis. The diameters of the inguinal masses in this CUP group vary between 1 and 9 cm. Local pain and discomfort occur in roughly 50% of cases, and lymphedema is rare.

Careful evaluation of the anorectal region, a meticulous gynecological examination, and cystoscopy are necessary investigations in attempts to localize a primary tumor (17). Inguinal lymph node dissection, with or without local radiotherapy, is the recommended treatment for this CUP cohort with inguinal lymphadenopathy and metastatic SCC. Long-term survival after definitive local therapy has been reported in a few patients. The role of systemic chemotherapy has not been evaluated prospectively, but its emerging role as part of a combined therapy for other squamous cancers in the same region (e.g., in the anus, cervix, and bladder) suggests a future role for this treatment modality.

PATIENTS WITH CUP AND BLASTIC BONE METASTASES.

Osteoblastic bone metastases (Fig. 10) in men raise the suspicion of prostatic carcinoma, and this neoplasm can be confirmed by observing elevated serum

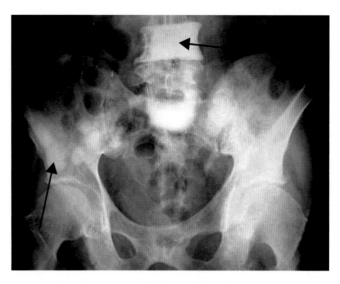

FIGURE 10 Bone X-ray. Multiple osteoblastic bone metastases.

PSA levels or demonstrating PSA in tumor tissue. Osteoblastic bone metastases also are an indication for an empiric trial of hormonal treatment, regardless of other clinicopathologic findings (19). Even when other clinical features do not suggest the presence of prostate carcinoma, elevated PSA levels in serum or positive immunostains for that marker justify the use of hormonal therapy (125, 126).

Osteoblastic metastases can be seen in other CUP cases as well, particularly those in which the tumor proves to be a well-differentiated neuroendocrine carcinoma ("carcinoid"), a breast carcinoma, or a pancreatic carcinoma (127–129). For this reason, serum tumor marker studies for chromogranin-A (130), CA15-3, and CA19-9 may be prudent in this scenario.

Recently, several radiopharmaceutical agents with an affinity for bone have been developed, including (186)Re-HEDP, (153)Sm-EDTMP, and (89)SrCl(2). They may be used in the palliative treatment of osseous metastases in lieu of, or in addition to, conventional radiotherapy (131, 132).

PDC WITH A MIDLINE DISTRIBUTION (EXTRAGONADAL GERM CELL TUMOR SYNDROME).

Initial observations that led to the definition of a unique CUP subset in 1979 were based on retrospective data from a small group of young male patients. They presented with malignancies that were difficult to characterize, but which were felt to represent undifferentiated carcinomas or PDAs of unknown origin. Despite those histological diagnoses, the cases were characterized by an excellent response to chemotherapy (3, 133). A subsequent pathological review of the tumors revealed features of germ cell malignancies, and many of the patients had abnormal β-HCG and AFP serum levels; some had testicular masses. Thus, the "extragonadal germ cell tumor syndrome" (EGCTS) was born. In the early 1980s, the clinical definition of this subgroup included a histological diagnosis of PDA or undifferentiated CUP site, age <50 years, tumor primarily located in the midline of the body, elevated serum levels of β-HCG and AFP, clinical evidence of rapid tumor growth, or tumor responsiveness to previous radiotherapy and/or chemotherapy. After 1982, Greco et al. abandoned these stipulations and included all young patients with PDAs or undifferentiated CUPs in EGCTS treatment protocols (134). In the largest reported series of 220 patients who were treated with cisplatin-based combination chemotherapy, an overall response rate of 62% was observed with a 10-year actuarial survival of 16% (135). However, a more recent study of 337 patients by Lenzi et al. could not confirm good survival or universal chemoresponsiveness of young patients with PDA (136). Although it is suggestive of EGCTS, chemosensitivity of poorly differentiated malignancies in young people is not diagnostic by itself. That characteristic may also be seen with lymphomas or neuroendocrine carcinomas.

The most common symptoms of the EGCTS–CUP subset include chest or back pain and shortness of breath. Weight loss, chills, and fever are less frequently reported than in CUP patients in unfavorable-prognosis subgroups. Most cases show tumor involvement of multiple anatomic sites at presentation, although the bulk of disease is, by definition, midline. The anterior mediastinum is the most frequent site of tumor growth (Fig. 11), followed by the lung fields, retroperitoneum, and supraclavicular and cervical lymph nodes. Some cases show involvement of the brain, bones, pleura, or pericardium (133).

Pathological evaluation is crucial to the proper classification of poorly differentiated epithelioid neoplasms, such as those in the EGCTS. The histological differential diagnosis includes carcinoma—both germ cell and somatic—as well as sarcoma, melanoma, and malignant lymphoma. Pathological evaluations to identify tumor lineage usually include immunostains for keratin, vimentin, CD45, CD20, CD3, S100 protein, and placental alkaline phosphatase (PLAP—a germ cell tumor–related marker). Once the diagnosis of carcinoma has been established, further assessment can focus on the anatomic site of origin. Lineage- or site-selective antibodies, such as TTF-1, PSA, GCDFP-15, CD56, and PLAP, can be employed at this point. Hainsworth et al. conducted a retrospective study to assess the clinical utility of immunostaining in 87 patients with poorly differentiated neoplasms with unknown primary sources (137). They reported that immunophenotyping confirmed the diagnosis of PDA in 56% of cases and yielded an alternative or more specific interpretation in 18% of cases. These included melanoma, lymphoma, prostatic carcinoma, and neuroendocrine carcinoma. In 28%, immunopathologic results were inconclusive.

Cytogenetic or molecular biological analyses may also be useful for young patients with midline PDCs of uncertain histology. In reference to germ cell tumors, Motzer et al. performed genetic analyses on 40 PDCs with a midline distribution. They showed abnormalities of chromosome 12 (e.g., i[12p]; del[12p]; multiple copies of 12p) in 12 of those cases, providing substantiation for a diagnosis of germ cell tumor (138). Other specific cytogenetic abnormalities were diagnostic of melanoma (two cases), lymphoma (one), primitive neuroectodermal tumor (one), and desmoplastic small round cell tumor (one).

The clinical evaluation of patients with midline PDCs includes CT scans of the chest, abdomen, and pelvis (17). Testicular ultrasonography and β-HCG and AFP serum levels are recommended for men in this CUP subset. However, Motzer et al. showed that AFP and HCG are most often normal in cases with midline tumors (138). Also, elevated serum levels of germ cell tumor markers do not predict the response to platinum-based chemotherapy in CUP patients (133, 139).

Patients with midline PDCs should be managed analogously to poor-prognosis germ cell tumor cases, using platinum-based chemotherapy (134, 140). Responses in >50% of patients has been reported, with 15% to 25% complete responders and 10% to 15% long-term disease-free survivors.

Few studies have focused specifically on primary mediastinal nonseminomatous germ cell tumors (MGCTs). These uncommon neoplasms have been said to have a particularly poor prognosis compared with

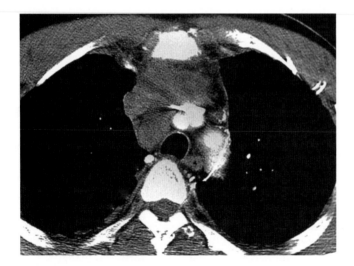

FIGURE 11 Chest CT scan. A mass in the anterior mediastinum represents an extragonadal germ cell tumor.

nonseminomatous germ cell tumors arising in other locations. The most common clinical symptoms of MGCTs include chest pain and shortness of breath. Weight loss, chills and fever, and the superior vena cava syndrome are possible (141). Forty percent of MGCT cases will go on to long-term survival after modern cisplatin-based chemotherapy, followed by surgical resection of residual masses (142).

POORLY DIFFERENTIATED NEUROENDOCRINE CARCINOMAS. Neuroendocrine carcinomas of un-known primary origin represent a broad spectrum of malignancies. Three clinicopathologic subsets of such lesions have been described. The first is that of low-grade neuroendocrine carcinomas (i.e., "carcinoids" or pancre-atic "islet cell tumors"), which usually secondarily involve the liver and sometimes produce symptoms that are associated with the secretion of vasoactive peptides. The second subset is that of small cell "anaplastic" carcinoma (poorly differentiated neuroendocrine carcinoma, small cell type), with a histological appearance and clinical behavior that is similar to that of small cell lung cancer or extrapulmonary small cell carcinoma. The third group represents PDCs or PDAs with "occult" neuroendocrine differentiation; that is to say, neuroendocrine features that are demonstrable only at immunohistologic or ultra-structural levels of pathological evaluation (143).

Metastatic "classical" carcinoid tumors with an unknown anatomic origin have been well described; they usually present in the liver and an occult GI primary site is suspected. The clinical behavior and treatment of carci-noidal CUPs are identical to those of metastatic GI carcinoids with a defined primary tumor (144). The mean age at diagnosis is 59 years. Presenting symptoms include abdominal pain (60%), diarrhea (51%), flushing (36%), enteric-obstructive symptoms (19%), and cardiac valvular disease (11%). The hormone levels seen with carcinoidal CUPs are not significantly different from those attending metastatic midgut carcinoids. Investigations to localize a primary tumor usually include CT scans of the abdomen and nuclear imaging with labelled octreotide (145). Van Tuyl et al. also showed that video capsule endoscopy can be useful in detecting primary carcinoids in the small intestine in this context (146).

Well-differentiated neuroendocrine carcinoma CUPs are typically indolent and do not respond well to chemo-therapy; however, octreotide may be helpful in controlling symptoms. The survival of patients with such tumors is similar to that of patients with metastatic midgut carcinoids; the 10-year survivals of these two groups are 22% and 28%, respectively.

Small cell carcinoma is now known to arise potentially in many organ sites. Cells with "neuroendocrine" features have been identified throughout the body, especially in the lungs, GI tract, and prostate. Therefore, it is not surprising that tumors with neuroendocrine features can also originate at many anatomic locations (147–149). So-called extrapulmonary small cell ("oat cell") carcinomas can arise in the GI tract, ear, nose, and throat, genitourinary system, biliary tract, pancreas, internal genitalia, upper respiratory system, kidneys, thymus, skin, and peritoneum (150–152). Metastatic small cell carcinoma CUP cases account for 10% of patients with extrapulmonary small cell carcinomas. Because all these tumors have the potential for rapid growth and early dissemination, diagnosis at an advanced stage of disease is frequent and one-third of patients have extensive tumor burdens. In all metastatic small cell carcinoma CUP cases, a primary site should first be sought in the lung, and then in the various documented locations for extrapulmonary small cell carcinoma. Regardless of their anatomic sources, small cell carcinoma CUPs are usually fatal, with a 13% five-year survival rate (150).

Finally, there is a subset of poorly differentiated tumors with "occult" neuroendocrine differentiation, identifiable only with electron microscopy or immunohis-tochemistry. This cohort of tumors represents 13% of PDC-CUPs (134). Most patients have clinical evidence of a high-grade malignancy with metastases in several sites (153). The median age at diagnosis is 54 years, with a male predominance. Most patients are smokers. The retroperitoneum (28%), lymph nodes (24%), and media-stinum (10%) are most frequently involved by PDC-CUPs with occult neuroendocrine features, and 6% of cases show metastatic tumors at two or more sites. Other possible locations for metastases include bones, liver, peritoneum, subcutaneous tissue, and the pharynx. Symptoms suggesting a hormonal syndrome are very unusual in this subset, consistent with the poorly differ-entiated nature of the tumors.

Many high-grade neuroendocrine carcinomas are very sensitive to chemotherapy (153, 154). In recent studies, responses to platinum-based or paclitaxel/carboplatine-based chemotherapy were reported to be as high as 50% to 70%, with >25% complete responses and 10% to 15% long-term survivors.

PATIENTS WITH SINGLE, SMALL, POTENTIALLY RESECTABLE METASTASES. In situations where only one apparent site of metastasis is identified (e.g., one lymph node group or one large mass), the possibility that an unusual primary tumor is *simulating* metastatic disease must be considered. Several neoplasms may present in this fashion, including Merkel cell carcinomas (Fig. 12) and cutaneous adnexal carcinomas, as well as sarcomas, melanomas, or lymphomas that are mistakenly interpreted as carcinomas on pathological and clinical grounds.

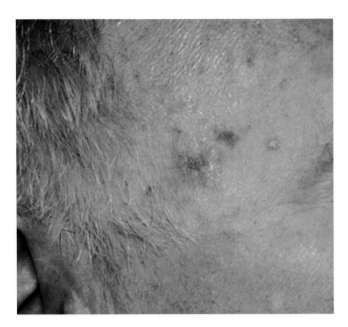

FIGURE 12 Potentially resectable Merkel cell carcinoma.

Usually, patients with "one" site of involvement do have metastatic carcinoma, and many other metastases are really present but are not detectable at that point in time.

There is no standard for the specific evaluation of patients in this CUP subset (17). French guidelines would lead one to consider whole-body CT scanning and bone scintigraphy as options. FDG–PET scans may also provide valuable information when local treatment is being considered (155). Further evaluation of these diagnostic measures, as well as cost–benefit analyses, are warranted.

In the absence of any other documented disease, patients with presumed unifocal metastasis should be treated with aggressive local therapy, including resection, radiation therapy, or both. A minority will enjoy long-term disease-free survival (19).

■ PROGNOSTIC AND PREDICTIVE FACTORS

Prognostic Factors in the General Population of CUP Patients

For malignant diseases, predictions concerning tumor behavior and choice of optimal therapy are based on the primary tumor site. Thus, in CUP cases, the *absence* of a known tumor source poses major uncertainties and generates anxiety for both patients and physicians. CUPs are a heterogeneous group of tumors with widely variable natural histories, but in aggregate, CUP patients historically have a poor survival rate. In nonrandomized clinical studies, median survivals range from 8 to 13 months, and

one-year survivals vary from 15% to 29% (156–161). These data are similar to those attending chemotherapy-treated metastases of lung, pancreatic, and gastric carcinomas, among others (162).

In patients who are evaluated for treatment at tertiary CCs, median survival ranges from 9 to 11 months (16). However, in tumor registry data, CUP cases have a poorer median survival of three to four months, with <15% being alive one year after diagnosis (1, 2, 20). Sève et al. observed important differences between patients being evaluated at CCs and those evaluated at other medical centers (20). Non-CC patients are significantly older, with more severe comorbidity and adverse functional status. The prognosis is indeed poorer in these individuals, with a three-week median survival. These data support the presence of a strong referral bias, and explain the better outcomes reported in CC-based studies. In this context, the ability to assign patients to prognostic subgroups using a simple, reliable classification scheme would be an important tool. It would help the oncologist to refine the management of CUP patients, to assess published treatment results, and to design clinical research studies.

As discussed, some CUP patients belong to more favorable subgroups that may respond to specific therapy. However, the majority of CUP cases fall outside such subsets and seldom respond to treatment. For them, a number of studies have been performed to identify adverse prognostic factors.

No prospective studies or meta-analyses of prognostic factors in CUP cases have been published. We have included here those recent studies with multivariate statistical analysis that have included more than 100 patients (Table 5).

Abbruzzese et al. studied the prognosis of 657 unselected CUP patients referred to the M.D. Anderson Cancer Center from 1987 to 1992 (16). It should be pointed out that cases in favorable subsets were also included in this study. Univariate analysis identified two favorable characteristics: isolated lymph nodal involvement and pathological diagnoses of carcinoma (not further specified), squamous carcinoma, and neuroendocrine carcinoma. Adverse characteristics included male sex; adenocarcinomatous histology; metastases to the brain, bones, liver, lungs, and pleura; and a multiplicity of metastatic sites, with survival being inversely related to the number of metastatic locations. Age, race, and the presence of cutaneous or peritoneal metastases did not significantly affect outcome in the univariate model. However, *multivariate* analysis identified lymph nodal and peritoneal metastases and neuroendocrine histology as independent predictors of longer survival. Male sex, a large number of metastatic sites, adenocarcinomatous

Table 5 Published studies of prognostic factors in patients with CUP

Reference	No. of Patients	Adverse Prognostic Variables	
		Univariate Analysis	Multivariate Analysis
Abbruzzese et al. (16)	657	Male sex	Male sex
		Adenocarcinoma histological type	Adenocarcinoma histological type
		No. of metastatic sites >1	No. of metastatic sites >1
		Lung metastases	Liver metastases
		Liver metastases	
		Bone metastases	
		Pleura metastases	
		Brain metastases	
Lortholary et al. (163)	311	Male sex	Male sex
		Adenocarcinoma histological type	Adenocarcinoma histological type
		No. of metastatic sites >1	No. of metastatic sites >1
		Poor PS	Poor PS
		Primary identified	
Culine et al. (33)	150	PS (0–1, 2–3)	PS (0–1, 2–3)
		No. of metastatic sites >1	LDH
		Liver metastases	
		CEA	
		CA-125	
		Alkaline phosphatase	
		LDH	
Sève et al. (20)	389	Age (0≥65 yr)	PS ≥ 2
		PS ≥ 2	Liver metastases

(Continued)

■ **Table 5** Published studies of prognostic factors in patients with CUP (*Continued*)

| Reference | No. of Patients | Adverse Prognostic Variables | |
		Univariate Analysis	Multivariate Analysis
		ACE-27 grade ≥2 adenocarcinoma histological type	Peritoneal metastases
		Liver metastases	ACE-27 grade ≥2
		Peritoneal metastases	
		Lack of lymph node metastases	
		No. of metastatic sites >1	
		LDH[a]	
Sève et al. (164)	317	PS ≥ 2	PS ≥ 2
		ACE-27 (3, < 2)	ACE-27 (3, < 2)
		Liver metastases	Liver metastases
		Peritoneal involvement	LDH
		No. of metastatic sites >1	Low serum albumin lymphopenia
		Alkaline phosphatase	
		LDH	
		Anemia	
		Thrombocytosis	
		Low serum albumin lymphopenia	

[a]Because of missing data, LDH level was not incorporated in the multivariate analysis.

Abbreviations: PS, performance status; LDH, lactate dehydrogenases; CEA, carcinoembryonic antigen; ACE-27, Adult Comorbidity Evaluation 27.

tumor type, and hepatic metastases were again confirmed as unfavorable indicators. Supraclavicular lymph node involvement was also found to be a significantly negative prognostic factor.

Lortholary et al. studied prognostic factors among 311 unselected CUP patients referred to one French CC between 1980 and 1995 (163). Patients belonging to favorable CUP subsets were not excluded. Univariate analysis of the data identified several favorable character-istics—female sex, a PS of <2, histological tumor types of

squamous or undifferentiated carcinoma, eventual identi-fication of a primary tumor source, and only one site of metastasis. Multivariate analysis by the Cox method resulted in four positive prognostic factors—female sex, PS <2, squamous carcinomatous histology, and only one site of metastasis.

In 1999, Hess et al. published a regression tree analysis of 1000 consecutive CUP cases seen at the M.D. Anderson Cancer Center between 1987 and 1994. It produced 10 subgroups that had median survivals ranging from five to 40 months (32). Several clinicopathologic variables, including age, sex, ethnicity, histopathologic tumor type and degree of differentiation, the number of metastatic sites, the number and locations of lymph nodal metastases, and involvement of specific nodal and extranodal sites were evaluated. The subgroup with the longest median survival comprised 127 patients with only one to two metastatic sites, histology other than adenocarcinoma, and no involvement of the adrenals, bones, liver, or pleura. The subset with the second best survival (24 months) was represented by 28 patients with isolated hepatic metastases of neuroendocrine carcinoma. One of the worst prognosis groups, with a median survival of only five months, included 153 patients who were older than 61.5 years, or with histology other than neuroendocrine carcinoma, or hepatic metastases. Another adverse category comprised 23 patients with adrenal metastases. An additional, previously undescribed subgroup was constituted by 76 patients with dominant pleural involvement and a median survival of nine months.

Two alternative prognosis "trees" were created in that study, using an initial separation centering on histological tumor type and lymph node involvement. The groups generated by a subsequent division of the lymph node variable included a "best survival" group of 99 patients with nonadenocarcinomatous histology, only one or two metastatic sites, and lymph node involvement; these individuals had a median survival of 45 months. The two groups with the shortest survival (five months) were characterized by nonneuroendocrine histology, hepatic involvement, and no nodal disease (117 patients); or by adrenal involvement, lymph nodal metastases, and two or more sites of metastasis (39 patients). This study confirmed the prognostic importance of hepatic and lymph nodal metastases, tumor histology, and the number of metastatic sites. However, the applicability of this model in daily practice is admittedly limited by its complexity.

Culine et al. developed a simple prognostic model that stressed the importance of PS and serum lactate dehydrogenases (LDH), in a study of 150 CUP patients evaluated at a French CC. Pathologically favorable tumor subsets were excluded in this assessment (33). By univariate analysis, adverse prognostic factors included a PS of 2 to 3, the presence of hepatic metastases, and two or more metastatic sites. The value of PS and hepatic involvement were confirmed as independently significant prognostic variables after multivariate analysis. The authors then evaluated blood levels of alkaline phosphatase, carcinoembryonic antigen (CEA), CA19.9, CA-125, CA15.3, and LDH that were seen prior to treatment. Of those, elevated LDH levels had independent adverse significance after multivariate analysis. Additional multiparametric studies including both clinical and biological variables

showed that only a PS of 2 to 3 and elevated LDH retained significance. The authors subsequently identified good-risk and poor-risk patients with median respective survivals of 11.7 and 3.9 months, by focusing on these two adverse prognostic factors. One-year survival rates in these cohorts were 45% and 11%, respectively. These results were subsequently validated with an independent data set of 116 patients who were enrolled in two prospective clinical trials.

More recently, Sève et al. conducted a Canadian retrospective study to assess the impact of comorbidity on prognosis in patients with CUP (20). This was done using the Adult Comorbidity Evaluation-27 (ACE-27) protocol at the time of diagnosis. The authors reviewed clinical data in 389 cases with a diagnosis of CUP in the Northern Alberta Cancer Registry, as seen between 2000 and 2003. In univariate analysis, short survival was significantly related to age ≥65 yrs, PS ≥2, an ACE-27 grade ≥2, adenocarcinomatous histology, the presence of hepatic or peritoneal metastases, lack of lymph nodal involvement, two or more metastatic sites, and a high serum LDH level. Multivariate analyses of these factors found that PS ≥2, the presence of hepatic or peritoneal metastases, a high comorbidity score, and two or more metastatic sites were independently significant predictors of survival. Because of incomplete data, LDH levels were not incorporated into the multivariate analysis. The impact of comorbidities on survival was limited to those patients with a low PS.

The same authors subsequently performed a retrospective study of consecutive CUP cases that were evaluated at the Cross Cancer Institute of Edmonton (Canada) between 1998 and 2004. The goal was to investigate whether lymphopenia and low serum albumin levels might be related to the prognosis of CUP patients (164). By univariate analysis, adverse prognostic factors included PS ≥2, an ACE-27 grade of 3 (vs. ACE-27 grades of <2), the presence of hepatic or peritoneal involvement, two or more metastatic sites, a high level of alkaline phosphatase or LDH, anemia, thrombocytosis, a low level of serum albumin, and lymphopenia (defined as an absolute peripheral blood lymphocyte count of ≤0.7 ×10^9/L). Multivariate analysis showed that patients with PS of ≥2, hepatic metastases, high overall comorbidity scores by ACE-27, elevated LDH levels, lymphopenia, and low serum albumin levels had a worse prognosis. Because of the observation that liver metastasis and low serum albumin levels were the most powerful adverse prognostic factors, with a hazard ratio for death of >2, a subsequent classification scheme was delineated. The "good-risk" group was that with no hepatic metastases and a normal serum albumin level, whereas the "poor-risk" group had the converse. Their respective median survivals were 371 days and 103 days (p < 0.0001). This classification was further validated in an independent data set of 124 patients evaluated at two French CCs, among whom median survivals were 378 days in the good-risk group and 90 days in the poor-risk subset ($p < 0.0001$). Interestingly, this prognostic model substantially outperformed the previous standard paradigm devised by Culine et al. This improvement was largely due to the impact of elevated LDH levels in cases classified as good-risk in the "new" prognostic model. Because of its potential lack of specificity in the CUP population, and its lesser prognostic value, the authors concluded that LDH is probably inferior to serum albumin for predicting survival in CUP cases.

Measurement of other biological variables, such as C-reactive protein and inflammatory cytokines, appears to predict survival in some populations of cancer patients. Hence, it is of interest in CUP cases as well (164). Prospective studies that include both clinical and biological variables are warranted to best determine the individual prognosis of CUP patients and design more tailored treatments.

Prognostic Factors in CUP Patients with PDC (Not Further Specified) and PDA

The preceding section considered prognostic studies on the general population of CUP patients. Others, however, have focused specifically on the prognosis of CUP patients with PDC and PDA.

Hainsworth et al. studied a prospectively compiled group of 220 patients who were treated with cisplatin-based chemotherapy over a period of 12 years, at Vanderbilt University (135). In selected patients, pathological diagnoses were revised at intervals after entry into the study, because of additional information obtained by rebiopsy, autopsy, or retrospective pathological evaluation using adjunctive methods such as immunohistochemistry. The final diagnoses were those of PDC (97 patients); PDA (70 patients); PDC with neuroendocrine features (25 patients); melanoma (eight patients); lymphoma (six patients); poorly differentiated SCC or sarcoma (five each); and yolk-sac tumor, primitive neuroectodermal tumor, mixed PDA/neuroendocrine carcinoma, and prostatic adenocarcinoma (one each). The authors assessed various clinicopathologic features in this case group as potential prognostic indicators, including age, sex, smoking history, histological diagnosis, the number of metastatic sites, the dominant site of tumor, serum LDH and CEA levels, and the chemotherapy regimen that was used. Univariate analysis showed only one favorable characteristic: a dominant tumor location in the retroperitoneum or peripheral lymph nodes. Three adverse characteristics were identified—a history of cigarette smoking, more than two metastatic sites, and elevated serum levels of LDH

and/or CEA. When these factors were assessed in Cox multivariate analysis, the independently favorable prognosticators were predominant tumor location in the retroperitoneum or peripheral lymph nodes; tumor limited to one or two metastatic sites; a negative smoking history; and young age. Saliently, histopathologic classification of the tumors as PDC or PDA was not prognostically important.

Van der Gaast et al. developed a simple prognostic model stressing the importance of PS and alkaline phosphatase, based on a population of 79 CUP patients with PDA and PDC. They were evaluated at a Dutch CC (165). The authors assessed demographic, clinical, and laboratory variables for possible significance as prognostic factors. In univariate analysis, PS ≥1, histological classification as adenocarcinoma versus undifferentiated carcinoma, the presence of bone and liver metastases, and serum levels of alkaline phosphatase and aspartate aminotransferase were found to be adverse prognostic indicators. Poor PS and the alkaline phosphatase level were confirmed as independently significant by multivariate analysis. "Good-prognosis" patients, with a PS of 0 and an alkaline phosphatase level <1.25 the upper limit of normal, had a median survival of >4 years. "Intermediate-prognosis" patients, with either PS ≤1 or an alkaline phosphatase level of >1.25× the upper limit of normal, had a median survival of 10 months and a 4-year survival rate of 15%. The "poor prognosis" group, with both a PS score of ≤1 and an alkaline phosphatase level of >1.25× the upper limit of normal, had a median survival of only four months and no survivors beyond 14 months.

To evaluate the prevalence of PDC and PDA in an unselected population of CUP patients, and to see whether favorable treatment-response profiles in PDC/PDA patients could be confirmed in a large consecutive series, Lenzi et al. studied 957 unselected CUP patients for whom comprehensive pathological evaluations had been done (136). The authors found that 140 cases were diagnosed as PDC and 197 as PDA. No clinical differences were identified among patients with PDC or PDA, or those with other histological types of carcinoma. Median survival for the PDC cases was 13 months, and for those with PDA it was 9 months, with PDC histology being statistically significant by univariate analysis. In multivariate analysis, however, there was no significant survival advantage in this histological subset. Variables that predicted survival in the PDC/PDA group included lymph nodal metastases, female sex, less than three metastatic sites, the histological carcinoma subtype, and age <64 years. The findings of this study appear to be supported by results of more recent phase II trials. In those assessments, patients with well-differentiated carcinomas and PDC histology had similar response rates with the same platinum-based regimen (156, 158).

■ CONCLUSIONS

CUPs are metastatic carcinomas for which a primary site cannot be identified during pretreatment assessments. These tumors are characterized by their slow local development and a high metastatic potential. The organ of origin remains unknown in 20% to 50% of CUP patients, but results from autopsies show that the primary tumors are most often located in the pancreas, lungs, gut, or kidneys. CUP is a common clinical syndrome that accounts for 2% to 5% of all cancer patients. With the ever-increasing sophistication of pathological and radiological techniques, this frequency will probably decline in the future. In referral centers, the median age of CUP patients at presentation is approximately 60 years, with a marginally higher frequency in men. However, in populations described by tumor registries, they are 10 years older and the number of women is greater.

Clinical presentations of CUPs are usually nonspecific and include a short history of local or constitutional symptoms. Major sites of metastases include the lymph nodes, liver, bones, and lungs. Roughly 30% of patients present with involvement of three or more organs. In most instances, the primary tumor remains unidentified throughout life.

The author proposes a general approach to diagnosis in patients with possible CUPs as outlined in Figure 13 (17, 36, 37, 166–168). The first step is procurement of a complete medical history and physical examination. One must also pay attention to past biopsy results, any history of surgery, the nature of any excised or regressed lesions, and a history of cigarette smoking. Family history is also important, and may, for example, suggest the possibility of the hereditary nonpolyposis colon carcinoma syndrome or hereditary breast carcinoma. The physical examination should include careful palpation of the thyroid, breasts, lymph nodes, prostate, and pelvic organs. Findings at that step can guide the physician to look for a specific primary tumor. For example, the presence of left supraclavicular lymphadenopathy (Virchow's node) (169) or periumbilical cutaneous tumor nodules (Sister Mary Joseph's nodules) (170) should prompt a thorough investigation of the GI tract. In addition,

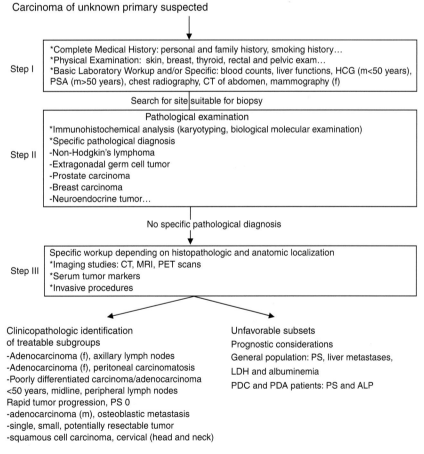

FIGURE 13 Steps in the diagnosis of patients with carcinoma of unknown primary origin. *Abbreviations*: HCG, human chorionic gonadotrophin; PSA, prostate-specific antigen; m, male; f, female; PS, performance status; LDH, lactate dehydrogenase level; PDC, poorly differentiated carcinoma; PDA, poorly differentiated adenocarcinoma; ALP, alkaline phosphatase. *Source*: From Refs. 17, 36, 37, 166–168.

a perianal mass may suggest the presence of a carcinoma at that site in a patient who presents with inguinal lymphadenopathy or isolated hepatic metastases.

The most important step in the diagnostic sequence is biopsy of the most accessible lesion for pathological examination. Therefore, noninvasive tests intended to search for the primary tumor are comparatively unhelpful and often cause significant delay in diagnosis and treatment (171). Pathological evaluation is important, to make certain that the patient in question does have a malignancy; 5% of cases referred to CUP clinics do not. Pathological examination, including immunohistochemistry, electron microscopy, and, in selected cases, cytogenetic and molecular–biological studies, are essential to exclude noncarcinomatous tumors such as lymphomas, melanomas, or sarcomas. It is also capable of positively identifying metastatic prostatic, breast, germ cell, and neuroendocrine tumors. Therefore, the pathologist may guide further clinical assessment to localize a primary neoplasm (17).

The third step is a diagnostic evaluation for possible identification of the primary tumor site and staging. The role of diagnostic radiology, including PET scanning, and the diagnostic value of serum tumor markers are discussed in other specific chapters in this book. Similarly, invasive procedures used for similar purposes are discussed in another chapter. Their use should be tailored to the particular clinical presentation of each patient. Physicians must use their discretion in submitting a patient to many procedures, especially if results would not change the overall treatment plan. This is particularly true for individuals with poor functional status.

At this point, the clinician can identify favorable and treatable CUP subsets. These include women with isolated axillary lymphadenopathy and adenocarcinoma (treated as AJCC stage II or III breast carcinoma), women with isolated peritoneal carcinomatosis (treated as metastatic ovarian carcinoma), young men with suspected EGCT syndrome, men with isolated blastic bone metastases (usually treated as metastatic prostate carcinoma), patients with a single potentially resectable tumor mass, and others with high cervical lymphadenopathy and SCC, for whom lymph node dissection and radiotherapy can result in long-term survival.

Patients not belonging to these subsets should be stratified according to known prognostic factors. Two prognostic models have been developed and validated in the general population of CUP patients. These respectively include one clinical variable (PS and liver metastases) and one biological variable (elevated serum LDH and low serum albumin) and can help the oncologist choose optimal treatment. In patients with PDC and PDA, the PS and serum alkaline phosphatase levels are additional prognostic factors.

In the future, we can expect that studies on the basic biology of carcinomas will allow us to better understand the clinical heterogeneity of CUPs and improve our ability to determine their prognoses. With recent techniques such as microarray technology (see Chapter 7), more accurate diagnostic and prognostic profiles are already being identified, which allows for better patient selection before deciding on a mode of treatment.

■ REFERENCES

1. Levi F, Te VC, Erler G, Randimbison L, La Vecchia C. Epidemiology of unknown primary tumours. *Eur J Cancer* 2002; 38(13):1810–2.
2. van de Wouw AJ, Janssen-Heijnen ML, Coebergh JW, Hillen HF. Epidemiology of unknown primary tumours; incidence and population-based survival of 1285 patients in Southeast Netherlands, 1984–1992. *Eur J Cancer* 2002; 38(3):409–13.
3. Stewart JF, Tattersall MH, Woods RL, Fox RM. Unknown primary adenocarcinoma: incidence of overinvestigation and natural history. *Br Med J* 1979; 1(6177):1530–3.
4. Nystrom JS, Weiner JM, Heffelfinger-Juttner J, Irwin LE, Bateman JR, Wolf RM. Metastatic and histologic presentations in unknown primary cancer. *Semin Oncol* 1977; 4(1):53–8.
5. Le Chevalier T, Cvitkovic E, Caille P, et al. Early metastatic cancer of unknown primary origin at presentation. A clinical study of 302 consecutive autopsied patients. *Arch Intern Med* 1988; 148(9):2035–9.
6. Blaszyk H, Hartmann A, Bjornsson J. Cancer of unknown primary: clinicopathologic correlations. *Apmis* 2003; 111(12): 1089–94.
7. Kirsten F, Chi CH, Leary JA, Ng AB, Hedley DW, Tattersall MH. Metastatic adeno or undifferentiated carcinoma from an unknown primary site—natural history and guidelines for identification of treatable subsets. *Q J Med* 1987; 62(238):143–61.
8. van de Wouw AJ, Jansen RL, Griffioen AW, Hillen HF. Clinical and immunohistochemical analysis of patients with unknown primary tumour. A search for prognostic factors in UPT. *Anticancer Res* 2004; 24(1):297–301.
9. Hamilton CS, Langlands AO. ACUPS (adenocarcinoma of unknown primary site): a clinical and cost benefit analysis. *Int J Radiat Oncol Biol Phys* 1987; 13(10):1497–503.
10. Jordan WE 3rd, Shildt RA. Adenocarcinoma of unknown primary site. The Brooke Army Medical Center experience. *Cancer* 1985; 55(4):857–60.
11. Lenzi R, Raber MN, Frost P, Schmidt S, Abbruzzese JL. Phase II study of cisplatin, 5-fluorouracil and folinic acid in patients with carcinoma of unknown primary origin. *Eur J Cancer* 1993; 29A(11):1634.
12. Holmes FF, Fouts TL. Metastatic cancer of unknown primary site. *Cancer* 1970; 26(4):816–20.
13. Didolkar MS, Fanous N, Elias EG, Moore RH. Metastatic carcinomas from occult primary tumors. A study of 254 patients. *Ann Surg* 1977; 186(5):625–30.
14. Osteem RT, Kopf G, Wilson RE. In pursuit of the unknown primary. *Am J Surg* 1978; 135(4):494–7.
15. Moertel CG, Hanley JA. Combination chemotherapy trials in metastatic carcinoid tumor and the malignant carcinoid syndrome. *Cancer Clin Trials* 1979; 2(4):327–34.
16. Abbruzzese JL, Abbruzzese MC, Hess KR, Raber MN, Lenzi R, Frost P. Unknown primary carcinoma: natural history and

prognostic factors in 657 consecutive patients. *J Clin Oncol* 1994; 12(6):1272–80.

17. Bugat R, Bataillard A, Lesimple T, et al. Summary of the standards, options and recommendations for the management of patients with carcinoma of unknown primary site (2002). *Br J Cancer* 2003; 89(Suppl. 1):S59–66.

18. Hainsworth JD, Greco FA. Treatment of patients with cancer of an unknown primary site. *N Engl J Med* 1993; 329(4):257–63.

19. Greco FA, Hainsworth JD. Cancer of unknown primary site. In: De Vita HS, Rosenberg SA, eds. *Cancer: Principles and Practice of Oncology*, 6th ed. Philadelphia: Lippincott-Raven, 2001, pp. 2537–60.

20. Sève P, Sawyer M, Hanson J, Broussolle C, Dumontet C, Mackey JR. The influence of comorbidities, age, and performance status on the prognosis and treatment of patients with metastatic carcinomas of unknown primary site: a population-based study. *Cancer* 2006; 106(9):2058–66.

21. Coates M, Armstrong B. NSW Central Cancer Registry. Cancer in New South Wales. Incidence and Mortality. *NSW Cancer Council.* NSW, 1995.

22. Komov DV, Komarov IG, Podrguliskii KR, et al. Cancer metastases from an unestablished primary tumor (clinical aspects, diagnosis, treatment). *Sov Med Rev F Oncol* 1991; 4(1–33).

23. Neumann G. The impact of cancer with unspecified site. *Off Gesundheitswes* 1988; 50:13–9.

24. Muir C. Cancer of unknown primary site. *Cancer* 1995; 75 (Suppl. 1):353–6.

25. Jemal A, Murray T, Samuels A, Ghafoor A, Ward E, Thun MJ. Cancer statistics, 2003. *CA Cancer J Clin* 2003; 53(1):5–26.

26. Parkin D, Muir C, Whelan S. Cancer incidence in five continents. *IARC Sci Publ Lyon: IARC*, 1992, pp. 45–173.

27. Parkin D, Whelan S, Ferlay J, Raymond L, Young J. Cancer incidence in five continents, 143 ed. *Lyon: IARC*, 1991.

28. Visser O, Coebergh JWW, Schouten LJ. Incidence of Cancer in the Netherlands 1993. *Utrecht: TNC Registry*, 1993.

29. Silverberg E, Lubera J. Cancer statistics, 1987. *CA Cancer J Clin* 1987; 37(1):2–19.

30. Visser O, van Wijnen JH, van Leeuwen FE. Incidence of cancer in the area around Amsterdam Airport Schiphol in 1988–2003: a population-based ecological study. *BMC Public Health* 2005; 5:127.

31. Jemal A, Siegel R, Ward E, et al. Cancer statistics, 2006. *CA Cancer J Clin* 2006; 56(2):106–30.

32. Hess KR, Abbruzzese MC, Lenzi R, Raber MN, Abbruzzese JL. Classification and regression tree analysis of 1000 consecutive patients with unknown primary carcinoma. *Clin Cancer Res* 1999; 5(11):3403–10.

33. Culine S, Kramar A, Saghatchian M, et al. Development and validation of a prognostic model to predict the length of survival in patients with carcinomas of an unknown primary site. *J Clin Oncol* 2002; 20(24):4679–83.

34. Ayoub JP, Hess KR, Abbruzzese MC, Lenzi R, Raber MN, Abbruzzese JL. Unknown primary tumors metastatic to liver. *J Clin Oncol* 1998; 16(6):2105–12.

35. Gaber AO, Rice P, Eaton C, Pietrafitta JJ, Spatz E, Deckers PJ. Metastatic malignant disease of unknown origin. *Am J Surg* 1983; 145(4):493–7.

36. Sève P, Stankovic K, Charbon A, Broussolle C. Carcinoma of unknown primary site. *Rev Med Intern* 2006; 27(7):532–45.

37. Lesimple T, Voigt JJ, Bataillard A, Coindre JM, Culine S, Lortholary A, et al. Clinical practice guidelines: standards, options and recommendations for the diagnosis of carcinomas of unknown primary site. *Bull Cancer* 2003; 90(12):1071–96.

38. Pouessel D, Thezenas S, Culine S, Becht C, Senesse P, Ychou M. Hepatic metastases from carcinomas of unknown primary site. *Gastroenterol Clin Biol* 2005; 29(12):1224–32.

39. Hess KR, Varadhachary GR, Taylor SH, Wei W, Raber MN, Lenzi R, et al. Metastatic patterns in adenocarcinoma. *Cancer* 2006; 106(7):1624–33.

40. Sears D, Hajdu SI. The cytologic diagnosis of malignant neoplasms in pleural and peritoneal effusions. *Acta Cytol* 1987; 31(2):85–97.

41. Antony V, Loddenkemper R, Astoul P, et al. Management of malignant pleural effusions. *Eur Respir J* 2001; 18:402–19.

42. Harwood TR, Gracey DR, Yokoo H. Pseudomesotheliomatous carcinoma of the lung. A variant of peripheral lung cancer. *Am J Clin Pathol* 1976; 65(2):159–67.

43. Attanoos RL, Gibbs AR. "Pseudomesotheliomatous" carcinomas of the pleura: a 10-year analysis of cases from the Environmental Lung Disease Research Group, Cardiff. *Histopathology* 2003; 43(5):444–52.

44. Kobashi Y, Matsushima T, Irei T. Clinicopathological analysis of lung cancer resembling malignant pleural mesothelioma. *Respirology* 2005; 10(5):660–5.

45. Ordonez NG. What are the current best immunohistochemical markers for the diagnosis of epithelioid mesothelioma? A review and update. *Hum Pathol* 2007; 38(1):1–16.

46. Bonnefoi H, Smith IE. How should cancer presenting as a malignant pleural effusion be managed? *Br J Cancer* 1996; 74(5):832–5.

47. Berrettoni BA, Carter JR. Mechanisms of cancer metastasis to bone. *J Bone Joint Surg Am* 1986; 68(2):308–12.

48. Vandecandelaere M, Flipo RM, Cortet B, Catanzariti L, Duquesnoy B, Delcambre B. Bone metastases revealing primary tumors. Comparison of two series separated by 30 years. *Joint Bone Spine* 2004; 71(3):224–9.

49. Maillefert JF, Tebib J, Aho S, et al. Bone metastasis of hepatocellular carcinoma. Apropos of 22 cases. *Rev Rhum Ed Fr* 1993; 60(12):907–12.

50. Vinceneux P, Cramer E, Grossin M, Kahn MF. Diagnosis of bone metastases. Value of the guided puncture and the posterior iliac crest systematic puncture-biopsy. *Presse Med* 1983; 12(14):873–6.

51. Katagiri H, Takahashi M, Inagaki J, Sugiura H, Ito S, Iwata H. Determining the site of the primary cancer in patients with skeletal metastasis of unknown origin: a retrospective study. *Cancer* 1999; 86(3):533–7.

52. Simon MA, Bartucci EJ. The search for the primary tumor in patients with skeletal metastases of unknown origin. *Cancer* 1986; 58(5):1088–95.

53. Rougraff BT, Kneisl JS, Simon MA. Skeletal metastases of unknown origin. A prospective study of a diagnostic strategy. *J Bone Joint Surg Am* 1993; 75(9):1276–81.

54. Nguyen LN, Maor MH, Oswald MJ. Brain metastases as the only manifestation of an undetected primary tumor. *Cancer* 1998; 83(10):2181–4.

55. Nussbaum ES, Djalilian HR, Cho KH, Hall WA. Brain metastases. Histology, multiplicity, surgery, and survival. *Cancer* 1996; 78(8):1781–8.

56. Lagerwaard FJ, Levendag PC, Nowak PJ, Eijkenboom WM, Hanssens PE, Schmitz PI. Identification of prognostic factors in patients with brain metastases: a review of 1292 patients. *Int J Radiat Oncol Biol Phys* 1999; 43(3):795–803.

57. Giordana MT, Cordera S, Boghi A. Cerebral metastases as first symptom of cancer: a clinico-pathologic study. *J Neurooncol* 2000; 50(3):265–73.

58. Eapen L, Vachet M, Catton G, et al. Brain metastases with an unknown primary: a clinical perspective. *J Neurooncol* 1988; 6(1):31–5.

59. Bartelt S, Lutterbach J. Brain metastases in patients with cancer of unknown primary. *J Neurooncol* 2003; 64(3):249–53.

60. Sadeghi B, Arvieux C, Glehen O, et al. Peritoneal carcinomatosis from non-gynecologic malignancies: results of the EVOCAPE 1 multicentric prospective study. *Cancer* 2000; 88(2):358–63.

61. Chu DZ, Lang NP, Thompson C, Osteen PK, Westbrook KC. Peritoneal carcinomatosis in nongynecologic malignancy. A prospective study of prognostic factors. *Cancer* 1989; 63(2):364–7.

62. Fromm GL, Gershenson DM, Silva EG. Papillary serous carcinoma of the peritoneum. *Obstet Gynecol* 1990; 75(1):89–95.

63. Kannerstein M, Churg J, McCaughey WT, Hill DP. Papillary tumors of the peritoneum in women: mesothelioma or papillary carcinoma. *Am J Obstet Gynecol* 1977; 127(3):306–14.

64. Jacobs IJ, Kobler MF, Wlseman RW, et al. Clonal origin of epithelial ovarian carcinoma: analysis by loss of heterozygosity, p53 mutation, and x-chromosome inactivation. *J Natl Cancer Inst* 1992; 84:1793–8.

65. Eltabbakh GH, Piver MS. Extraovarian primary peritoneal carcinoma. *Oncology* 1998; 12:813–9.

66. Muto MG, Welch WR, Mol SCH, et al. Evidence for a multifocal origin of papillary serous carcinoma of the peritoneum. *Cancer Res* 1995; 55:490–2.

67. Karlan BY, Baldwin RL, Lopez-Lucvanos E, et al. Peritoneal serous papillary carcinoma, a phenotypic variant of familiary ovarian carcinoma cancer; Implications for ovarian cancer screening. *Am J Obstet Gynecol.* 1999; 18:917–28.

68. Bloss JD, Shu-Yuan L, Buller RE, et al. Extraovarian peritoneal serous papillary carcinoma: a case-control retrospective comparison to papillary adenocarcinoma of the ovary. *Gynecol Oncol* 1993; 5:347–51.

69. Swerdlow M. Mesothelioma of the pelvic peritoneum resembling papillary cystadenocarcinoma of the ovary; case report. *Am J Obstet Gynecol* 1959; 77(1):197–200.

70. Gooneratne S, Sassone M, Blaustein A, Talerman A. Serous surface papillary carcinoma of the ovary: a clinicopathologic study of 16 cases. *Int J Gynecol Pathol* 1982; 1(3):258–69.

71. Hochster H, Wernz JC, Muggia FM. Intra-abdominal carcinomatosis with histologically normal ovaries. *Cancer Treat Rep* 1984; 68(6):931–2.

72. Chen KT, Flam MS. Peritoneal papillary serous carcinoma with long-term survival. *Cancer* 1986; 58(6):1371–3.

73. Lele SB, Piver MS, Matharu J, Tsukada Y. Peritoneal papillary carcinoma. *Gynecol Oncol* 1988; 31(2):315–20.

74. Strnad CM, Grosh WW, Baxter J, et al. Peritoneal carcinomatosis of unknown primary site in women. A distinctive subset of adenocarcinoma. *Ann Intern Med* 1989; 111(3):213–7.

75. Dalrymple JC, Bannatyne P, Russell P, et al. Extraovarian peritoneal serous papillary carcinoma. A clinicopathologic study of 31 cases. *Cancer* 1989; 64(1):110–5.

76. Ransom DT, Patel SR, Keeney GL, Malkasian GD, Edmonson JH. Papillary serous carcinoma of the peritoneum. A review of 33 cases treated with platin-based chemotherapy. *Cancer* 1990; 66(6):1091–4.

77. Piver MS, Eltabbakh GH, Hempling RE, Recio FO, Blumenson LE. Two sequential studies for primary peritoneal carcinoma: induction with weekly cisplatin followed by either cisplatin-doxorubicin-cyclophosphamide or paclitaxel-cisplatin. *Gynecol Oncol* 1997; 67(2):141–6.

78. Halperin R, Zehavi S, Langer R, Hadas E, Bukovsky I, Schneider D. Primary peritoneal serous papillary carcinoma: a new epidemiologic trend? A matched-case comparison with ovarian serous papillary cancer. *Int J Gynecol Cancer* 2001; 11(5):403–8.

79. Tobacman JK, Greene MH, Tucker MA, Costa J, Kase R, Fraumeni JF Jr. Intra-abdominal carcinomatosis after prophylactic oophorectomy in ovarian-cancer-prone families. *Lancet* 1982; 2(8302):795–7.

80. Schorge JO, Muto MG, Welch WR, et al. Molecular evidence for multifocal papillary serous carcinoma of the peritoneum in patients with germline BRCA1 mutations. *J Natl Cancer Inst* 1998; 90(11):841–5.

81. Jermann M, Vogt P, Pestalozzi BC. Peritoneal carcinoma in a male patient. *Oncology* 2003; 64(4):468–72.

82. Jaaback KS, Ludeman L, Clayton NL, Hirschowitz L. Primary peritoneal carcinoma in a UK cancer center: comparison with advanced ovarian carcinoma over a 5-year period. *Int J Gynecol Cancer* 2006; 16(Suppl. 1):123–8.

83. Piura B, Meirovitz M, Bartfeld M, Yanai-Inbar I, Cohen Y. Peritoneal papillary serous carcinoma: study of 15 cases and comparison with stage III-IV ovarian papillary serous carcinoma. *J Surg Oncol* 1998; 68(3):173–8.

84. Nam JH, Kim YM, Jung MH, et al. Primary peritoneal carcinoma: experience with cytoreductive surgery and combination chemotherapy. *Int J Gynecol Cancer* 2006; 16(1):23–8.

85. Pickhardt PJ, Bhalla S. Primary neoplasms of peritoneal and subperitoneal origin: CT findings. *Radiographics* 2005; 25(4):983–95.

86. Ayhan A, Taskiran C, Yigit-Celik N, et al. Long-term survival after paclitaxel plus platinum-based combination chemotherapy for extraovarian peritoneal serous papillary carcinoma: is it different from that for ovarian serous papillary cancer? *Int J Gynecol Cancer* 2006; 16(2):484–9.

87. Barnetson RJ, Burnett RA, Downie I, Harper CM, Roberts F. Immunohistochemical analysis of peritoneal mesothelioma and primary and secondary serous carcinoma of the peritoneum: antibodies to estrogen and progesterone receptors are useful. *Am J Clin Pathol* 2006; 125(1):67–76.

88. Kowalski LD, Kanbour AI, Price FV, et al. A case-matched molecular comparison of extraovarian versus primary ovarian adenocarcinoma. *Cancer* 1997; 79(8):1587–94.

89. Chen LM, Yamada SD, Fu YS, Baldwin RL, Karlan BY. Molecular similarities between primary peritoneal and primary ovarian carcinomas. *Int J Gynecol Cancer* 2003; 13(6):749–55.

90. Mulhollan TJ, Silva EG, Tornos C, Guerrieri C, Fromm GL, Gershenson D. Ovarian involvement by serous surface papillary carcinoma. *Int J Gynecol Pathol* 1994; 13(2):120–6.

91. Dubernard G, Morice P, Rey A, et al. Prognosis of stage III or IV primary peritoneal serous papillary carcinoma. *Eur J Surg Oncol* 2004; 30(9):976–81.

92. Killackey MA, Davis AR. Papillary serous carcinoma of the peritoneal surface: matched-case comparison with papillary serous ovarian carcinoma. *Gynecol Oncol* 1993; 51(2):171–4.

93. Rothacker D. Uncertain malignant peritoneal tumors in 28 years of autopsy. Histologic reclassification. *Pathologe* 1991; 12(3):138–44.

94. Mills SF, Andersen WA, Foohner RE, et al. Serous surface papillary carcinoma. A clinicopathologic study of 1 cases and comparison with stage III-IV ovarian serous carcinoma. *Am J Surg Pathol* 1988; 12:827–34.

95. Look M, Chang C, Sugarbaker PH. Long-term results of cytoreductive surgery for advanced and recurrent epithelial ovarian cancers and papillary serous carcinoma of the peritoneum. *Int J Gynocol Cancer* 2004; 14:35–41.

96. Nowack R, Gobel U, Klooker P, Hergesell O, Andrassy K, van der Woude FJ. Mycophenolate mofetil for maintenance therapy of Wegener's granulomatosis and microscopic polyangiitis: a pilot study in 11 patients with renal involvement. *J Am Soc Nephrol* 1999; 10(9):1965–71.

97. Khandelwal AK, Garguilo GA. Therapeutic options for occult breast cancer: a survey of the American Society of Breast Surgeons and review of the literature. *Am J Surg* 2005; 190(4):609–13.

98. Halsted W. The results of radical operations for the cure of carcinoma of the breast. *Ann Surg* 1907; 46:1–19.

99. Rasponi A, Costa A, Clemente C, Merson M, Marchini S, Andreoli C. Lymphnodal metastases from unknown primary tumors. *Neoplasma* 1982; 29(5):631–8.

100. van Ooijen B, Bontenbal M, Henzen-Logmans SC, Koper PC. Axillary nodal metastases from an occult primary consistent with breast carcinoma. *Br J Surg* 1993; 80(10):1299–300.

101. Scoggins CR, Vitola JV, Sand;er MP. Occult breast carcinoma presenting as an axillary mass. *Am J Surg* 1999; 65:1–5.

102. Vlastos G, Jean ME, Mirza AN, et al. Feasibility of breast preservation in the treatment of occult primary carcinoma presenting with axillary metastases. *Ann Surg Oncol* 2001; 8(5):425–31.

103. Haagensen C. *Diseases of the Breast*, 3rd ed. Philadelphia: Saunders, 1986, pp. 516–45.

104. de Andrade JM, Marana HR, Sarmento Filho JM, Murta EF, Velludo MA, Bighetti S. Differential diagnosis of axillary masses. *Tumori* 1996; 82(6):596–9.

105. Campana F, Fourquet A, Ashby MA, et al. Presentation of axillary lymphadenopathy without detectable breast primary (T0 N1b breast cancer): experience at Institut Curie. *Radiother Oncol* 1989; 15(4):321–5.

106. Sakorafas GH, Tsiotou AG. Occult breast cancer: a challenge from a surgical perspective. *Surg Oncol* 1999; 8:27–33.

107. Vicini FA, Antonucci JV, Wallace M, et al. Long-term efficacy and patterns of failure after accelerated partial breast irradiation: a molecular assay-based clonality evaluation. *Int J Radiat Oncol Biol Phys* 2007.

108. Tench D, Page D. The unknown primary presenting with axillary lymphadenopathy. In: Bland KCM, ed. *The Breast: Comprehensive Management of Benign and Malignant Disease.* London: Saunders, 1991, pp. 1041–5.

109. Knapper WH. Management of occult breast cancer presenting as an axillary metastasis. *Semin Surg Oncol* 1991; 7(5):311–3.

110. Bhatia SK, Saclarides TJ, Witt TR, Bonomi PD, Anderson KM, Economou SG. Hormone receptor studies in axillary metastases from occult breast cancers. *Cancer* 1987; 59(6):1170–2.

111. Jackson B, Scott-Conner C, Moulder J. Axillary metastasis from occult breast carcinoma: diagnosis and management. *Am Surg* 1995; 61(5):431–4.

112. Lee WJ, Chu JS, Chang KJ, Chen KM. Occult breast carcinoma–use of color Doppler in localization. *Breast Cancer Res Treat* 1996; 37(3):299–302.

113. Gundry KR. The application of breast MRI in staging and screening for breast cancer. *Oncology (Williston Park)* 2005; 19(2):159–69; discussion 70, 73–74, 77.

114. Orel SG, Weinstein SP, Schnall MD, et al. Breast MR imaging in patients with axillary node metastases and unknown primary malignancy. *Radiology* 1999; 212(2):543–9.

115. Olson JA Jr, Morris EA, Van Zee KJ, Linehan DC, Borgen PI. Magnetic resonance imaging facilitates breast conservation for occult breast cancer. *Ann Surg Oncol* 2000; 7(6):411–5.

116. Morris EA. Cancer staging with breast MR imaging. *Magn Reson Imaging Clin N Am* 2001; 9(2):333–44, vi-vii.

117. Zangheri B, Messa C, Picchio M, Gianolli L, Landoni C, Fazio F. PET/CT and breast cancer. *Eur J Nucl Med Mol Imag* 2004; 31(Suppl. 1):S135–42.

118. Foroudi F, Tiver KW. Occult breast carcinoma presenting as axillary metastases. *Int J Radiat Oncol Biol Phys* 2000; 47(1):143–7.

119. Jereczek-Fossa BA, Jassem J, Orecchia R. Cervical lymph node metastases of squamous cell carcinoma from an unknown primary. *Cancer Treat Rev* 2004; 30(2):153–64.

120. Grau C, Johansen LV, Jakobsen J, Geertsen P, Andersen E, Jensen BB. Cervical lymph node metastases from unknown primary tumours. Results from a National Survey by the Danish Society for Head and Neck Oncology. *Radiother Oncol* 2000; 55(2):121–9.

121. Rusthoven KE, Koshy M, Paulino AC. The role of fluorodeoxyglucose positron emission tomography in cervical lymph node metastases from an unknown primary tumor. *Cancer* 2004; 101(11):2641–9.

122. Feinmesser R, Miyazaki I, Cheung R, Freeman JL, Noyek AM, Dosch HM. Diagnosis of nasopharyngeal carcinoma by DNA amplification of tissue obtained by fine-needle aspiration. *N Engl J Med* 1992; 326(1):17–21.

123. Nieder C, Gregoire V, Ang KK. Cervical lymph node metastases from occult squamous cell carcinoma: cut down a tree to get an apple? *Int J Radiat Oncol Biol Phys* 2001; 50(3):727–33.

124. Guarischi A, Keane TJ, Elhakim T. Metastatic inguinal nodes from an unknown primary neoplasm. A review of 56 cases. *Cancer* 1987; 59(3):572–7.

125. Gentile PS, Carloss HW, Huang TY, Yam LT, Lam WK. Disseminated prostatic carcinoma simulating primary lung cancer. Indications for immunodiagnostic studies. *Cancer* 1988; 62(4):711–5.

126. Tell DT, Khoury JM, Taylor HG, Veasey SP. Atypical metastasis from prostate cancer. Clinical utility of the immunoperoxidase technique for prostate-specific antigen. *JAMA* 1985; 253(24):3574–5.

127. Giordano N, Nardi P, Vigni P, Palumbo F, Battisti E, Gennari C. Osteoblastic metastases from carcinoid tumor. *Clin Exp Rheumatol* 1994; 12(2):228–9.

128. Joffe N, Antonioli DA. Osteoblastic bone metastases secondary to adenocarcinoma of the pancreas. *Clin Radiol* 1978; 29(1):41–6.

129. Cochrane LB, Heselson NG, Freson M. Semilunar osteoblastic metastases in breast carcinoma. A new radiological sign. *J Belge Radiol* 1989; 72(6):497–500.

130. Eriksson B, Oberg K, Stridsberg M. Tumor markers in neuroendocrine tumors. *Digestion* 2000; 62(Suppl. 1):33–8.

131. Pandit-Taskar N, Batraki M, Divgi CR. Radiopharmaceutical therapy for palliation of bone pain from osseous metastases. *J Nucl Med* 2004; 45(8):1358–65.

132. Hoegler D. Radiotherapy for palliation of symptoms in incurable cancer. *Curr Probl Cancer* 1997; 21(3):129–83.

133. Richardson RL, Schoemacher RA, Fer ME, et al. The unrecognized extragonadal germ cell cancer syndrome. *Ann Intern Med* 1981; 94:181–6.

134. Greco FA, Vaughn WK, Hainsworth JD. Advanced poorly differentiated carcinoma of unknown primary site: recognition of a treatable syndrome. *Ann Intern Med* 1986; 104(4):547–553.

135. Hainsworth JD, Johnson DH, Greco FA. Cisplatin-based combination chemotherapy in the treatment of poorly differentiated carcinoma and poorly differentiated adenocarcinoma of unknown primary site: results of a 12-year experience. *J Clin Oncol* 1992; 10(6):912–22.

136. Lenzi R, Hess KR, Abbruzzese MC, Raber MN, Ordonez NG, Abbruzzese JL. Poorly differentiated carcinoma and poorly differentiated adenocarcinoma of unknown origin: favorable subsets of patients with unknown-primary carcinoma? *J Clin Oncol* 1997; 15(5):2056–66.

137. Hainsworth JD, Wright EP, Johnson DH, Davis BW, Greco FA. Poorly differentiated carcinoma of unknown primary site: clinical usefulness of immunoperoxidase staining. *J Clin Oncol* 1991; 9(11):1931–8.

138. Motzer RJ, Rodriguez E, Reuter VE, Bosl GJ, Mazumdar M, Chaganti RS. Molecular and cytogenetic studies in the diagnosis of patients with poorly differentiated carcinomas of unknown primary site. *J Clin Oncol* 1995; 13(1):274–82.

139. Currow DC, Findlay M, Cox K, Harnett PR. Elevated germ cell markers in carcinoma of uncertain primary site do not predict response to platinum based chemotherapy. *Eur J Cancer* 1996; 32A(13):2357–9.

140. van der Gaast A, Verweij J, Henzen-Logmans SC, Rodenburg CJ, Stoter G. Carcinoma of unknown primary: identification of a treatable subset? *Ann Oncol* 1990; 1(2):119–22.

141. Moran CA, Suster S, Koss MN. Primary germ cell tumors of the mediastinum: III. Yolk sac tumor, embryonal carcinoma, choriocarcinoma, and combined nonteratomatous germ cell tumors of the mediastinum—a clinicopathologic and immunohistochemical study of 64 cases. *Cancer* 1997; 80(4):699–707.

142. Fizazi K, Culine S, Droz JP, et al. Primary mediastinal non-seminomatous germ cell tumors: results of modern therapy including cisplatin-based chemotherapy. *J Clin Oncol* 1998; 16(2):725–32.

143. Cerilli LA, Ritter JH, Mills SE, Wick MR. Neuroendocrine neoplasms of the lung. *Am J Clin Pathol* 2001; 116(Suppl): S65–96.

144. Kirshbom PM, Kherani AR, Onaitis MW, Feldman JM, Tyler DS. Carcinoids of unknown origin: comparative analysis with foregut, midgut, and hindgut carcinoids. *Surgery* 1998; 124(6):1063–70.

145. Fuster D, Navasa M, Pons F, et al. In-111 octreotide scan in a case of a neuroendocrine tumor of unknown origin. *Clin Nucl Med* 1999; 24(12):955–8.

146. van Tuyl SA, van Noorden JT, Timmer R, Stolk MF, Kuipers EJ, Taal BG. Detection of small-bowel neuroendocrine tumors by video capsule endoscopy. *Gastrointest Endosc* 2006; 64(1):66–72.

147. Volante M, Rindi G, Papotti M. The grey zone between pure (neuro)endocrine and non-(neuro)endocrine tumours: a comment on concepts and classification of mixed exocrine-endocrine neoplasms. *Virchows Arch* 2006; 449(5):499–506.

148. di Sant' Agnese PA. Divergent neuroendocrine differentiation in prostatic carcinoma. *Semin Diagn Pathol* 2000; 17(2):149–161.

149. Foley EF, Gaffey MJ, Frierson HF Jr. The frequency and clinical significance of neuroendocrine cells within stage III adenocarcinomas of the colon. *Arch Pathol Lab Med* 1998; 122(10): 912–4.

150. Galanis E, Frytak S, Lloyd RV. Extrapulmonary small cell carcinoma. *Cancer* 1997; 79(9):1729–36.

151. Lo Re G, Canzonieri V, Veronesi A, et al. Extrapulmonary small cell carcinoma: a single-institution experience and review of the literature. *Ann Oncol* 1994; 5(10):909–13.

152. Ibrahim NB, Briggs JC, Corbishley CM. Extrapulmonary oat cell carcinoma. *Cancer* 1984; 54(8):1645–61.

153. Hainsworth JD, Johnson DH, Greco FA. Poorly differentiated neuroendocrine carcinoma of unknown primary site. A newly recognized clinicopathologic entity. *Ann Intern Med* 1988; 109 (5):364–71.

154. Mitry E, Baudin E, Ducreux M, et al. Treatment of poorly differentiated neuroendocrine tumours with etoposide and cisplatin. *Br J Cancer* 1999; 81(8):1351–5.

155. Seve P, Billotey C, Broussolle C, Dumontet C, Mackey JR. The role of 2-deoxy-2-[F-18]fluoro-D-glucose positron emission tomography in disseminated carcinoma of unknown primary site. *Cancer* 2007; 109(2):292–9.

156. Greco FA, Hainsworth JD. One-hour paclitaxel, carboplatin, and extended-schedule etoposide in the treatment of carcinoma of unknown primary site. *Semin Oncol* 1997; 24(6Suppl. 19): S19-101–S19-115.

157. Greco FA, Gray J, Burris HA 3rd, Erland JB, Morrissey LH, Hainsworth JD. Taxane-based chemotherapy for patients with carcinoma of unknown primary site. *Cancer J* 2001; 7(3):203–12.

158. Briasoulis E, Kalofonos H, Bafaloukos D, et al. Carboplatin plus paclitaxel in unknown primary carcinoma: a phase II Hellenic Cooperative Oncology Group Study. *J Clin Oncol* 2000; 18(17): 3101–7.

159. Greco FA, Hainsworth JD. The evolving role of paclitaxel for patients with carcinoma of unknown primary site. *Semin Oncol* 1999; 26(1Suppl. 2):129–33.

160. Greco FA, Erland JB, Morrissey LH, et al. Carcinoma of unknown primary site: phase II trials with docetaxel plus cisplatin or carboplatin. *Ann Oncol* 2000; 11(2):211–5.

161. Greco FA, Burris HA 3rd, Erland JB, et al. Carcinoma of unknown primary site. *Cancer* 2000; 89(12):2655–60.

162. Greco FA, Burris HA 3rd, Litchy S, et al. Gemcitabine, carboplatin, and paclitaxel for patients with carcinoma of unknown primary site: a Minnie Pearl Cancer Research Network study. *J Clin Oncol* 2002; 20(6):1651–6.

163. Lortholary A, Abadie-Lacourtoisie S, Guerin O, Mege M, Rauglaudre GD, Gamelin E. Cancers of unknown origin: 311 cases. *Bull Cancer* 2001; 88(6):619–27.

164. Sève P, Ray-Coquard I, Trillet-Lenoir V, et al. Low serum albumin levels and liver metastasis are powerful prognostic markers for survival in patients with carcinomas of unknown primary site. *Cancer* 2006; 107(11):2698–705.

165. van der Gaast A, Verweij J, Planting AS, Hop WC, Stoter G. Simple prognostic model to predict survival in patients with undifferentiated carcinoma of unknown primary site. *J Clin Oncol* 1995; 13(7):1720–5.

166. Bugat R, Bataillard A, Lesimple T, et al. Standards, options and recommendations for the management of patient with carcinoma of unknown primary site. *Bull Cancer* 2002; 89(10):869–75.

167. Pavlidis N, Briasoulis E, Hainsworth J, Greco FA. Diagnostic and therapeutic management of cancer of an unknown primary. *Eur J Cancer* 2003; 39(14):1990–2005.

168. Pavlidis N, Fizazi K. Cancer of unknown primary (CUP). *Crit Rev Oncol Hematol* 2005; 54(3):243–50.

169. Mizutani M, Nawata S, Hirai I, Murakami G, Kimura W. Anatomy and histology of Virchow's node. *Anat Sci Int* 2005; 80(4):193–8.

170. Schneider V, Smyczek B. Sister Mary Joseph's nodule. Diagnosis of umbilical metastases by fine needle aspiration. *Acta Cytol* 1990; 34(4):555–8.

171. Farag SS, Green MD, Morstyn G, Sheridan WP, Fox RM. Delay by internists in obtaining diagnostic biopsies in patients with suspected cancer. *Ann Intern Med* 1992; 116(6):473–8.

2

Paraneoplastic Syndromes Associated with MCUOs

Neurological Paraneoplasias

MARIEKE T. DE GRAAF

PETER A. E. SILLEVIS SMITT

■ INTRODUCTION

Paraneoplastic syndromes are defined as remote effects of cancer that are not caused by invasion of the tumor or its metastases, nor by infection, ischemia, metabolic and nutritional deficits, surgery, or other forms of tumor treatment (1, 2). Paraneoplastic syndromes can present with a plethora of symptoms affecting many organ systems (Table 1).

The incidence of paraneoplastic syndromes varies widely both by the type of syndrome and by the underlying cancer. Cachexia, anorexia, and weight loss are for instance extremely common in advanced cancer patients. On the other hand, most of the antibody-associated paraneoplastic neurological syndromes (PNSs) are very rare, with an incidence of well below 1% of cancer patients (2).

Several mechanisms may be involved in the pathogenesis of paraneoplastic syndromes, including factors secreted by the tumors and other immunological mechanisms (Table 2). Most systemic, endocrine and metabolic, and cutaneous paraneoplastic syndromes are caused by tumor-secreted substances. Examples include the secretion of parathyroid hormone–related peptide by the tumor, resulting in hypercalcemia or the secretion of ACTH, resulting in Cushing's syndrome. Immunological factors on the other hand appear to be important in the pathogenesis of most PNSs and some cutaneous syndromes such as paraneoplastic pemphigus.

The precise pathogenesis of many paraneoplastic disorders is not yet known. Some disorders, once thought to be paraneoplastic, are not; e.g., progressive multifocal leukoencephalopathy, once considered paraneoplastic, has proven to be an opportunistic infection caused by a papovavirus.

The diagnosis of paraneoplastic syndromes is straightforward when they develop in a patient known to have cancer, once metastatic complications have been ruled out. However, the majority of paraneoplastic syndromes occur in patients not yet diagnosed with cancer. In this situation, detection of paraneoplastic autoantibodies can help direct the search toward an underlying tumor. In a patient with carcinoma of unknown origin, the type of antibody can also give a clue to the most likely site of the primary tumor.

When the paraneoplastic syndrome is caused by factors secreted by the tumor, symptoms often respond favorably to treatment of the underlying tumor. However, in immune-mediated paraneoplastic syndromes, the response to antitumor treatment and/or immunosuppressive or immunomodulatory treatment is usually less satisfying.

■ NEUROLOGICAL PARANEOPLASTIC SYNDROMES

In the pathogenesis of PNSs, immunologic factors are believed to be important because antibodies and T-cell responses against nervous system antigens have been defined for many of these disorders (1). Hypothetically, the immunologic response is elicited by the ectopic

■ **Table 1** Paraneoplastic syndromes associated with carcinomas

Neurological	Hematologic	Endocrine/metabolic (*continued*)
Central nervous system	Anemia[a]	Hypertension
Encephalomyelitis[b]	Dysproteinemia (amyloidosis)	Hyperthyroidism
Limbic encephalitis[b]	Eosinophilia	Hypoglycemia
Brainstem encephalitis	Hypercoagulability	Hyponatremia[a]
Subacute cerebellar degeneration[b]	Leukocytosis/leukoerythroblastic reaction	Hypophosphatemia
Opsoclonus–myoclonus	Polycythemia	Hypouricemia
Stiff-person syndrome	Thrombocytopenic purpura	Lactic acidosis
Paraneoplastic visual syndromes		
Cancer-associated retinopathy	**Renal**	**Cutaneous**
Melanoma-associated retinopathy	Glomerulopathies	Acanthosis nigrans
Paraneoplastic optic neuropathy	Tubulointerstitial disorders	Acquired hypertrichosis lanuginose
Motor neuron syndromes		Acquired ichthyosis
Subacute motor neuronopathy	**Systemic**	Acquired palmoplantar keratoderma
Other motor neuron syndromes	Cachexia, anorexia, weight loss[a]	Acrokeratosis (Bazex's syndrome)
Peripheral nervous system	Fever	Clubbing[a]
Subacute sensory neuronopathy[b]	Nonbacterial thrombotic endocarditis	Dermatomyositis
Acute sensorimotor neuropathy	Orthostatic hypotension	Erythema annulare centrifugum
Chronic sensorimotor neuropathy[a]		Erythema gyratum repens
Association with M-proteins		Exfoliative dermatitis
Subacute autonomic neuropathy	**Endocrine/metabolic**	Florid cutaneous papillomatosis
Paraneoplastic peripheral nerve vasculitis	Acromegaly	Hypertrophic pulmonary osteoarthropathy
Neuromuscular junction and muscle	Carcinoid syndrome	Pemphigus vulgaris
Lambert-Eaton myasthenic syndrome[a,b]	Cushing's syndrome	Pityriasis rotunda
Myasthenia gravis	Galactorrhea	Pruritus
Neuromyotonia	Gynecomastia	Sign of Leser-Trélat
Dermatomyositis[b]	Hyperamylasemia	Superficial thrombophlebitis[a]
Acute necrotizing myopathy	Hypercacitonemia	Sweet's syndrome
Cachectic myopathy[a]	Hypercalcemia[a]	Tripe palms
	Hyperglycemia	Vasculitis

[a]Indicates more common paraneoplastic syndromes.
[b]Classical paraneoplastic neurological syndromes.

expression of neuronal antigens by the tumor. Expression of these "onconeural" antigens is limited to the tumor and the nervous system and sometimes also the testis. At the time of presentation of the neurological symptoms, most patients have not yet been diagnosed with cancer (3–6). Detection of paraneoplastic antibodies can help diagnose

■ **Table 2** Pathogenetic mechanisms in paraneoplastic syndromes

Mechanism	Example of Paraneoplastic Syndrome
Toxic substance released by tumor	ACTH release by SCLC causes Cushing's syndrome
	Cytokine release by tumor or immune system (TNF-α, IL-1, IL-6, IFN-γ) causes cachectic myopathy
Competition for substrate	Carcinoid tumors compete for tryptophan, causing pellagra
	Sarcomas competing for glucose cause hypoglycemia
Autoimmune process	Lambert-Eaton myasthenic syndrome caused by autoantibodies against VGCC
	Paraneoplastic pemphigus caused by autoantibodies against desmoglein

Abbreviations: ACTH, adrenocorticotropic hormone; SCLC, small cell lung cancer; VGCC, voltage-gated calcium channels.

the neurological syndrome as paraneoplastic and may direct the search for an underlying neoplasm. In patients known to have cancer, the presentation of a PNS may presage the recurrence of the tumor or a second tumor. In these patients, however, metastatic complications of the known cancer must first be ruled out. Despite the presumed autoimmune etiology of PNS, the results of various forms of immunotherapy have been disappointing, with some exceptions (3–6). Rapid detection and immediate treatment of the underlying tumor appears to offer the best chance of stabilizing the patient and preventing further neurological deterioration (3–6).

Pathogenesis

The discovery of paraneoplastic antineuronal autoantibodies resulted in the general belief that PNSs are immune-mediated disorders triggered by aberrant expression of "onconeural" antigens in the tumor. Support for this hypothesis comes from the fact that the target paraneoplastic antigens are expressed both in the tumor and in the affected parts of the nervous system. Furthermore, the tumors are usually small and heavily infiltrated with inflammatory cells, and spontaneous remissions at the time of neurological presentation have also been described (7, 8). These findings suggest that some PNSs without identifiable tumor may result from immune-mediated eradication of the tumor (7, 8). In keeping with this hypothesis, one study found more limited disease distribution and better oncologic outcome in small cell lung cancer (SCLC) patients with paraneoplastic autoantibodies (9).

Although the paraneoplastic antibodies are synthesized intrathecally (10–12), a pathogenic role could only be proven for those paraneoplastic autoantibodies that are directed against easily accessible antigens located at the cell surface. Examples of such antigens are the acetylcholine receptor (anti-AChR muscle type in myasthenia gravis and neuronal ganglionic type in autonomic neuropathy), P/Q type voltage-gated calcium channels [VGCC in Lambert-Eaton myasthenic syndrome (LEMS)], voltage-gated potassium channels (anti-VGPC in neuromyotonia), and the metabotropic glutamate receptor mGluR1 (anti-mGluR1 in paraneoplastic cerebellar degeneration) (1, 13). Most paraneoplastic antigens are located in the cytoplasm (e.g., the Yo antigen) or nucleus (e.g., the Hu and Ri antigens) and a pathogenic role for the respective antibodies could not be demonstrated (14). In these disorders, indirect lines of evidence support the view that the cellular immune response against these antigens is responsible for the neurological damage (15–17). The relative contribution of the cellular and humoral immunity to the clinical and pathological manifestations has not been resolved (15–18). The paraneoplastic antibodies may, in these cases, be surrogate markers for T-lymphocyte activation (19).

Incidence and Diagnosis

The incidence of PNS varies with the neurological syndrome and with the tumor. In solid tumors, the more common neurological syndromes are myasthenia gravis, which occurs in 15% of patients with a thymoma, and LEMS, which affects 3% of patients with SCLC. For other solid tumors, the incidence of PNS is less than 1%.

Neurological syndromes are never pathognomonic for a paraneoplastic etiology and a high index of clinical suspicion is important. Some syndromes such as limbic encephalitis and sub-acute cerebellar degeneration associate relatively often with cancer. These are called "classical" paraneoplastic syndromes and are presented in Table 1 (20). Other syndromes such as sensorimotor polyneuropathy are much more prevalent, and the association with cancer may be by chance. Detection of a "well-characterized" paraneoplastic antibody is extremely helpful because it proves the paraneoplastic etiology of the neurological syndrome. The paraneoplastic antibodies are generally divided into three categories (Table 3) (20). The well-characterized antibodies are reactive with molecularly defined onconeural antigens (Fig. 1). These antibodies are strongly associated with cancer and have been detected unambiguously by several laboratories in a reasonable number of patients with well-defined neurological syndromes (20). The partially characterized antibodies are those with an unidentified target antigen and those that have been either described by a single group of investigators or reported in only a few patients. The third group consists of antibodies that are associated with specific disorders but do not differentiate between paraneoplastic and nonparaneoplastic cases.

Diagnosing a neurological syndrome as paraneoplastic requires the exclusion of other possible causes by a reasonably complete workup. Because of the difficulties in diagnosis, an international panel of neurologists has established diagnostic criteria that divide patients with a suspected paraneoplastic syndrome into "definite" and "probable" categories. These criteria are based on the presence or absence of cancer, the presence of "well-characterized" antibodies, and the type of clinical syndrome (Table 4) (20). Unfortunately, almost 50% of patients with a definite PNS do not have any of the "well-characterized" paraneoplastic antibodies (20). In these patients, early diagnosis of the tumor is often difficult, resulting in delay of tumor treatment.

Once a paraneoplastic diagnosis has been established or is suspected, rapid identification of the tumor becomes essential but may be difficult because most paraneoplastic syndromes develop in the early stages of cancer. The workup generally starts with a detailed history including smoking habits, weight loss, night sweats, and fever. A thorough physical examination should include palpation

■ **Table 3** Antibodies, paraneoplastic neurological syndromes, and associated tumors		
Antibody	**Clinical Syndromes**	**Associated Tumors**
Well-characterized paraneoplastic antibodies		
Anti-Hu (ANNA-1)	Encephalomyelitis, limbic encephalitis, sensory neuronopathy, subacute cerebellar degeneration, autonomic neuropathy	SCLC, neuroblastoma, prostate
Anti-Yo (PCA-1)	Subacute cerebellar degeneration	Ovary, breast
Anti-CV2 (CRMP5)	Encephalomyelitis, chorea, limbic encephalitis, sensory neuronopathy, sensorimotor neuropathy, optic neuritis, subacute cerebellar degeneration, autonomic neuropathy	SCLC, thymoma
Anti-Ri (ANNA-2)	Opsoclonus–myoclonus, brainstem encephalitis	Breast, SCLC
Anti-Ma2 (Ta)[a]	Limbic/diencephalic/brainstem encephalitis, subacute cerebellar degeneration	Testicle, lung
Anti-amphiphysin	Stiff-person syndrome, encephalomyelitis, subacute sensory neuronopathy, sensorimotor neuropathy	Breast, SCLC
Anti-recoverin	Cancer associated retinopathy	SCLC
Partially characterized antibodies		
Anti-Tr (PCA-Tr)	Subacute cerebellar degeneration	Hodgkin's disease
Anti-NMDAR	Limbic encephalitis	Teratoma
ANNA-3	Encephalomyelitis, subacute sensory neuronopathy	SCLC
PCA-2	Encephalomyelitis, subacute cerebellar degeneration	SCLC
Anti-Zic4	Subacute cerebellar degeneration	SCLC
Anti-mGluR1	Subacute cerebellar degeneration	Hodgkin's disease
Antibodies that occur with and without cancer		
Anti-VGCC	Lambert-Eaton myasthenic syndrome, subacute cerebellar degeneration	SCLC
Anti-AchR	Myasthenia gravis	Thymoma
Anti-nAChR	Subacute autonomic neuropathy	SCLC
Anti-VGKC	Limbic encephalitis, neuromyotonia	Thymoma, SCLC

[a]Patients with brainstem encephalitis or subacute cerebellar degeneration usually associate with tumors other than testicular cancer and their sera also react with Ma1 protein.

Abbreviations: ANNA, antineuronal nuclear antibody; SCLC, small cell lung carcinoma; VGCC, voltage-gated calcium channels; PCA, Purkinje cytoplasmic antibody; mGluR1, metabotropic glutamate receptor type 1; nAChR, nicotinic acetylcholine receptor; VGKC, voltage-gated potassium channel.

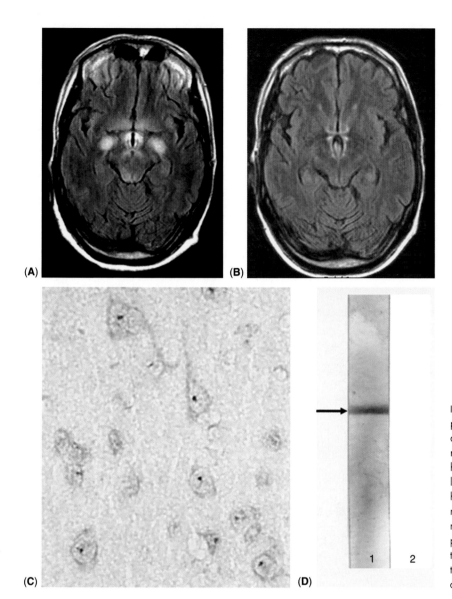

FIGURE 1 Ma2-encephalitis. A 41-year-old man presented with severe limbic encephalitis. Biopsy from a para-aortal mass showed undifferentiated carcinoma. (**A**) MRI of the brain showed on FLAIR images hyperintense abnormalities in the medial temporal lobes and around the third ventricle. The patient had high titer anti-Ma2 antibodies reactive with cytoplasmic and nuclear antigens in rat cortex (**C**) and purified recombinant Ma2 protein (**D**). He subsequently tested positive for AFP and β-HCG serum markers and was treated for presumed testicular cancer. During chemotherapy, the limbic encephalitis improved clinically and radiologically (**B**).

for pathological lymph nodes, rectal and pelvic examination, and palpation of breasts and testis. Often, the tumor is detected by high-resolution computed tomography (CT) of chest, abdomen, and pelvis. If the CT scan remains negative, whole body fluorodeoxyglucose positron emission tomography (FDG-PET) or PET/CT is recommended to detect an occult tumor or its metastases (21–23). In addition, the type of antibody and paraneoplastic syndrome may suggest a specific underlying tumor and indicate further diagnostic tests such as mammography (may be replaced by MRI) or ultrasound of the testes or pelvis (Table 3). When all tests remain negative, repeat evaluation at three- to six-month intervals for two to three years is recommended.

Treatment and Prognosis

Despite the immunological etiology of most of the PNSs, the results of immunotherapy have been disappointing (24). Exceptions are the neurological syndromes associated with paraneoplastic antibodies that are directed against antigens that are located at the surface of the cell (i.e., antigens that are accessible to circulating antibodies). These include not only disorders of the peripheral nervous system (LEMS, myasthenia gravis, and neuromyotonia) but also anti-mGluR1–associated paraneoplastic cerebellar degeneration and antiamphiphysin-associated stiff-person syndrome (13, 25). Immunotherapy modalities that are recommended for these disorders include plasma

■ **Table 4** Diagnostic criteria for paraneoplastic neurological syndromes

Definite paraneoplastic neurological syndrome

1. A classical syndrome (i.e., encephalomyelitis, limbic encephalitis, subacute cerebellar degeneration, opsoclonus–myoclonus, subacute sensory neuronopathy, chronic gastro-intestinal pseudo-obstruction, LEMS, or dermatomyositis) and cancer that develops within 5 years of the diagnosis of the neurological disorder, regardless of the presence of paraneoplastic antibodies
2. A nonclassical syndrome that objectively improves or resolves after cancer treatment, provided that the syndrome is not susceptible to spontaneous remission
3. A nonclassical syndrome with paraneoplastic antibodies (well-characterized or not) and cancer that develops within 5 years of the diagnosis of the neurological disorder
4. A neurological syndrome (classical or not) with well-characterized paraneoplastic antibodies (i.e., anti-Hu, Yo, Ri, amphiphysin, CV2 or Ma2)

Possible paraneoplastic neurological syndrome

1. A classical syndrome without paraneoplastic antibodies and no cancer, but at high risk of having an underlying tumor (e.g., smoking habit)
2. A neurological syndrome (classical or not) without cancer but with partially characterized paraneoplastic antibodies
3. A nonclassical neurological syndrome, no paraneoplastic antibodies, and cancer that presents within 2 years of the neurological syndrome

Source: From Ref. 20.

exchange, immunoadsorption (extraction of patient IgG over a protein A column), steroids, and intravenous immunoglobulins (IVIG).

For most PNSs, where the antigen is cytoplasmic or nuclear, the nervous dysfunction is probably not caused by functional interference of antibodies with the target antigen. In disorders with intracellular target antigens and a strong cellular immune reaction, plasma exchange and immunoadsorption are not expected to give much benefit. In these cases, a trial of a treatment that modulates the activation and function of effector T cells makes more sense, but to date there is only limited evidence that steroids, cyclophosphamide, IVIG, or other immunosuppressive therapies are effective (26).

Hence, the first goal of treatment for paraneoplastic neurological disorders is control of the tumor. In addition, antitumor therapy has been demonstrated to stop the paraneoplastic neurological deterioration and leave the patients, on average, in a better condition (4, 5, 27). In severely debilitated patients, e.g., the elderly and bed-ridden, treatment of an underlying tumor is often withheld because of the very small chance of clinically relevant neurological improvement.

■ CLINICAL DESCRIPTION

PNS may affect any level of the nervous system (central or peripheral nervous system including neuromuscular junction and muscle). Most PNSs are rapidly progressive, often leaving the patient severely debilitated within weeks or months (3–5, 27). However, slow progression, relapses, or a benign course does not exclude the diagnosis. This section describes the classical PNSs.

Encephalomyelitis

Paraneoplastic encephalomyelitis is characterized by involvement of several areas of the nervous system, including the temporal lobes and limbic system (limbic encephalitis), brainstem (brainstem encephalitis), cerebellum (subacute cerebellar degeneration), spinal cord (myelitis), dorsal root ganglia (subacute sensory neuronopathy), and autonomous nervous system (autonomic neuropathy) (28, 29). Patients with predominant involvement of one area but clinical evidence of only mild involvement of other areas are usually classified according to the predominant clinical syndrome. Symptoms of limbic encephalitis, subacute cerebellar degeneration, subacute sensory neuronopathy, and autonomic neuropathy are described below. Symptoms of brainstem encephalitis can include diplopia, dysarthria, dysphagia, gaze abnormalities (nuclear, internuclear or supranuclear), facial numbness, and subacute hearing loss.

Underlying Tumor

Although virtually all cancer types have been associated with paraneoplastic encephalomyelitis, approximately 75% of patients have an underlying SCLC (3, 4, 28–30). More than 70% of the patients are not known to have cancer when the neurological symptoms present, and the SCLC may be difficult to demonstrate due to its small size. When anti-Hu antibodies are detected or when the patient is at risk for lung cancer (smoking, age >50 years) a careful and repeated search for an underlying SCLC is warranted. When CT scan is negative, a total body FGD-PET scan or FDG-PET/CT may detect the neoplasm (21, 22).

Diagnostic Evaluation

MRI or CT of the brain is normal or shows nonspecific changes in most paraneoplastic encephalomyelitis patients, with two exceptions (29). In 65% to 80% of patients with predominant limbic encephalitis, MRI and CT scans show temporal lobe abnormalities (31, 32), and in patients with a predominant cerebellar syndrome, MRI and CT will ultimately show cerebellar atrophy. Cerebrospinal fluid (CSF) is abnormal in most patients with elevated protein, mild mononuclear pleocytosis, elevated IgG index, or oligoclonal bands (29).

Antineuronal Antibodies

Patients with paraneoplastic encephalomyelitis and SCLC often have anti-Hu antibodies (also called antineuronal nuclear autoantibodies or ANNA-1) in their serum and CSF (3, 4, 29, 30). Other less-frequent antibodies are anti-CRMP5/CV2 (19), antiamphiphysin (33), and the less well-characterized ANNA-3 (34) and PCA-2 antibody (35).

Treatment and Prognosis

Tumor treatment offers the best chance of stabilizing the patient's neurological condition while immunotherapy does not appear to modify the outcome of paraneoplastic encephalomyelitis (3, 4, 24). Because of incidental reports of neurological improvement following various forms of immunosuppressive treatment, a trial of one or two immunosuppressive modalities may be warranted in a single patient. Because of the limited efficacy of plasma exchange, IVIG, and corticosteroids (3, 4, 24) and the presumed role of cellular immunity, more aggressive immunosuppression with cyclophosphamide, tacrolimus,

or cyclosporine may be considered. To limit toxicity, these more aggressive immunosuppressive approaches should probably be reserved for patients who are not receiving chemotherapy. The overall functional outcome is bad, and more than 50% of patients are confined to bed or chair in the chronic phase of the disease (3, 4, 24).

Limbic Encephalitis

Limbic encephalitis is characterized by the subacute onset (in days to a few months) of short-term memory loss, seizures, confusion, and psychiatric symptoms, suggesting involvement of the limbic system (28, 36). Hypothalamic dysfunction may occur with somnolence, hyperthermia, and endocrine abnormalities. Approximately two-thirds of patients with paraneoplastic limbic encephalitis develop involvement of other areas of the nervous system during the course of the disease (i.e., encephalomyelitis). Several specific antibody-related clinical syndromes have been identified (32, 37–39).

Underlying Tumor

More than half of the patients presenting with limbic encephalitis will have an underlying neoplasm (32). The associated tumor is a lung tumor in 50% to 60% of the patients, usually SCLC (40–55%) and testicular germ-cell tumors in 20% (31, 32, 40). Other tumors include breast cancer, thymoma, Hodgkin's disease, and teratomas (31, 32).

Diagnostic Evaluation

The diagnosis is often difficult, especially when the patient presents with psychiatric symptoms, because there are no specific clinical markers and symptoms usually precede the diagnosis of cancer (32, 41). An MRI scan may show increased signal on T2-weighted and fluid attenuated inversion recovery (FLAIR) images of one or both medial temporal lobes, hypothalamus, and brainstem in 65% to 80% of the patients (31, 32). Early in the course of the disease, the MRI may be normal, and repeat imaging may be indicated. Coregistration of FDG-PET may further improve the sensitivity of imaging (42). CSF examination is abnormal in 80% of the patients, showing transient mild lymphocytic pleocytosis with increased protein, IgG, or oligoclonal bands (31, 32).

Antineuronal Antibodies

Several antibody-related clinical syndromes have been identified that vary with the associated tumors. The first group consists of patients with anti-Hu antibodies and lung cancer (usually SCLC). Patients may also have antiamphiphysin (SCLC) or anti-CV2/CRMP5 (SCLC or thymoma) antibodies (19). Limbic encephalitis is part of paraneoplastic encephalomyelitis, and patients have involvement of other areas outside the limbic system and brainstem. These patients are older (median age 62 years), usually smoke, and are more often female (32, 40).

The second group consists of young males with testicular cancer and anti-Ma2 antibodies (Fig. 1) (43). The median age is 34 years, and symptoms are usually confined to the limbic system, hypothalamus, and brainstem. Patients with anti-Ma2 and anti-Ma1 antibodies are significantly older and are more often female (44). Anti-Ma1 patients are more likely to develop cerebellar dysfunction and usually harbor tumors other than testicular cancer.

The third group consists of young women with ovarian teratomas who harbor antibodies reactive to the N-methyl-D-aspartate (NMDA) receptor (37–39). The patients develop subacute psychiatric symptoms, seizures, and hypopnea, requiring mechanical ventilation. Patients may also develop choreic or dystonic movements. The CSF invariably shows signs of inflammation including lympho-cytosis, and increased protein and oligoclonal banding. The anti-NMDA receptor antibodies are sometimes only detectable in CSF (and not in serum).

The fourth group has antibodies reactive to voltage-gated potassium channels (anti-VGKC) that can be associated either with paraneoplastic limbic encephal-itis and thymoma or with nonparaneoplastic limbic encephalitis (45, 46). Most patients present with or develop seizures that may progress into nonconvulsive status epilepticus. Patients may have concomitant autonomic or peripheral nerve dysfunction (neuromyo-tonia) and rapid eye movement sleep behavior abnor-malities. Hyponatremia is frequent while the CSF is usually acellular.

The last group has no antineuronal antibodies (approximately 20–40% of patients with paraneoplastic limbic encephalitis) (31, 32). In these patients, the symptoms are more often confined to the limbic system, the median age is around 57 years, and the associated tumor is often located in the lung (32, 40).

Treatment and Prognosis

Spontaneous complete recovery has been described, although very rarely (40, 47). Immunotherapy is largely ineffective in patients with antibodies reactive to intra-cellular antigens (anti-Hu, Ma2, amphiphysin, or CV2/CRMP5) (32), but multiple cases benefiting from anti-tumor treatment have been reported (32, 40, 48). Therefore, all efforts should be directed at identifying and treating the underlying tumor. If no tumor is found, the search should be repeated every three to six months for a total of two to three years. Irrespective of treatment, partial neurological recovery was seen in 38% of anti-Hu patients, 30% of anti-Ta (Ma2) patients, and 64% of patients without antibodies (32).

In contrast, patients with antibodies reactive to easily accessible cell-surface antigens often respond dramatically to immunotherapy and antitumor treatment. Ovarian teratoma patients often clinically improve following resec-tion of the tumor and/or treatment with corticosteroids, IVIG, or plasma exchange (38). In patients with anti-VGKC–associated limbic encephalitis, treatment with corticosteroids, IVIG, or plasma exchange results in significant improvement in 70% to 80% of the cases (45).

Cerebellar Degeneration

Paraneoplastic cerebellar degeneration is one of the most common and characteristic paraneoplastic syndromes (5, 28). In a study of 137 consecutive patients with antibody-associated paraneoplastic syndromes, 50 (37%) patients presented with subacute cerebellar degeneration (5). Paraneoplastic cerebellar degeneration usually starts acutely with nausea, vomiting, dizziness, and slight incoordination of walking, evolving rapidly over weeks to a few months with progressive ataxia of gait, limbs and trunk, dysarthria, and often nystagmus associated with oscillopsia. The disease reaches its peak within months and then stabilizes. By this time, most patients are severely debilitated. They are generally unable to walk or sit without support, writing is often impossible, and feeding themselves is quite difficult.

The symptoms and signs are limited to the cerebellum and cerebellar pathways, but other mild neurological abnormalities may be found on careful examination. These include hearing loss, dysphagia, pyramidal and extrapyramidal tract signs, mental status change, and peripheral neuropathy (6, 49, 50).

Underlying Tumor

Paraneoplastic cerebellar degeneration can be associated with any cancer, but the most common tumors are lung cancer (usually SCLC), ovarian cancer, and lymphomas (particularly Hodgkin's lymphoma). In 60% to 70% of the patients, the neurological symptoms precede the diagnosis of the cancer by a few months to two to three years and lead to its detection (5, 6, 51).

Diagnostic Evaluation

Subacute cerebellar degeneration is a rare disorder in cancer patients. On the other hand, 50% of patients presenting with acute or subacute nonfamilial ataxia are estimated to have an underlying malignancy (28). MRI and CT scans are initially normal but often reveal cerebellar atrophy later in the course of the disease. FDG-PET scan and SPECT may show cerebellar hypermetabolism and increased perfusion during the acute stage of the illness (52). CSF examination shows mild lymphocytic pleocytosis, with elevation of protein and IgG levels in the first weeks to months.

Oligoclonal bands may be present. The diagnosis of paraneoplastic cerebellar degeneration is established by demonstration of specific antineuronal antibodies.

Antineuronal Antibodies

Paraneoplastic cerebellar degeneration can be associated with various antineuronal autoantibodies (Table 3). Anti-Yo (also called anti-Purkinje cell antibody type 1 or PCA-1), anti-Tr (PCA-Tr), and anti-mGluR1 are associated with relatively "pure" cerebellar syndromes. Anti-Yo antibodies are associated with breast cancer and tumors of the ovaries, endometrium, and fallopian tubes (5, 6, 53). These antibodies are directed against the calcium-dependent regulator (cdr) proteins that are expressed by Purkinje cells and the associated tumors (53, 54). Cdr-2–specific cytotoxic T cells have been identified in the serum from patients with paraneoplastic cerebellar degeneration, suggesting a pathogenic role for the cellular immune response in this paraneoplastic syndrome (16). Anti-Tr (PCA-Tr) antibodies are directed against an unidentified cytoplasmic Purkinje cell antigen and appear to be specific for Hodgkin's disease (51). Anti-mGluR1 antibodies have been found in two patients with paraneoplastic cerebellar degeneration and Hodgkin's disease. Passive transfer of patient anti-mGluR1 IgG into CSF of mice induced severe, transient ataxia (13).

Approximately 50% of patients with cerebellar degeneration and an underlying SCLC have high titer anti-Hu antibodies (55). The remaining patients are likely to have anti P/Q-type VGCC antibodies. These antibodies were present in all patients who had LEMS and in some patients with cerebellar degeneration without LEMS. In patients with antiamphiphysin or anti-CV2/CRMP5 antibodies, the cerebellar degeneration is often part of the paraneoplastic encephalomyelitis syndrome, and more widespread neurological symptoms and signs are usually found.

The more recently discovered Purkinje cell antibody (PCA-2) and the ANNA-3 antibody are associated with lung cancer and a variety of neurological syndromes including cerebellar degeneration (35). The anti-Zic4 antibodies are strongly associated with SCLC, and most patients have paraneoplastic encephalomyelitis often presenting with cerebellar dysfunction (56). These patients often have concurrent anti-Hu or anti-CV2/CRMP5 antibodies. Patients with isolated anti-Zic4 antibodies are more likely to develop cerebellar symptoms.

Treatment and Prognosis

The outcome of paraneoplastic cerebellar degeneration is generally poor and the best chance to at least stabilize the syndrome is to treat the underlying tumor (5). Incidental improvement has been reported either spontaneously or in association with plasma exchange, steroids, IVIG, or rituximab (57). In patients with anti-Yo–associated cerebellar degeneration, the prognosis is better for patients with breast cancer than for those with gynecologic cancer (6). The prognosis is better in patients with paraneoplastic cerebellar degeneration associated with Hodgkin's disease and anti-Tr (PCA-Tr) or anti-mGluR1 antibodies. With successful treatment of the tumor and/or immunotherapy, symptoms may disappear and the antibodies vanish (13, 51).

Opsoclonus–Myoclonus

Opsoclonus is a disorder of ocular motility that consists of involuntary, arrhythmic, high-amplitude conjugate saccades in all directions. Opsoclonus may occur intermittently or, if more severe, constantly, and it does not remit in the darkness or when the eyes are closed. Opsoclonus is often associated with diffuse or focal myoclonus, the "dancing eyes and dancing feet syndrome," and other cerebellar and brainstem signs (58–60). An excessive startle response reminiscent of hyperexplexia may also occur in opsoclonus–myoclonus (61). In contrast to most paraneoplastic syndromes, the course of opsoclonus–myoclonus may be remitting and relapsing (60).

Underlying Tumor

Approximately 20% of adult patients with opsoclonus–myoclonus have a previously undiscovered malignancy (59). The most commonly associated neoplasms are SCLC and breast and gynecologic cancers (61, 62).

Almost 50% of children with opsoclonus–myoclonus have an underlying neuroblastoma. Conversely, approximately 2% to 3% of children with neuroblastoma have paraneoplastic opsoclonus–myoclonus (63, 64). Tumors in children with paraneoplastic opsoclonus–myoclonus apparently have a better prognosis than tumors in patients without this paraneoplastic syndrome.

Diagnostic evaluation

MRI is usually normal but may show hyperintensities in the brainstem on T2-weighted images (65). Examination of the CSF may show mild pleocytosis and protein elevation. Adult patients with paraneoplastic opsoclonus–myoclonus are older (median age 66 years) than patients with the idiopathic syndrome (median age 40 years). In adult patients, the tumor search should be directed at the most common underlying tumors, i.e., high-resolution CT of the chest and abdomen and gynecological examination and mammography (or MRI of the breasts) (62). When this is negative, FDG-PET should be considered (23, 66).

In children, nonparaneoplastic opsoclonus–myoclonus occurs as a self-limited illness and is probably the result of a viral infection of the brainstem. The search for an occult neuroblastoma should include imaging of chest and abdomen (CT scan or MRI), urine catecholamine measurements, and metaiodobenzylguanidine scan (67).

Antineuronal Antibodies

Specific antibodies are found in only a minority of patients with paraneoplastic opsoclonus–myoclonus (62). In women, anti-Ri antibodies (or antineuronal nuclear autoantibody type 2, ANNA-2) are mostly associated with breast and gynecologic tumors. Anti-Ri has occasionally been found in bladder cancer and SCLC and may then occur in male patients (58, 68). Paraneoplastic opsoclonus–myoclonus can also be associated with anti-Hu antibodies, usually as part of a more widespread paraneoplastic encephalomyelitis.

In children presenting with opsoclonus–myoclonus, the detection of anti-Hu antibodies is diagnostic of an underlying neuroblastoma (69). The frequency of anti-Hu antibodies in neuroblastoma with paraneoplastic opsoclonus–myoclonus is approximately 10% (69–71). This finding differs little from the 4% to 15% of anti-Hu positive sera in children with neuroblastoma who do not have opsoclonus–myoclonus (69, 70).

Treatment and Prognosis

In contrast to most of the other paraneoplastic syndromes, paraneoplastic opsoclonus–myoclonus may remit either spontaneously, following treatment of the tumor, or in association with clonazepam or thiamine treatment. Most patients with idiopathic opsoclonus–myoclonus make a good recovery that seems to be accelerated by steroids or IVIG. Paraneoplastic opsoclonus–myoclonus usually has a more severe clinical course, and treatment with steroids or IVIG appears ineffective. In a series of 14 patients with paraneoplastic opsoclonus–myoclonus, eight patients whose tumors were treated showed complete or partial neurological recovery. In contrast, five of the six patients whose tumors were not treated died of the neurological syndrome despite steroids, IVIG, or plasma exchange (62). However, improvement following the administration of steroids, cyclophosphamide, azathioprine, IVIG, plasma exchange, or plasma filtration with a protein A column has been described in single cases (61, 72–74).

In children, paraneoplastic opsoclonus–myoclonus may improve following treatment with adrenocorticotropic hormone (ACTH), prednisone, azathioprine, or IVIG, but residual central nervous system signs are frequent (64, 75, 76). Treatment of the tumor with chemotherapy is the most important predictor of good neurological recovery (77).

Subacute Sensory Neuronopathy

The symptoms of subacute sensory neuronopathy begin with pain and paraesthesia (78, 79). Clumsiness and unsteady gait then develop and usually become predominant. The distribution of symptoms is often asymmetrical or multifocal. The upper limbs are often affected first and are almost invariably involved with evolution. Sensory loss may also affect the face, chest, or abdomen. On examination, all sensory modalities are affected, but the most striking abnormality is loss of deep sensation, causing sensory ataxia with pseudoathetosis of the hands. Tendon reflexes are depressed or absent. In most patients, the disease progresses rapidly over weeks to months, leaving the patient severely disabled. In a few patients, the neuronopathy remains stable for months with mild neurological deficits (80). Subacute sensory neuronopathy occurs in approximately 75% of patients with paraneoplastic encephalomyelitis, is predominant in 50% of patients and clinically pure in 25% of the patients (3, 4). Autonomic neuropathy including gastrointestinal pseudoobstruction is common.

Underlying Tumor

Subacute sensory neuronopathy is probably paraneoplastic in about 20% of patients. In 70% to 80% of patients, subacute sensory neuronopathy is associated with SCLC (3, 4, 30). Other associated tumors include breast cancer, ovarian cancer, sarcoma, and Hodgkin's lymphoma (78, 79). Subacute sensory neuronopathy usually predates the diagnosis of cancer with a median delay of 3.5 to 4.5 months (3, 4).

Diagnostic Evaluation

Electrophysiology shows absence or marked reduction of sensory nerve action potentials with normal or mildly reduced motor conduction velocities. Early in the course of the disease, CSF examination shows mild pleocytosis, with an elevated IgG and oligoclonal bands (4, 78, 79). Sural nerve biopsy is rarely required for the diagnosis but may differentiate from vasculitic neuropathy.

Antineuronal Antibodies

Anti-Hu is the most frequent paraneoplastic antibody in subacute sensory neuronopathy (3, 4, 29, 30). In this setting, anti-Hu antibody detection has a specificity of 99% and sensitivity of 82% (81). The absence of anti-Hu antibodies does not rule out an underlying cancer. Anti-CRMP5/CV2 antibodies also occur with paraneoplastic peripheral neuropathies (82). These patients usually have a sensory or sensorimotor neuropathy with less frequent involvement of the arms, but it is often associated with cerebellar ataxia (19, 82, 83). Anti-CRMP5/CV2 antibodies are usually associated with SCLC, neuroendocrine tumors, and thymoma. Antiamphiphysin antibodies are associated with multifocal paraneoplastic encephalomyelitis, and symptoms often include sensory or sensorimotor neuropathy (33, 84, 85). Associated tumors (mostly limited) are mainly SCLC, breast cancer, and melanoma.

Treatment and Prognosis

Immunotherapy consisting of plasma exchange, steroids, and IVIG is ineffective, with only some exceptions (24, 27, 86, 87). In one study, two out of ten patients stabilized in a relatively good clinical condition following intensive treatment with a combination of steroids, cyclophosphamide, and IVIG (24). Early detection and treatment of the underlying neoplasm, usually SCLC, appears to offer the best chance of stabilizing the neurological symptoms (4, 27). In patients with an identifiable tumor, antitumor treatment is recommended. In the absence of a tumor, antitumor treatment may be considered in patients with anti-Hu antibodies, age >50 years, and a history of smoking. In patients not receiving antitumor therapy, a short course of immunotherapy can be considered. Symptomatic treatment is directed at neuropathic pain and dysautonomic symptoms such as orthostatic hypotension.

Lambert-Eaton Myasthenic Syndrome

LEMS presents with proximal weakness of the lower extremities and fatigability. Bulbar symptoms may occur more frequently than previously reported (88) but are generally milder than in myasthenia gravis. Respiratory weakness can occur. Deep tendon reflexes, especially those in the legs, are diminished or absent but may reappear after exercise. Autonomic features ultimately develop in 95% of patients, especially dryness of the mouth, impotence, and mild/moderate ptosis (88, 90). In some patients, LEMS may develop in association with other paraneoplastic syndromes, including paraneoplastic cerebellar degeneration and encephalomyelitis (55).

Underlying Tumor

Approximately 70% of patients have cancer, almost always SCLC (89, 91). Other tumors include small cell carcinomas of the prostate and cervix, lymphomas, and adenocarcinomas. The prevalence of LEMS in SCLC is estimated to be around 3% (90, 92). Clinically and serologically, the 30% without an identifiable tumor are indistinguishable from the paraneoplastic LEMS patients, although LEMS may have a more progressive course in patients with SCLC (88). In patients presenting with LEMS, smoking history and absence of the HLA-B8 genotype strongly predict an underlying SCLC (88). Patients with SCLC and LEMS survive significantly longer than SCLC patients who do not have the paraneoplastic syndrome (88).

Diagnostic Evaluation

The typical pattern of electromyographic abnormalities is the hallmark of LEMS. This includes a low compound muscle action potential at rest with a decreased response at low rates of repetitive stimulation (3 Hz) and an incremental response at high rates of repetitive stimulation (50 Hz) or 15 to 30 seconds of maximal voluntary contraction (Fig. 2) (93).

Antineuronal Antibodies

Most patients with LEMS have antibodies against P/Q type calcium channels that are located presynaptically in the neuromuscular junction (93). About 20% have anti-MysB antibodies reactive to the β-subunit of neuronal calcium channels (94).

Treatment and Prognosis

Treatment of LEMS must be tailored to the individual based on severity of the symptoms, underlying disease, life expectancy, and previous response to treatment. In patients with paraneoplastic LEMS, treatment of the tumor frequently leads to neurological improvement (95). Symptomatic treatment is with drugs that facilitate the release of acetylcholine from motor nerve terminals such as 3,4-diaminopyridine (DAP) (96). In a placebo-controlled randomized trial, DAP (5–20 mg tid-qid) was effective for long-term therapy, alone or in combination with other treatments (97). The maximum recommended daily dose of DAP is 80 mg; at higher doses, seizures occur (97). Cholinesterase inhibitors (pyridostigmine, 30–60 mg, q6h) may improve dryness of mouth but rarely relieve weakness. If these treatments are not effective enough, it must be decided if immunosuppressive therapy with steroids, azathioprine, or cyclosporine is in order. Removal of the pathogenic anti-P/Q type calcium channel antibodies by plasma exchange (98) and IVIG can give quick but transient relief (89, 99). LEMS responds less favorably to immunotherapy than myasthenia gravis.

Dermatomyositis

In dermatomyositis, the characteristic heliotrope rash (purplish discoloration of the eyelids) (Fig. 3) often precedes the appearance of proximal muscle weakness. Other manifestations include arthralgia, myocarditis and congestive heart failure, and interstitial lung disease. Clinical, electromyographical, and pathological findings of dermatomyositis are similar in patients with and without cancer.

Underlying Tumor

The standardized incidence ratio for a malignant disease in dermatomyositis is 6.2 (95% confidence interval 3.9–10.0) (100). Dermatomyositis is associated with cancer of the ovary, lung, pancreas, stomach, colorectum, and breast, and with non-Hodgkin's lymphoma (101).

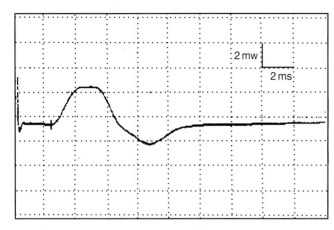

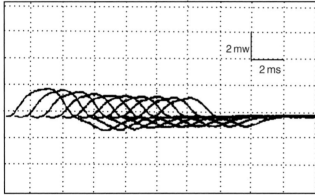

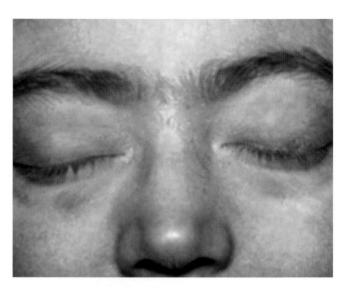

FIGURE 3 Dermatomyositis. This 50-year-old woman presented with proximal muscle weakness and tenderness and reddish skin eruption on the face. Similar lesions were present over the dorsal fingers. A breast carcinoma was subsequently found.

myopathy and in selecting an appropriate biopsy site. Muscle or skin biopsy is the definitive diagnostic procedure and shows inflammatory infiltrates (102).

Antineuronal Antibodies

Antibodies to the Mi-2 protein complex are specific for dermatomyositis and are present in high titers in about 35% of cases (103).

Treatment and Prognosis

Treatment of paraneoplastic dermatomyositis is generally the same as for patients without a tumor. Nearly all patients respond to corticosteroids (104). Refractory patients and patients requiring a lower dose of steroids can be treated with azathioprine, methotrexate, or cyclophosphamide (104).

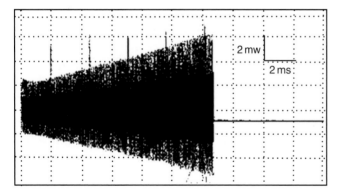

FIGURE 2 Electromyography results: Lambert-Eaton myasthenic syndrome. This compound muscular action potential from an ulnar nerve, collected from the abductor muscle of the fifth finger, shows an amplitude of 1.6 mV (*top*). Repetitive stimulation at 3 Hz yields a decremental response (*center*), whereas repetitive stimulation at 20 Hz demonstrates potentiation (*bottom*). The patient was a 63-year-old man with small cell neuroendocrine carcinoma of the lung.

Diagnostic Evaluation

Most patients have elevated serum creatine kinase levels and electromyographic evidence of myopathy. Muscle imaging (CT or MRI) may help in confirming the diagnosis and determining the type of inflammatory

■ REFERENCES

1. Darnell JC, Posner JB. Paraneoplastic syndromes involving the nervous system. *N Engl J Med* 2003; 349:1543–54.
2. de Beukelaar JW, Sillevis Smitt PA. Managing paraneoplastic neurological disorders. *Oncologist* 2006; 11:292–305.
3. Graus F, Keime-Guibert F, Rene R, et al. Anti-Hu-associated paraneoplastic encephalomyelitis: analysis of 200 patients. *Brain* 2001; 124:1138–48.
4. Sillevis Smitt P, Grefkens J, De Leeuw B, et al. Survival and outcome in 73 anti-Hu positive patients with paraneoplastic encephalomyelitis/sensory neuronopathy. *J Neurol* 2002; 249: 745–53.

5. Shams'ili S, Grefkens J, de Leeuw B, et al. Paraneoplastic cerebellar degeneration associated with antineuronal antibodies: analysis of 50 patients. *Brain* 2003; 126:1409–18.

6. Rojas I, Graus F, Keime-Guibert F, et al. Long-term clinical outcome of paraneoplastic cerebellar degeneration and anti-Yo antibodies. *Neurology* 2000; 55:713–5.

7. Darnell RB, DeAngelis LM. Regression of small-cell lung carcinoma in patients with paraneoplastic neuronal antibodies. *Lancet* 1993; 341:21–2.

8. Byrne T, Mason WP, Posner JB, Dalmau J. Spontaneous neurological improvement in anti-Hu associated encephalomyelitis. *J Neurol Neurosurg Psychiatry* 1997; 62:276–8.

9. Graus F, Dalmau J, Rene R, et al. Anti-Hu antibodies in patients with small-cell lung cancer: association with complete response to therapy and improved survival. *J Clin Oncol* 1997; 15:2866–72.

10. Rauer S, Kaiser R. Demonstration of anti-HuD specific oligoclonal bands in the cerebrospinal fluid from patients with paraneoplastic neurological syndromes. Qualitative evidence of anti-HuD specific IgG-synthesis in the central nervous system. *J Neuroimmunol* 2000; 111:241–4.

11. Stich O, Graus F, Rasiah C, Rauer S. Qualitative evidence of anti-Yo-specific intrathecal antibody synthesis in patients with paraneoplastic cerebellar degeneration. *J Neuroimmunol* 2003; 141: 165–9.

12. Stich O, Rauer S. Qualitative evidence of anti-Ri specific intrathecal antibody synthesis and quantification of anti-Ri antibodies in serial samples from a patient with anti-Ri syndrome. *J Neurol Neurosurg Psychiatry* 2006; 77:282–3.

13. Sillevis Smitt P, Kinoshita A, DeLeeuw B, et al. Paraneoplastic cerebellar ataxia due to autoantibodies against a glutamate receptor. *N Engl J Med* 2000; 342:21–7.

14. Sillevis Smitt PAE, Manley GT, Posner JP. Immunization with the paraneoplastic encephalomyelitis antigen HuD does not cause neurologic disease in mice. *Neurology* 1995; 45:1873–8.

15. Benyahia B, Liblau R, Merle-Beral H, Tourani JM, Dalmau J, Delattre JY. Cell-mediated autoimmunity in paraneoplastic neurological syndromes with anti-Hu antibodies. *Ann Neurol* 1999; 45:162–7.

16. Albert ML, Austin LM, Darnell RB. Detection and treatment of activated T cells in the cerebrospinal fluid of patients with paraneoplastic cerebellar degeneration. *Ann Neurol* 2000; 47: 9–17.

17. Tanaka M, Tanaka K, Tokiguchi S, Shinozawa K, Tsuji S. Cytotoxic T cells against a peptide of Yo protein in patients with paraneoplastic cerebellar degeneration and anti-Yo antibody. *J Neurol Sci* 1999; 168:28–31.

18. De Beukelaar J, Verjans GM, van Norden Y, et al. No evidence for circulating HuD-specific CD8+ T cells in patients with paraneoplastic neurological syndromes and Hu antibodies. *Cancer Immunol Immunother.* In Press.

19. Yu Z, Kryzer TJ, Griesmann GE, Kim K, Benarroch EE, Lennon VA. CRMP-5 neuronal autoantibody: marker of lung cancer and thymoma-related autoimmunity. *Ann Neurol* 2001; 49:146–54.

20. Graus F, Delattre JY, Antoine JC, et al. Recommended diagnostic criteria for paraneoplastic neurological syndromes. *J Neurol Neurosurg Psychiatry* 2004; 75:1135–40.

21. Antoine JC, Cinotti L, Tilikete C, et al. [18F]fluorodeoxyglucose positron emission tomography in the diagnosis of cancer in patients with paraneoplastic neurological syndrome and anti-Hu antibodies. *Ann Neurol* 2000; 48:105–8.

22. Rees JH, Hain SF, Johnson MR, et al. The role of [18F]fluoro-2-deoxyglucose-PET scanning in the diagnosis of paraneoplastic neurological disorders. *Brain* 2001; 124:2223–31.

23. Younes-Mhenni S, Janier MF, Cinotti L, et al. FDG-PET improves tumour detection in patients with paraneoplastic neurological syndromes. *Brain* 2004; 127:2331–8.

24. Keime-Guibert F, Graus F, Fleury A, et al. Treatment of paraneoplastic neurological syndromes with antineuronal antibodies (Anti-Hu, anti-Yo) with a combination of immunoglobulins, cyclophosphamide, and methylprednisolone. *J Neurol Neurosurg Psychiatry* 2000; 68:479–82.

25. Sommer C, Weishaupt A, Brinkhoff J, et al. Paraneoplastic stiffperson syndrome: passive transfer to rats by means of IgG antibodies to amphiphysin. *Lancet* 2005; 365:1406–11.

26. Vernino S, O'Neill BP, Marks RS, O'Fallon JR, Kimmel DW. Immunomodulatory treatment trial for paraneoplastic neurological disorders. *Neuro-Oncol* 2004; 6:55–62.

27. Keime-Guibert F, Graus F, Broet P, et al. Clinical outcome of patients with anti-Hu-associated encephalomyelitis after treatment of the tumor. *Neurology* 1999; 53:1719–23.

28. Henson RA, Urich H. *Cancer and the Nervous System: The Neurologic Complications of Systemic Malignant Disease.* Oxford: Blackwell Scientific, 1982.

29. Dalmau J, Graus F, Rosenblum MK, Posner JB. Anti-Hu-associated paraneoplastic encephalomyelitis/sensory neuronopathy. A clinical study of 71 patients. *Medicine* 1992; 71:59–72.

30. Lucchinetti CF, Kimmel DW, Lennon VA. Paraneoplastic and oncologic profiles of patients seropositive for type 1 antineuronal nuclear autoantibodies. *Neurology* 1998; 50:652–7.

31. Lawn ND, Westmoreland BF, Kiely MJ, Lennon VA, Vernino S. Clinical, magnetic resonance imaging, and electroencephalographic findings in paraneoplastic limbic encephalitis. *Mayo Clin Proc* 2003; 78:1363–8.

32. Gultekin SH, Rosenfeld MR, Voltz R, Eichen J, Posner JB, Dalmau J. Paraneoplastic limbic encephalitis: neurological symptoms, immunological findings and tumour association in 50 patients. *Brain* 2000; 123:1481–94.

33. Dropcho EJ. Antiamphiphysin antibodies with small-cell lung carcinoma and paraneoplastic encephalomyelitis. *Ann Neurol* 1996; 39:659–67.

34. Chan KH, Vernino S, Lennon VA. ANNA-3 anti-neuronal nuclear antibody: marker of lung cancer-related autoimmunity. *Ann Neurol* 2001; 50:301–11.

35. Vernino S, Lennon VA. New Purkinje cell antibody (PCA-2): marker of lung cancer-related neurological autoimmunity. *Ann Neurol* 2000; 47:297–305.

36. Corsellis JAN, Goldberg GJ, Norton AR. "Limbic encephalitis" and its association with cancer. *Brain* 1968; 91:481–96.

37. Ances BM, Vitaliani R, Taylor RA, et al. Treatment-responsive limbic encephalitis identified by neuropil antibodies: MRI and PET correlates. *Brain* 2005; 128:1764–77.

38. Dalmau J, Tuzun E, Wu HY, et al. Paraneoplastic anti-N-methyl-D-aspartate receptor encephalitis associated with ovarian teratoma. *Ann Neurol* 2007; 61:25–36.

39. Vitaliani R, Mason W, Ances B, Zwerdling T, Jiang Z, Dalmau J. Paraneoplastic encephalitis, psychiatric symptoms, and hypoventilation in ovarian teratoma. *Ann Neurol* 2005; 58:594–604.

40. Alamowitch S, Graus F, Uchuya M, Reñé R, Bescansa E, Delattre JY. Limbic encephalitis and small cell lung cancer. Clinical and immunological features. *Brain* 1997; 120:923–8.

41. Voltz R. Neuropsychological symptoms in paraneoplastic disorders. *J Neurol* 2007; 254(Suppl. 2):1184–6.

42. Kassubek J, Juengling FD, Nitzsche EU, Lucking CH. Limbic encephalitis investigated by 18FDG-PET and 3D MRI. *J Neuroimag* 2001; 11:55–9.

43. Voltz R, Gultekin SH, Rosenfeld MR, et al. A serologic marker of paraneoplastic limbic and brain-stem encephalitis in patients

with testicular cancer [see comments]. *N Engl J Med* 1999; 340: 1788–95.

44. Dalmau J, Graus F, Villarejo A, et al. Clinical analysis of anti-Ma2-associated encephalitis. *Brain* 2004; 127:1831–44.

45. Vincent A, Buckley C, Schott JM, et al. Potassium channel antibody-associated encephalopathy: a potentially immunotherapy-responsive form of limbic encephalitis. *Brain* 2004; 127: 701–12.

46. Pozo-Rosich P, Clover L, Saiz A, Vincent A, Graus F. Voltage-gated potassium channel antibodies in limbic encephalitis. *Ann Neurol* 2003; 54:530–3.

47. Taylor RB, Mason W, Kong K, Wennberg R. Reversible paraneoplastic encephalomyelitis associated with a benign ovarian teratoma. *Can J Neurol Sci* 1999; 26:317–20.

48. Rosenfeld MR, Eichen JG, Wade DF, Posner JB, Dalmau J. Molecular and clinical diversity in paraneoplastic immunity to Ma proteins. *Ann Neurol* 2001; 50:339–48.

49. Hammack J, Kotanides H, Rosenblum MK, Posner JB. Paraneoplastic cerebellar degeneration. II. Clinical and immunologic findings in 21 patients with Hodgkin's disease. *Neurology* 1992; 42:1938–43.

50. Posner JB. Paraneoplastic cerebellar degeneration. *Can J Neurol Sci* 1993; 20:S117–22.

51. Bernal F, Shams'ili S, Rojas I, et al. Anti-Tr antibodies as markers of paraneoplastic cerebellar degeneration and Hodgkin's disease. *Neurology* 2003; 60:230–4.

52. Choi KD, Kim JS, Park SH, Kim YK, Kim SE, Smitt PS. Cerebellar hypermetabolism in paraneoplastic cerebellar degeneration. *J Neurol Neurosurg Psychiatry* 2006; 77:525–8.

53. Furneaux HM, Rosenblum MK, Dalmau J, et al. Selective expression of Purkinje-cell antigens in tumor tissue from patients with paraneoplastic cerebellar degeneration. *N Engl J Med* 1990; 322:1844–51.

54. Fathallah-Shaykh H, Wolf S, Wong E, Posner JB, Furneaux HM. Cloning of a leucine-zipper protein recognized by the sera of patients with antibody-associated paraneoplastic cerebellar degeneration. *Proc Natl Acad Sci USA* 1991; 88:3451–4.

55. Mason WP, Graus F, Lang B, et al. Small-cell lung cancer, paraneoplastic cerebellar degeneration and the Lambert-Eaton myasthenic syndrome. *Brain* 1997; 120:1279–300.

56. Bataller L, Wade DF, Graus F, Stacey HD, Rosenfeld MR, Dalmau J. Antibodies to Zic4 in paraneoplastic neurologic disorders and small-cell lung cancer. *Neurology* 2004; 62: 778–82.

57. Shams'ili S, Sillevis Smitt P. Paraneoplasia. In: Schiff D, O'Neill BP, eds. *Principles of Neuro-Oncology*. New York: McGraw-Hill, 2005:649–79.

58. Posner JB. Paraneoplastic syndromes. *Neurologic Complications of Cancer*. Philadelphia: FA Davis, 1995:353–85.

59. Digre KB. Opsoclonus in adults. Report of three cases and review of the literature. *Arch Neurol* 1986; 43:1165–75.

60. Anderson NE, Budde-Steffen C, Rosenblum MK, et al. Opsoclonus, myoclonus, ataxia, and encephalopathy in adults with cancer: a distinct paraneoplastic syndrome. *Medicine* 1988; 67:100–9.

61. Wirtz PW, Sillevis Smitt PA, Hoff JI, et al. Anti-Ri antibody positive opsoclonus-myoclonus in a male patient with breast carcinoma. *J Neurol* 2002; 249:1710–12.

62. Bataller L, Graus F, Saiz A, Vilchez JJ. Clinical outcome in adult onset idiopathic or paraneoplastic opsoclonus-myoclonus. *Brain* 2001; 124:437–43.

63. Altman AJ, Baehner RL. Favorable prognosis for survival in children with coincident opso-myoclonus and neuroblastoma. *Cancer* 1976; 37:846–52.

64. Rudnick E, Khakoo Y, Antunes NL, et al. Opsoclonus-myoclonus-ataxia syndrome in neuroblastoma: clinical outcome and antineuronal antibodies-a report from the Children's Cancer Group Study. *Med Pediatr Oncol* 2001; 36:612–22.

65. Hormigo A, Dalmau J, Rosenblum MK, River ME, Posner JB. Immunological and pathological study of anti-Ri-associated encephalopathy. *Ann Neurol* 1994; 36:896–902.

66. Linke R, Schroeder M, Helmberger T, Voltz R. Antibody-positive paraneoplastic neurologic syndromes: value of CT and PET for tumor diagnosis. *Neurology* 2004; 63:282–6.

67. Swart JF, de Kraker J, van der Lely N. Metaiodobenzylguanidine total-body scintigraphy required for revealing occult neuroblastoma in opsoclonus-myoclonus syndrome. *Eur J Pediatr* 2002; 161:255–8.

68. Prestigiacomo CJ, Balmaceda C, Dalmau J. Anti-Ri-associated paraneoplastic opsoclonus-ataxia syndrome in a man with transitional cell carcinoma. *Cancer* 2001; 91:1423–8.

69. Dalmau J, Graus F, Cheung NK, et al. Major histocompatibility proteins, anti-Hu antibodies and paraneoplastic encephalomyelitis in neuroblastoma and small cell lung cancer. *Cancer* 1995; 75: 99–109.

70. Antunes NL, Khakoo Y, Matthay KK, et al. Antineuronal antibodies in patients with neuroblastoma and paraneoplastic opsoclonus-myoclonus. *J Pediatr Hematol Oncol* 2000; 22: 315–20.

71. Pranzatelli MR, Tate ED, Wheeler A, et al. Screening for autoantibodies in children with opsoclonus-myoclonus-ataxia. *Pediatr Neurol* 2002; 27:384–7.

72. Jongen JL, Moll WJ, Sillevis Smitt PA, Vecht CJ, Tijssen CC. Anti-Ri positive opsoclonus-myoclonus-ataxia in ovarian duct cancer. *J Neurol* 1998; 245:691–2.

73. Dropcho EJ, Kline LB, Riser J. Antineuronal (anti-Ri) antibodies in a patient with steroid-responsive opsoclonus-myoclonus. *Neurology* 1993; 43:207–11.

74. Nitschke M, Hochberg F, Dropcho E. Improvement of paraneoplastic opsoclonus-myoclonus after protein A column therapy. *N Engl J Med* 1995; 332:192.

75. Hayward K, Jeremy RJ, Jenkins S, et al. Long-term neurobehavioral outcomes in children with neuroblastoma and opsoclonus-myoclonus-ataxia syndrome: relationship to MRI findings and anti-neuronal antibodies. *J Pediatr* 2001; 139:552–9.

76. Mitchell WG, Davalos-Gonzalez Y, Brumm VL, et al. Opsoclonus-ataxia caused by childhood neuroblastoma: developmental and neurologic sequelae. *Pediatrics* 2002; 109:86–98.

77. Russo C, Cohn SL, Petruzzi MJ, de Alarcon PA. Long-term neurologic outcome in children with opsoclonus-myoclonus associated with neuroblastoma: a report from the Pediatric Oncology Group. *Med Pediatr Oncol* 1997; 28:284–8.

78. Chalk CH, Windebank AJ, Kimmel DW, McManis PG. The distinctive clinical features of paraneoplastic sensory neuronopathy. *Can J Neurol Sci* 1992; 19:346–51.

79. Horwich MS, Cho L, Porro RS, et al. Subacute sensory neuropathy: a remote effect of carcinoma. *Ann Neurol* 1977; 2: 7–19.

80. Graus F, Bonaventura I, Uchuya M, et al. Indolent anti-Hu-associated paraneoplastic sensory neuropathy. *Neurology* 1994; 44:2258–61.

81. Molinuevo JL, Graus F, Serrano C, Rene R, Guerrero A. Utility of anti-Hu antibodies in the diagnosis of paraneoplastic sensory neuropathy. *Ann Neurol* 1998; 44:976–80.

82. Antoine JC, Honnorat J, Camdessanche JP, et al. Paraneoplastic anti-CV2 antibodies react with peripheral nerve and are associated with a mixed axonal and demyelinating peripheral neuropathy. *Ann Neurol* 2001; 49:214–21.

83. Honnorat J, Antoine JC, Derrington E, Aguera M, Belin MF. Antibodies to a subpopulation of glial cells and a 66 kDa developmental protein in patients with paraneoplastic neurological syndromes. *J Neurol Neurosurg Psychiatry* 1996; 61:270–8.

84. Pittock SJ, Lucchinetti CF, Parisi JE, et al. Amphiphysin autoimmunity: paraneoplastic accompaniments. *Ann Neurol* 2005; 58:96–107.

85. Saiz A, Dalmau J, Butler MH, et al. Anti-amphiphysin I antibodies in patients with paraneoplastic neurological disorders associated with small cell lung carcinoma. *J Neurol Neurosurg Psychiatry* 1999; 66:214–7.

86. Uchuya M, Graus F, Vega F, Rene R, Delattre J-Y. Intravenous immunoglobulin treatment in paraneoplastic neurological syndromes with antineuronal autoantibodies. *J Neurol Neurosurg Psychiatry* 1996; 60:388–92.

87. Oh SJ, Dropcho EJ, Claussen GC. Anti-Hu-associated paraneoplastic sensory neuropathy responding to early aggressive immunotherapy: report of two cases and review of literature. *Muscle Nerve* 1997; 20:1576–82.

88. Wirtz PW, Willcox N, van der Slik AR, et al. HLA and smoking in prediction and prognosis of small cell lung cancer in autoimmune Lambert-Eaton myasthenic syndrome. *J Neuroimmunol* 2005; 159:230–7.

89. O'Neill JH, Murray NM, Newsom-Davis J. The Lambert-Eaton myasthenic syndrome. A review of 50 cases. *Brain* 1988; 111: 577–96.

90. Elrington GM, Murray NM, Spiro SG, Newsom-Davis J. Neurological paraneoplastic syndromes in patients with small cell lung cancer. A prospective survey of 150 patients. *J Neurol Neurosurg Psychiatry* 1991; 54:764–7.

91. Wirtz PW, Willcox N, Roep BO, et al. HLA-B8 in patients with the Lambert-Eaton myasthenic syndrome reduces likelihood of associated small cell lung carcinoma. *Ann NY Acad Sci* 2003; 998:200–1.

92. Hawley RJ, Cohen MH, Saini N, Armbrustmacher VW. The carcinomatous neuromyopathy of oat cell lung cancer. *Ann Neurol* 1980; 7:65–72.

93. Motomura M, Johnston I, Lang B, Vincent A, Newsom-Davis J. An improved diagnostic assay for Lambert-Eaton myasthenic syndrome. *J Neurol Neurosurg Psychiatry* 1995; 58:85–7.

94. Rosenfeld MR, Wong E, Dalmau J, et al. Cloning and characterization of a Lambert-Eaton myasthenic syndrome antigen. *Ann Neurol* 1993; 33:113–20.

95. Chalk CH, Murray NMF, Newsom-Davis J, O'Neill JH, Spiro SG. Response of the Lambert-Eaton myasthenic syndrome to treatment of associated small-cell lung carcinoma. *Neurology* 1990; 40:1552–6.

96. McEvoy KM, Windebank AJ, Daube JR, Low PA. 3,4-Diaminopyridine in the treatment of Lambert-Eaton myasthenic syndrome. *N Engl J Med* 1989; 321:1567–71.

97. Sanders DB, Massey JM, Sanders LL, Edwards LJ. A randomized trial of 3,4-diaminopyridine in Lambert-Eaton myasthenic syndrome. *Neurology* 2000; 54:603–7.

98. Newsom-Davis J, Murray NM. Plasma exchange and immunosuppressive drug treatment in the Lambert-Eaton myasthenic syndrome. *Neurology* 1984; 34:480–5.

99. Bird SJ. Clinical and electrophysiologic improvement in Lambert-Eaton syndrome with intravenous immunoglobulin therapy. *Neurology* 1992; 42:1422–3.

100. Buchbinder R, Forbes A, Hall S, Dennett X, Giles G. Incidence of malignant disease in biopsy-proven inflammatory myopathy. A population-based cohort study. *Ann Intern Med* 2001; 134: 1087–95.

101. Hill CL, Zhang Y, Sigurgeirsson B, et al. Frequency of specific cancer types in dermatomyositis and polymyositis: a population-based study. *Lancet* 2001; 357:96–100.

102. Mastaglia FL, Garlepp MJ, Phillips BA, Zilko PJ. Inflammatory myopathies: clinical, diagnostic and therapeutic aspects. *Muscle Nerve* 2003; 27:407–25.

103. Targoff IN. Update on myositis-specific and myositis-associated autoantibodies. *Curr Opin Rheumatol* 2000; 12:475–81.

104. Griggs RC, Mendell JR, Miller RG. *Evaluation and Treatment of Myopathies. Contemporary Neurology Series.* Philadelphia: FA Davis Company, 1995.

Dermatologic Paraneoplasias

JAMES W. PATTERSON

■ INTRODUCTION

The word *paraneoplastic* is derived from the Greek roots *para*, meaning "to, at, or from the side of," *neo*, meaning "new," and *plasma*, meaning "formation," and is used to refer to changes in tissue remote from a tumor or its metastases (1). Neoplasms, of course, can be both benign and malignant. As commonly used, the term *paraneoplastic* usually refers to syndromes associated with malignant tumors, though as it happens a number of these conditions are also associated with the development of benign tumors. The focus in this chapter is on conditions that are, or can be, associated with malignancy.

Paraneoplastic conditions of the skin are particularly important. From an academic standpoint, the accessibility of diseased skin can provide insights into basic tumor biology. This has certainly been the case, for example, in understanding some tumors associated with paraneoplastic pemphigus. In more practical terms, and in contrast to most internal disorders, changes involving the skin are often readily identifiable at an early stage. Patients can sometimes pinpoint the time of onset of a skin lesion and relate it to the development of other symptoms. As a result, cutaneous lesions can serve as the harbinger of a malignant process, allowing for earlier detection and treatment and increasing the likelihood of a favorable outcome. Although it is uncommon for the pathologist to make a definitive diagnosis of a paraneoplastic condition based upon biopsy findings alone, it can occur, as in the case of necrolytic migratory erythema (glucagonoma), acanthosis nigricans (gastrointestinal adenocarcinoma), or paraneoplastic pemphigus (non-Hodgkin's lymphoma). Since the microscopic changes of these and other paraneoplastic syndromes can be seen in the absence of neoplasia (the latter arising either at the time of diagnosis or later), the role of the pathologist is more often to suggest heightened surveillance for a malignant process. Other conditions are either less predictably associated with malignancy (e.g., dermatomyositis, exfoliative dermatitis, multicentric reticulohistiocytosis) or lack specific histopathologic findings, even though the clinical features are particularly suggestive of paraneoplasia (e.g., acrokeratosis paraneoplastica, erythema gyratum repens, the sign of Leser-Trélat). In such cases, good communication between pathologist and clinician can comprise a powerful diagnostic tool that may well prove to be lifesaving.

The following discussion is divided into five sections. The first considers those paraneoplastic syndromes in which the skin findings are potentially diagnostic of an underlying neoplasm, either through histopathology or clinicopathologic correlation. The second section deals with genetic syndromes that link cutaneous lesions of varying degrees of specificity to internal malignancy. In the third, a miscellaneous group of dermatoses is discussed that may be associated with a variety of underlying conditions, one of which (not necessarily the most common) may be neoplastic. The fourth section includes a few genetic disorders featuring cutaneous findings that alone would be considered quite nonspecific (e.g., granulomas, eczematous dermatitis, altered pigmentation), but in the context of a particular syndrome have a known association with malignancy. The fifth and final category includes several specific dermatologic conditions that are not generally considered paraneoplastic and the diagnosis of which would not ordinarily prompt a search for malignancy, but a review of the literature shows that malignant tumors have been encountered from time to time and this occurrence may be more than coincidental.

■ PARANEOPLASTIC SYNDROMES WITH SKIN FINDINGS THAT ARE POTENTIALLY DIAGNOSTIC

Necrolytic Migratory Erythema (Glucagonoma Syndrome)

Clinical Findings

This syndrome features anemia, weight loss, glossitis, and adult onset diabetes mellitus. The characteristic cutaneous feature is a migrating annular erythema with erosions and crusting. It is concentrated in intertriginous areas of the trunk, groin, buttocks, and thighs, and perioral lesions may occur (2, 3). Necrolytic migratory erythema is most often associated with a glucagon-secreting islet cell tumor of the pancreas (2, 3). In a typical case, elevated glucagon levels and reduced plasma amino acids are detected. However, the identical skin changes have also been seen in association with neuroendocrine hepatic tumors (4) and hepatic cirrhosis (5)—other situations in which glucagons can be elevated—as well as jejunal and rectal adeno-carcinoma, myelodysplastic syndrome (5), inflammatory bowel disease, pancreatitis, and malabsorption disorders. The occurrence of necrolytic migratory erythema in the absence of a pancreatic tumor is sometimes called the pseudoglucagonoma syndrome (6). Skin lesions resolve with treatment of the underlying tumor and/or correction of nutritional deficiencies. There appears to be no clear consensus regarding the pathogenesis of necrolytic migratory erythema, but amino acid deficiency due to the catabolic effects of elevated glucagon levels, other nutritional deficiencies (such as zinc and fatty acids), and the effects of certain inflammatory mediators, including arachidonic acid, may all play a part (6, 7).

Histopathology

There is often some degree of acanthosis, which may range from mild to marked and psoriasiform. Confluent parakeratosis overlies distinctly vacuolated keratinocytes in the upper portion of the epidermis (Fig. 1) (8). Necrosis may ensue, with coalescence of vacuoles and neutrophil accumulation, at times producing spongiform pustulation. Subcorneal pustules occasionally form and may be the principal histopathologic finding (9). Within the superficial to mid dermis, there is a perivascular infiltrate comprised mainly of lymphocytes but sometimes including neutrophils.

Specificity of Findings and Differential Diagnosis

The presence of confluent parakeratosis overlying vacuolated superficial keratinocytes is quite characteristic of necrolytic migratory erythema and should raise suspicions

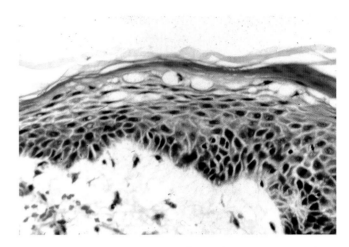

FIGURE 1 Microscopic image of necrolytic migratory erythema (glucagonoma syndrome), showing parakeratosis, vacuolated changes of the epidermal surface, and an absent granular cell layer.

of the diagnosis. However, other nutritional deficiency disorders, such as zinc deficiency (acrodermatitis enteropathica), biotin deficiency, and pellagra can have similar microscopic changes (10, 11). In general, biopsies showing parakeratosis and pallor or vacuolization of superficial keratinocytes should suggest a nutritional deficiency disorder and prompt investigations in this regard. The clinical presentations of biotin deficiency, pellagra, and childhood acrodermatitis enteropathica should be sufficiently distinctive, but adult onset zinc deficiency could be difficult to distinguish from necrolytic migratory erythema in the absence of laboratory data. There is another condition resembling necrolytic migratory erythema but occurring in an acral distribution, particularly on the legs, termed *necrolytic acral erythema*. This entity is virtually identical histopathologically to necrolytic migratory erythema of the glucagonoma syndrome, but it has a strong association with hepatitis C infection (12, 13). In this instance, knowledge of the clinical distribution of the lesions would be important, and laboratory studies would be essential.

Psoriasiform varieties of necrolytic migratory erythema could be difficult to distinguish from true psoriasis. Vacuolization of superficial keratinocytes is not typical of psoriasis in the absence of spongiform pustulation—spongiotic change in superficial portions of the epidermis associated with accumulations of neutrophils. But the latter change can occur in both conditions. Among the other dermatoses characterized by spongiform pustulation, candidiasis would be expected to show organisms at the surface epidermis with PAS or silver methenamine stains. Unfortunately, coexistence of necrolytic migratory erythema and candidiasis has been reported (14), so the diagnosis of the former cannot be entirely excluded if organisms are found. The occasional case presenting with purely subcorneal pustules would be quite difficult to distinguish from subcorneal pustular dermatosis. However, the variant of IgA pemphigus manifesting as subcorneal pustules could be recognized through direct immunofluorescence study; in that case, intraepidermal intercellular IgA deposition would be detected.

Acrokeratosis Paraneoplastica (Bazex's Syndrome)

Clinical Findings

Individuals with this condition display psoriasiform or eczematous lesions that are concentrated over acral surfaces, including the hands, feet, knees, ears, nose and cheeks (15, 16). Brittle nails with surrounding psoriasis-like changes can occur. The skin lesions often have a distinctly violaceous color (17). Bullous lesions are uncommon but have been reported (18).

Acrokeratosis paraneoplastica is associated with malignancy in virtually all cases, particularly those arising in supradiaphragmatic locations and associated with the aerodigestive tract. Examples include carcinomas of the tongue, pharynx, soft palate, esophagus, and lung (18). Some recently reported tumor associations include carcinoma of the breast (19), metastatic thymic carcinoma (20), and liposarcoma (21). The development of acrokeratosis paraneoplastica typically precedes initial symptoms or diagnosis of the underlying malignancy by an average of 11 months (18). Occasionally, the skin lesions may serve as a harbinger of recurrent or metastatic tumor. In most cases, cutaneous lesions improve following treatment of the malignancy. Although the precise cause is yet to be determined, possibilities include a host immune response directed toward shared tumor antigens, or tumor-induced inflammatory mediators such as transforming growth factor-alpha (TGF-α) (18, 22).

Histopathology

Microscopic findings include focal parakeratosis, hyperkeratosis, and acanthosis (23). Varying degrees of vacuolar alteration and formation of apoptotic keratinocytes have been detected (16, 17). Within the superficial dermis is a mild perivascular lymphocytic infiltrate. Bullous lesions could result from lichen planus–like clefting along the basement membrane zone or from a superimposed, "second-hit" bullous disorder, possibly due to epitope spreading (18).

Specificity of Findings and Differential Diagnosis

In the absence of a clinical history, the microscopic findings must be regarded as nonspecific. The constellation of features would ordinarily raise the differential diagnosis of psoriasis versus psoriasiform spongiotic dermatitis, a common issue in diagnostic dermatopathology. It is also not unusual for some dermatoses to feature spongiotic changes as well as a degree of vacuolar alteration of the basilar layer; this can be seen, for example, in drug reactions. However, neutrophil accumulations within the stratum corneum, forming Munro microabscesses or spongiform pustules, have not been emphasized as a feature in acrokeratosis paraneoplastica, and their absence would tend to militate against a confident diagnosis of psoriasis. Acrokeratosis paraneoplastica showing significant hyperkeratosis and minimal inflammatory or spongiotic changes could also mimic ichthyosis, and in fact, coexistence of these two paraneoplastic signs has been reported (24). Formation of bullae within these lesions would make specific diagnosis extremely difficult.

However, the clinical presentation of acrokeratosis paraneoplastica is quite characteristic, and in that context, the microscopic findings can be strongly supportive of the diagnosis. Clearly, a high index of suspicion and good communication with the clinician would be essential to making the diagnosis. Recent onset of a spongiotic or psoriasiform dermatitis in an acral location, with the enumerated microscopic features, should at least raise the possibility of this uncommon but specific paraneoplastic disorder.

Papuloerythroderma of Ofuji

Clinical Findings

First described by Ofuji in 1984 (25), papuloerythroderma is another clinically distinctive dermatosis that often lacks specific histopathologic features. This condition typically presents in elderly males. Widespread erythema and solid, red-brown papules develop, with dramatic sparing of flexural folds—a finding often termed the "deck chair sign" (Fig. 2). Eosinophilia and lymphopenia may accompany the dermatosis (26). Papuloerythroderma has a strong association with malignancy, especially lymphoma. The most common lymphoproliferative disorder is T-cell lymphoma, particularly cutaneous T-cell lymphoma (27–33). In some cases, cutaneous T-cell lymphoma has actually presented with the clinical appearance of papuloerythroderma (28, 31), while in other instances, papuloerythroderma has apparently evolved from a nonspecific histopathologic picture to one of mycosis fungoides (34). Nonepidermotropic peripheral T-cell lymphoma (35), Hodgkin's disease (36), and acute myeloid leukemia (37) have also been reported. Solid tumors have included gastric carcinoma (38, 39), adenocarcinoma of the colon (40), and hepatocellular carcinoma (41). Despite the apparently strong cancer association, some patients have not

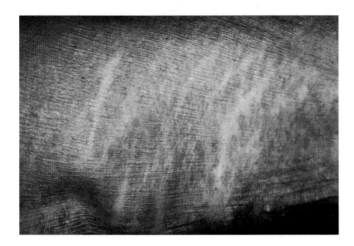

FIGURE 2 Papuloerythroderma of Ofuji, showing the "deck chair sign."

developed malignancy during a limited period of follow-up, while sporadic cases have been related to HIV infection (42) and choledocholithiasis with secondary sepsis (43). Therapies that have been effective for the dermatosis include ultraviolet light, both UVB and PUVA, and oral or topical corticosteroids (30).

Histopathology

The findings include parakeratosis, varying degrees of acanthosis, and spongiosis (Fig. 3). There is a moderately intense perivascular and interstitial inflammatory infiltrate, concentrated in the upper to mid dermis, comprised mainly of lymphocytes, though scattered eosinophils and plasma cells can also be observed. Varying numbers of Langerhans cells can be identified within the dermis (40).

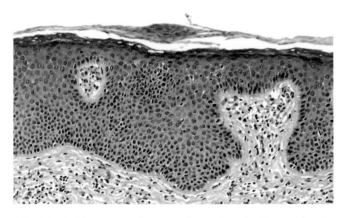

FIGURE 3 Microscopic features of papuloerythroderma, showing parakeratosis, acanthosis, spongiosis, and a moderately intense superficial dermal inflammatory infiltrate.

Specificity of Findings and Differential Diagnosis

None of the microscopic changes enumerated above are considered to be specific. In fact, these findings can be encountered in a wide variety of spongiotic dermatitides, including forms of eczematous dermatitis (e.g., contact dermatitis, nummular dermatitis) and erythroderma. In the authors' experience, the diagnosis is largely a clinical one, with histopathology playing mainly a supportive role. Clinically, the "deck chair sign" is far more distinctive than any of the histopathologic features. However, the microscopic findings can be crucial in those few cases that clinically resemble papuloerythroderma but in reality represent cutaneous T-cell lymphoma. In those circumstances, the observation of significant epidermotropism, Pautrier microabscesses, haloed lymphocytes, and wiry papillary dermal collagen can be decisive, prompting further study via immunohistochemistry or gene rearrangement testing (31).

Paraneoplastic Pemphigus

Clinical Findings

Although there had been a number of reports of an association between pemphigus and cancer, dating back to at least 1910, it was Anhalt et al. who in 1990 defined the disorder that has come to be known as paraneoplastic pemphigus (44). Patients develop erosions of the lips and oropharynx, pseudomembranous conjunctivitis, and pruritic, polymorphous skin lesions with blisters and erosions (44). Some lesions have an iris, or target-like configuration, and these combined with the mucous membrane changes can be quite suggestive of erythema multiforme, including the Stevens-Johnson syndrome.

Paraneoplastic pemphigus has a strong association with lymphoproliferative disorders, including both T- and B-cell lymphomas, thymoma, chronic lymphocytic leukemia, and Castleman's disease (44–46). Several other tumors have been identified as well, comprising 16% of all cases in a recent review (46). These include carcinomas, sarcomas, and malignant melanoma. In typical cases associated with lymphoma, the neoplastic process is already established at the time of onset of paraneoplastic pemphigus, and thus the prognosis is usually poor. Unusual cases have also been reported in which no tumor was detected (47), or in which other factors may have been involved, e.g., radiation therapy (48, 49).

Patients with paraneoplastic pemphigus have been shown to develop circulating antibodies to a variety of keratinocyte-derived proteins, particularly desmoplakin I (250 kd), bullous pemphigoid antigen (230 kd), envoplakin (210 kd), and periplakin (190 kd) (50, 51), important desmosome-related proteins. Presumably, autoantibodies directed toward tumors cross-react with epithelia that contain related antigens (44). Zhang et al. recently reported that B-lymphocyte clones from Castleman's tumors in patients with paraneoplastic pemphigus specifically react to epidermal proteins (52).

Histopathology

The microscopic image combines features of erythema multiforme with those of pemphigus vulgaris. There are vacuolar alteration of the basilar layer, apoptotic keratinocytes that may be found at all levels of the epidermis, and a superficial dermal infiltrate comprised mainly of lymphocytes, but with some eosinophils and neutrophils. All of these changes can be seen in erythema multiforme. In addition, suprabasilar acantholysis with cleft formation is often but not invariably present (53, 54). It is possible that the exposure of antigens resulting from lichenoid dermatitis could promote the development of autoimmunity and the subsequent acantholytic changes of pemphigus; this could be considered an example of a phenomenon termed "epitope spreading" (55). Direct immunofluorescence shows a combination of intercellular epidermal deposits of IgG and C3 and linear-granular basement membrane zone staining for C3 and/or IgG, a combination of findings also observed in the disorder pemphigus erythematosus (56). Positive intercellular IgG is also found by indirect immunofluorescence using the traditional monkey esophagus substrate, as would also be the case for nonparaneoplastic forms of pemphigus. In addition, sera from patients with paraneoplastic pemphigus show antibody binding to simple epithelia such as that found in murine bladder, a finding not encountered in ordinary pemphigus. However, negative results do not exclude the diagnosis of paraneoplastic pemphigus (57).

Specificity of Findings and Differential Diagnosis

The microscopic findings in paraneoplastic are potentially diagnostic, even without full clinical data. If not often predictive of malignancy (since, as mentioned previously, lymphomas associated with these cases are usually well established when skin disease develops), at least the pathologist has the opportunity to provide an explanation for a clinically puzzling dermatosis. The best opportunity for a specific diagnosis arises when interface (lichenoid) changes, sometimes resembling erythema multiforme, coexist with suprabasilar acantholysis. Supportive evidence is provided by direct immunofluorescent study, in which both intracellular and basement membrane zone fluorescence are often noted. Although these immunofluorescent changes could also be seen in pemphigus erythematosus, the histopathologic image of the latter is quite different, showing more superficial acantholytic changes (through

the region of the granular cell layer) and an absence of interface changes. If possible to accomplish, positive staining of rat bladder epithelium would generally clinch the diagnosis of paraneoplastic pemphigus.

Diagnostic problems can arise when no acantholytic changes are identified (53, 54). The differential diagnosis would include a variety of interface or lichenoid dermatoses, particularly erythema multiforme but also (in the absence of clinical information) graft versus host disease or fixed drug eruption. A clinical description of the lesions and/or history of malignancy would then prompt a recommendation for direct immunofluorescent studies. If positive intercellular staining were to be found, paraneoplastic pemphigus would be a strong consideration. At times, biopsy findings may show only suprabasilar acantholysis, without lichenoid tissue changes, a circumstance that has been reported in 27% of cases (58). Pemphigus would then be the leading consideration; securing the diagnosis of paraneoplastic pemphigus would require indirect immunofluorescence using rat bladder or comparable murine epithelium, and/or detection of the characteristic spectrum of circulating antibodies to keratinocyte-related proteins.

Dermatomyositis

Clinical Findings

Dermatomyositis is a well-known condition combining the features of polymyositis with inflammatory skin lesions. Some patients present with identical skin lesions in the absence of clinical and laboratory findings of myositis. When this situation continues for over two years, it is called "amyopathic dermatomyositis" (59). Internal malignancy has been reported in 15% to 25% of cases of dermatomyositis (60), including amyopathic cases (61). On the other hand, polymyositis alone may not have an increased risk for malignancy (62). The association with malignancy is strongest among older adults. The neoplastic process may precede, develop concurrently with, or follow the onset of dermatomyositis with approximately equal frequencies (63). Furthermore, the types of malignant lesions occur with a frequency mirroring that in the general population (63). Thus, carcinomas of breast or lung are among the most common, but a complete spectrum of tumors has been encountered, including lymphomas, melanoma, and sarcomas. The literature suggests that a diagnosis of dermatomyositis should not, by itself, prompt a detailed evaluation for malignancy; instead, such an evaluation should be guided by specifically suggestive findings resulting from history, physical examination, and/or routine laboratory studies (64). Treatment of the underlying malignancy may or may not result in improvement in the muscular or cutaneous disease (63).

The most common clinical features include violaceous erythema and scale, particularly in the head and neck regions or over extensor surfaces of the extremities, often with poikiloderma (variegated pigmentation and telangiectasia) and a degree of atrophy. "Heliotrope" eyelids are classic signs but are not always found. Papules or plaques involving skin overlying the interphalangeal joints (Gottron's papules) are often seen, and there may be nailfold telangiectasias or ragged-appearing cuticles (Samitz's sign). Photosensitivity, sometimes with a burning painful sensation, and plaque-like calcifications may also occur (65). When coexistent with myositis, proximal muscle weakness, elevated muscle enzymes, and a variety of circulating autoantibodies may be found.

Histopathology

The most typical presentation is that of a lichenoid tissue reaction, with vacuolar alteration of the basilar layer of the epidermis and formation of apoptotic keratinocytes. Often the features are those of poikiloderma atrophicans vasculare: basilar vacuolar change in the face of an atrophic epidermis, vasodilatation, and pigmentary incontinence. Basement membrane zone thickening has been reported. The superficial dermal infiltrate tends to be mild, lymphocytic, and perivascular. A lymphoplasmacytic panniculitis can be seen, but in the authors' experience, it is uncommon. Dermal mucin deposition is frequently identified with colloidal iron or alcian blue staining (Fig. 4) (66). Clinically apparent subepidermal blister formation is rare, but the few cases with this finding were associated with malignancy and poor

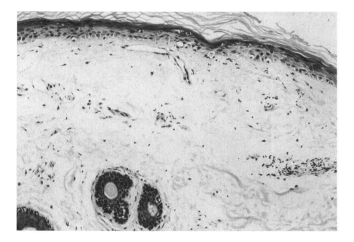

FIGURE 4 Typical microscopic findings of dermatomyositis, including epidermal atrophy, vacuolar alteration of the basilar layer, and marked dermal mucin deposition.

outcome (67, 68). Direct immunofluorescent studies tend to be negative, except for the presence of apoptotic (Civatte) bodies that stain positively for IgM and C3.

Specificity of Findings and Differential Diagnosis

Interface dermatitis in general raises a broad differential diagnosis, but skin biopsies showing features of poikiloderma atrophicans vasculare, particularly when arising in adult life, suggest three major possibilities: dermatomyositis, lupus erythematosus, and the early poikilodermatous phase of mycosis fungoides. There is considerable overlap of the changes in lupus erythematosus and dermatomyositis, and a distinct differentiation is not always possible. However, in addition to the epidermal changes, lupus erythematosus often shows a prominent perivascular and periadnexal infiltrate, which (in the case of follicles) is typically accompanied by vacuolar alteration of basilar outer root sheath epithelium. Thinning of lateral follicular walls occurs particularly in the discoid form of lupus erythematosus. When present, lupus panniculitis can be distinctive, with mixed septal-lobular arrangement, pools of mucin, focal hyalinizing change, and nodular aggregates of lymphocytes and plasma cells. Direct immunofluorescence of skin biopsies can be helpful in that only lupus erythematosus would be expected to show basement membrane deposits of complement and immunoglobulin. However, a false-negative study (which could result from lesion selection, the site chosen for biopsy, or sampling of very early or very late lesions) could be problematic. Correlation with clinical and laboratory findings would then be essential, because overlap or mixed connective tissue diseases also occur. Mycosis fungoides would be expected to show atypical lymphocytes, exocytosis with formation of haloed cells or Pautrier microabscesses in the epidermis, possibly abnormal immunophenotyping, or positive T-cell receptor gene rearrangement studies.

Diffuse (Normolipemic) Plane Xanthoma

Clinical Findings

In this xanthomatous condition, patchy or diffuse orange-yellow discoloration of the skin develops over the face and trunk and particularly in intertriginous areas such as the axillae (69, 70). Most patients with this syndrome are normolipemic, though plane xanthomas themselves can certainly occur in hyperlipoproteinemias of types 2 through 4. This condition has a strong association with multiple myeloma (69, 71). There are also reports of plane xanthomatosis associated with chronic lymphocytic leukemia (72) and rectal adenocarcinoma (73). Clinical and histopathologic links have been suggested between diffuse plane xanthoma and necrobiotic xanthogranuloma, another dermatosis associated with paraproteinemia (74, 75).

Histopathology

The findings include clusters of foamy macrophages scattered through the dermis, in the absence of fibrosis. Lymphocytic inflammation is typically sparse or absent (76, 77).

Specificity of Findings and Differential Diagnosis

The distribution of foam-laden macrophages, minimal degree of inflammation, and lack of fibrosis would be suggestive of plane xanthoma. Clinical correlation would then be necessary in order to confirm the "diffuseness" of the process. In addition to the hyperlipoproteinemias mentioned above, plane xanthomas can also accompany biliary cirrhosis. Cases showing foci of degenerated connective tissue or multinucleated cells can resemble necrobiotic xanthogranuloma.

Erythema Gyratum Repens

Clinical Findings

Erythema gyratum repens is surely one of the most dramatic clinical presentations in all of dermatology. In this condition, arcuate erythematous bands, sometimes with a trailing edge of scale, migrate over the skin surface. In some cases, this produces intricate patterns resembling the grain of wood (78, 79). Involvement is concentrated over the trunk and proximal extremities. This condition has a strong association with cancers, including lung (80, 81), breast (78), and undifferentiated carcinomas (79, 82). However, though most closely associated with malignancy, the same changes have accompanied nonneoplastic conditions such as cystic hypertrophy of the breast (83) and pulmonary tuberculosis (84), and have arisen in apparently normal individuals (85). When associated with malignancy, the eruption has been reported to occur either before or after the detection of the cancer. As is the case with a number of other cutaneous paraneoplastic syndromes, erythema gyratum repens may result from lymphokines secreted by the tumors, such as epidermal growth factor (80).

Histopathology

The microscopic findings include foci of parakeratosis and spongiosis and a moderately intense, perivascular infiltrate concentrated around vessels of the superficial to mid-dermis, comprised of lymphocytes and "histiocytes" (macrophages) (78, 86). In some reports, the infiltrates have been more diffuse (82) or have contained eosinophils (79). On direct immunofluorescence, granular IgG and C3 deposition were seen along the dermal–epidermal junction (86), the significance of which is not entirely clear.

Specificity of Findings and Differential Diagnosis

The histopathologic image of this entity is quite nonspecific. Basically, a diagnosis of erythema gyratum repens depends upon the clinical presentation, which as mentioned is usually quite striking. However, the microscopic findings can be supportive of the diagnosis. The combination of focal parakeratosis, spongiosis, and a superficial perivascular lymphocytic and macrophagic infiltrate can also be seen in the superficial variant of erythema annulare centrifugum (EAC), another less complex annular erythema that is not usually associated with internal cancer. It is interesting to note that in some case reports, erythema gyratum repens has begun as a more localized annular erythema with the clinical features of EAC. However, microscopic evaluation can be important in excluding other annular erythemas that might be clinical mimics of erythema gyratum repens, such as dermatophyte infection (organisms should be detectable in the stratum corneum with PAS or silver methenamine stains) or subacute cutaneous lupus erythematosus (interface rather than spongiotic dermatitis, often with dermal mucin deposition).

Sweet's Syndrome (Acute Febrile Neutrophilic Dermatosis)

Clinical Findings

Although often described as a rare entity, Sweet's syndrome is encountered from time to time, particularly in academic and referral centers, and it is even more often included in the differential diagnosis of puzzling dermatoses with neutrophilic components. In this condition, erythematous plaques and nodules develop over the face, trunk, or extremities. These are often described as painful (87). Characteristically, the lesions arise rather suddenly, are accompanied by fever and leukocytosis, and are particularly responsive to treatment with systemic corticosteroids. Multiple disease associations have been reported; these can be placed in the following groups: autoimmune inflammatory, including inflammatory bowel disease (88, 89), infection (90, 91), therapeutic agents (92, 93), and pregnancy related (94). Idiopathic cases definitely occur.

The other significant disease category is malignancy. Sweet's syndrome has been associated with malignancy in about 10% of cases (95). Leukemia has been the most frequent condition in this category, particularly acute myeloid or myelomonocytic leukemia (96–99). Sweet's syndrome has also accompanied chronic myeloid leukemia, in apparently uncomplicated disease (100), preceding blast crisis (101), or with use of the tyrosine kinase inhibitor imatinib mesylate (102, 103). Other leukemia-related associations have included hairy cell leukemia (104) and myelodysplastic syndrome (105). There are also reports of Sweet's syndrome occurring with lymphoma

(106), myeloma (107), and solid tumors. Most recent examples of the latter category are carcinomas of the bladder and prostate (108) and cervix (109).

Histopathology

The findings include pronounced papillary dermal edema and a dense neutrophilic infiltrate in the upper to mid-dermis (Fig. 5). Leukocytoclasis is usually apparent, but leukocytoclastic vasculitis typically cannot be demonstrated (110, 111). A neutrophil-poor variant has been described (112), but this is sufficiently unusual that reconsideration of the diagnosis would be warranted. A histiocytoid variant may suggest that "histiocytes" (macrophages) are prominent, while in fact, the cells in question are most likely immature myeloid forms (113). There have been other reports of immature or leukemic cells in lesions of Sweet's syndrome (114, 115).

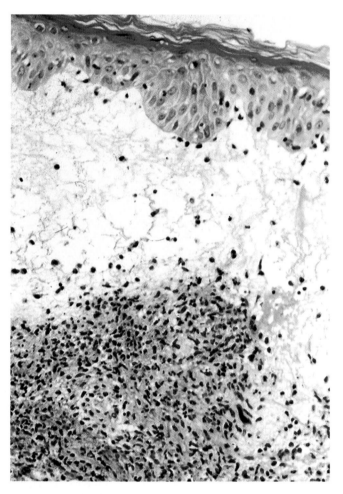

FIGURE 5 The characteristic features of Sweet's syndrome include papillary dermal edema and a dense neutrophilic infiltrate, with leukocytoclasis, occupying the upper to mid-dermis.

Specificity of Findings and Differential Diagnosis

The microscopic findings in Sweet's syndrome are quite characteristic and often diagnostic. There is some overlap with the early stages of pyoderma gangrenosum, and it has been suggested that these conditions are parts of a spectrum of neutrophilic skin disorders (116). However, early lesions of pyoderma gangrenosum often show evidence for acute folliculitis (117), and it is not typical for lesions of Sweet's syndrome to evolve into ulcers. The lesions of erythema elevatum diutinum can have overlapping microscopic features. However, they are of longer duration, have a typical distribution over extensor portions of distal extremities, can show true vasculitis microscopically, and resolve with fibrosis, sometimes with lipid deposition. A condition termed "rheumatoid neutrophilic dermatosis" also bears a close resemblance, but in the authors' experience, it tends to show deep as well as superficial dermal involvement, demonstrates a lesser degree of leukocytoclasis, and may be associated with the changes of interstitial granulomatous dermatitis (118).

Once a diagnosis of Sweet's syndrome has been made, clinical and laboratory investigations are in order to determine what, if any, disease association might be detected. Neoplasm is among the possibilities, but the majority of cases will not be associated with a malignant process. Although there are few microscopic clues that would lead the pathologist to specifically suspect an underlying malignancy, the detection of primitive myeloid forms should certainly prompt an investigation into the possibility of leukemia.

Superficial Thrombophlebitis

The association between superficial migratory thrombophlebitis and malignancy was first described by Trousseau in 1865, and therefore it is sometimes referred to as Trousseau's syndrome (119). Nodules or cords appear on the lower legs or elsewhere, conveying the impression of "migration." Although an association with Behcet's or Buerger's diseases is known, there is also often an association with an underlying cancer, particularly involving the pancreas, stomach, lung, prostate, or hematopoietic system (120). The hypercoagulable state associated with these malignancies likely predisposes patients to the syndrome (121–123). Microscopically, a vein at the dermal–subcutaneous interface shows thrombosis, with an inflammatory infiltrate consisting mainly of neutrophils at first, followed by lymphocytes and granulomatous elements. The infiltrates are concentrated in the immediate vicinity of the involved vessel (124). Although veins are traditionally distinguished from arteries by the finding of an internal elastic lamina in the latter, veins can also possess an elastic lamina. A recent paper by Dalton et al. indicates that the smooth muscle pattern of the vessel wall may be more diagnostic: arteries have a circumferential smooth muscle pattern, while that in veins is more haphazard and "cobblestoned" in appearance (Fig. 6) (125). In the absence of another explanation, biopsy changes of superficial thrombophlebitis should at least prompt the consideration of internal malignancy, particularly carcinoma of the body or tail of the pancreas.

Hypertrichosis Lanuginosa (Malignant Down)

Clinical Findings

This acquired condition consists of extensive growth of lanugo hairs that cover the face and can progress to the neck, trunk, and extremities (126, 127). Most reported patients have had a malignancy, usually carcinoma. These have included carcinomas of the lung, colon, gallbladder, rectum, uterus, breast, endometrium, and prostate; one lymphoma has also been reported (127–132). In the majority of reported patients, the malignancy was known to be present when the lanugo hair growth occurred, but in a few cases, hair growth preceded identification of the cancer (131, 132). Resolution of the condition has occasionally been reported to follow treatment of the underlying malignancy (128, 130). The pathogenesis of hypertrichosis lanuginosa is unclear, and an endocrinologic mechanism has not been discovered.

Histopathology

A histopathologic study by Hegedus and Schorr described the presence of mantle hair follicles in hypertrichosis lanuginosa. The follicular mantle is a poorly recognized

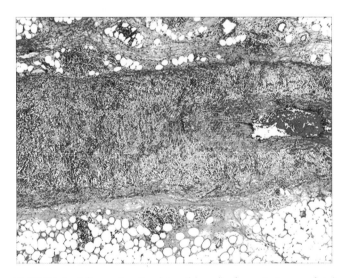

FIGURE 6 Inflammation involving the wall of a vein in superficial thrombophlebitis. Note the haphazard, "cobblestoned" appearance of the smooth muscle in this vessel.

structure championed by Pinkus (133). It consists of cords of basaloid cells that extend downward around the follicular infundibulum with a resemblance in tissue sections to a set of parentheses. They sometimes contain sebaceous cells and are believed to give rise to sebaceous glands. Most reported cases of hypertrichosis lanuginosa have not included histopathologic descriptions, so it remains to be seen if this is truly a characteristic finding of the disorder.

Specificity of Findings and Differential Diagnosis

Mantle hair follicles can occasionally be seen as an incidental finding in biopsies done for other reasons, so their identification does not "make" a diagnosis of hypertrichosis lanuginosa. The condition is so striking clinically that the diagnosis is often made without resorting to histopathology. However, the pathologist might be called upon to support the diagnosis, which could be accomplished by finding increased numbers of lanugo hairs per unit area (best accomplished with horizontal sectioning of a biopsy specimen), together with the detection of mantle hair follicles (best identified in vertically oriented sections).

Acanthosis Nigricans

Clinical Findings

Acanthosis nigricans is perhaps best known as a sign of malignancy, but it also accompanies a group of endocrinologic disorders, particularly those associated with insulin resistance (134), may be associated with obesity (sometimes termed pseudoacanthosis nigricans), presents as an autosomal dominant familial disorder (135), or may be caused by certain medications, including corticosteroids, nicotinic acid, and triazinate (136).

"Malignant" acanthosis nigricans (so-called because of its association with malignancy; the skin disease itself has no propensity toward malignant change) is mainly a disorder of adults. It is most closely associated with gastrointestinal carcinoma, but has been seen with carcinomas of the lung, kidney, and bladder as well as with mycosis fungoides (137). There have been recent cases reporting an association with carcinomas of the ovary (138) and pancreas (139). According to the classic studies by Curth, changes of acanthosis nigricans preceded the detection of malignancy in 17% of cases, appeared more or less simultaneously with the cancer in 60% of cases, and followed the development of cancer by variable periods of time in 22% of cases (140). The changes have been reported to regress, at least temporarily, when the tumor has been resected (141). Although the mechanism for development of acanthosis nigricans has not been completely worked out, it is likely that growth factors produced by the tumors may be responsible, particularly in view of the probable role for insulin in endocrinologic forms of the disorder (142).

All forms of the disorder feature pigmented, velvety plaques concentrated in flexures, such as the neck, axillae, and groin (Fig. 7) (143). The palms may be hyperkeratotic and develop a "honeycomb" appearance. Cases have been reported that link acanthosis nigricans to tripe palms, mucosal papillomas, and the sign of Leser-Trélat (138, 144, 145).

Histopathology

The findings in acanthosis nigricans are characteristic, if not pathognomonic, and include marked papillomatosis with "finger-like" projections of rete ridges, associated with hyperkeratosis that tends to be basket-woven rather than compact. Acanthosis is mild, usually limited to the valleys between papillomatous formations (Fig. 8). Basilar melanization is often mild, except in dark-skinned individuals, and it is believed that in most instances, the pigmentation perceived clinically is primarily due to hyperkeratosis (146).

Specificity of Findings and Differential Diagnosis

The changes of acanthosis nigricans are characteristic but not entirely specific. Similar combinations of hyperkeratosis and papillomatosis can be seen in confluent and reticulated papillomatosis (a hyperkeratotic condition most commonly seen on the trunk of younger individuals, unassociated with malignancy), some seborrheic keratoses, and epidermal nevi. Seborrheic keratoses may also

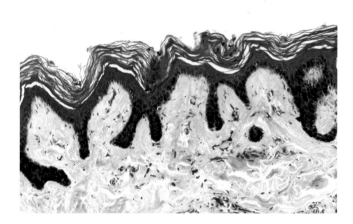

FIGURE 8 Microscopic findings of acanthosis nigricans include hyperkeratosis, papillomatosis, and "finger-like" elongations of rete ridges. Acanthosis is mild. In this particular case, hyperpigmentation is evident.

have horn cysts and a greater degree of acanthosis, while the changes in confluent and reticulated papillomatosis are generally less pronounced. Obviously, the clinical history and physical examination have a great bearing on the diagnosis in many cases. Once a diagnosis of acanthosis nigricans is established, there is still a need to determine the underlying cause. In the absence of a family history, endocrinologic syndrome, obesity, or relevant medications, the development of this condition in an adult should prompt a search for malignancy, particularly of the gastrointestinal tract.

Tripe Palms

Clinical Findings

"Tripe palms" represents a form of acquired palmar keratoderma in which the palms take on what is most commonly described as a *rugose* (wrinkled) appearance, resembling the luminal surface of the small bowel. It is sometimes observed together with acanthosis nigricans or the sign of Leser-Trélat (see below) (138, 139, 144), but it can also appear as an isolated finding. Despite some earlier literature contaminated with cases of acanthosis nigricans and keratoderma not necessarily featuring the typical "tripe palm" appearance, the evidence suggests that tripe palms constitute an independent sign of internal malignancy. Carcinomas of the lung and stomach appear to be most common (144, 147, 148). Ovarian and pancreatic carcinomas have also been reported (138, 139, 149). A recent interesting case was associated with systemic mastocytosis, elevated TGF-α levels, and detection of TGF-α in mast cells; treatment with interferon-alfa therapy resulted in decreased TGF-α levels and regression of the tripe palms (150).

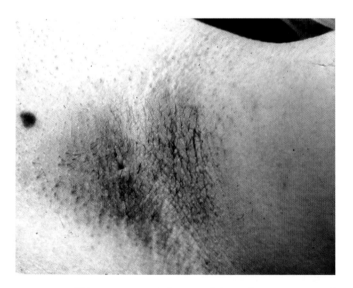

FIGURE 7 Velvety pigmented changes of the axilla in a patient with acanthosis nigricans.

Histopathology

Little has been written about the histopathology of tripe palms. In some instances, only "hyperkeratosis" has been emphasized (150). However, a study by Requena et al. demonstrated an undulant (wavy) epidermis featuring hyperkeratosis, papillomatosis, and acanthosis (149).

Specificity of Findings and Differential Diagnosis

Additional histopathologic studies will be necessary to determine if the changes that have been described are specific for the diagnosis of tripe palms. It certainly seems likely that there would be considerable overlap with other forms of palmar keratoderma, most of which are not associated with malignancy. However, an appreciation of undulation of the epidermis could be diagnostically useful. Proper evaluation of this feature would require sufficient sampling to enable inspection of a reasonable stretch of epidermis, and it might also be dependent upon the orientation of the specimen (i.e., whether parallel or perpendicular to the surface undulation). Again, clinical correlation would be decisive in most cases.

The Sign of Leser-Trélat

Clinical Findings

The sign of Leser-Trélat consists of the rapid increase in the number and/or size of seborrheic keratoses, particularly on the trunk, in association with an internal malignancy. Inflammation of seborrheic keratoses may be a part of this process (151), and it is conceivable that a host inflammatory response directed toward existing but subtle seborrheic keratoses could account for the "rapid increase" of lesions seen in some cases. Since multiple seborrheic keratoses are prevalent among older adults, and rapidity of onset may be questionable in any given case, a determination that the sign is present may be problematic. In addition, purists do not accept the development of multiple keratoses in the setting of erythroderma, even if that erythroderma is a manifestation of cutaneous T-cell lymphoma, i.e., Sézary syndrome (Fig. 9). As mentioned previously, coexistence of this sign with acanthosis nigricans has been reported.

The malignancies associated with the sign of Leser-Trélat include gastrointestinal carcinomas and lymphomas (152–156). Recent papers have reported an association with pancreatic carcinoma (157) and anaplastic ependymoma (158). The eruption of seborrheic keratoses can precede recognition of the cancer, or it can follow or develop concurrently (156, 159). The seborrheic keratoses may resolve following treatment of the primary tumor (159). A role for growth factors in the production of these lesions has been suggested, including epidermal growth factor and TGF-α (160).

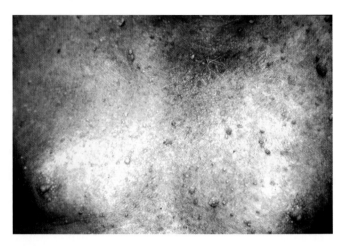

FIGURE 9 Multiple seborrheic keratoses in a patient with Sézary syndrome.

Histopathology

The microscopic findings have differed somewhat from case to case, ranging from typical seborrheic keratoses to foci of hyperkeratosis with variable degrees of papillomatosis (156, 161). Although regression of lesions was associated with mononuclear cell infiltration in one case (162), inflammation may be an integral part of the development (or appearance) of these seborrheic keratoses, at least in some cases. This has been observed in a case in which a patient presented with both the sign of Leser-Trélat and tripe palms (Fig. 10).

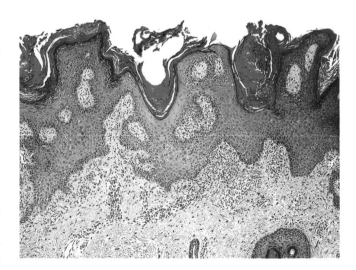

FIGURE 10 Inflamed seborrheic keratosis from a patient with the sign of Leser-Trélat. This patient also had tripe palms.

Specificity of Findings and Differential Diagnosis

Unfortunately, seborrheic keratoses, including inflamed seborrheic keratoses, are quite common, and this histopathologic finding by itself is not diagnostic of the sign. However, in the context of rapidly eruptive seborrheic keratoses (particularly if other changes, such as acanthosis nigricans or tripe palms, are also present), the microscopic features can be supportive of the diagnosis of the sign of Leser-Trélat.

Cushing's Syndrome or Disease

There are numerous cutaneous changes in Cushing's syndrome or disease, including changes in distribution of body fat, striae, hirsutism, addisonian pigmentation, and steroid acne. The pigmentation occurs with pituitary tumors, nonpituitary ACTH-secreting tumors, or in Nelson's syndrome following bilateral adrenalectomy. In steroid acne, there is an eruption of papules and pustules in the same stages of development; comedones and cystic lesions as seen in typical acne vulgaris do not occur. Nevertheless, none of these conditions produces very specific microscopic findings, and clinical data rather than cutaneous histopathology are likely to create a suspicion of Cushing's syndrome or disease and lead to detection of an underlying tumor.

Carcinoid Syndrome

Carcinoid syndrome is another endocrinologic disorder in which skin manifestations can accompany the underlying tumor. This syndrome is seen in about 10% of cases of patients with carcinoid tumors (163). It is associated with flushing and rosacea-like dermatitis. With chronicity, changes resembling pellagra or scleroderma can occur (163); the former results because tryptophan metabolism by tumor cells is diverted toward serotonin at the expense of nicotinic acid formation. None of these changes in isolation would be sufficiently specific microscopically to suggest carcinoid syndrome in the absence of clinical data, though biopsy findings could be supportive of the diagnosis. Rarely, carcinoid tumors have arisen primarily in the skin (164).

■ GENETIC SYNDROMES WITH SKIN FINDINGS THAT ARE POTENTIALLY DIAGNOSTIC

Multiple Endocrine Neoplasia

Clinical Findings

The multiple endocrine neoplasia (MEN) syndromes include MEN 1, MEN 2a, and MEN 2b. Two of these, MEN 1 and MEN 2b, are associated with significant cutaneous findings. In MEN 1, there are tumors of the pituitary, pancreatic islets, adrenal cortex, and parathyroid glands; gastrinomas also occur. The cutaneous lesions include facial angiofibromas of the type seen in tuberous sclerosis, collagenomas, lipomas, café au lait spots, and hypopigmented macules (165, 166). This syndrome results from a germline mutation of the MEN 1 gene on chromosome 11 (166). Microscopic confirmation of these types of cutaneous tumors, in the setting of endocrinologic disorders, should raise the possibility of MEN 1. MEN 2a, also known as the Sipple's syndrome, is associated with medullary carcinoma of the thyroid, parathyroid hyperplasia, and bilateral pheochromocytoma. It lacks significant cutaneous findings, with the exception of notalgia paresthetica, a pruritic condition of the scapular region that can be associated with macular amyloidosis (167, 168). MEN 2a is associated with a mutation in exon 10 or 11 of the RET proto-oncogene on chromosome 10.

MEN 2b is characterized by marfanoid habitus, characteristic facies, and multiple mucosal neuromas. These patients have thick, everted lips and thickened eyelids. Numerous neuromas are found on the lips, oral commissures, tongue, gingivae, and buccal mucosa (169, 170). These patients develop medullary carcinoma of the thyroid, the most frequent ages of incidence being between 8 and 18 years (171). Since the characteristic facial changes can be detected at an early age (172), preemptive management of the thyroid gland is possible. These patients also develop pheochromocytomas and intestinal ganglioneuromatosis. There is a mutation of the RET proto-oncogene on chromosome 10, affecting the tyrosine kinase domain (173).

Histopathology

The mucosal neuromas of MEN 2b feature fascicles of Schwann cells and axons in haphazard array. This may take on the appearance of tortuous, hypertrophied nerves within the dermis or lamina propria that resemble traumatic neuromas (174).

Specificity of Findings and Differential Diagnosis

The finding of one or more mucosal neuromas with the above microscopic features, particularly in a young individual and in the absence of a history of trauma, should raise suspicions of MEN 2b and prompt further investigations for thyroid carcinoma or other abnormalities associated with the syndrome.

Neurofibromatosis

One of the best-known neurocutaneous syndromes is type 1 neurofibromatosis, or von Recklinghausen's disease. This dominantly inherited trait is characterized by multiple cutaneous and subcutaneous neurofibromas, café au lait spots, axillary freckling, Lisch nodules of the iris, and other findings (175). The responsible gene, the NF1 gene, is found on chromosome 17 (176). In addition to malignant peripheral nerve sheath tumor, neurofibromatosis has been linked to a number of other tumors, including pheochromocytoma (177, 178), somatostatinoma (177, 179), osteosarcoma (180), xanthoastrocytoma (181), and (possibly) malignant melanoma (182).

Microscopically, neurofibromas are usually readily identifiable, featuring spindled cells with "buckled" or S-shaped nuclei, small vessels, and numerous mast cells in a delicate, sometimes mucinous stroma. This diagnosis is not especially challenging, and sporadic neurofibromas are certainly common. Nevertheless, a diagnosis of neurofibroma (especially when occurring in the setting of multiple cutaneous lesions in a young individual) can trigger careful patient evaluation for the possibility of neurofibromatosis and therefore promote surveillance for the development of other associated tumors. Although it is now known that the plexiform neurofibroma is not pathognomonic for neurofibromatosis (183), the association is nevertheless a strong one.

Xeroderma Pigmentosum

Clinical Findings

This genodermatosis is a classic example of an "experiment of nature," in which a relatively specific genetic abnormality—inability to repair ultraviolet-damaged DNA—results in a proneness to epithelial malignancy, resembling the situation in chronically sun-exposed skin of older adults. It is an autosomal recessive disorder associated with development in early childhood of severe sunburns, freckling, and atrophy, and the formation of actinic keratoses, squamous cell carcinomas, and basal cell carcinomas (Fig. 11). Other malignancies include malignant melanomas, keratoacanthomas, and atypical fibroxanthomas (184, 185).

Xeroderma pigmentosum has been organized into eight or more complementation groups, originally determined though hybridization studies in which cultured fibroblasts from two different patients corrected each other's DNA repair defects (186). These groups show varying degrees of deficiency in the ability to perform excision repair of ultraviolet-damaged DNA at the endonuclease step. Some of them are associated with neurologic abnormalities, including mental retardation; this is particularly the case in the De Sanctis-Cacchione syndrome (187). There is also a variant form, originally termed *pigmented xerodermoid* but now often referred to as the *XP variant*, in which excision repair is normal but there is defective postreplication repair, resulting from an abnormality in converting low- to high-molecular weight

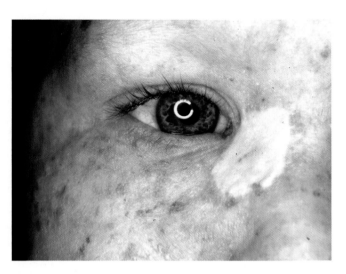

FIGURE 11 Young patient with xeroderma pigmentosum. Note freckling, atrophy, and formation of keratoses. The graft site denotes previous excision and repair of a squamous cell carcinoma.

DNA following ultraviolet irradiation (188). The responsible genes have been cloned for most of the complementation groups (189). The gene responsible for the XP variant has been determined to be the POLH gene, located on chromosome 6p21.1–6p12 (188). Aggressive prevention of ultraviolet injury is a significant part of the clinical management of these individuals (190).

Histopathology

The initial changes may be subtle and are often appreciated only in retrospect. However, there is hyperkeratosis, with irregularly distributed areas of epidermal atrophy and rete ridge elongation and variable degrees of basilar hypermelanosis (185, 191). Eventually, foci of basilar keratinocyte atypia can be identified, and the various types of tumors associated with the syndrome begin to appear (Fig. 12).

Specificity of Findings and Differential Diagnosis

The key to making a diagnosis of xeroderma pigmentosum is the recognition that tumors commonly associated with adults—especially squamous cell carcinomas and basal cell carcinomas—are appearing in childhood. When faced with that possibility, it would be important to confirm the age of the patient (misprints do occur on accession forms!). Facial tumors with a surprising lack or sparsity of solar elastosis might provide some corroborating evidence. For those individuals who develop mainly basal cell carcinomas, particularly in complementation groups C and E, basal cell nevus syndrome would have to be considered in the clinical differential diagnosis.

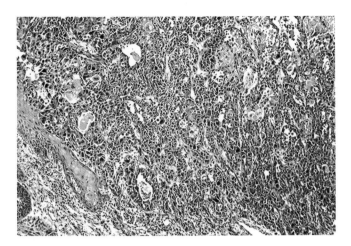

FIGURE 12 A moderately to poorly differentiated squamous cell carcinoma of the skin that arose in the patient shown in Figure 11.

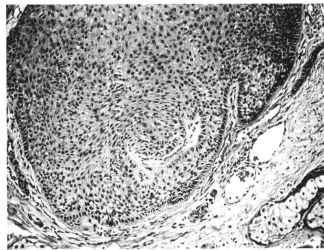

FIGURE 13 Trichilemmoma, one of the tumors commonly seen in Cowden's syndrome. Note the lobulation, exaggerated palisading of the basilar layer, and cuticular basement membrane zone.

Cowden's Syndrome (Multiple Hamartoma Syndrome)

Clinical Findings

Cowden's syndrome is an autosomal dominant disorder in which a variety of benign cutaneous and subcutaneous tumors are associated with carcinomas of the breast, thyroid gland, and other sites (192). Among the more common mucocutaneous lesions are trichilemmomas and tumors of the follicular infundibulum, particularly involving the facial region (193), oral fibromas, nonspecific keratoses of the dorsa of hands and wrists, and punctate keratoses of the palms. Other specific lesions that have been identified in Cowden's syndrome include inverted follicular keratoses (194), sclerotic fibromas of skin and oral mucosa (195), and a sclerotic lipoma (196). The syndrome has been linked to a mutation in a tumor suppressor gene known as PTEN on chromosome 10 (197). The Bannayan-Riley-Ruvalcaba syndrome, consisting of macrocephaly, lipomas, and delayed development, is associated with mutations of the same gene. It has been proposed that this may be the same disorder, but with a different expression and onset in childhood (198).

Histopathology

Trichilemmomas are lobulated epithelial tumors displaying outer root sheath differentiation. They feature clear cells, slightly exaggerated palisading of the basilar layer, and an underlying cuticular basement membrane zone (Fig. 13) (199). The surfaces of these tumors may be wart-like, but evidence for HPV infection in these lesions is lacking (200). The tumor of the follicular infundibulum consists of a subepidermal, plate-like epithelial structure often showing multiple connections to the overlying epidermis. Follicular units may merge with the lower surface of the plate-like epithelial growth, which itself may have some features resembling trichilemmoma (201). Inverted follicular keratoses resemble irritated seborrheic keratoses and include spongiosis as well as squamous eddy formation, but in contrast to that lesion, they have an endophytic growth pattern (194). The sclerotic fibroma consists of nodular aggregates of laminated homogeneous, eosinophilic collagen with a "wood grain" appearance, and low cellularity (Fig. 14) (202). The sclerotic lipoma is a subcutaneous tumor featuring adipocytes within a fibrosclerotic matrix (196, 203).

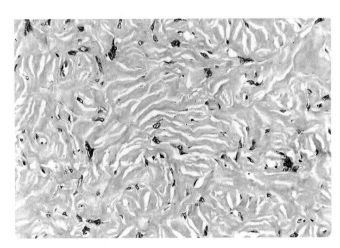

FIGURE 14 Detail of a sclerotic fibroma, showing the "wood grain" appearance of dermal collagen.

Although characteristic of Cowden's syndrome, none of the above-mentioned tumors, in isolation, would be specific for that diagnosis. The pathologist is most likely to contribute to recognition of the syndrome through the realization that multiple such tumors exist. This may happen because an astute clinician recognizes that there are multiple similar cutaneous lesions, or because the pathologist has diagnosed multiple trichilemmomas, sclerotic fibromas, and so on, in the same individual or his/her relatives.

Gardner's Syndrome

Clinical Findings

Gardner's syndrome is an autosomal dominant disorder characterized by colonic and rectal polyps, in association with epidermal cysts, desmoid tumors, fibromas, and other noncutaneous anomalies that include osteomatosis, dental abnormalities, and congenital hypertrophy of retinal pigment epithelium (204, 205).

The gastrointestinal polyps are adenomatous, and carcinomas develop in 50% of patients (206). Gastric, duodenal, and small intestinal polyps may also develop. The epidermal cysts may be large and disfiguring and are often located on the face. Abdominal and extra-abdominal desmoid tumors are seen, as is the lesion termed *nuchal fibroma*, which typically presents as an area of induration on the posterior neck. However, in Gardner's syndrome, these may be multiple and found in other areas such as the back, face, scalp, and chest wall (207).

Gardner's syndrome and familial polyposis of the colon result from mutations in the adenomatosis-polyposis gene (APC gene), a tumor suppressor gene located on chromosome 5q21 (208).

Histopathology

The epidermal cysts of Gardner's syndrome may be unique, because they sometimes show pilomatrixoma-like changes. These consist of portions of cyst wall–containing basaloid cells that show intraluminal transition to eosinophilic "shadow" cells with loss of nuclei—evidence for primitive hair matrix differentiation (Fig. 15) (209, 210). Fibromas of the nuchal fibroma type display thick collagen bundles that are continuous with the lower dermis and largely replace the subcutaneous adipose tissue (211). These lesions are typically paucicellular, but the cells that are present often express CD34 (212).

Specificity of Findings and Differential Diagnosis

Since both the nuchal-type fibromas and the cysts with pilomatrical changes can occur in childhood, these may represent sentinel signs of Gardner's syndrome, and

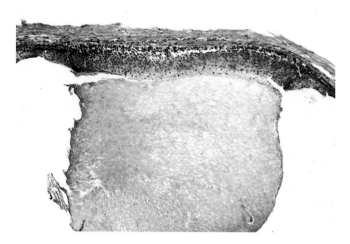

FIGURE 15 A portion of the wall of an epidermal cyst from a patient with Gardner's syndrome. Projecting into the lumen is a column of shadow cells, underlain by a band of basaloid cells. This represents evidence for primitive hair matrix differentiation as seen in pilomatrixoma.

therefore their recognition may trigger an investigation for intestinal polyposis at an early stage. A provisional diagnosis of Gardner's syndrome (later proven to be correct) has also been made on the basis of finding a large epidermal cyst and desmoid tumor in a particular patient.

Peutz-Jeghers Syndrome

Clinical Findings

Peutz-Jeghers syndrome is a well-recognized, autosomal dominant disorder combining periorificial and acral pigmented macules with gastrointestinal polyposis, melena, and intussusception. There does not appear to be as high an incidence of gastrointestinal cancer as is the case in Gardner's syndrome, in part because the polyps are largely hamartomatous rather than adenomatous. However, malignancies are well documented, especially above the ligament of Treitz and in the colon (213, 214). In addition, cancers of other sites have been reported, including the breast, lung, kidney, uterus, and cervix (214).

The pigmented macules are present at birth or during childhood and are located over the vermilion borders of the lips (Fig. 16), oral mucosa, perianal area, and the fingers and toes (215). Pigmented streaks are also found on the nails (216). These features can be quite similar to those of a sporadic or familial condition known as the Laugier-Hunziker syndrome, though pigmentation in the latter begins after puberty, and the systemic abnormalities associated with Peutz-Jeghers syndrome are not observed (217, 218). In Peutz-Jeghers syndrome, the pigmented macules on the face fade with age.

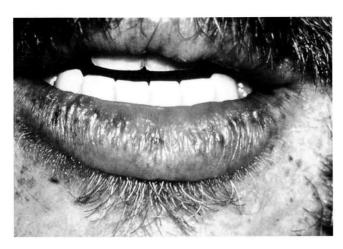

FIGURE 16 Pigmented macules of the lips in a patient with Peutz-Jeghers syndrome.

In many, but not all, cases of Peutz-Jeghers syndrome, there is aberrant expression of the tumor suppressor gene STK11 located on chromosome 19 (219).

Histopathology

The skin and mucosal lesions show basilar hypermelanosis, though there is controversy over the issue of whether or not melanocytes are increased per unit area (220, 221). There may also be regional variations in pigment transfer from melanocytes to keratinocytes as discerned ultrastructurally (220).

Specificity of Findings and Differential Diagnosis

It is doubtful that the pathologist would be in a position to diagnose, or even to suggest the diagnosis of, Peutz-Jeghers syndrome based upon biopsy findings alone, but certainly the microscopic findings could provide corroborative evidence when interpreted in the light of the clinical findings. Not only could the lesions microscopically resemble those of Laugier-Hunziker syndrome, and probably those of Cronkhite-Canada or multiple lentigines syndromes, but they would also have features similar to isolated lentigines or labial melanotic macules, sporadic lesions also characterized by basilar hypermelanosis.

Muir-Torre Syndrome

Clinical Findings

The Muir-Torre syndrome was first recognized in the late 1960s. It is an autosomal dominant disorder in which sebaceous tumors are associated with carcinomas, particularly of the gastrointestinal and genitourinary tracts (222, 223). The visceral tumors may show a surprisingly indolent clinical course (224, 225). Recognition of the cutaneous lesions can either precede or follow the first manifestations of internal malignancy.

The sebaceous tumors are most often classified as sebaceous adenomas or sebaceomas, but also seen are basal cell carcinomas with sebaceous differentiation, sebaceous carcinomas, and sebaceous tumors that are difficult to categorize (226). Keratoacanthomas have also been reported in the syndrome (227). Microsatellite instability is detected in the cutaneous tumors, resulting from inactivating mutations of DNA mismatch repair genes (228).

Histopathology

The microscopic features of the sebaceous tumors often closely resemble those of their sporadic counterparts. Thus, the sebaceous adenomas show circumscribed lobules of sebaceous cells with a greater proportion of basaloid, germinative cells than would be encountered in normal sebaceous glands (Fig. 17) (229). The sebaceoma features islands of predominantly basaloid cells with randomly scattered sebaceous cells (230). Sebaceous carcinomas show dermal infiltration by atypical basaloid or squamoid cells, some of which exhibit the vacuolated cytoplasm of sebaceous cells (229). Yet, a number of these tumors are difficult to classify, and may show cystic foci, solid sheets of basaloid cells, or other changes (231). The "keratoacanthomas" associated with the syndrome are not quite typical either, and may contain sebaceous elements not observed in sporadic keratoacanthoma (231). In tumors where the sebaceous aspect is difficult to discern, staining for epithelial membrane antigen or

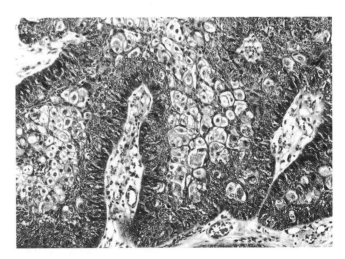

FIGURE 17 Microscopic features of sebaceous adenoma, a lesion frequently encountered in Muir-Torre syndrome. Note the prominence of the basaloid, germinative cells.

androgen receptor may be helpful (232). Lipid stains are worthwhile only when the diagnosis is anticipated and/or frozen sections are available.

The presence of a mutation in one of the mismatch repair genes, a fundamental feature of Muri-Torre syndrome, can be exploited immunohistochemically. Stains for MLH1, MSH2, or MSH6 are most often employed for this purpose. Lack of expression of one of these antigens, with appropriate controls, can confirm the presence of a mutation and closely correlates with microsatellite instability (233–235).

Specificity of Findings and Differential Diagnosis

It has been suggested that the finding of one sebaceous adenoma should raise concerns regarding the Muir-Torre syndrome. Certainly the entire spectrum of established sebaceous tumors can occur sporadically, with no apparent association with visceral malignancy. However, pathologists can clearly play an important role in the early recognition of this syndrome, either through the realization that there have been multiple such tumors in a patient, or through recognition of sebaceous tumors with unusual configurations (e.g., cystic or solid basaloid forms) (236). When suspicions have been raised, staining for expression of mismatch repair genes can confirm the diagnosis of Muir-Torre syndrome and initiate cancer surveillance.

■ PARANEOPLASTIC SYNDROMES WITH GENERALLY NONDIAGNOSTIC SKIN FINDINGS

AIDS

AIDS has been associated with a variety of cutaneous manifestations, including infectious diseases (molluscum contagiosum, lesions induced by human papillomavirus, mycobacterial infection, candidosis, scabies), neoplasms (with infection, in the case of Kaposi's sarcoma), and inflammatory dermatoses (exacerbations of psoriasis and seborrheic dermatitis, and eosinophilic folliculitis). It has also been linked to a number of malignancies. Some of these are termed "AIDS-defining" malignancies, and include Kaposi's sarcoma, non-Hodgkin's lymphoma, and cervical cancer (237). The lymphomas include diffuse large B-cell lymphoma, Burkitt's lymphoma (238), and two conditions that are relatively specific for HIV infection: primary effusion lymphoma and plasmablastic lymphoma of the oral cavity (239). Tumors that are not considered "AIDS-defining" but are significantly related to HIV infection include Hodgkin's disease, carcinomas of the lung and anus, nonmelanocytic skin cancers, and testicular germ cell tumors (237). As survivals have improved with antiretroviral therapy, there may be an increasing incidence of these non-AIDS-defining cancers (240). Through the detection of opportunistic infections, Kaposi's sarcoma, or severe dermatoses in previously healthy individuals, the pathologist may suggest the possibility of virally mediated immunosuppression, leading to early diagnosis and therapy of HIV-infected individuals and close surveillance for the possible development of malignancy.

Amyloidosis

It is well known that multiple myeloma can be associated with amyloid deposits in the skin. These present as waxy papules and plaques, particularly in the periorbital areas, but they also appear on other parts of the face, scalp, and neck. Hemorrhage occurs with minor trauma, a finding often referred to as pinch purpura. On biopsy, deposits of eosinophilic, amorphous, fissured material are seen within the dermis and subcutis, often surrounding vessels or adipocytes ("amyloid rings"). Subcutaneous deposits can be found in apparently uninvolved abdominal skin, with a high yield of positive results among those with systemic amyloidosis (241). The amyloid material stains positively with Congo red (with the characteristic apple-green birefringence under polarized light), stains metachromatically with crystal violet, and shows greenish fluorescence with thioflavin T. In contrast to secondary amyloidosis, the amyloid of primary amyloidosis retains its affinity for Congo red despite pretreatment of sections with potassium permanganate (242). The amyloid can be shown to be light chain derived. The finding of amyloid deposits in skin with these characteristics should raise the possibility of primary systemic amyloidosis and/or multiple myeloma. One possible confounding problem might be created by the lesions of nodular amyloidosis confined to skin; these also contain light chain–derived amyloid, and monoclonality of the associated plasma cells has been reported (243, 244). The other primary cutaneous amyloid deposits, manifesting as macular amyloidosis and lichen amyloidosus, are keratin derived.

Cryoglobulinemia

Cryoglobulinemia, particularly the monoclonal or type 1 variant, is associated chiefly with multiple myeloma, but it also occurs with macroglobulinemia of Waldenström and chronic lymphocytic leukemia (245). An essential form also exists. Cutaneous lesions include purpura, ulcerations, and livedo reticularis; a case of generalized livedo reticularis has recently been reported (246). Type 2, or mixed cryoglobulinemia, contains a monoclonal component with antibody activity against polyclonal IgG (247). Type 3 cryoglobulins are comprised of mixed polyclonal immunoglobulins that may be combined with nonimmunoglobulin molecules (247). Mixed cryoglobulinemia is most often associated with autoimmune and viral diseases, but type 2 cryoglobulins are sometimes identified in patients with macroglobulinemia of Waldenström. Palpable purpura, polyarthralgia, and glomerulonephritis have been associated with the mixed form of the disease (248). On biopsy, monoclonal cryoglobulinemia shows deposits of amorphous, eosinophilic material within dermal vessels, while mixed cryoglobulinemia shows changes of leukocytoclastic vasculitis (249). Combinations of intravascular deposits and vasculitic changes have been observed in some examples of cryoglobulinemia, but have also been seen in vasculitis due to infection: specifically, gonococcemia. Rarely, crystal formation can occur within small vessels. This phenomenon, called cryocrystalglobulinemia, has a strong association with myeloma or monoclonal gammopathy.

There are numerous possible causes of cutaneous vasculitis and/or thrombosis, and cryoglobulinemia is not the most common among these. Nevertheless, this disorder should always be considered within the differential diagnosis, leading in some cases to appropriate laboratory studies and (particularly in the case of monoclonal cryoglobulinemia) to a consideration of monoclonal gammopathy.

Erythema Multiforme

Although malignancy has rarely been linked to erythema multiforme (250), there are few well-documented cases, and it may well be that past examples of this association actually represented paraneoplastic pemphigus, which is now known to have considerable clinical and histopathologic resemblances to erythema multiforme. Histopathologic changes have been reported resembling erythema multiforme in patients with underlying lymphoma (among other disease associations), but these patients presented clinically with exfoliative dermatitis; their skin disease might better be categorized as exfoliative lichenoid dermatitis (251). Erythema multiforme has also developed secondary to radiation therapy for malignancy (252, 253).

Exfoliative Dermatitis

Exfoliative dermatitis, or erythroderma, has been reported in association with lymphomas, leukemias, and Hodgkin's disease (Fig. 18) (254). However, the best-documented association with malignancy is seen in cutaneous T-cell lymphoma, where erythroderma is an integral part of the Sézary syndrome (255). In fact, it has been argued that cases of erythroderma that had been linked to chronic lymphocytic leukemia were most likely examples of the Sézary syndrome (256). However, there are well-documented associations with Hodgkin's disease and even

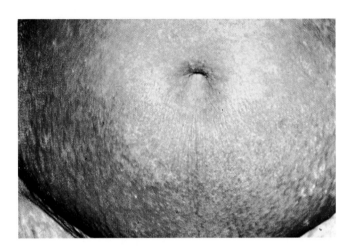

FIGURE 18 Exfoliative dermatitis (erythroderma) with involvement of the abdominal region. This condition can accompany malignancy, but can also be associated with drug reaction or a preexisting dermatosis, such as psoriasis or contact dermatitis.

(rarely) with solid tumors, including carcinomas of the stomach, liver, prostate, lung, thyroid, and gall bladder (254, 257). Exfoliative dermatitis can precede, follow, or present at the same time as the underlying malignancy. In some cases, removal of a solid tumor has resulted in clearing of the dermatitis (257).

But exfoliative dermatitis develops even more commonly in patients who do not have malignancies. In fact, it is most often associated with drug reaction or a preexisting dermatosis, such as psoriasis, contact dermatitis, or stasis dermatitis, and a number of cases are idiopathic (258, 259). Lymphadenopathy commonly accompanies exfoliative dermatitis and is not necessarily an indicator of underlying malignancy. Microscopically, there are usually parakeratosis, acanthosis with mild spongiosis, vasodilatation, and a chronic inflammatory infiltrate—findings that are suggestive of exfoliative dermatitis but are otherwise nonspecific (Fig. 19). Occasionally, a lichenoid tissue reaction pattern can be identified (251). Atypical lymphocytes and/or Pautrier microabscesses would provide a clue to the diagnosis of Sézary syndrome, or occasionally the changes may be sufficiently specific to suggest an underlying dermatosis such as psoriasis. Certainly, the development of a persistent exfoliative dermatitis, in the absence of a clear explanation, should prompt investigations into the possibility of an underlying malignancy, particularly Sézary syndrome.

Herpes Zoster

Herpes zoster infection appears to have an association with malignancy, particularly Hodgkin's disease, non-Hodgkin's lymphoma, and chronic lymphocytic leukemia,

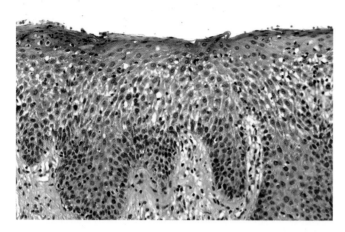

FIGURE 19 Histopathologic features in a case of exfoliative dermatitis. Note the focal lack of stratum corneum, spongiosis, and acanthosis. These changes would be considered nonspecific; they could accompany malignancy, but might also be encountered in cases that are idiopathic or the result of an underlying eczematous dermatitis.

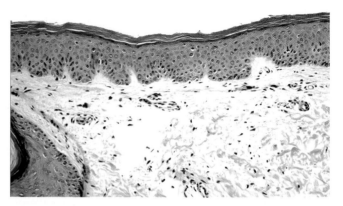

FIGURE 20 Microscopic findings in a case of acquired ichthyosis. Note the compact orthokeratosis and markedly attenuated granular cell layer.

in addition to carcinoma of the breast subjected to radiation therapy. A recent retrospective study from Malaysia has shown an incidence of 5% among children with malignancy, particularly leukemia (260). However, a number of studies have failed to demonstrate that herpes zoster is a marker for occult malignancy (261–263). Disseminated zoster does accompany malignancy and may be explained in part by immunosuppression, including reduction in circulating antibody levels against the varicella-zoster virus (264).

Ichthyosis

Acquired ichthyosis in adults is frequently associated with malignancy. The malignant process is most often a lymphoma, Hodgkin's disease being more common than non-Hodgkin's lymphomas (265). It has also been reported in association with lymphomatoid papulosis (266), multiple myeloma (267), and uncommonly with solid tumors such as carcinoma of breast and lung (268). Ichthyosis in this setting usually arises in patients with established malignant disease, although it may occasionally be the initial manifestation. However, there are other causes of acquired ichthyosis, including malnutrition, hypothyroidism, sarcoidosis, and drugs such as nicotinic acid and clofazimine.

Microscopically, skin biopsies show compact orthokeratosis, a lack of spongiosis unless secondary eczematization has occurred, and minimal dermal inflammation. The granular cell layer is often attenuated or absent, mimicking the image of the genodermatosis, ichthyosis vulgaris (Fig. 20). Some cases of ichthyosis associated with myeloma have also presented with follicular keratotic

spicules; biopsy of such lesions has demonstrated intercellular deposition of cryoproteins (267). Certainly, ichthyosiform biopsy changes in adults, in the absence of a long-term or familial history, should raise the possibility of underlying malignancy, though as noted above, there are other possible explanations for this finding.

Insect Bite-Like Reactions in Hematologic Malignancies

The development of lesions resembling arthropod bites, though without the typical history or clinical course of true arthropod bites, has been reported in patients with leukemias and lymphomas. Best known as an accompaniment of chronic lymphocytic leukemia, these reactions have also been seen in acute lymphoblastic leukemia, acute monocytic leukemia, large cell lymphoma, myelofibrosis (269), and mantle cell lymphoma (269–271). These lesions most often arise in patients with established malignancy, but they can precede the diagnosis of lymphoma/leukemia by several years, and on occasion, their development has even led to the diagnosis of malignancy (270). Microscopically, there are varying degrees of spongiosis, sometimes with intraepidermal vesicle formation, along with papillary dermal edema and a perivascular, periadnexal, and interstitial dermal infiltrate containing mononucleated cells and eosinophils (Fig. 21) (271). The infiltrating lymphocytes predominantly mark as T cells, and clonality has only rarely been detected in the lesions (269). In one case, dapsone was employed in the clinical management of the skin lesions (272). Although the microscopic findings alone would not generally elicit a suspicion of underlying malignancy, lesions of long duration without a supportive history of arthropod injury may raise the possibility of a hematologic neoplasm.

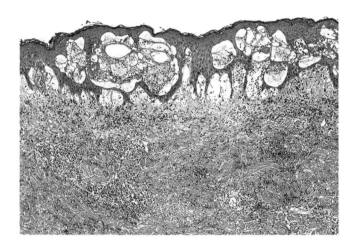

FIGURE 21 Insect bite-like reaction in a patient with chronic lymphocytic leukemia. There is marked spongiosis with intraepidermal vesiculation, and a dermal inflammatory infiltrate containing eosinophils.

Tylosis

Tylosis, or *keratosis palmaris et plantaris*, can occur in a wide variety of genetic disorders. It can also arise as an acquired disease in a number of ways, e.g., following arsenic exposure, as keratoderma climactericum, or as an accompaniment of other dermatoses such as pityriasis rubra pilaris. Clinically the hyperkeratosis can be diffuse, focal or nummular, or punctate (Fig. 22). Acquired tylosis can also be associated with internal malignancies of varying types, ranging from lymphoma (273) to bronchogenic carcinoma (274). In fact, tripe palms may be regarded as a variant of palmar keratoderma.

Tylosis has also been associated with gastrointestinal carcinoma as part of a familial syndrome. The best known is the Howel-Evans syndrome, associating tylosis with the development of esophageal carcinoma (275). The genetic locus for tylosis with esophageal cancer has been mapped to a 500 kb region on chromosome 17q25, though work continues on identification of the precise locus of the responsible gene (276–278). In 1984, Bennion and Patterson reported on a family with punctate keratoderma of palms and soles and carcinomas of the colon and pancreas (279). Microscopically, forms of keratoderma show orthokeratosis, variable parakeratosis, hypergranulosis, and acanthosis. In punctate variants, a degree of keratin plugging can also be observed (280). Underlying malignancy should be included in the differential diagnosis of conditions associated with acquired keratoderma of palms and soles, though it is not the most common. Although Howel-Evans keratoderma begins in childhood, it tends to be later in onset than is the case for benign hereditary keratoderma.

■ SELECTED GENETIC SYNDROMES WITH GENERALLY NONDIAGNOSTIC SKIN FINDINGS

Common Variable Immunodeficiency

Common variable immunodeficiency (CVID) can demonstrate both autosomal dominant and autosomal recessive inheritance. It is characterized by late onset (defined as occurring after 24 months of age, but in reality often beginning in young adult life) of deficient humoral immune function. This manifests as susceptibility to infections and reduced responses to polysaccharide vaccines. Most infections are sinopulmonary, but there are also gastrointestinal symptoms such as bloating, diarrhea, and malabsorption, and autoimmune phenomena including disorders resembling rheumatoid arthritis or lupus erythematosus (281–283). These patients are also at risk for developing malignancy, particularly non-Hodgkin's lymphoma, though Hodgkin's disease and solid tumors have also been reported. Low serum levels of IgG and other immunoglobulins can be demonstrated. Testing is available for the TACI and ICOS genes, found in a minority of individuals with the syndrome. Tumor necrosis factor-α is elevated in these patients, and its inhibition may be helpful in ameliorating the disease (284).

The most frequently reported cutaneous lesions associated with CVID are granulomas, which are described as sarcoidal or caseating in appearance (285–287), with

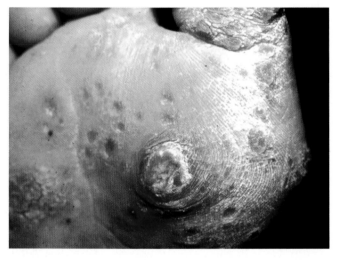

FIGURE 22 Tylosis (*keratosis palmaris et plantaris*), punctate type. In this case, there was a family history of both gastrointestinal carcinoma and tylosis.

some exceptions (288). Alopecia universalis is regarded as one of the autoimmune phenomena that can occur in this disorder. Other reported conditions include lesions of epidermodysplasia verruciformis (289), pityriasis lichenoides (290), and myofibroblastic tumors (291). It is unlikely that the disorder would first be discovered by diagnosing one of these cutaneous lesions, but certainly such findings, in the context of recurrent sinopulmonary infections, would lend support to a diagnosis of CVID.

Wiskott-Aldrich Syndrome

This is an X-linked recessively inherited disorder consisting of a widespread eczematous dermatitis, thrombocytopenia, and a propensity for recurrent viral, bacterial, and fungal infections. Serum IgM levels are low and there may be elevated levels of IgA and IgE. About 12% of patients develop malignancy, primarily immunoblastic large cell lymphomas, although Hodgkin's disease and leukemias have also been reported (292). The genetic defect is located on Xp11.22–23 and affects a protein termed the Wiskott-Aldrich syndrome protein (WASp) (293). This protein may act as a bridge between signaling and movement of actin filaments in the cytoskeleton, affecting a variety of cellular functions in cells of hematopoietic lineage. The microscopic features of the eczematous dermatitis are spongiotic in nature, closely resembling those of atopic dermatitis, and in the absence of other data, they would not be regarded as being diagnostic of the syndrome.

■ SPECIFIC DERMATOSES SOMETIMES ASSOCIATED WITH MALIGNANCY

Bullous Pemphigoid

Pemphigoid is a blistering eruption that occurs typically, but not exclusively (294), in elderly adults. It is characterized by tense bullae arising on erythematous or normal skin, particularly over the trunk, intertriginous areas, and flexural surfaces (Fig. 23). Urticarial lesions also occur and may precede the development of bullae. Autoantibodies develop to components of the epidermal basement membrane zone, particularly to 230 and 180 kd antigens. Microscopically, the characteristic finding is that of a subepidermal blister with a dermal infiltrate that often contains numerous eosinophils (Fig. 24), though inflammatory infiltrates can also be sparse to virtually absent. Direct immunofluorescence shows linear deposits of IgG and C3 along the dermal–epidermal junction.

Malignancies of a variety of types have been reported among patients with pemphigoid, including lymphomas (295) and solid tumors (296, 297). This has raised the

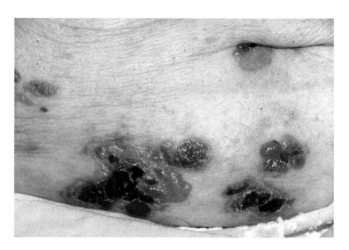

FIGURE 23 Clinical features in a case of bullous pemphigoid.

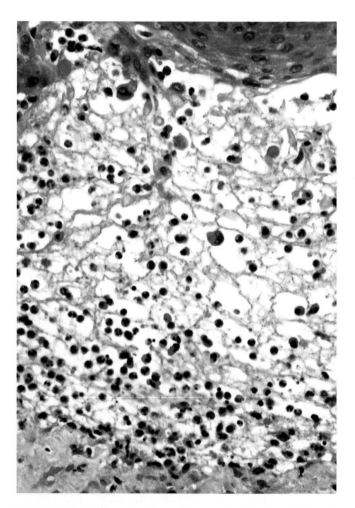

FIGURE 24 Medium power magnification of a subepidermal blister in a case of bullous pemphigoid. The base of the epidermis can be seen at the top of this photomicrograph. Numerous eosinophils are identified in the blister cavity.

question of whether the disorder might be a paraneoplastic phenomenon. Interest in this possible association increased when it was recognized in some studies that the incidence of malignancy in pemphigoid seemed to be increased among those with negative serology (negative indirect immunofluorescent studies) (298, 299). However, a study by Ahmed and Amerian failed to confirm this association (300), and other studies have not shown an increased incidence of internal malignancy in pemphigoid patients when compared to the general population matched for age and sex (301). It seems likely that the reported associations with tumors may simply reflect the advanced age of many of the patients with pemphigoid. Based upon the evidence to date, the diagnosis of pemphigoid, by itself, should not prompt an extensive search for malignant neoplasms.

Herpes Gestationis

Now more commonly termed *pemphigoid gestationis* in view of its close relationship to bullous pemphigoid, this is a vesiculobullous dermatosis associated with pregnancy. It typically begins in the second or third trimester as urticarial plaques with the evolution of blisters over the trunk and extremities (Fig. 25). Although it usually subsides shortly after delivery, it can sometimes persist for months or years (302). An IgG_1 circulating antibody is directed against a 180 kd antigen shared by placental matrix and the epidermal basement membrane zone (303). Microscopic findings include pronounced papillary dermal edema, subepidermal separation, and an infiltrate containing eosinophils (Fig. 26). Direct immunofluorescence studies show linear C3 and, sometimes, IgG deposition along the dermal–epidermal junction.

An association between herpes gestationis and choriocarcinoma, though rare, has been reported on a number of occasions (304–307). While a diagnosis of herpes gestationis should not automatically generate a search for this malignancy, other clinical findings may raise the possibility. This is underscored by a recent case of a biopsy received from a young woman with the microscopic and immunofluorescent characteristics of pemphigoid. Her young age led us to suggest the possibility of herpes gestationis, despite the initial history that she was not pregnant. Further inquiry disclosed that she had recently experienced an aborted pregnancy, and a subsequent workup demonstrated the presence of a choriocarcinoma; the tumor was treated successfully.

Dermatitis Herpetiformis

Dermatitis herpetiformis is a blistering dermatosis that presents as extremely pruritic, grouped vesicles over extensor surfaces (Fig. 27). It has a strong association with gluten-sensitive enteropathy. IgA antibodies, perhaps formed in the gut, are believed to bind to microfibrillar bundles in the papillary dermis, resulting in complement activation and attraction of neutrophils (308, 309). The characteristic microscopic changes are neutrophilic microabscesses in the dermal papillae with subepidermal clefting (Fig. 28). On direct immunofluorescence, granular IgA deposition is identified in the dermal papillae.

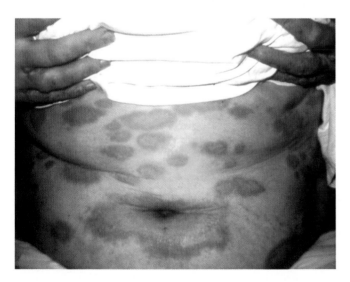

FIGURE 25 Herpes gestationis. Urticarial plaques with early blister formation are present on the trunk.

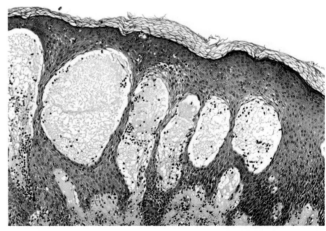

FIGURE 26 Microscopic image of herpes gestationis. Note the marked papillary dermal edema, sufficient to produce subepidermal separation.

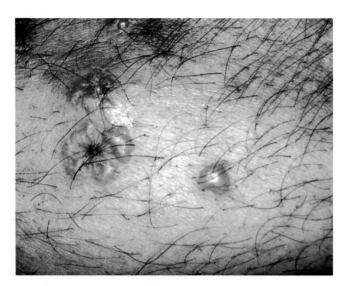

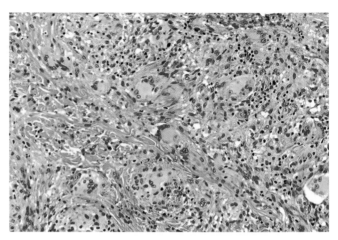

FIGURE 29 In multicentric reticulohistiocytosis, there are mono- and multinucleated cells with ground glass cytoplasm and nuclei with distinct chromatin rims and prominent nucleoli.

FIGURE 27 Dermatitis herpetiformis. Grouped blisters with erythema are present on an extensor surface.

Malignancy has been reported in dermatitis herpetiformis, the most significant type being enteropathy-associated non-Hodgkin's lymphoma, as also seen in patients with celiac disease who do not have dermatitis herpetiformis (310, 311). Recent population studies seem to indicate, at most, only a slightly increased cancer risk among patients with dermatitis herpetiformis and an actual decrease in mortality (312, 313). There is good evidence for a protective role for gluten-free diet (310, 311, 314, 315). For this disease, the surgical pathologist's role is mainly one of establishing or substantiating the diagnosis of dermatitis herpetiformis; this in turn sets up the appropriate treatment and long-term clinical surveillance for possible complications, including lymphoma.

Multicentric Reticulohistiocytosis

This uncommon histiocytic proliferative disorder is associated with a widespread papulonodular eruption and a severe arthritis, involving particularly the interphalangeal joints of the hands. Microscopically, the cutaneous lesions show a dermal infiltrate of mono- and multi-nucleated cells with eosinophilic "ground glass" cytoplasm and nuclei with distinct chromatin rims and prominent nucleoli (Fig. 29). These cells express macrophagic markers such as CD68 and HAM-56, and are sometimes factor XIIIa positive (316). Spontaneous regression may occur after a period of years, though residual damage to joints may persist.

Malignancies have been reported in up to 25% to 30% of cases. There have been a variety of types, including mesothelioma (317), carcinoma of the breast (318), and papillary serous carcinoma of the endometrium (319). However, multicentric reticulohistiocytosis has not been established as a paraneoplastic disorder (319), probably, at least in part, due to a selection bias introduced by those cases that appear in the literature.

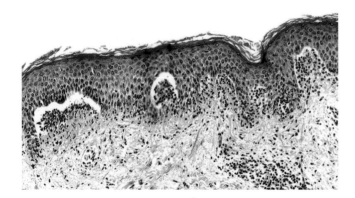

FIGURE 28 Classic (but not entirely pathognomonic) microscopic changes of dermatitis herpetiformis: papillary neutrophilic microabscesses with formation of subepidermal clefts.

■ REFERENCES

1. *Dorland's Illustrated Medical Dictionary*. 27th ed. Philadelphia: W.B. Saunders, 1988.
2. Vandersteen PR, Scheithauer BW. Glucagonoma syndrome. A clinicopathologic, immunocytochemical, and ultrastructural study. *J Am Acad Dermatol* 1985; 12(6):1032–9.
3. Leichter SB. Clinical and metabolic aspects of glucagonoma. *Medicine (Baltimore)* 1980; 59(2):100–13.
4. Marko PB, Miljkovic J, Zemljic TG. Necrolytic migratory erythema associated with hyperglucagonemia and neuroendocrine

hepatic tumors. *Acta Dermatovenerol Alp Panonica Adriat* 2005; 14(4):161–164, 166.

5. Technau K, Renkl A, Norgauer J, Ziemer M. Necrolytic migratory erythema with myelodysplastic syndrome without glucagonoma. *Eur J Dermatol* 2005; 15(2):110–2.

6. Tierney EP, Badger J. Etiology and pathogenesis of necrolytic migratory erythema: review of the literature. *MedGenMed* 2004; 6(3):4.

7. Peterson LL, Shaw JC, Acott KM, Mueggler PA, Parker F. Glucagonoma syndrome: in vitro evidence that glucagon increases epidermal arachidonic acid. *J Am Acad Dermatol* 1984; 11(3): 468–73.

8. Franchimont C, Pierard GE, Luyckx AS, Gerard J, Lapiere CM. Angioplastic necrolytic migratory erythema. Unique association of necrolytic migratory erythema, extensive angioplasia, and high molecular weight glucagon-like polypeptide. *Am J Dermatopathol* 1982; 4(6):485–95.

9. Kheir SM, Omura EF, Grizzle WE, Herrera GA, Lee I. Histologic variation in the skin lesions of the glucagonoma syndrome. *Am J Surg Pathol* 1986; 10(7):445–53.

10. Hendricks WM. Pellagra and pellagralike dermatoses: etiology, differential diagnosis, dermatopathology, and treatment. *Semin Dermatol* 1991; 10(4):282–92.

11. Gonzalez JR, Botet MV, Sanchez JL. The histopathology of acrodermatitis enteropathica. *Am J Dermatopathol* 1982; 4(4): 303–11.

12. Nofal AA, Nofal E, Attwa E, El-Assar O, Assaf M. Necrolytic acral erythema: a variant of necrolytic migratory erythema or a distinct entity? *Int J Dermatol* 2005; 44(11):916–21.

13. Abdallah MA, Ghozzi MY, Monib HA, et al. Histological study of necrolytic acral erythema. *J Ark Med Soc* 2004; 100(10): 354–5.

14. Katz R, Fischmann AB, Galotto J, et al. Necrolytic migratory erythema, presenting as candidiasis, due to a pancreatic glucagonoma. *Cancer* 1979; 44(2):558–63.

15. Bazex A. Syndrome paraneoplastique a type d'hyperkeratose des extremites: guerison apres le traitement de l'epithelioma larynges. *Bull Soc Fr Dermatol Syph* 1965; 72:182.

16. Bazex A, Griffiths A. Acrokeratosis paraneoplastica—a new cutaneous marker of malignancy. *Br J Dermatol* 1980; 103(3):301–6.

17. Jacobsen FK, Abildtrup N, Laursen SO, Brandrup F, Jensen NK. Acrokeratosis paraneoplastica (Bazex's syndrome). *Arch Dermatol* 1984; 120(4):502–4.

18. Bolognia JL, Brewer YP, Cooper DL. Bazex syndrome (acrokeratosis paraneoplastica). An analytic review. *Medicine (Baltimore)* 1991; 70(4):269–80.

19. Akhyani M, Mansoori P, Taheri A, Asadi Kani Z. Acrokeratosis paraneoplastica (Bazex syndrome) associated with breast cancer. *Clin Exp Dermatol* 2004; 29(4):429–30.

20. Chave TA, Bamford WM, Harman KE. Acrokeratosis paraneoplastica associated with recurrent metastatic thymic carcinoma. *Clin Exp Dermatol* 2004; 29(4):430–2.

21. Sator PG, Breier F, Gschnait F. Acrokeratosis paraneoplastica (Bazex's syndrome): association with liposarcoma. *J Am Acad Dermatol* 2006; 55(6):1103–5.

22. Lucker GP, Steijlen PM. Acrokeratosis paraneoplastica (Bazex syndrome) occurring with acquired ichthyosis in Hodgkin's disease. *Br J Dermatol* 1995; 133(2):322–5.

23. Richard M, Giroux JM. Acrokeratosis paraneoplastica (Bazex' syndrome). *J Am Acad Dermatol* 1987; 16(1 Pt 2):178–83.

24. Braverman IM. Skin Signs of Systemic Disease. Philadelphia: W. B. Saunders, 1998:35.

25. Ofuji S, Furukawa F, Miyachi Y, Ohno S. Papuloerythroderma. *Dermatologica* 1984; 169(2):125–30.

26. Wakeel RA, Keefe M, Chapman RS. Papuloerythroderma. Another case of a new disease. *Arch Dermatol* 1991; 127(1): 96–8.

27. Tay YK, Tan KC, Ong BH. Papuloerythroderma of Ofuji and cutaneous T-cell lymphoma. *Br J Dermatol* 1997; 137(1):160–1.

28. Shah M, Reid WA, Layton AM. Cutaneous T-cell lymphoma presenting as papuloerythroderma—a case and review of the literature. *Clin Exp Dermatol* 1995; 20(2):161–3.

29. Suh KS, Kim HC, Chae YS, Kim ST. Ofuji papuloerythroderma associated with follicular mucinosis in mycosis fungoides. *J Dermatol* 1998; 25(3):185–9.

30. Bech-Thomsen N, Thomsen K. Ofuji's papuloerythroderma: a study of 17 cases. *Clin Exp Dermatol* 1998; 23(2):79–83.

31. Hur J, Seong JY, Choi TS, et al. Mycosis fungoides presenting as Ofuji's papuloerythroderma. *J Eur Acad Dermatol Venereol* 2002; 16(4):393–6.

32. Pereiro M Jr, Sanchez-Aguilar D, Pereiro Ferreiros MM, Amrouni B, Toribio J. Cutaneous T-cell lymphoma: an expression of papuloerythroderma of Ofuji. *J Eur Acad Dermatol Venereol* 2003; 17(2):240–1.

33. Martinez-Barranca ML, Munoz-Perez MA, Garcia-Morales I, Fernandez-Crehuet JL, Segura J, Camacho F. Ofuji papuloerythroderma evolving to cutaneous T-cell lymphoma. *J Eur Acad Dermatol Venereol* 2005; 19(1):104–6.

34. Dwyer CM, Chapman RS, Smith GD. Papuloerythroderma and cutaneous T cell lymphoma. *Dermatology* 1994; 188(4):326–8.

35. Grob JJ, Collet-Villette AM, Horchowski N, Dufaud M, Prin L, Bonerandi JJ. Ofuji papuloerythroderma. Report of a case with T cell skin lymphoma and discussion of the nature of this disease. *J Am Acad Dermatol* 1989; 20(5 Pt 2):927–31.

36. de Vries HJ, Koopmans AK, Starink TM, Mekkes JR. Ofuji papuloerythroderma associated with Hodgkin's lymphoma. *Br J Dermatol* 2002; 147(1):186–7.

37. Wong CL, Houghton JB, Andrew S, Griffiths CE. Papuloerythroderma of Ofuji associated with acute myeloid leukaemia. *Clin Exp Dermatol* 2003; 28(3):277–9.

38. Sunami K, Taniguchi H, Moriyama T, et al. Papuloerythroderma associated with gastric cancer; report of a case. *Nippon Shokakibyo Gakkai Zasshi* 1995; 92(9):1285–8.

39. Nazzari G, Crovato F, Nigro A. Papuloerythroderma (Ofuji): two additional cases and review of the literature. *J Am Acad Dermatol* 1992; 26(3 Pt 2):499–501.

40. Schepers C, Malvehy J, Azon-Masoliver A, Navarra E, Ferrando J, Mascaro JM. Papuloerythroderma of Ofuji: a report of 2 cases including the first European case associated with visceral carcinoma. *Dermatology* 1996; 193(2):131–5.

41. Nishijima S. Papuloerythroderma associated with hepatocellular carcinoma. *Br J Dermatol* 1998; 139(6):1115–6.

42. Lonnee ER, Toonstra J, van der Putte SC, van Weelden H, van Vloten WA. Papuloerythroderma of Ofuji in a HIV-infected patient. *Br J Dermatol* 1996; 135(3):500–1.

43. Azon-Masoliver A, Casado J, Brunet J, Martinez MA, del Castillo D. Ofuji's papuloerythroderma following choledocholithiasis with secondary sepsis: complete resolution with surgery. *Clin Exp Dermatol* 1998; 23(2):84–6.

44. Anhalt GJ, Kim SC, Stanley JR, et al. Paraneoplastic pemphigus. An autoimmune mucocutaneous disease associated with neoplasia. *N Engl J Med* 1990; 323(25):1729–35.

45. Camisa C, Helm TN, Liu YC, et al. Paraneoplastic pemphigus: a report of three cases including one long-term survivor. *J Am Acad Dermatol* 1992; 27(4):547–53.

46. Kaplan I, Hodak E, Ackerman L, Mimouni D, Anhalt GJ, Calderon S. Neoplasms associated with paraneoplastic pemphigus: a review with emphasis on non-hematologic malignancy

and oral mucosal manifestations. *Oral Oncol* 2004; 40(6): 553–62.

47. Ostezan LB, Fabre VC, Caughman SW, Swerlick RA, Korman NJ, Callen JP. Paraneoplastic pemphigus in the absence of a known neoplasm. *J Am Acad Dermatol* 1995; 33(2 Pt 1):312–5.

48. Lee MS, Kossard S, Ho KK, Barnetson RS, Ravich RB. Paraneoplastic pemphigus triggered by radiotherapy. *Australas J Dermatol* 1995; 36(4):206–10.

49. Fried R, Lynfield Y, Vitale P, Anhalt G. Paraneoplastic pemphigus appearing as bullous pemphigoid-like eruption after palliative radiation therapy. *J Am Acad Dermatol* 1993; 29(5 Pt 2): 815–7.

50. de Bruin A, Muller E, Wyder M, Anhalt GJ, Lemmens P, Suter MM. Periplakin and envoplakin are target antigens in canine and human paraneoplastic pemphigus. *J Am Acad Dermatol* 1999; 40 (5 Pt 1):682–5.

51. Oursler JR, Labib RS, Ariss-Abdo L, Burke T, O'Keefe EJ, Anhalt GJ. Human autoantibodies against desmoplakins in paraneoplastic pemphigus. *J Clin Invest* 1992; 89(6):1775–82.

52. Zhang B, Zheng R, Wang J, Bu D, Zhu X. Epitopes in the linker subdomain region of envoplakin recognized by autoantibodies in paraneoplastic pemphigus patients. *J Invest Dermatol* 2006; 126 (4):832–40.

53. Mehregan DR, Oursler JR, Leiferman KM, Muller SA, Anhalt GJ, Peters MS. Paraneoplastic pemphigus: a subset of patients with pemphigus and neoplasia. *J Cutan Pathol* 1993; 20(3):203–10.

54. Horn TD, Anhalt GJ. Histologic features of paraneoplastic pemphigus. *Arch Dermatol* 1992; 128(8):1091–5.

55. Bowen GM, Peters NT, Fivenson DP, et al. Lichenoid dermatitis in paraneoplastic pemphigus: a pathogenic trigger of epitope spreading? *Arch Dermatol* 2000; 136(5):652–6.

56. Hashimoto T, Amagai M, Watanabe K, et al. Characterization of paraneoplastic pemphigus autoantigens by immunoblot analysis. *J Invest Dermatol* 1995; 104(5):829–34.

57. Helou J, Allbritton J, Anhalt GJ. Accuracy of indirect immuno-fluorescence testing in the diagnosis of paraneoplastic pemphigus. *J Am Acad Dermatol* 1995; 32(3):441–7.

58. Joly P, Richard C, Gilbert D, et al. Sensitivity and specificity of clinical, histologic, and immunologic features in the diagnosis of paraneoplastic pemphigus. *J Am Acad Dermatol* 2000; 43(4): 619–26.

59. Schmid MH, Trueb RM. Juvenile amyopathic dermatomyositis. *Br J Dermatol* 1997; 136(3):431–3.

60. Callen JP, Wortmann RL. Dermatomyositis. *Clin Dermatol* 2006; 24(5):363–73.

61. Gerami P, Schope JM, McDonald L, Walling HW, Sontheimer RD. A systematic review of adult-onset clinically amyopathic dermatomyositis (dermatomyositis sine myositis): a missing link within the spectrum of the idiopathic inflammatory myopathies. *J Am Acad Dermatol* 2006; 54(4):597–613.

62. Callen JP. Relationship of cancer to inflammatory muscle diseases. Dermatomyositis, polymyositis, and inclusion body myositis. *Rheum Dis Clin North Am* 1994; 20(4):943–53.

63. Richardson JB, Callen JP. Dermatomyositis and malignancy. *Med Clin North Am* 1989; 73(5):1211–20.

64. Callen JP. The value of malignancy evaluation in patients with dermatomyositis. *J Am Acad Dermatol* 1982; 6(2):253–9.

65. Ichiki Y, Akiyama T, Shimozawa N, Suzuki Y, Kondo N, Kitajima Y. An extremely severe case of cutaneous calcinosis with juvenile dermatomyositis, and successful treatment with diltiazem. *Br J Dermatol* 2001; 144(4):894–7.

66. Janis JF, Winkelmann RK. Histopathology of the skin in dermatomyositis. A histopathologic study of 55 cases. *Arch Dermatol* 1968; 97(6):640–50.

67. McCollough ML, Cockerell CJ. Vesiculo-bullous dermatomyositis. *Am J Dermatopathol* 1998; 20(2):170–4.

68. Kubo M, Sato S, Kitahara H, Tsuchida T, Tamaki K. Vesicle formation in dermatomyositis associated with gynecologic malignancies. *J Am Acad Dermatol* 1996; 34(2 Pt 2):391–4.

69. Moschella SL. Plane xanthomatosis associated with myelomatosis. *Arch Dermatol* 1970; 101(6):683–7.

70. Wilkinson SM, Atkinson A, Neary RH, Smith AG. Normolipaemic plane xanthomas: an association with increased vascular permeability and serum lipoprotein(a) concentration. *Clin Exp Dermatol* 1992; 17(3):211–3.

71. Jones RR, Baughan AS, Cream JJ, Levantine A, Whicher JT. Complement abnormalities in diffuse plane xanthomatosis with paraproteinaemia. *Br J Dermatol* 1979; 101(6):711–6.

72. Derrick EK, Price ML. Plane xanthomatosis with chronic lymphatic leukaemia. *Clin Exp Dermatol* 1993; 18(3):259–60.

73. Broeshart JH, Prens EP, Habets WJ, de Bruijckere LM. Normolipemic plane xanthoma associated with adenocarcinoma and severe itch. *J Am Acad Dermatol* 2003; 49(1):119–22.

74. Nestle FO, Hofbauer G, Burg G. Necrobiotic xanthogranuloma with monoclonal gammopathy of the IgG lambda type. *Dermatology* 1999; 198(4):434–5.

75. Williford PM, White WL, Jorizzo JL, Greer K. The spectrum of normolipemic plane xanthoma. *Am J Dermatopathol* 1993; 15 (6):572–5.

76. Altman J, Winkelmann RK. Diffuse normolipemic plane xanthoma. Generalized xanthelasma. *Arch Dermatol* 1962; 85: 633–40.

77. Fleischmajer R, Hyman AB, Weidman AI. Normolipemic plane xanthomas. *Arch Dermatol* 1964; 89:319–23.

78. Gammel JA. Erythema gyratum repens; skin manifestations in patient with carcinoma of breast. *AMA Arch Derm Syphilol* 1952; 66(4):494–505.

79. Leavell UW Jr, Winternitz WW, Black JH. Erythema gyratum repens and undifferentiated carcinoma. *Arch Dermatol* 1967; 95 (1):69–72.

80. Caux F, Lebbe C, Thomine E, et al. Erythema gyratum repens. A case studied with immunofluorescence, immunoelectron microscopy and immunohistochemistry. *Br J Dermatol* 1994; 131(1): 102–7.

81. Loske KD, Ragunath M, Sunderkotter C, Metze D. Atypical erythema gyratum repens secondary to bronchogenic carcinoma. *J Dtsch Dermatol Ges* 2003; 1(3):216–8.

82. Skolnick M, Mainman ER. Erythema gyratum repens with metastatic adenocarcinoma. *Arch Dermatol* 1975; 111(2):227–9.

83. Shelley WB, Hurley HJ. An unusual autoimmune syndrome. Erythema annulare centrifugum, generalized pigmentation and breast hypertrophy. *Arch Dermatol* 1960; 81:889–97.

84. Barber PV, Doyle L, Vickers DM, Hubbard H. Erythema gyratum repens with pulmonary tuberculosis. *Br J Dermatol* 1978; 98(4): 465–8.

85. Garrett SJ, Roenigk HH Jr. Erythema gyratum repens in a healthy woman. *J Am Acad Dermatol* 1992; 26(1):121–2.

86. Holt PJ, Davies MG. Erythema gyratum repens—an immunologically mediated dermatosis? *Br J Dermatol* 1977; 96(4): 343–7.

87. Sweet RD. Acute febrile neutrophilic dermatosis—1978. *Br J Dermatol* 1979; 100(1):93–9.

88. Beitner H, Nakatani T, Hammar H. A case report of acute febril neutrophilic dermatosis (Sweet's syndrome) and Crohn's disease. *Acta Derm Venereol* 1991; 71(4):360–3.

89. Choi JW, Chung KY. Sweet's syndrome with systemic lupus erythematosus and herpes zoster. *Br J Dermatol* 1999; 140(6): 1174–5.

90. Choonhakarn C, Chetchotisakd P, Jirarattanapochai K, Mootsikapun P. Sweet's syndrome associated with non-tuberculous mycobacterial infection: a report of five cases. *Br J Dermatol* 1998; 139(1):107–10.

91. Tan E, Yosipovitch G, Giam YC, Tan SH. Bullous Sweet's syndrome associated with acute hepatitis B infection: a new association. *Br J Dermatol* 2000; 143(4):914–6.

92. Thibault MJ, Billick RC, Srolovitz H. Minocycline-induced Sweet's syndrome. *J Am Acad Dermatol* 1992; 27(5 Pt 2):801–4.

93. Johnson ML, Grimwood RE. Leukocyte colony-stimulating factors. A review of associated neutrophilic dermatoses and vasculitides. *Arch Dermatol* 1994; 130(1):77–81.

94. Satra K, Zalka A, Cohen PR, Grossman ME. Sweet's syndrome and pregnancy. *J Am Acad Dermatol* 1994; 30(2 Pt 2):297–300.

95. von den Driesch P. Sweet's syndrome (acute febrile neutrophilic dermatosis). *J Am Acad Dermatol* 1994; 31(4):535–56; quiz 557–60.

96. Salmon-Ehr V, Esteve E, Serpier H, Cambie MP, Pignon B, Kalis B. Acute febrile pustular and bullous neutrophilic dermatosis (Sweet syndrome) disclosing acute myeloblastic leukemia. *Rev Med Interne* 1995; 16(5):347–50.

97. Pirard C, Delannoy A. Sweet syndrome and acute myeloid leukemia. *Ann Dermatol Venereol* 1977; 104(2):160–1.

98. del Pozo J, Martinez W, Pazos JM, Yebra-Pimentel MT, Garcia Silva J, Fonseca E. Concurrent Sweet's syndrome and leukemia cutis in patients with myeloid disorders. *Int J Dermatol* 2005; 44 (8):677–80.

99. Al-Saad K, Khanani MF, Naqvi A, Krafchik B, Grant R, Pappo A. Sweet syndrome developing during treatment with all-trans retinoic acid in a child with acute myelogenous leukemia. *J Pediatr Hematol Oncol* 2004; 26(3):197–9.

100. Cohen PR, Kurzrock R. Chronic myelogenous leukemia and Sweet syndrome. *Am J Hematol* 1989; 32(2):134–7.

101. Rauh G, Gresser U, Meurer M, Dorfler H. Sweet syndrome in chronic myeloid leukemia. *Klin Wochenschr* 1989; 67(9):506–10.

102. Liu D, Seiter K, Mathews T, Madahar CJ, Ahmed T. Sweet's syndrome with CML cell infiltration of the skin in a patient with chronic-phase CML while taking Imatinib Mesylate. *Leuk Res* 2004; 28 (Suppl. 1):S61–3.

103. Ayirookuzhi SJ, Ma L, Ramshesh P, Mills G. Imatinib-induced sweet syndrome in a patient with chronic myeloid leukemia. *Arch Dermatol* 2005; 141(3):368–70.

104. Levy RM, Junkins-Hopkins JM, Turchi JJ, James WD. Sweet syndrome as the presenting symptom of relapsed hairy cell leukemia. *Arch Dermatol* 2002; 138(12):1551–4.

105. Choi HJ, Chang SE, Lee MW, Choi JH, Moon KC, Koh JK. A case of recurrent Sweet's syndrome in an 80-year-old man: a clue to an underlying malignancy. *Int J Dermatol* 2006; 45(4):457–9.

106. Krolikowski FJ, Reuter K, Shultis EW. Acute febrile neutrophilic dermatosis (Sweet's syndrome) associated with lymphoma. *Hum Pathol* 1985; 16(5):520–2.

107. Berth-Jones J, Hutchinson PE. Sweet's syndrome and malignancy: a case associated with multiple myeloma and review of the literature. *Br J Dermatol* 1989; 121(1):123–7.

108. Hussein K, Nanda A, Al-Sabah H, Alsaleh QA. Sweet's syndrome (acute febrile neutrophilic dermatosis) associated with adenocarcinoma of prostate and transitional cell carcinoma of urinary bladder. *J Eur Acad Dermatol Venereol* 2005; 19(5):597–9.

109. Culp L, Crowder S, Hatch S. A rare association of Sweet's syndrome with cervical cancer. *Gynecol Oncol* 2004; 95(2): 396–9.

110. Jordaan HF. Acute febrile neutrophilic dermatosis. A histo-pathological study of 37 patients and a review of the literature. *Am J Dermatopathol* 1989; 11(2):99–111.

111. Greer KE, Cooper PH. Sweet's syndrome (acute febrile neutrophilic dermatosis). *Clin Rheum Dis* 1982; 8(2):427–41.

112. Smith HR, Ashton RE, Beer TW, Theaker JM. Neutrophil-poor Sweet's syndrome with response to potassium iodide. *Br J Dermatol* 1998; 139(3):555–6.

113. Requena L, Kutzner H, Palmedo G, et al. Histiocytoid Sweet syndrome: a dermal infiltration of immature neutrophilic granulocytes. *Arch Dermatol* 2005; 141(7):834–42.

114. Piette WW, Trapp JF, O'Donnell MJ, Argenyi Z, Talbot EA, Burns CP. Acute neutrophilic dermatosis with myeloblastic infiltrate in a leukemia patient receiving all-trans-retinoic acid therapy. *J Am Acad Dermatol* 1994; 30(2 Pt 2):293–7.

115. Tomasini C, Aloi F, Osella-Abate S, Dapavo P, Pippione M. Immature myeloid precursors in chronic neutrophilic dermatosis associated with myelodysplastic syndrome. *Am J Dermatopathol* 2000; 22(5):429–33.

116. Davies MG, Hastings A. Sweet's syndrome progressing to pyoderma gangrenosum—a spectrum of neutrophilic skin disease in association with cryptogenic cirrhosis. *Clin Exp Dermatol* 1991; 16(4):279–82.

117. Hurwitz RM, Haseman JH. The evolution of pyoderma gangrenosum. A clinicopathologic correlation. *Am J Dermatopathol* 1993; 15(1):28–33.

118. Magro CM, Crowson AN, Regauer S. Granuloma annulare and necrobiosis lipoidica tissue reactions as a manifestation of systemic disease. *Hum Pathol* 1996; 27(1):50–6.

119. James WD. Trousseau's syndrome. *Int J Dermatol* 1984; 23(3): 205–6.

120. Sack GH Jr, Levin J, Bell WR. Trousseau's syndrome and other manifestations of chronic disseminated coagulopathy in patients with neoplasms: clinical, pathophysiologic, and therapeutic features. *Medicine (Baltimore)* 1977; 56(1):1–37.

121. Samlaska CP, James WD. Superficial thrombophlebitis. II. Secondary hypercoagulable states. *J Am Acad Dermatol* 1990; 23(1):1–18.

122. Samlaska CP, James WD. Superficial thrombophlebitis. I. Primary hypercoagulable states. *J Am Acad Dermatol* 1990; 22 (6 Pt 1):975–89.

123. Miller SP, Sanchez-Avalos J, Stefanski T, Zuckerman L. Coagulation disorders in cancer. I. Clinical and laboratory studies. *Cancer* 1967; 20(9):1452–65.

124. Montgomery H, O'Leary PA, Barker NW. Nodular vascular diseases of the legs. *JAMA* 1945; 128:335–41.

125. Dalton SR, Fillman EP, Ferringer T, Tyler W, Elston DM. Smooth muscle pattern is more reliable than the presence or absence of an internal elastic lamina in distinguishing an artery from a vein. *J Cutan Pathol* 2006; 33(3):216–9.

126. van der Lught L, de Wit CD. Hypertrichosis lanuginosa acquisita. *Dermatologica* 1973; 146(1):46–54.

127. Fretzin DF. Malignant down. *Arch Dermatol* 1967; 95(3):294–7.

128. Wyatt JP, Anderson HF, Greer KE, Cordoro KM. Acquired hypertrichosis lanuginosa as a presenting sign of metastatic prostate cancer with rapid resolution after treatment. *J Am Acad Dermatol* 2007; 56(Suppl. 2):S45–7.

129. Hegedus SI, Schorr WF. Acquired hypertrichosis lanuginosa and malignancy. A clinical review and histopathologic evaluation with special attention to the "mantle" hair of Pinkus. *Arch Dermatol* 1972; 106(1):84–8.

130. Kaiser IH, Perry G, Yoonessi M. Acquired hypertrichosis lanuginosa associated with endometrial malignancy. *Obstet Gynecol* 1976; 47(4):479–82.

131. Samson MK, Buroker TR, Henderson MD, Baker LH, Vaitkevicius VK. Acquired hypertrichosis languiginosa. Report of two new cases and a review of the literature. *Cancer* 1975; 36(4): 1519–21.

132. Wadskov S, Bro-Jorgensen A, Sondergaard J. Acquired hypertrichosis lanuginosa. A skin marker of internal malignancy. *Arch Dermatol* 1976; 112(10):1442–4.

133. de Viragh PA. The "mantle hair of Pinkus." A review on the occasion of its centennial. *Dermatology* 1995; 191(2):82–7.

134. Rendon MI, Cruz PD Jr, Sontheimer RD, Bergstresser PR. Acanthosis nigricans: a cutaneous marker of tissue resistance to insulin. *J Am Acad Dermatol* 1989; 21(3 Pt 1):461–9.

135. Tasjian D, Jarratt M. Familial acanthosis nigricans. *Arch Dermatol* 1984; 120(10):1351–4.

136. Elgart ML. Acanthosis nigricans and nicotinic acid. *J Am Acad Dermatol* 1981; 5(6):709–10.

137. Schweitzer WJ, Goldin HM, Bronson DM, Brody PE. Acanthosis nigricans associated with mycosis fungoides. *J Am Acad Dermatol* 1988; 19(5 Pt 2):951–3.

138. Kebria MM, Belinson J, Kim R, Mekhail TM. Malignant acanthosis nigricans, tripe palms and the sign of Leser-Tre'lat, a hint to the diagnosis of early stage ovarian cancer: a case report and review of the literature. *Gynecol Oncol* 2006; 101(2):353–5.

139. McGinness J, Greer K. Malignant acanthosis nigricans and tripe palms associated with pancreatic adenocarcinoma. *Cutis* 2006; 78(1):37–40.

140. Curth HO. Dermatoses and malignant internal tumors. *AMA Arch Derm* 1955; 71(1):95–107.

141. Moller H, Eriksson S, Holen O, Waldenstrom JG. Complete reversibility of paraneoplastic acanthosis nigricans after operation. *Acta Med Scand* 1978; 203(4):245–6.

142. Flier JS, Eastman RC, Minaker KL, Matteson D, Rowe JW. Acanthosis nigricans in obese women with hyperandrogenism. Characterization of an insulin-resistant state distinct from the type A and B syndromes. *Diabetes* 1985; 34(2):101–7.

143. Flier JS. Metabolic importance of acanthosis nigricans. *Arch Dermatol* 1985; 121(2):193–4.

144. Pentenero M, Carrozzo M, Pagano M, Gandolfo S. Oral acanthosis nigricans, tripe palms and sign of Leser-Trélat in a patient with gastric adenocarcinoma. *Int J Dermatol* 2004; 43(7):530–2.

145. Kleikamp S, Bohm M, Frosch P, Brinkmeier T. Acanthosis nigricans, papillomatosis mucosae and "tripe palms" in a patient with metastasized gastric carcinoma. *Dtsch Med Wochenschr* 2006; 131(21):1209–13.

146. Brown J, Winkelmann RK. Acanthosis nigricans: a study of 90 cases. *Medicine (Baltimore)* 1968; 47(1):33–51.

147. Lo WL, Wong CK. Tripe palms: a significant cutaneous sign of internal malignancy. *Dermatology* 1992; 185(2):151–3.

148. Patel A, Teixeira F, Redington AE. Palmoplantar keratoderma ("tripe palms") associated with primary pulmonary adenocarcinoma. *Thorax* 2005; 60(11):976.

149. Requena L, Aguilar A, Renedo G, et al. Tripe palms: a cutaneous marker of internal malignancy. *J Dermatol* 1995; 22(7):492–5.

150. Chosidow O, Becherel PA, Piette JC, Arock M, Debre P, Frances C. Tripe palms associated with systemic mastocytosis: the role of transforming growth factor-alpha and efficacy of interferon-alfa. *Br J Dermatol* 1998; 138(4):698–703.

151. Barth G, Basten O, Ruschoff J, Rompel R. Clinical and histopathological characteristics of early Leser-Trélat syndrome. *Hautarzt* 2001; 52(7):649–52.

152. Sperry K, Wall J. Adenocarcinoma of the stomach with eruptive seborrheic keratoses: the sign of Leser-Trélat. *Cancer* 1980; 45(9):2434–7.

153. McCrary ML, Davis LS. Sign of Leser-Trélat and mycosis fungoides. *J Am Acad Dermatol* 1998; 38(4):644.

154. Holdiness MR. On the classification of the sign of Leser-Trélat. *J Am Acad Dermatol* 1988; 19(4):754–7.

155. Venencie PY, Perry HO. Sign of Leser-Trélat: report of two cases and review of the literature. *J Am Acad Dermatol* 1984; 10(1):83–8.

156. Elewski BE, Gilgor RS. Eruptive lesions and malignancy. *Int J Dermatol* 1985; 24(10):617–29.

157. Ohashi N, Hidaka N. Pancreatic carcinoma associated with the Leser-Trélat sign. *Int J Pancreatol* 1997; 22(2):155–60.

158. Hamada Y, Iwaki T, Muratani H, Imayama S, Fukui M, Tateishi J. Leser-Trélat sign with anaplastic ependymoma—an autopsy case. *Acta Neuropathol (Berl)* 1997; 93(1):97–100.

159. Liddell K, White JE, Caldwell IW. Seborrhoeic keratoses and carcinoma of the large bowel. Three cases exhibiting the sign of Lester-Trélat. *Br J Dermatol* 1975; 92(4):449–52.

160. Ellis DL, Kafka SP, Chow JC, et al. Melanoma, growth factors, acanthosis nigricans, the sign of Leser-Trélat, and multiple acrochordons. A possible role for alpha-transforming growth factor in cutaneous paraneoplastic syndromes. *N Engl J Med* 1987; 317(25):1582–7.

161. Halevy S, Feuerman EJ. The sign of Leser-Trélat. A cutaneous marker for internal malignancy. *Int J Dermatol* 1985; 24(6):359–61.

162. Berman A, Winkelmann RK. Seborrheic keratoses: appearance in course of exfoliative erythroderma and regression associated with histologic mononuclear cell inflammation. *Arch Dermatol* 1982; 118(8):615–8.

163. Bell HK, Poston GJ, Vora J, Wilson NJ. Cutaneous manifestations of the malignant carcinoid syndrome. *Br J Dermatol* 2005; 152(1):71–5.

164. Cokonis CD, Green JJ, Manders SM. Primary carcinoid tumor of the skin. *J Am Acad Dermatol* 2004; 51(Suppl. 5):S146–8.

165. Darling TN, Skarulis MC, Steinberg SM, Marx SJ, Spiegel AM, Turner M. Multiple facial angiofibromas and collagenomas in patients with multiple endocrine neoplasia type 1. *Arch Dermatol* 1997; 133(7):853–7.

166. Pack S, Turner ML, Zhuang Z, et al. Cutaneous tumors in patients with multiple endocrine neoplasia type 1 show allelic deletion of the MEN1 gene. *J Invest Dermatol* 1998; 110(4):438–40.

167. Gagel RF, Levy ML, Donovan DT, Alford BR, Wheeler T, Tschen JA. Multiple endocrine neoplasia type 2a associated with cutaneous lichen amyloidosis. *Ann Intern Med* 1989; 111(10):802–6.

168. Nunziata V, Giannattasio R, Di Giovanni G, D'Armiento MR, Mancini M. Hereditary localized pruritus in affected members of a kindred with multiple endocrine neoplasia type 2A (Sipple's syndrome). *Clin Endocrinol (Oxf)* 1989; 30(1):57–63.

169. Walker DM. Oral mucosal neuroma-medullary thyroid carcinoma syndrome. *Br J Dermatol* 1973; 88(6):599–603.

170. Brown RS, Colle E, Tashjian AH Jr. The syndrome of multiple mucosal neuromas and medullary thyroid carcinoma in childhood. Importance of recognition of the phenotype for the early detection of malignancy. *J Pediatr* 1975; 86(1):77–83.

171. Gagel RF, Melvin KE, Tashjian AH Jr, et al. Natural history of the familial medullary thyroid carcinoma-pheochromocytoma syndrome and the identification of preneoplastic stages by screening studies: a five-year report. *Trans Assoc Am Phys* 1975; 88:177–91.

172. Khairi MR, Dexter RN, Burzynski NJ, Johnston CC Jr. Mucosal neuroma, pheochromocytoma and medullary thyroid carcinoma: multiple endocrine neoplasia type 3. *Medicine (Baltimore)* 1975; 54(2):89–112.

173. Hofstra RM, Landsvater RM, Ceccherini I, et al. A mutation in the RET proto-oncogene associated with multiple endocrine

neoplasia type 2B and sporadic medullary thyroid carcinoma. *Nature* 1994; 367(6461):375–6.

174. Harkin J, Reed, RJ. *Neurocutaneous Phakomatosis Tumors of the Peripheral Nervous System*, vol. 3, second series. Washington, DC: Armed Forces Institute of Pathology, 1969:97.

175. Otsuka F, Kawashima T, Imakado S, Usuki Y, Hon-Mura S. Lisch nodules and skin manifestation in neurofibromatosis type 1. *Arch Dermatol* 2001; 137(2):232–3.

176. Koivunen J, Yla-Outinen H, Korkiamaki T, et al. New function for NF1 tumor suppressor. *J Invest Dermatol* 2000; 114(3):473–9.

177. Caiazzo R, Mariette C, Piessen G, Jany T, Carnaille B, Triboulet JP. Type I neurofibromatosis, pheochromocytoma and somatostatinoma of the ampulla. *Literature review. Ann Chir* 2006; 131 (6–7):393–7.

178. Erem C, Onder Ersoz H, Ukinc K, et al. Neurofibromatosis type 1 associated with pheochromocytoma: a case report and a review of the literature. *J Endocrinol Invest* 2007; 30(1):59–64.

179. Cappelli C, Agosti B, Braga M, et al. Von Recklinghausen's neurofibromatosis associated with duodenal somatostatinoma. A case report and review of the literature. *Minerva Endocrinol* 2004; 29(1):19–24.

180. Hatori M, Hosaka M, Watanabe M, Moriya T, Sasano H, Kokubun S. Osteosarcoma in a patient with neurofibromatosis type 1: a case report and review of the literature. *Tohoku J Exp Med* 2006; 208(4):343–8.

181. Saikali S, Le Strat A, Heckly A, Stock N, Scarabin JM, Hamlat A. Multicentric pleomorphic xanthoastrocytoma in a patient with neurofibromatosis type 1. Case report and review of the literature. *J Neurosurg* 2005; 102(2):376–81.

182. Salvi PF, Lombardi A, Puzzovio A, et al. Cutaneous melanoma with neurofibromatosis type 1: rare association? A case report and review of the literature. *Ann Ital Chir* 2004; 75 (1):91–5.

183. Fisher DA, Chu P, McCalmont T. Solitary plexiform neurofibroma is not pathognomonic of von Recklinghausen's neurofibromatosis: a report of a case. *Int J Dermatol* 1997; 36(6):439–42.

184. Patterson JW, Jordan WP Jr. Atypical fibroxanthoma in a patient with xeroderma pigmentosum. *Arch Dermatol* 1987; 123(8):1066–70.

185. Lynch HT, Anderson DE, Smith JL Jr, Howell JB, Krush AJ. Xeroderma pigmentosum, malignant melanoma, and congenital ichthyosis. A family study. *Arch Dermatol* 1967; 96 (6):625–35.

186. Kraemer KH, Lee MM, Scotto J. Xeroderma pigmentosum. Cutaneous, ocular, and neurologic abnormalities in 830 published cases. *Arch Dermatol* 1987; 123(2):241–50.

187. Hessel A, Siegle RJ, Mitchell DL, Cleaver JE. Xeroderma pigmentosum variant with multisystem involvement. *Arch Dermatol* 1992; 128(9):1233–7.

188. Gratchev A, Strein P, Utikal J, Sergij G. Molecular genetics of Xeroderma pigmentosum variant. *Exp Dermatol* 2003; 12(5):529–36.

189. Itoh T, Linn S, Ono T, Yamaizumi M. Reinvestigation of the classification of five cell strains of xeroderma pigmentosum group E with reclassification of three of them. *J Invest Dermatol* 2000; 114(5):1022–9.

190. Robbins JH, Kraemer KH, Lutzner MA, Festoff BW, Coon HG. Xeroderma pigmentosum. An inherited diseases with sun sensitivity, multiple cutaneous neoplasms, and abnormal DNA repair. *Ann Intern Med* 1974; 80(2):221–48.

191. Kraemer KH, Slor H. Xeroderma pigmentosum. *Clin Dermatol* 1985; 3(1):33–69.

192. Uppal S, Mistry D, Coatesworth AP. Cowden disease: a review. *Int J Clin Pract* 2007; 61(4):645–52.

193. Cribier B, Grosshans E. Tumor of the follicular infundibulum: a clinicopathologic study. *J Am Acad Dermatol* 1995; 33(6):979–84.

194. Ruhoy SM, Thomas D, Nuovo GJ. Multiple inverted follicular keratoses as a presenting sign of Cowden's syndrome: case report with human papillomavirus studies. *J Am Acad Dermatol* 2004; 51(3):411–5.

195. Alawi F, Freedman PD. Sporadic sclerotic fibroma of the oral soft tissues. *Am J Dermatopathol* 2004; 26(3):182–7.

196. Laskin WB, Fetsch JF, Michal M, Miettinen M. Sclerotic (fibroma-like) lipoma: a distinctive lipoma variant with a predilection for the distal extremities. *Am J Dermatopathol* 2006; 28 (4):308–16.

197. Kubo Y, Urano Y, Hida Y, et al. A novel PTEN mutation in a Japanese patient with Cowden disease. *Br J Dermatol* 2000; 142 (6):1100–5.

198. Lachlan KL, Lucassen AM, Bunyan DJ, Temple IK. Cowden syndrome and Bannayan-Riley-Ruvalcaba syndrome represent one condition with variable expression and age-related penetrance: a clinical study of 42 individuals with PTEN mutations. *J Med Genet* 2007.

199. Brownstein MH, Shapiro L. Trichilemmoma. Analysis of 40 new cases. *Arch Dermatol* 1973; 107(6):866–9.

200. Leonardi CL, Zhu WY, Kinsey WH, Penneys NS. Trichilemmomas are not associated with human papillomavirus DNA. *J Cutan Pathol* 1991; 18(3):193–7.

201. Mehregan AH. Infundibular tumors of the skin. *J Cutan Pathol* 1984; 11(5):387–95.

202. Rapini RP, Golitz LE. Sclerotic fibromas of the skin. *J Am Acad Dermatol* 1989; 20(2 Pt 1):266–71.

203. Zelger BG, Zelger B, Steiner H, Rutten A. Sclerotic lipoma: lipomas simulating sclerotic fibroma. *Histopathology* 1997; 31 (2):174–81.

204. Traboulsi EI, Krush AJ, Gardner EJ, et al. Prevalence and importance of pigmented ocular fundus lesions in Gardner's syndrome. *N Engl J Med* 1987; 316(11):661–7.

205. Traboulsi EI, Maumenee IH, Krush AJ, et al. Congenital hypertrophy of the retinal pigment epithelium predicts colorectal polyposis in Gardner's syndrome. *Arch Ophthalmol* 1990; 108 (4):525–6.

206. Weary PE, Linthicum A, Cawley EP, Coleman CC Jr., Graham GF. Gardner's syndrome. A family group study and review. *Arch Dermatol* 1964; 90:20–30.

207. Wehrli BM, Weiss SW, Yandow S, Coffin CM. Gardner-associated fibromas (GAF) in young patients: a distinct fibrous lesion that identifies unsuspected Gardner syndrome and risk for fibromatosis. *Am J Surg Pathol* 2001; 25(5):645–51.

208. Rustgi AK. Hereditary gastrointestinal polyposis and nonpolyposis syndromes. *N Engl J Med* 1994; 331(25):1694–702.

209. Leppard BJ, Bussey HJ. Gardner's syndrome with epidermoid cysts showing features of pilomatrixomas. *Clin Exp Dermatol* 1976; 1(1):75–82.

210. Cooper PH, Fechner RE. Pilomatricoma-like changes in the epidermal cysts of Gardner's syndrome. *J Am Acad Dermatol* 1983; 8(5):639–44.

211. Michal M, Fetsch JF, Hes O, Miettinen M. Nuchal-type fibroma: a clinicopathologic study of 52 cases. *Cancer* 1999; 85(1):156–63.

212. Diwan AH, Graves ED, King JA, Horenstein MG. Nuchal-type fibroma in two related patients with Gardner's syndrome. *Am J Surg Pathol* 2000; 24(11):1563–7.

213. Giardiello FM, Welsh SB, Hamilton SR, et al. Increased risk of cancer in the Peutz-Jeghers syndrome. *N Engl J Med* 1987; 316 (24):1511–4.

214. Linos DA, Dozois RR, Dahlin DC, Bartholomew LG. Does Peutz-Jeghers syndrome predispose to gastrointestinal malignancy? A later look. *Arch Surg* 1981; 116(9):1182–4.

215. Pereira CM, Coletta RD, Jorge J, Lopes MA. Peutz-Jeghers syndrome in a 14-year-old boy: case report and review of the literature. *Int J Paediatr Dent* 2005; 15(3):224–8.

216. Valero A, Sherf K. Pigmented nails in Peutz-Jeghers syndrome. *Am J Gastroenterol* 1965; 43:56–8.

217. Sabesan T, Ramchandani PL, Peters WJ. Laugier-Hunziker syndrome: a rare cause of mucocutaneous pigmentation. *Br J Oral Maxillofac Surg* 2006; 44(4):320–1.

218. Makhoul EN, Ayoub NM, Helou JF, Abadjian GA. Familial Laugier-Hunziker syndrome. *J Am Acad Dermatol* 2003; 49 (2 Suppl Case Reports):S143–5.

219. Tseng CJ, Chen SF, Liou SI, et al. Lack of STK11 gene expression in homozygous twins with Peutz-Jeghers syndrome. *Ann Clin Lab Sci* 2004; 34(2):154–8.

220. Yamada K, Matsukawa A, Hori Y, Kukita A. Ultrastructural studies on pigmented macules of Peutz-Jeghers syndrome. *J Dermatol* 1981; 8(5):367–77.

221. Blank AA, Schneider BV, Panizzon R. Pigment spot polyposis (Peutz-Jeghers syndrome). *Hautarzt* 1981; 32(6):296–300.

222. Cohen PR, Kohn SR, Kurzrock R. Association of sebaceous gland tumors and internal malignancy: the Muir-Torre syndrome. *Am J Med* 1991; 90(5):606–13.

223. Torre D. Multiple sebaceous tumors. *Arch Dermatol* 1968; 98(5):549–51.

224. Warschaw KE, Eble JN, Hood AF, Wolverton SE, Halling KC. The Muir-Torre syndrome in a black patient with AIDS: histopathology and molecular genetic studies. *J Cutan Pathol* 1997; 24 (8):511–8.

225. Kanitakis J, Petiot-Roland A, Souillet AL, Faure M, Claudy A. Sebaceous adenomas with atypical immunohistochemical features in the Muir-Torre syndrome [letter]. *Br J Dermatol* 1999; 140(4):749–50.

226. Graham R, McKee P, McGibbon D, Heyderman E. Torre-Muir syndrome. An association with isolated sebaceous carcinoma. *Cancer* 1985; 55(12):2868–73.

227. Schwartz RA. Keratoacanthoma: a clinico-pathologic enigma. *Dermatol Surg* 2004; 30(2 Pt 2):326–33;discussion 333.

228. Halling KC, Honchel R, Pittelkow MR, Thibodeau SN. Microsatellite instability in keratoacanthoma. *Cancer* 1995; 76 (10):1765–71.

229. Rulon DB, Helwig EB. Cutaneous sebaceous neoplasms. *Cancer* 1974; 33(1):82–102.

230. Troy JL, Ackerman AB. Sebaceoma. A distinctive benign neoplasm of adnexal epithelium differentiating toward sebaceous cells. *Am J Dermatopathol* 1984; 6(1):7–13.

231. Burgdorf WH, Pitha J, Fahmy A. Muir-Torre syndrome. Histologic spectrum of sebaceous proliferations. *Am J Dermatopathol* 1986; 8(3):202–8.

232. Bayer-Garner IB, Givens V, Smoller B. Immunohistochemical staining for androgen receptors: a sensitive marker of sebaceous differentiation. *Am J Dermatopathol* 1999; 21(5):426–31.

233. Ponti G, Losi L, Pedroni M, et al. Value of MLH1 and MSH2 mutations in the appearance of Muir-Torre syndrome phenotype in HNPCC patients presenting sebaceous gland tumors or keratoacanthomas. *J Invest Dermatol* 2006; 126(10):2302–7.

234. Ponti G, Losi L, Di Gregorio C, et al. Identification of Muir-Torre syndrome among patients with sebaceous tumors and keratoacanthomas: role of clinical features, microsatellite instability, and immunohistochemistry. *Cancer* 2005; 103(5):1018–25.

235. Marazza G, Masouye I, Taylor S, et al. An illustrative case of Muir-Torre syndrome: contribution of immunohistochemical analysis in identifying indicator sebaceous lesions. *Arch Dermatol* 2006; 142(8):1039–42.

236. Curry ML, Eng W, Lund K, Paek D, Cockerell CJ. Muir-Torre syndrome: role of the dermatopathologist in diagnosis. *Am J Dermatopathol* 2004; 26(3):217–21.

237. Lim ST, Levine AM. Non-AIDS-defining cancers and HIV infection. *Curr HIV/AIDS Rep* 2005; 2(3):146–53.

238. Navarro WH, Kaplan LD. AIDS-related lymphoproliferative disease. *Blood* 2006; 107(1):13–20.

239. Carbone A, Gloghini A. AIDS-related lymphomas: from pathogenesis to pathology. *Br J Haematol* 2005; 130(5):662–70.

240. Bower M, Palmieri C, Dhillon T. AIDS-related malignancies: changing epidemiology and the impact of highly active antiretroviral therapy. *Curr Opin Infect Dis* 2006; 19(1):14–9.

241. Lee DD, Huang CY, Wong CK. Dermatopathologic findings in 20 cases of systemic amyloidosis. *Am J Dermatopathol* 1998; 20 (5):438–42.

242. Wright JR, Calkins E. Clinical-pathologic differentiation of common amyloid syndromes. *Medicine (Baltimore)* 1981; 60(6):429–48.

243. Hagari Y, Mihara M, Konohana I, Ueki H, Yamamoto O, Koizumi H. Nodular localized cutaneous amyloidosis: further demonstration of monoclonality of infiltrating plasma cells in four additional Japanese patients. *Br J Dermatol* 1998; 138(4):652–4.

244. Hagari Y, Mihara M, Hagari S. Nodular localized cutaneous amyloidosis: detection of monoclonality of infiltrating plasma cells by polymerase chain reaction. *Br J Dermatol* 1996; 135(4):630–3.

245. Heim LR. Cryoglobulins: characterization and classification. *Cutis* 1979; 23(3):259–66.

246. Requena L, Kutzner H, Angulo J, Renedo G. Generalized livedo reticularis associated with monoclonal cryoglobulinemia and multiple myeloma. *J Cutan Pathol* 2007; 34(2):198–202.

247. Brouet JC, Clauvel JP, Danon F, Klein M, Seligmann M. Biologic and clinical significance of cryoglobulins. A report of 86 cases. *Am J Med* 1974; 57(5):775–88.

248. Boom BW, Brand A, Bavinck JN, Eernisse JG, Daha MR, Vermeer BJ. Severe leukocytoclastic vasculitis of the skin in a patient with essential mixed cryoglobulinemia treated with high-dose gamma-globulin intravenously. *Arch Dermatol* 1988; 124 (10):1550–3.

249. Cohen SJ, Pittelkow MR, Su WP. Cutaneous manifestations of cryoglobulinemia: clinical and histopathologic study of seventy-two patients. *J Am Acad Dermatol* 1991; 25(1 Pt 1):21–7.

250. Horiuchi Y, Kunii T, Hidaka Y, Ogata K, Urata Y. Erythema multiforme-like eruptions associated with adenocarcinoma of the stomach in a patient with generalized prurigo simplex of two years duration. *J Dermatol* 1999; 26(4):264–6.

251. Patterson JW, Berry AD 3rd, Darwin BS, Gottlieb A, Wilkerson MG. Lichenoid histopathologic changes in patients with clinical diagnoses of exfoliative dermatitis. *Am J Dermatopathol* 1991; 13(4):358–64.

252. Yoshitake T, Nakamura K, Shioyama Y, et al. Erythema multiforme and Stevens-Johnson syndrome following radiotherapy. *Radiat Med* 2007; 25(1):27–30.

253. Ridgway HB, Miech DJ. Erythema multiforme (Stevens-Johnson syndrome) following deep radiation therapy. *Cutis* 1993; 51(6):463–4.

254. Nicolis GD, Helwig EB. Exfoliative dermatitis. A clinicopathologic study of 135 cases. *Arch Dermatol* 1973; 108(6): 788–97.

255. Vonderheid EC, Bigler RD, Kotecha A, et al. Variable CD7 expression on T cells in the leukemic phase of cutaneous T cell lymphoma (Sézary syndrome). *J Invest Dermatol* 2001; 117(3): 654–62.

256. Edelson RL, Kirkpatrick CH, Shevach EM, et al. Preferential cutaneous infiltration by neoplastic thymus-derived lymphocytes. Morphologic and functional studies. *Ann Intern Med* 1974; 80 (6):685–92.

257. Kameyama H, Shirai Y, Date K, Kuwabara A, Kurosaki R, Hatakeyama K. Gallbladder carcinoma presenting as exfoliative dermatitis (erythroderma). *Int J Gastrointest Cancer* 2005; 35(2): 153–5.

258. Pal S, Haroon TS. Erythroderma: a clinico-etiologic study of 90 cases. *Int J Dermatol* 1998; 37(2):104–7.

259. Botella-Estrada R, Sanmartin O, Oliver V, Febrer I, Aliaga A. Erythroderma. A clinicopathological study of 56 cases. *Arch Dermatol* 1994; 130(12):1503–7.

260. Menon BS, Wan Maziah WM. Herpes zoster in children with cancer. *Malays J Pathol* 2001; 23(1):47–8.

261. Fueyo MA, Lookingbill DP. Herpes zoster and occult malignancy. *J Am Acad Dermatol* 1984; 11(3):480–2.

262. Ragozzino MW, Melton LJ 3rd, Kurland LT, Chu CP, Perry HO. Population-based study of herpes zoster and its sequelae. *Medicine (Baltimore)* 1982; 61(5):310–6.

263. Buntinx F, Wachana R, Bartholomeeusen S, Sweldens K, Geys H. Is herpes zoster a marker for occult or subsequent malignancy? *Br J Gen Pract* 2005; 55(511):102–7.

264. Mazur MH, Whitley RJ, Dolin R. Serum antibody levels as risk factors in the dissemination of herpes zoster. *Arch Intern Med* 1979; 139(12):1341–5.

265. Sneddon IB. Acquired ichthyosis in Hodgkin's disease. *Br Med J* 1955; 1(4916):763–4.

266. Yokote R, Iwatsuki K, Hashizume H, Takigawa M. Lymphomatoid papulosis associated with acquired ichthyosis. *J Am Acad Dermatol* 1994; 30(5 Pt 2):889–892.

267. Bork K, Bockers M, Pfeifle J. Pathogenesis of paraneoplastic follicular hyperkeratotic spicules in multiple myeloma. Follicular and epidermal accumulation of IgG dysprotein and cryoglobulin. *Arch Dermatol* 1990; 126(4):509–13.

268. Van D. Ichthyosiform atrophy of the skin associated with internal malignant diseases. *Dermatologica* 1963; 127:413–28.

269. Barzilai A, Shpiro D, Goldberg I, et al. Insect bite-like reaction in patients with hematologic malignant neoplasms. *Arch Dermatol* 1999; 135(12):1503–7.

270. Dodiuk-Gad RP, Dann EJ, Bergman R. Insect bite-like reaction associated with mantle cell lymphoma: a report of two cases and review of the literature. *Int J Dermatol* 2004; 43 (10):754–8.

271. Khamaysi Z, Dodiuk-Gad RP, Weltfriend S, et al. Insect bite-like reaction associated with mantle cell lymphoma: clinicopathological, immunopathological, and molecular studies. *Am J Dermatopathol* 2005; 27(4):290–5.

272. Ulmer A, Metzler G, Schanz S, Fierlbeck G. Dapsone in the management of "insect bite-like reaction" in a patient with chronic lymphocytic leukaemia. *Br J Dermatol* 2007; 156(1): 172–4.

273. Trattner A, Katzenelson V, Sandbank M. Palmoplantar keratoderma in a noncutaneous T-cell lymphoma. *Int J Dermatol* 1991; 30(12):871–2.

274. Murata Y, Kumano K, Tani M, Saito N, Kagotani K. Acquired diffuse keratoderma of the palms and soles with bronchial carcinoma: report of a case and review of the literature. *Arch Dermatol* 1988; 124(4):497–8.

275. Howel-Evans W, McConnell RB, Clarke CA, Sheppard PM. Carcinoma of the oesophagus with keratosis palmaris et plantaris (tylosis): a study of two families. *Q J Med* 1958; 27: 413–29.

276. Langan JE, Cole CG, Huckle EJ, et al. Novel microsatellite markers and single nucleotide polymorphisms refine the tylosis with oesophageal cancer (TOC) minimal region on 17q25 to 42.5 kb: sequencing does not identify the causative gene. *Hum Genet* 2004; 114(6):534–40.

277. McRonald FE, Liloglou T, Xinarianos G, et al. Down-regulation of the cytoglobin gene, located on 17q25, in tylosis with oesophageal cancer (TOC): evidence for trans-allele repression. *Hum Mol Genet* 2006; 15(8):1271–7.

278. Iwaya T, Maesawa C, Kimura T, et al. Infrequent mutation of the human envoplakin gene is closely linked to the tylosis oesophageal cancer locus in sporadic oesophageal squamous cell carcinomas. *Oncol Rep* 2005; 13(4):703–7.

279. Bennion SD, Patterson JW. Keratosis punctata palmaris et plantaris and adenocarcinoma of the colon. A possible familial association of punctate keratoderma and gastrointestinal malignancy. *J Am Acad Dermatol* 1984; 10(4):587–91.

280. Rubenstein DJ, Schwartz RA, Hansen RC, Payne CM. Punctate hyperkeratosis of the palms and soles. An ultrastructural study. *J Am Acad Dermatol* 1980; 3(1):43–9.

281. Santaella ML, Font I, Disdier O. Common variable immunodeficiency: experience in Puerto Rico. *P R Health Sci J* 2005; 24 (1):7–10.

282. Cunningham-Rundles C, Bodian C. Common variable immunodeficiency: clinical and immunological features of 248 patients. *Clin Immunol* 1999; 92(1):34–48.

283. Cunningham-Rundles C. Common variable immunodeficiency. *Curr Allergy Asthma Rep* 2001; 1(5):421–9.

284. Smith KJ, Skelton H. Common variable immunodeficiency treated with a recombinant human IgG, tumour necrosis factor-alpha receptor fusion protein. *Br J Dermatol* 2001; 144(3):597–600.

285. Pierson JC, Camisa C, Lawlor KB, Elston DM. Cutaneous and visceral granulomas in common variable immunodeficiency. *Cutis* 1993; 52(4):221–2.

286. Pujol RM, Nadal C, Taberner R, Diaz C, Miralles J, Alomar A. Cutaneous granulomatous lesions in common variable immunodeficiency: complete resolution after intravenous immunoglobulins. *Dermatology* 1999; 198(2):156–8.

287. Torrelo A, Mediero IG, Zambrano A. Caseating cutaneous granulomas in a child with common variable immunodeficiency. *Pediatr Dermatol* 1995; 12(2):170–3.

288. Abdel-Naser MB, Wollina U, El Hefnawi MA, Habib MA, El Okby M. Non-sarcoidal, non-tuberculoid granuloma in common variable immunodeficiency. *J Drugs Dermatol* 2006; 5(4): 370–2.

289. Goldes JA, Filipovich AH, Neudorf SM, et al. Epidermodysplasia verruciformis in a setting of common variable immunodeficiency. *Pediatr Dermatol* 1984; 2(2):136–9.

290. Pasic S, Pavlovic M, Vojvodic D, Abinun M. Pityriasis lichenoides in a girl with the granulomatous form of common variable immunodeficiency. *Pediatr Dermatol* 2002; 19(1):56–9.

291. Yalcin I, Somer A, Akcay A, Buyukbabani N, Salman N, Guler N. Myofibroblastic tumors involving bilateral adrenal glands and skin in a patient with common variable immunodeficiency. *J Pediatr Surg* 2002; 37(1):124–6.

292. Cotelingam JD, Witebsky FG, Hsu SM, Blaese RM, Jaffe ES. Malignant lymphoma in patients with the Wiskott-Aldrich syndrome. *Cancer Invest* 1985; 3(6):515–22.

293. Peacocke M, Siminovitch KA. Wiskott-Aldrich syndrome: new molecular and biochemical insights. *J Am Acad Dermatol* 1992; 27(4):507–19.

294. Bourdon-Lanoy E, Roujeau JC, Joly P, et al. Bullous pemphigoid in young patients: a retrospective study of 74 cases. *Ann Dermatol Venereol* 2005; 132(2):115–22.

295. Iranzo P, Lopez I, Robles MT, Mascaro JM Jr, Campo E, Herrero C. Bullous pemphigoid associated with mantle cell lymphoma. *Arch Dermatol* 2004; 140(12):1496–9.

296. Gul U, Kilic A, Demirel O, Cakmak SK, Gonul M, Oksal A. Bullous pemphigoid associated with breast carcinoma. *Eur J Dermatol* 2006; 16(5):581–2.

297. Yanagi T, Kato N, Yamane N, Osawa R. Bullous pemphigoid associated with dermatomyositis and colon carcinoma. *Clin Exp Dermatol* 2007; 32(3):291–4.

298. Venencie PY, Rogers RS 3rd, Schroeter AL. Bullous pemphigoid and malignancy: relationship to indirect immunofluorescent findings. *Acta Derm Venereol* 1984; 64(4):316–9.

299. Hodge L, Marsden RA, Black MM, Bhogal B, Corbett MF. Bullous pemphigoid: the frequency of mucosal involvement and concurrent malignancy related to indirect immunofluorescence findings. *Br J Dermatol* 1981; 105(1):65–9.

300. Ahmed AR, Amerian ML. Correlation of serum anti-basement membrane zone antibody and malignancy in bullous pemphigoid. *Dermatologica* 1985; 171(2):82–5.

301. Ortiz LJ, Vazquez M, Sanchez JL. Bullous pemphigoid and malignancy. *Bol Asoc Med P R* 1990; 82(10):458–9.

302. Fine JD, Omura EF. Herpes gestationis. Persistent disease activity 11 years post partum. *Arch Dermatol* 1985; 121(7):924–6.

303. Kelly SE, Black MM. Pemphigoid gestationis: placental interactions. *Semin Dermatol* 1989; 8(1):12–7.

304. Slazinski L, Degefu S. Herpes gestationis associated with choriocarcinoma. *Arch Dermatol* 1982; 118(6):425–8.

305. Halkier-Sorensen L, Beck HI, Sogaard H. Herpes gestationis in association with neoplasma malignum generalisata. A case report. *Acta Derm Venereol Suppl (Stockh)* 1985; 120:96–100.

306. do Valle Chiossi MP, Costa RS, Ferreira Roselino AM. Titration of herpes gestationis factor fixing to C3 in pemphigoid herpes gestationis associated with choriocarcinoma. *Arch Dermatol* 2000; 136(1):129–30.

307. Djahansouzi S, Nestle-Kraemling C, Dall P, Bender HG, Hanstein B. Herpes gestationis may present itself as a paraneoplastic syndrome of choriocarcinoma—a case report. *Gynecol Oncol* 2003; 89(2):334–7.

308. Hall RP. The pathogenesis of dermatitis herpetiformis: recent advances. *J Am Acad Dermatol* 1987; 16(6):1129–44.

309. Katz SI, Strober W. The pathogenesis of dermatitis herpetiformis. *J Invest Dermatol* 1978; 70(2):63–75.

310. Fry L. Dermatitis herpetiformis. *Baillieres Clin Gastroenterol* 1995; 9(2):371–93.

311. Hervonen K, Vornanen M, Kautiainen H, Collin P, Reunala T. Lymphoma in patients with dermatitis herpetiformis and their first-degree relatives. *Br J Dermatol* 2005; 152(1):82–6.

312. Viljamaa M, Kaukinen K, Pukkala E, Hervonen K, Reunala T, Collin P. Malignancies and mortality in patients with coeliac disease and dermatitis herpetiformis: 30-year population-based study. *Dig Liver Dis* 2006; 38(6):374–80.

313. Askling J, Linet M, Gridley G, Halstensen TS, Ekstrom K, Ekbom A. Cancer incidence in a population-based cohort of individuals hospitalized with celiac disease or dermatitis herpetiformis. *Gastroenterology* 2002; 123(5):1428–35.

314. Leonard JN, Tucker WF, Fry JS, et al. Increased incidence of malignancy in dermatitis herpetiformis. *Br Med J (Clin Res Ed)* 1983; 286(6358):16–8.

315. Bose SK, Lacour JP, Bodokh I, Ortonne JP. Malignant lymphoma and dermatitis herpetiformis. *Dermatology* 1994; 188 (3):177–81.

316. Zelger B, Cerio R, Soyer HP, Misch K, Orchard G, Wilson-Jones E. Reticulohistiocytoma and multicentric reticulohistiocytosis. Histopathologic and immunophenotypic distinct entities. *Am J Dermatopathol* 1994; 16(6):577–84.

317. Coupe MO, Whittaker SJ, Thatcher N. Multicentric reticulohistiocytosis. *Br J Dermatol* 1987; 116(2):245–7.

318. Valencia IC, Colsky A, Berman B. Multicentric reticulohistiocytosis associated with recurrent breast carcinoma. *J Am Acad Dermatol* 1998; 39(5 Pt 2):864–6.

319. Malik MK, Regan L, Robinson-Bostom L, Pan TD, McDonald CJ. Proliferating multicentric reticulohistiocytosis associated with papillary serous carcinoma of the endometrium. *J Am Acad Dermatol* 2005; 53(6):1075–9.

Nonneurological, Nondermatologic Paraneoplasias

MARK R. WICK

MARIEKE T. DE GRAAF

PETER A. E. SILLEVIS SMITT

INTRODUCTION

Paraneoplastic (Greek, "from a new creature") syndromes constitute one of the most fascinating topics in oncology, if not all of medicine (1–17). They comprise a constellation of pathologic changes seen in patients with malignancies, which are not related directly to tumor growth in a mechanical or topographical sense. Instead, such alterations represent the elaboration of diverse exportable molecules by the neoplastic cells—many of which are still poorly characterized—that have physiological effects on distant organs or tissues. Those changes may precede or postdate overt manifestations of the responsible tumor, and, as such, are important not only to treating oncologists but to all other physicians caring for the patients in question. Moreover, paraneoplastic phenomena can be the overwhelmingly *dominant* expression of a malignancy; for example, rather small, localized neuroendocrine carcinomas (NECs) that synthesize adrenocorticotrophic hormone (ACTH) may nonetheless produce florid changes of Cushing's syndrome (18).

In the context of this monograph, regarding metastatic carcinomas of unknown origin (MCUO), paraneoplasias are germane in three respects. First, particular types of paraneoplastic syndromes (PSs) may be linked preferentially to relatively narrowly defined subsets of MCUO. Therefore, they can provide possible clues to the site of primary tumor growth. Second, reflecting the fact that the PSs themselves may be the major sources of clinical morbidity, one must always remember to screen patients with such disorders for underlying malignancies. Finally, paraneoplasias often complicate the choice of therapy offered to MCUO patients, because their physiological effects may overlap with those produced by various medications and other interventions.

VETERINARY PARALLELS OF HUMAN PARANEOPLASIA

PSs are not unique to human beings; many reports have also been made in the veterinary literature of similar conditions in nonhuman vertebrates (19–25). In specific reference to carcinomas in such hosts, paraneoplastic hypoglycemia has been documented—owing to tumor production of insulin-like peptides—in dogs with hepatocellular carcinoma (26), and in horses and dogs with renal cell carcinoma (RCC) (27, 28). Pancreatic endocrine tumors in cats and dogs are capable of synthesizing insulin itself, with comparable clinical results (29). Tumor-related hypercalcemia has appeared in connection with apocrine carcinoma in dogs and pulmonary carcinomas of several histotypes in cats (30, 31). Various hematologic disorders and coagulopathies may accompany malignant renal, hepatic, or lung tumors in vertebrate animals in various genera, as may paraneoplastic pemphigus, necrolytic dermatitis, scleroderma, and hypertrophic osteoarthropathy (HOA) (19, 20, 23, 32–35). Finally, Stauffer's syndrome, also known as paraneoplastic hepatopathy, has been associated with RCC in dogs (36), as it is in humans.

As is true in people, paraneoplasias in animals do not necessarily manifest themselves at a clinical level in concurrence with the responsible tumor, but may instead produce metachronous symptoms and signs. Pathophysiological mechanisms for the assorted paraneoplastic conditions cited above also appear to be comparable between organisms in different genera and species. These similarities are certainly biologically intriguing. They also provide possible substrates for models of human paraneoplastic conditions, including those that are seen in the context of MCUO, which could be utilized in future studies of pathophysiologic mechanisms and treatment.

SPECIFIC CATEGORIES OF HUMAN PSs

Human PSs can be categorized into several mechanistic or organ system–related groups. Any or all of them may affect patients with MCUO.

Systemic Paraneoplasias

Several paraneoplastic conditions are systemic, in the sense that their symptoms and signs do not have an etiology in a clearly defined anatomic site. Moreover, the mechanisms of such problems are rather vague, and they may well relate to more than one pathophysiological pathway.

Paraneoplastic Fever

Fever—in the absence of a definable infection—represents a relatively common paraneoplastic condition in patients with malignancies (37–42). It may be continuous or assume a cyclic pattern, appearing at relatively the same time each day and remitting spontaneously in the interim. On the other hand, several days or weeks may separate febrile from afebrile periods. The fever in malignancy is typically not above 101°F or 102°F, and it may or may not be accompanied by rigors and sweats (38).

As should be done for any other fever of unknown origin, a thorough clinical evaluation must be undertaken that includes evaluations for infection, a survey of medications, and clinicopathologic assessments for possible collagen vascular disease or vascular thrombosis. Only if all of these are negative is it permissible to label a patient as having paraneoplastic pyrexia (43).

Underlying tumors are relatively varied in nature; indeed, virtually any neoplasm may cause the problem in question. Overall, paraneoplastic fever is most closely linked with lymphohematologic malignancies. Among solid neoplasms, however, cancers of the head and neck, kidney, lung, and breast most often cause elevations in temperature (38).

The mechanism of paraneoplastic pyrexia is still poorly characterized. Nevertheless, because fever in this context is reproducibly ameliorated by nonsteroidal anti-inflammatory medications (44, 45), a cytokine-induced pathway is generally accepted at this point. It is unknown whether the tumors themselves or secondarily recruited inflammatory cells are responsible for release of the putative mediators.

The principal differential diagnosis for paraneoplastic fever in MCUO cases is with infection. Penel et al. have addressed this issue specifically (46, 47), with regard to laboratory tests that might distinguish between the two possibilities. They found that neither C-reactive protein nor procalcitonin serum levels were capable of making this separation, and that conventional microbiological testing is still necessary to do so.

The treatment of paraneoplastic pyrexia is, as stated earlier, predicated on the use of nonsteroidal anti-inflammatory drugs (NSAIDs) such as naproxen, indomethacin, diclophenac, and ibuprofen (45). Indeed, these agents are effective enough for a successful therapeutic trial involving them to have diagnostic weight in identifying a fever caused by malignancy (44).

Parageusia/Dysgeusia

Some patients with malignancies develop an altered taste for certain foods, such that it is distorted (dysgeusia) or unpleasant (parageusia) (48–51). Probably the most well-known among these phenomena is the distaste for meat that patients with carcinoma of the stomach may report (48). Another interesting and relatively specific dysgeusia, which is linked to hyponatremia, is the sensation of unpleasant perceived sweetness of many ingested foods. It is observed in patients with hyponatremia, owing to the syndrome of inappropriate secretion of antidiuretic hormone (SIADH) (49, 50). The problem is often—but not always—associated with small cell NEC of the lung.

The mechanisms for these problems are largely unknown. There has been some speculation that they relate to disturbances in trace elements, such as a deficiency of zinc (48). However, therapeutic replacement of such substances has been only inconstantly associated with an improvement in symptoms. Alternatively, dysgeusia and parageusia may represent neurologic paraneoplasias rather than deficiency states.

Alterations in taste may accompany any of a variety of occult carcinomas. Therefore, after eliminating the possibility that these complaints relate to drugs or oral-dental disorders, the presence of dys-/parageusias should prompt evaluation for a possible underlying malignancy.

Pruritus

Generalized itching, or pruritus, in the absence of a definable dermatosis, is one of the most maddening of the potential paraneoplasias for patients with MCUO and their physicians (Fig. 1) (52). It may be linked directly to an underlying hematopoietic or solid malignancy (53), but more often simply relates to xerosis (dry skin) or a reaction to a self-administered or prescribed medication (54). Chronic renal insufficiency and cholestatic hepatic disease are additional possible explanations for pruritus (55). If assessments of kidney and liver function are unrevealing, and dermatologic consultation fails to disclose a definable source for itching, a paraneoplasia must be suspected and appropriately evaluated.

The mechanisms for paraneoplastic pruritus are unknown. It is seen preferentially with carcinomas of the kidney, hepatobiliary system, pancreas, and lung, among other possibilities (52, 54). Symptomatic treatment includes optimal care of the skin, administration of antihistamines and tricyclic antidepressants, and ultra-violet cutaneous phototherapy (56, 57).

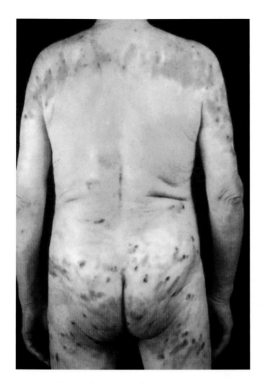

FIGURE 1 The effects of paraneoplastic pruritus are seen in this 60-year-old man with pancreatic carcinoma. Numerous excoriations are present in areas where the patient can reach his skin surfaces.

Anorexia/Cachexia

Cachexia is a common paraneoplasia in MCUO cases and in oncology patients in general (58–63). It is characterized by anorexia, involuntary weight loss, wasting, and weakness. The name is an appropriate one, derived from Greek *kakos* (bad) and *hexis* (condition) (63). Breast carcinoma is virtually the only solid tumor that is not associated with cachexia to any substantial degree. On the other hand, lung carcinomas and gastrointestinal cancers are linked to this problem in 60% to 80% of cases (64).

In some instances, the cause of cachexia is straightforward, such as a mechanical/functional inability to ingest food, obstruction of the alimentary tract, or profound depression with a loss of interest in eating. In other circumstances, however, marked loss of weight and wasting does appear to have a truly paraneoplastic underpinning. Cytokines such as tumor necrosis factor (TNF)-alpha, interleukin-1, interleukin-6 (IL6), and interferon-gamma have been implicated as mediators, and they may be synthesized by various tumors or in response to them (63). They possibly interfere with the activity of leptin, a fat-derived hormone that indirectly stimulates feeding centers in the hypothalamus (65, 66). Disruption of neuropeptide-Y signaling and melanocortin

regulation—which also affect appetite—are additional possibilities, as are alterations in the intrinsic nature of carbohydrate, protein, or lipid metabolism (67–69).

The loss of 10% of premorbid body weight is a minimal criterion for the assignment of the diagnosis of cachexia (63). Laboratory tests are of limited value in establishing its presence.

Symptomatic treatment includes parenteral nutrition or ingestion of high-calorie supplements (when possible). Administration of megestrol acetate, cannabinoids, thalidomide, or cyproheptadine—all of which stimulate appetite—is another option (63). Mirtazapine is an appetite-promoting antidepressant drug that also can be used when psychic depression is felt to be a contributing element (70).

Flushing

Flushing is defined as the relatively sudden appearance of intense cutaneous erythema—usually involving the skin of the head and neck (Fig. 2)—which can last for minutes, hours, or even days (71). It is usually associated with an unpleasant burning sensation in the skin, along with sweating or edema or both. Other extracutaneous symptoms and signs such as wheezing, lacrimation, and

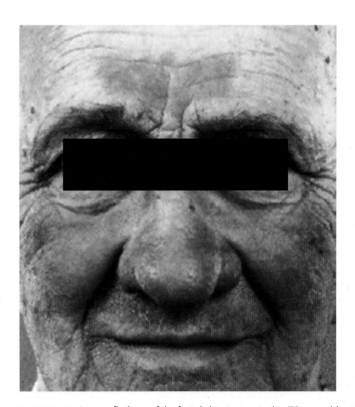

FIGURE 2 Intense flushing of the facial skin is seen in this 73-year-old man with metastatic ileal carcinoid tumor in the liver.

diarrhea may appear concurrently with flushing. In the long term, repeated episodes of facial erythema may lead to telangiectasia of the skin or overt rosacea.

The most well-known cause of cutaneous flushing is metastatic, well-differentiated NEC ("carcinoid"), usually taking origin in the mid-gut (small intestine, pancreas, and proximal colon) and secondarily involving the liver (Fig. 3) (72–74). However, primary NEC of the ovary, testis, and, rarely, the lung, may also produce similar symptoms and signs in the absence of metastasis. Medullary carcinoma of the thyroid and RCC are additional possible sources of paraneoplastic flushing syndromes (75, 76).

Various vasoactive molecules have been implicated in this problem, including serotonin, 5-hydroxytryptamine, prostaglandins, tachykinins, and histamine (72, 76). All of them are thought to be direct products of the underlying tumors.

In NEC-related flushing, several precipitating factors have been delineated empirically. They include exercise, alcohol intake, stress, and ingestion of certain spices, chocolate, cheese, avocados, plums, walnuts, cured sausages, and red wine. Intravenous administration of phentolamine is capable of blocking the response in many instances (77). In contrast, the precipitants just listed are not operative in flushing that is related to RCC. The latter tumor appears to synthesize prostaglandin-E2 instead of vasoactive amines, and such production is not influenced by dietary intake (75). Medullary thyroid carcinoma is an organ-specific form of NEC, and, as such, it may also make vasoactive substances. However, it also has the potential for prostaglandin synthesis (76).

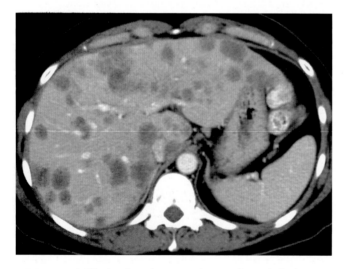

FIGURE 3 A CT taken from the patient shown in Figure 2 demonstrates innumerable tumor implants throughout the hepatic parenchyma.

Laboratory testing should include assessment of 5-hydroxyindoleacetic acid in urine, or serotonin in blood, or both. Levels of chromogranin-A, a protein that is part of the neurosecretory granule matrix in NECs, may also be elevated in plasma, as may those of substance-P and neurokinin-A (78, 79). Prostaglandins in serum must be measured *during* a flushing episode, and, in examples of RCC and other tumors that synthesize this molecular family, elevations may be observed (75, 76).

Treatment is tailored to the presumed chemical mediator(s) underlying attacks of flushing. Patients with tumors that produce vasoactive amines can be managed with a combination of somatostatin analogs (e.g., octreotide) and H1- and H2-type antihistamines (80–82). Cyproheptadine is sometimes effective in helping to control concomitant diarrhea (83). On the other hand, prostaglandin-mediated flushing is best treated with the prophylactic use of NSAIDs such as naproxen, ibuprofen, and indomethacin (80).

Endocrine Paraneoplasias

PSs that are caused by the tumor synthesis of peptide, amine, or steroid hormones are endocrine in nature. Underlying neoplasms may arise in a wide array of anatomic sites, and they may be small, despite producing dramatic physiologic abnormalities.

Cushing's Syndrome

One of the best-known endocrine PSs is Cushing's syndrome. One potential mechanism for this problem is the ectopic synthesis of ACTH or corticotrophin-releasing hormone (CRH) by a neoplasm, subsequently driving the adrenal cortex to release excessive corticosteroid (84–87). Another possible explanation is the *direct* production of corticosteroid, usually by an adrenocortical or gonadal stromal tumor (88–90).

The clinical findings of Cushing's syndrome are well known to most physicians. They include weight gain, redistribution of fat—with truncal obesity and a "moon" facies (Fig. 4)—hirsutism, glucose intolerance, proximal muscle weakness, osteoporosis, cutaneous striae, poor wound healing, hypokalemia, and hypertension (2, 85).

Unfortunately, because many malignant neoplasms that produce ectopic ACTH or CRH [including NECs of foregut structures; medullary thyroid carcinomas; pancreatic NECs (islet cell tumors); and nonendocrine carcinomas with "occult" neuroendocrine differentiation] are small, they may easily elude radiographic detection (91). In contrast, the adrenals are often found to be generous in size on imaging studies. The authors have seen several cases in which misdirected pituitary surgery or

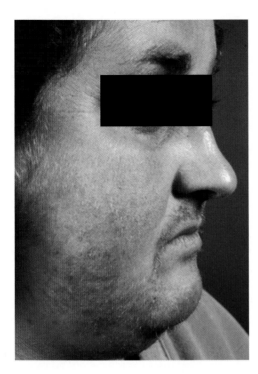

FIGURE 4 Cushing's syndrome in a 45-year-old woman with small cell neuroendocrine carcinoma of the lung. Facial fullness ("moon facies") and hirsutism are evident.

adrenalectomy was undertaken, only to have an ACTH/CRH-producing neoplasm in another location become apparent at a later date.

Initial laboratory assessment of possible ectopic Cushing's syndrome should include measurement of 24-hour urinary free cortisol, low-dose dexamethasone testing, salivary cortisol, and night-time plasma cortisol values (92). A dexamethasone CRH test can discriminate between Cushing's syndrome and those that simulate it (93). Several recent publications have also examined the role of bilateral simultaneous inferior petrosal sinus sampling (BSIPSS) for ACTH, after stimulation with exogenous CRH and desmopressin (94, 95). The "central" ACTH level in blood, as obtained in this way, is then compared in a ratio with peripheral blood levels. Ratios of ≥2 are thought to substantiate a pituitary source for hypercortisolism. Specifically, Tsagarakis et al. found that 98% of patients with hypophyseal Cushing's disease demonstrated such values, whereas no patient in their series with ectopic ACTH/CRH syndrome did so (94). BSIPSS is undeniably an invasive procedure, but when compared with the risk of morbidly unnecessary surgery, as mentioned above, the former intervention is felt to be justifiable.

Identification of the primary ACTH/CRH-producing tumor, and ablation of it, is obviously the best treatment of ectopic Cushing's syndrome. However, in MCUO

cases, that may not be possible. Alternatively, treatment with oral ketoconazole, metyrapone, aminoglutethimide, mifepristone, or ortho,para,dichlorodiphenyl dichloroethane (o,p′-DDD) may be useful in blunting or even eliminating many of the symptoms and signs of this PS (96, 97). Surgical adrenalectomy is reserved for those patients who do not respond to medical management. Probably because of endocrinopathy-related comorbidity, the prognosis of patients with ectopic Cushing's syndrome is said to be adverse, compared with that of cohorts who lack this condition (98).

Cushing's syndrome, which relates directly to cortisol synthesis by adrenocortical carcinomas, is accompanied by *low* ACTH/CRH levels. Steroid-producing tumors of this type can be treated using chemotherapy. o,p′-DDD (mitotane) is given when surgery is not possible or after incomplete resection of metastatic disease. Frequently employed therapeutic combinations are etoposide, doxorubicin, cisplatin, and mitotane, as well as streptozotocin and mitotane (99).

Syndrome of Inappropriate Secretion of Antidiuretic Hormone (SIADH)

SIADH, or the Schwartz-Bartter syndrome, is characterized by hyponatremia, and serum hypo-osmolality in the face of urine normo-osmolality or hyperosmolality. The serum sodium level is often below 130 mEq/L and hypouricemia is commonly observed as well (100).

The most common epithelial tumors that may ectopically synthesize antidiuretic hormone include small-cell NEC of the lung (by far, the most common); small-cell carcinomas of the thymus, head and neck, and pancreas; nonsmall-cell pulmonary carcinomas; squamous cell carcinoma of the oropharynx and larynx; adenoid cystic carcinoma of salivary glands and lung; prostatic adenocarcinoma; gastric adenocarcinoma; and mesothelioma (101–115). Electrolyte abnormalities may precede clinical recognition of such neoplasms by several months (114). Several nonneoplastic causes of SIADH exist as well, and only after these are excluded systematically should one assume that an occult malignancy likely is present (114).

Whether or not patients with SIADH manifest symptoms depends not only on the absolute sodium concentration in serum, but the rapidity with which it drops from a normal level. Hyponatremia may be slowly progressive and virtually asymptomatic for prolonged periods, but, conversely, it may appear suddenly and dramatically after chemotherapy of a malignancy commences. This phenomenon is felt to be a consequence of tumor lysis with massive spillage of antidiuretic hormone (110, 115). If the sodium level in serum drops below 125 mEq/L, fatigue, confusion, anorexia, muscle cramping, and nausea may appear, along with "sweet parageusia." Profound hyponatremia (<120 mEq/L) can produce seizure activity and coma (101).

Treatment of SIADH is predicated on the administration of oral sodium chloride (when possible) and intravenous slightly hypertonic saline, in conjunction with the judicious use of "loop" diuretics (e.g., furosemide) and restriction of oral water intake. One should not attempt to correct the serum sodium level abruptly, because a rebound phenomenon may subsequently yield a hyperosmolar state that is neurologically damaging (100, 117). Demeclocycline—a drug that appears to block the effect of antidiuretic hormone on the renal tubules—may also be helpful (117). In general, successful chemotherapy of underlying tumors will eliminate dysfunctional water metabolism in such cases; if and when the lesion recurs, SIADH may or may not reappear (101).

Tumor-Related Hypercalcemia

Hypercalcemia as a PS is a potential oncological emergency. The association between elevation of serum calcium and underlying malignancy—even in the absence of bone metastases—has been known for decades (118–124). Mild hypercalcemia is usually asymptomatic, at corrected serum calcium values <12 mEq/L. However, elderly patients may develop complaints at those levels nonetheless. Symptoms and signs may include nausea and vomiting; confusion, depression, or lethargy; headache; abdominal pain; constipation; weakness, and polyuria and polydipsia (119). However, patients with hypercalcemia presenting in the context of MCUO may inexplicably lack many of those complaints.

Humoral factors, principally tumor-derived parathyroid hormone (PTH) or parathyroid hormone-related peptide (PTHrP), play a major etiologic role in such cases (125, 126). However, increased osteoclastic activity and subsequent mobilization of osseous calcium may occur due to factors secreted by tumor cells in bone metastases, such as osteoclast activating factor (OAF), prostaglandins, TNF, and interleukin-1 (119, 120). Transforming growth factor-beta likewise is an operative factor in the increased bone resorption that is seen in conjunction with some tumors (2). Impaired renal clearance of calcium may also occur under the influence of PTH, PTHrP, and other factors secreted by malignancies; they cause increased tubular resorption of this mineral (127).

Essentially any solid tumor potentially may be associated with hypercalcemia. Lung carcinomas—of all histotypes—account for 25% to 35% of reported cases, and 30% to 40% are related to breast cancer. However, in the latter instance, the usual mechanism is that of calcium mobilization after *metastasis* to bone has occurred, with release of OAF or other locally acting factors by the neoplastic cells (128). PTH and PTHrP are not as often involved mechanistically in breast carcinoma cases, despite the fact that such tumors can indeed synthesize these peptides (129).

Diagnosis is established by assessing the possible presence of appropriate clinical findings of hypercalcemia, as well as measuring the "corrected" serum calcium (total serum calcium – serum albumin in g/dL + 4) (127). Acidosis decreases serum calcium levels, but these alterations are minor.

Leukocytosis may be seen concurrently with hypercalcemia in some cases, especially in association with lung carcinoma (121). However, combined PS is rare, affecting <1% of all cases.

The treatment of malignancy-related hypercalcemia is based on liberal intravenous fluid replacement; careful use of loop diuretics (if the serum calcium is >14 mg/dL, *forced* diuresis with normal saline and furosemide is indicated); and administration of calcitonin, corticosteroids, and bisphosphonates (130). Moreover, optimal responses to chemotherapy are capable, by themselves, of normalizing calcium levels as well. Finally, Sato et al. reported success in an animal model in treating hypercalcemia with an antibody to PTHrP (131).

Hypoglycemia and Hyperglycemia

Disturbances in glucose metabolism represent additional forms of PS. The most common of them is tumor-related hypoglycemia (Doege-Potter syndrome), reflecting the synthesis of insulin, proinsulin, or insulin-like growth factor peptides [ILGFs (types I and II)] by malignant solid neoplasms (132–141). NECs—especially those in the pancreas—may produce true insulin or proinsulin (142), but virtually all other epithelial malignancies may synthesize ILGFs and be the cause of hypoglycemia. Among the latter, hepatocellular carcinoma (Nadler-Wolfer-Elliott syndrome), RCC, gynecologic carcinomas, non–small-cell lung carcinomas, adrenocortical carcinomas (Anderson syndrome), and mesothelioma are most often implicated in paraneoplastic hypoglycemia (132–137, 139, 140, 143).

Symptoms and signs of low blood-glucose levels are several, including anxiety, nervousness, tremor, palpitations, sweating, pallor, clamminess, pupillary dilatation, hunger, borborygmi, nausea, confusion, changes in personality, irritability, fatigue, weakness, slurred speech, incoordination, paresthesiae, seizures, and loss of consciousness. These problems typically occur in an episodic fashion, such that affected patients complain of having "spells."

Traditionally, "Whipple's triad" (133) must be fulfilled for a diagnosis of bona fide hypoglycemia. It requires that case-specific symptoms and signs must be known to possibly be caused by low glucose levels; measured serum glucose must be below normal during a "spell"; and clinical complaints should be promptly and completely abolished by administration of intravenous or oral glucose. The laboratory definition of hypoglycemia is variable, but most observers agree that blood glucose levels of <60 mg/dL would qualify (144). Even more definitively, concomitantly normal or elevated serum values of insulin and/or proinsulin provide even more evidence for the presence of pathologic hypoglycemia (145).

Treatment of paraneoplastic hypoglycemia is rather difficult, if the responsible neoplasm cannot be ablated surgically or with other forms of treatment. Medical management includes administration of oral diazoxide (146) or octreotide (147), or both, as well as a diet that is rich in complex carbohydrates with frequent feedings.

Isolated tumor-related *hyper*glycemia appears to be much less frequent, probably because it is often asymptomatic. Underlying tumor types include NECs—again, favoring those that arise in the pancreas (148, 149)—as well as RCC (122), and, very rarely, non–small cell carcinoma of the lung. The mechanisms for elevation in blood glucose in such cases are much less well understood than those pertaining to paraneoplastic hypoglycemia. Pancreatic NECs synthesize glucagon (150)—a hyperglycemic peptide—but the hormonal mediators pertaining to other tumor types have been largely unstudied to date.

Symptoms and signs of tumor-related hyperglycemia parallel those of diabetes mellitus. If treatment is required, oral hypoglycemic agents or parenteral insulin are used.

"Carcinoid" Syndrome

As mentioned earlier in connection with cutaneous flushing, the "carcinoid" syndrome (CS) is associated with NECs virtually exclusively. In its complete form, in which facial and upper truncal erythema is accompanied by watery diarrhea, abdominal cramping, wheezing, and edema of the head and neck, CS typically is caused by NECs of the midgut—the portion of the intestinal tract from the ligament of Treitz to the mid-transverse colon (151). Moreover, those tumors must have metastasized to the liver (and possibly beyond as well), such that their vasoactive products can no longer be metabolized effectively by this organ. Much less commonly, tumors of the gonads—which are drained by caval rather than the portal venous system—also may produce the CS (152). Foregut and hindgut NECs may manifest with *partial* CS, but only extraordinarily demonstrate all of its constituents (153).

The underlying proposed mediators for the CS, and laboratory tests for them, have been discussed earlier in this chapter. In reality, more than one amine or peptide is probably operative in this context (154). From a radiographic perspective, imaging studies of the gut, pancreas, and liver are appropriate in such cases. The use of ^{111}In-pentetreotide scintigraphy or ^{123}I-metaiodobenzylguanidine (MIBG) scintigraphy is especially helpful, because these compounds localize themselves selectively in neuroendocrine tissues (Fig. 5) (155).

Two serious distant complications of CS may occur in some instances. The first concerns intimal sclerosis of medium-sized or large arteries, which is thought to be caused by vasoactive products of NECs. When it is located in a mesenteric vessel, this phenomenon may cause intestinal ischemia or even infarction (156). One extraordinary case, reported by Bourgault et al., also involved a patient with CS who developed coronary vasospasm as a consequence of the tumor (157). The second complication of CS also is cardiac in nature; namely, the evolution of right-sided valvular disease with fibroelastic scarring of the valve leaflets or cusps (Fig. 6). This process—termed "carcinoid heart disease"—yields tricuspid and pulmonic valvular orifices that are relatively fixed in size and shape, producing a combination of insufficiency and stenosis. Right-sided congestive heart failure may supervene (158–160).

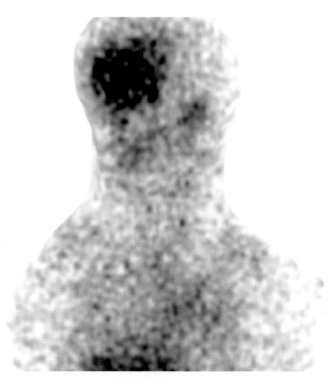

FIGURE 5 This MIBG (iodine-131-meta-iodobenzylguanidine) scintiscan was taken from a patient with neuroendocrine carcinoma of the lung. The radiotracer localizes in the cranial bones, corresponding to metastatic deposits.

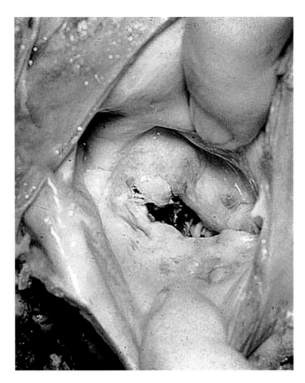

FIGURE 6 Carcinoid-induced valvular cardiac disease, showing partial fusion and fibrosis of the tricuspid valve leaflets.

Treatment of the CS may include surgical debulking of metastatic disease; chemo- or radioembolization of secondary lesions; alcohol-sclerotherapy, radioablation, or cryoablation of hepatic metastases; administration of MIBG, somatostatin analogs, or interferon-alpha; radiotherapy; or traditional chemotherapy with streptozotocin (151, 161). Patients with metastatic NEC in the setting of MCUO may have unexpectedly prolonged survivals, as discussed in other chapters in this book.

Verner-Morrison Syndrome

Vasoactive intestinal polypeptide (VIP) is also potentially synthesized by neuroendocrine tumors, particularly NECs (162). This mediator comprises 28 amino acids and acts to inhibit water and electrolyte absorption by the intestinal mucosa (142, 148, 162).

Pancreatic NECs are the most common source of tumor-related VIP production. The resulting clinico-pathologic complex, called the Verner-Morrison syndrome, features severe, persistent, watery diarrhea with associated hypokalemia and achlorhydria ("watery diarrhea-hypokalemia-achlorhydria syndrome") (142, 150, 162). Extreme dehydration may result, which explains another term for the syndrome; namely, "paraneoplastic cholera."

VIP can be measured in serum by radioimmunoassay to confirm the clinical diagnosis of the Verner-Morrison syndrome (163). Imaging studies of the pancreas and gut are recommended in MCUO cases for locating a primary tumor. Moreover, medullary carcinoma of the thyroid also may synthesize VIP, and lung carcinomas—both neuroendocrine and nonneuroendocrine—may do so as well. Some studies have suggested that VIP is a relatively common autocrine growth factor in the latter neoplasms (164).

The general treatment of VIP-producing tumors is comparable to that outlined for carcinoid tumors in the preceding section. Vigorous fluid replacement and potassium supplementation are also required (165).

Virilization and Feminization

Virilization in women and feminization in men are relatively uncommon forms of PS, and they commonly relate to an underlying steroid-producing carcinoma of the adrenal cortex or liver (80, 81, 166–168). Stromal tumors of the gonads are also a possibility, but these lesions do not enter this discussion of MCUO. More apropos to the topic being considered here, metastatic carcinomas affecting the ovaries may secondarily cause stromal hypersynthesis of sex hormones, producing the same results (169, 170).

Symptoms and signs of tumor-related virilization include hirsutism; facial acne (Fig. 7); menometrorrhagia, oligomenorrhea, or amenorrhea; and increased libido. Feminization is very rare in this context, and is typified by impotence, altered growth of facial hair, possible gynecomastia, and lessened sex drive (166–168).

Imaging of the abdomen by CT scanning or MRI characteristically demonstrates a large suprarenal mass in examples of adrenocortical carcinoma (Fig. 8). Measurement of sex steroids and their metabolites shows elevations thereof in the blood and urine, and serum levels of follicle-stimulating hormone and luteinizing hormone are usually conversely low (171, 172).

Chemotherapy of paraneoplastic feminization or virilization is again predicated on the use of o,p′-DDD, with or without cisplatin (173). Aromatase inhibitors may ameliorate the associated endocrinopathies; these agents include testolactone, anastrozole, letrozole, and fadrozole (174).

Isolated Gynecomastia

In males, isolated gynecomastia (Fig. 9) may be seen as a PS in MCUO cases, in the absence of other feminizing signs. This finding is seen in conjunction with carcinomas that synthesize beta-human chorionic gonadotrophin. These principally include not only germ-cell malignancies (175) but also somatic tumors such as non–small-cell carcinomas of the lung, transitional cell carcinoma of the bladder, adenocarcinoma of the stomach, and

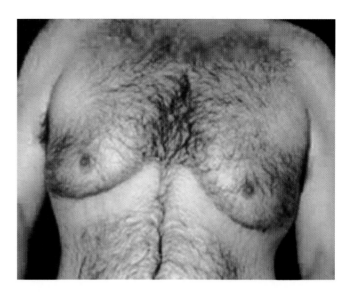

FIGURE 9 Gynecomastia is apparent in this 50-year-old man with transitional cell carcinoma of the bladder. The tumor secreted beta-human chorionic gonadotropin.

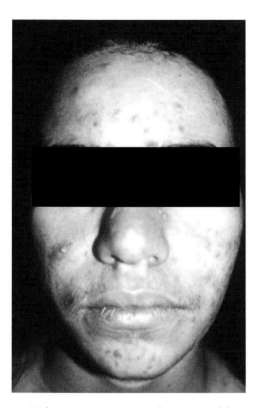

FIGURE 7 Virilization is apparent in this 31-year-old woman with adrenocortical carcinoma. She has male-pattern baldness and facial acne.

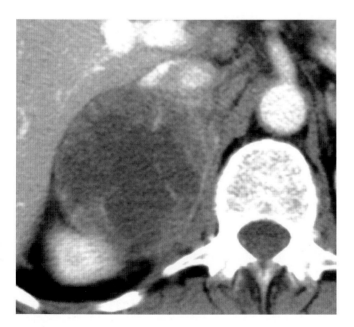

FIGURE 8 This CT scan, taken from the patient in Figure 7, demonstrates a large right suprarenal mass.

hepatocellular carcinoma (176–181). The diagnosis is confirmed by radioimmunoassay of serum for the peptide in question. Treatment of the gynecomastia is rarely undertaken in such cases.

Acromegaly

Ectopic acromegaly can be encountered as a PS, not only in cases involving NECs (usually of the foregut) but also with neuroendocrine and non-NECs of the lung, breast, and endometrium (182–194). This condition can be related either to tumor synthesis of growth hormone (GH) itself, or to growth hormone–releasing hormone (GHRH) (188, 192). Both of those eventualities are associated with increased serum levels of GH; however, in the second scenario (i.e., ectopic GHRH secretion), imaging studies of the pituitary may also demonstrate enlargement of the adenohypophysis. In contrast, it is normally sized when neoplastic synthesis of GH is applicable.

Symptoms and signs of ectopic acromegaly are identical to those attending the pituitary adenoma-driven form of the disorder (Fig. 10). They include coarsening of facial features; enlargement of the tongue, hands, and feet; arthritis; glucose intolerance or overt diabetes mellitus; hypertension; and cardiovascular disease, including cardiomyopathy and congestive heart failure (195). Laboratory assessment also may show hyperphosphatemia, hypercalciuria, and hypertriglyceridemia. ILGF-1 is commonly associated with elevations of GH, and high serum levels of the former marker can be used as an indirect indicator of disease severity (196).

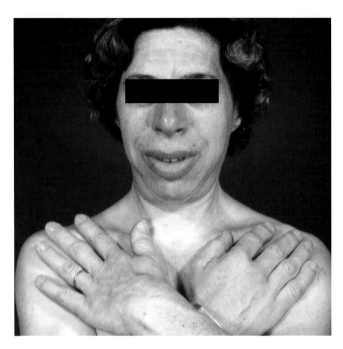

FIGURE 10 The changes of acromegaly are evident in this 52-year-old woman with a metastatic pancreatic neuroendocrine carcinoma. The tumor produced growth hormone–releasing hormone.

Treatment of this disorder is predicated on antineoplastic therapy for the underlying malignancy. When this is not feasible or is ineffective, palliative intervention with dopamine agonists and GH-blocking agents can be utilized. Those medications include bromocriptine, cabergoline, octreotide, and pegvisomant (197, 198).

Hypertension

Hypertension as a true PS is difficult to identify. This is because it is also seen as a complication of other tumor-related problems such as Cushing's syndrome and acromegaly. Furthermore, selected therapies can also produce elevations in blood pressure, and the psychic distress of some patients with MCUO may do so as well.

Only two neoplasms are directly associated with hypertension in a hormonal fashion; namely, adrenocortical carcinoma and RCC. The former may synthesize mineralocorticoids (aldosterone or related moieties), driving increased reabsorption of sodium and water by the kidneys (Conn's syndrome) (199). On the other hand, RCCs can produce either renin—a stimulant of aldosterone synthesis—or noradrenaline, raising blood pressure by either mechanism (200). Hypokalemia with alkalosis is a well-known clue to the diagnosis of aldosterone-mediated hypertension. Ultimately, however, measurements of renin, angiotensin, and aldosterone in the blood and urine are the most helpful, with and without

metoclopramide stimulation (201). A successful trial of spironolactone—an aldosterone inhibitor—may also provide corroborative diagnostic information if diastolic blood pressure decreases by at least 20 torr after the administration of the medication for a week (202). Imaging of the abdomen, perhaps necessitating angiographic examinations, can demonstrate the presence of adrenocortical or RCCs.

If antineoplastic therapy and the use of spironolactone or eplerenone (another aldosterone inhibitor) (203) are unsuccessful in reducing the blood pressure in patients with paraneoplastic hypertension and MCUO, other traditional antihypertensive medications are indicated. These include angiotensin–converting enzyme inhibitors, angiotensin receptor blockers, beta-blockers, centrally acting antihypertensives (e.g., clonidine), and potassium-sparing diuretics.

Nonneurologic and Nonhematologic Immunological Disorders

Immune dysfunction is another mechanism for the manifestation of PSs. Many disorders in this category affect the nervous system or skin, and they are considered in other sections of this chapter. Those that remain are discussed in the following sections.

Glomerulonephropathies

Several forms of glomerulopathy may be paraneoplastic in nature, the most prominent of which is membranous nephropathy (MN). This condition is the prototype of immune complex–mediated renal disease. In the specific context of MCUO, it is believed that tumor-specific antigens in selected cases idiosyncratically incite a humoral host response that culminates in the formation of circulating immune complexes (204–216). These then lodge in the glomerular basement membrane and compromise its integrity, such that passage of large macromolecules is allowed into the urine and glomerular damage accrues. Accordingly, tumor-related MN is associated with proteinuria, which may be severe (> 4 g in urine per 24 hours.) (211, 214). Renal biopsy demonstrates the classical findings of this condition (Fig. 11), without any nuances that would identify it as a PS. Indeed, the linkage between the kidney disease(s) in question and underlying malignancy is usually established in retrospect. Other symptoms and signs of the inciting tumor usually appear concurrently with proteinuria, and in cases where therapy is successful, they likewise subside contemporaneously (207, 217).

Clinical manifestations of MN relate to the loss of intravascular oncotic pressure; they principally include weight gain and dependent edema or anasarca. Associated

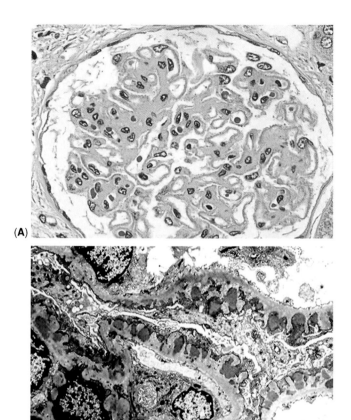

FIGURE 11 (**A**) Membranous nephropathy, seen in association with gastric adenocarcinoma. This glomerulus demonstrates subtle but definite thickening of its capillary basement membranes. (**B**) A corresponding electron micrograph shows subepithelial and intramembranous immune deposits in the capillary basement membrane. The nephropathy resolved after total gastrectomy.

carcinomas primarily occur in the lung and gastrointestinal tract, with less frequent tumor origin in the head and neck, kidney, and breast (211, 213). Other common epithelial malignancies, such as squamous carcinoma of the skin and adenocarcinoma of the endometrium, have only rarely been associated with MN (211, 218). However, virtually any carcinoma has the potential to cause this PS.

Other varieties of paraneoplastic renal disease include immunoglobulin A (IgA) nephropathy, rapidly progressive crescentic glomerulonephritis (RPGN), membranoproliferative glomerulonephritis, focal sclerosing glomerulonephropathy, and minimal-change disease (211, 213, 219–221). However, those disorders are much less common in this setting than is MN. Tumor antigens that have been implicated in the etiology of these disorders include carcinoembryonic antigen, prostate-specific antigen, renal-cell carcinoma–selective antigens, and other more nebulous tumor products (206, 208, 209, 212–215). All of these conditions are again principally characterized by proteinuria, with a similar immune complex–related pathogenesis.

The treatment of paraneoplastic glomerular disease is based on attempts at extirpating the underlying malignancy. Otherwise, interventions are palliative, including intravenous supplementation of plasma protein levels, administration of oral corticosteroids—possibly with tacrolimus or an alkylating agent (222)—and possible apheresis with plasma exchange for RPGN (223). Most of the time, patients with MCUO do not survive long enough for paraneoplastic nephropathies to become life limiting. Nevertheless, the latter conditions may add significantly to tumor-related morbidity.

Polymyositis, Systemic Lupus Erythematosus, Polyarthritis, and Systemic Sclerosis

Patients who are older than 45 years of age when they present with symptoms and signs of polymyositis, lupus, symmetrical polyarthritis, or scleroderma have a definite risk for causation of these conditions by an occult malignancy (224, 225). Carcinomas of the lungs, ovaries, kidneys, breasts, gastrointestinal tract, and nasopharynx have been implicated in that association (226–245), apropos to this discussion of MCUO.

The symptoms and signs of these paraneoplastic conditions are essentially the same as in their idiopathic versions (Figs. 12 and 13). However, the rapidity of disease progression in tumor-related rheumatologic disorders is often greater, and bone pain may be more prominent than in de novo polymyositis, lupus, or systemic sclerosis (241, 245).

The mechanisms for the neoplastic induction of the latter syndromes are largely speculative. It is thought that tumor-related antigens demonstrate sufficient structural homology to native proteins that autoimmunity is enabled (225, 238, 246).

Laboratory investigations may reveal circulating antibodies to single-stranded or double-stranded DNA, ribonucleoproteins, rheumatoid factor, nucleolar proteins, and muscle-related proteins (247). However, a recent study by Chinoy et al. (248) found that patients with paraneoplastic myositis often had negative results in "routine" laboratory testing for autoimmunity (for anti-Jo-1, -PM-Scl, -U1-RNP, -U3-RNP, -Ku antibodies). Moreover, in that analysis, the presence of antibodies against 155 and 140 kDa muscle proteins was common in paraneoplastic disease.

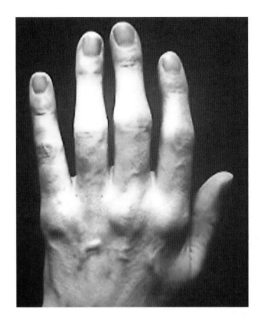

FIGURE 12 Symmetrical polyarthritis of the hands in a 49-year-old man with squamous cell carcinoma of the lung.

Treatment of the underlying carcinomas is predictably the primary approach to therapy of autoimmune PSs. The use of mycophenolate mofetil, corticosteroids, alkylating agents, and cyclosporine is also a possibility (249). Unfortunately, paraneoplastic rheumatologic syndromes appear to be more refractory to pharmacotherapy than their idiopathic counterparts (233).

Nonimmunological Rheumatologic Syndromes

Clubbing and HOA

HOA (Pierre Marie-Bamberger syndrome) is characterized by proliferation of the skin and osseous tissue in the distal extremities (Fig. 14) (250). HOA is, by far, most commonly associated with primary lung carcinomas (251–254), pulmonary infections, or right-to-left cardiac shunts. In patients with primary extrapulmonary carcinomas, it may also herald the presence of pulmonary metastases (255, 256). Clinical features of HOA include digital clubbing and periostosis of long tubular bones (Fig. 15) that is often painful and accompanied by synovial effusions. In some cases, the presenting symptom is a painful arthropathy that precedes clubbing and may be confused with inflammatory arthritis (251–254). In one study, clubbing was present in 29% of lung carcinoma patients (256a). This finding was more common in women than in men, and was more frequently seen in association with non–small-cell carcinoma as compared with small-cell lung cancer (256a).

The cause of HOA and digital clubbing is unknown. One explanation for nonneoplastic disorders could be the bypass of the pulmonary vascular bed by megakaryocytes and platelet clumps through right-to-left shunting, resulting in subsequent peripheral impaction of those elements and release of growth factors such as platelet-derived growth factor (256b). Alternatively, responsible tumors may secrete moieties that promote HOA, such as vascular endothelial growth factor (257), or inducers of bone morphogenetic protein and bone-derived growth factors (258). Effective ablation of the tumor or treatment of the other causes of HOA usually results in resolution of this problem (259, 260).

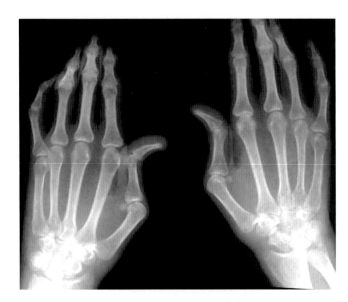

FIGURE 13 Bilateral mutilating arthritis in the small joints of the hands in a 55-year-old woman with ductal breast carcinoma.

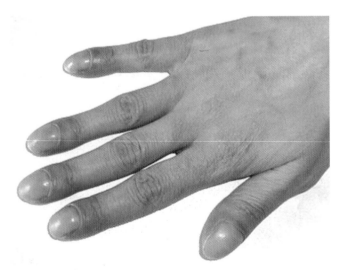

FIGURE 14 Digital clubbing of the distal fingers is apparent in this 58-year-old woman with adenocarcinoma of the lung.

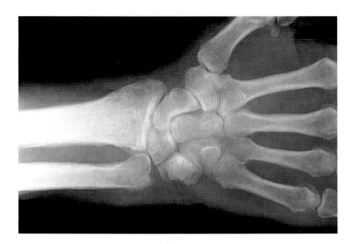

FIGURE 15 Hypertrophic osteoarthropathy of the distal radius in a 61-year-old woman with pulmonary adenocarcinoma. This disorder is reflected by proliferation of the bony cortex.

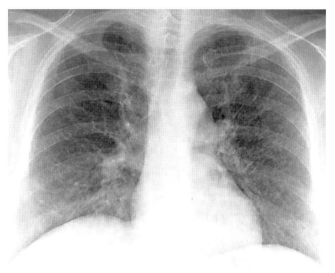

FIGURE 16 Nonspecific interstitial pneumonitis in a patient who had prior chemotherapy for small cell neuroendocrine carcinoma of the lung. Diffuse reticulonodular infiltrates are seen throughout the pulmonary interstitium.

Paraneoplastic Fasciitis-Polyarthritis

Some patients with primary carcinomas of the head and neck, gynecological tract, stomach, and breast may develop a rare PS featuring fasciitis in the distal extremities and polyarthritis (261–268). Flexion contractures may result from fibrosis of the fascia (269). Although an immunological mechanism for this process has been suggested, it has not been proven. Successful treatment of the underlying tumor may ameliorate the arthritic component of this syndrome, but usually not the fasciitis (265, 266).

Tumor-Associated Polymyalgia Rheumatica-Temporal Arteritis

Polymyalgia rheumatica (PR), in which marked proximal muscle weakness and limb girdle pain are present, may be associated with underlying carcinomas of the breast, kidney, colon, prostate, stomach, pancreas, and lung (241, 270–272). Symptoms and signs of temporal arteritis (headache, loss of visual acuity) also may be seen. The erythrocyte sedimentation rate is elevated in such cases, as are serum levels of C-reactive protein. However, no laboratory indicators of autoimmune disease are present.

Paraneoplastic PR should be suspected when the affected patients are < 50 years old, or when corticosteroid therapy of the condition is ineffective (271, 272). Symptoms and signs will persist unless the underlying tumor can be effectively treated (272).

Nonspecific Interstitial Pneumonitis

In rare cases of pulmonary carcinoma, patients may develop diffuse interstitial infiltrates throughout both lung fields (Fig. 16), accompanied by dyspnea and hypo-oxygenation with exercise. Biopsies of the lung parenchyma in such cases have shown a pattern of "nonspecific interstitial pneumonia" (273–275). Because the process is pan-pulmonary, rather than simply being limited to the tissue near the tumor, it is likely that the interstitial pneumonia represents a paraneoplastic response to the neoplasm. However, the cause is currently unclear, and no evidence of an autoimmune mechanism has been elucidated. Treatment with corticosteroids produces variable benefit (275).

Alimentary Tract–Related Paraneoplasias

Several paraneoplastic disorders principally affect the gut. Aside from the Verner-Morrison syndrome, as discussed earlier their etiologic mechanisms are undetermined at this point.

Sprue-Like Disorder

Very rarely, patients with a variety of carcinoma morphotypes may manifest a clinical syndrome simulating that of sprue (celiac disease) (276, 277). Symptoms and signs include weight loss, steatorrhea, and abdominal discomfort. Antibodies to gliadin and endomysial proteins may or may not be found through serologic testing in such cases, and radiographic studies show aberrations of the small intestinal mucosa (Fig. 17) (278, 279). Enforcement of a gluten-free diet has generally been effective in controlling this disorder, and doubts remain as to whether

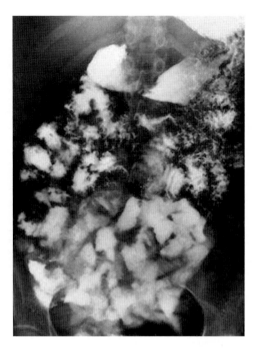

FIGURE 17 Barium follow-through study of the small intestine in a patient with breast carcinoma and new-onset malabsorption. This study shows irregular distribution of luminal barium, dilatation of the bowel lumen, and thickening of mucosal folds. A small-bowel biopsy demonstrated the changes of celiac disease.

it is actually paraneoplastic. The alternative is that true celiac disease has serendipitously developed in patients with carcinomas.

Protein-Losing Enteropathy

Selected cases of gastric or colonic carcinoma can be complicated by a protein-losing enteropathy (PLE), wherein excessive stool volumes are produced and a marked decrease is seen in plasma protein levels (280–283). The other main clinical manifestation of this disorder is peripheral edema. Alpha-1-antitrypsin in the stools is a helpful indicator of PLE (284). Mechanistically, some examples of this syndrome are possibly related to extensive lymphatic obstruction by tumor cell microemboli throughout the gut, or gross plasma seepage from an ulcerated neoplasm (281). In other instances, the pathogenesis of paraneoplastic PLE is uncertain. Symptomatic control of diarrhea, dietary protein supplementation, and intravenous administration of plasma comprise the therapeutic possibilities in this setting.

Pancreatic Fat Necrosis

In a small proportion of patients with primary pancreatic adenocarcinoma, indurated and tender subcutaneous nodules develop multifocally. These are usually concentrated over the extremities (Fig. 18) (285). In very rare cases, similar internal lesions develop in deep adipose tissues. Microscopically, such foci represent areas of liquefactive fat necrosis with secondary dystrophic calcification and minimal inflammation. The etiology of such lesions is vague. Some investigators believe that lipolytic enzymes, especially lipase, are released by the exocrine tissue around pancreatic carcinomas. These proteins enter lymphatics and are activated at distant anatomic locations including the skin (286). In some cases, however, cutaneous lesions are lacking, despite serum elevations of lipolytic enzymes; conversely, distant fat necrosis associated with pancreatic carcinoma may fail to show augmented circulating levels of lipase. Another explanatory hypothesis holds that tumor-related pancreatitis results in the release of cytokines such as TNF and interleukin-1 (287). These factors then activate neutrophils and endothelial cells, resulting in free radical generation and fat necrosis.

There is no effective direct therapy for the lesions of paraneoplastic fat necrosis. If the underlying pancreatic tumor can be ablated, they may become fibrotic and calcified, and the formation of new lesions will cease.

Collagenous Colitis

Examples of collagenous colitis have been reported in conjunction with colonic adenocarcinoma (288, 289). The latter condition typically presents itself with unremitting,

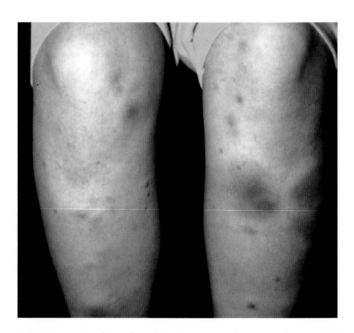

FIGURE 18 Tender, red, nodular lesions over the anterior legs in a 57-year-old woman with pancreatic carcinoma. Biopsy of the lesions showed fat necrosis in the subcutis.

watery, high-volume diarrhea, sometimes with abdominal cramping (290). Colon biopsies show an increase in intraepithelial lymphocytes, with or without a thickened subepithelial collagen mantle. Mucosal secretion of vascular endothelial growth factor, a fibrosis-enhancing peptide, has been increased in some cases of collagenous colitis (291). Symptomatic control of diarrhea may constitute sufficient treatment, along with therapy for the associated tumor. Corticosteroids and alkylating agents such as azathioprine have also been used to treat collagenous colitis (292).

Stauffer's Syndrome

Stauffer's syndrome is a rare paraneoplastic manifestation of RCC (293–296) [and, occasionally, with other tumors as well; e.g., prostatic adenocarcinoma (297)]. It is characterized by elevated serum levels of alkaline phosphatase, alpha-2-globulin, and gamma-glutamyl transferase; an increased erythrocyte sedimentation rate; thrombocytosis; prolongation of the prothrombin time, and enlargement of the liver and spleen in the absence of hepatic metastasis (294). Clinical cholestasis with jaundice may or may not be seen. The mechanism underlying these aberrations is unclear, although IL6 has been implicated as a possible mediator (298). If the underlying neoplasm can be effectively treated, all of the hepatic abnormalities will regress (295).

Hematologic Paraneoplasias

Hematologic abnormalities are among the most common paraneoplasias seen in clinical practice, although several of them may be relatively asymptomatic. Moreover, some overlap exists between hematologic abnormalities that are straightforward complications of malignancy (e.g., intestinal blood loss from an ulcerated colonic carcinoma, causing anemia; anemia of chronic disease in carcinoma cases with protracted courses; leukocytosis as a reflection of sepsis, etc.) and others that have more complex etiologies.

Aplastic Anemia

Marrow aplasia is, of course, most commonly encountered in oncology patients as a consequence of cytoablative chemotherapy. However, it may also be seen as a paraneoplastic condition, usually in association with carcinomas of the lung in reference to epithelial malignancies (299–302). The usual clinical symptoms and signs of pancytopenia are present in such cases, and bone marrow biopsies disclose a virtually acellular picture. Treatment may be tried with exogenous synthetic hematopoietic growth factors, but transfusion support is typically required, with concomitant chelation therapy. Antithymocyte globulin, cyclosporine, corticosteroids, and androgenic steroids may also be employed (303).

The mechanism of this condition is unknown. It may be true that certain tumor types share antigenic structures that are similar to those of hematopoietic elements, leading to an autoimmune response against the marrow by the host. However, this explanation is purely speculative.

Autoimmune Hemolytic Anemia

Autoimmune hemolytic anemia [AIHA; immune spherocytic anemia (Fig. 19)] is usually a paraneoplastic complication of non-Hodgkin's lymphoma (304). However, it may arise in association with solid tumors as well in selected instances (305, 305). Sokol et al. assessed 160 examples of this conjunction (307). They found that underlying neoplasms included carcinomas of the lung, breast, colon and rectum, and prostate; adenocarcinomas, squamous carcinomas, transitional cell carcinomas, and undifferentiated carcinomas were all represented. The operative autoantibodies included warm-acting moieties (usually of the IgG isotype), cold-acting immunoglobulins (usually IgM), and a mixture of the two, in individual cases.

Interestingly, because the tumor types just cited are relatively common, Sokol et al. tested the hypothesis that these neoplasms might be linked with AIHA merely through coincidence (307). However, that presumption was not affirmed by statistical analysis. It was concluded that erythrocyte autoantibodies were associated in a truly causal fashion with selected carcinomas, probably as a

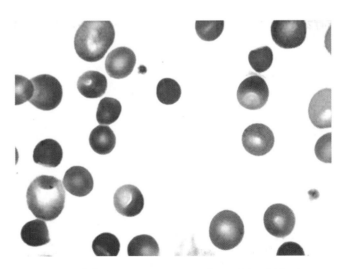

FIGURE 19 Spherocytes are present in this peripheral blood smear, taken from a 71-year-old man with squamous cell carcinoma of the lung and warm-acting autoimmune hemolytic anemia. The latter disorder was felt to be paraneoplastic.

reflection of systemic immune dysregulation. AIHA showed a preferential linkage with large tumor masses and metastatic disease, and had a poor prognosis in that setting.

Treatment of the anemia may require the use of corticosteroids or alkylating agents, splenectomy, or apheresis (308). Symptomatic blood transfusions are commonly ineffective because of accelerated erythrocyte loss.

Schistocytic (Microangiopathic) Anemias

Some carcinomas—usually of the stomach, breasts, pancreas, ovaries, colon, lungs, and prostate—may cause paraneoplastic thrombocytopenic purpura (PTTP), with circulating schistocytic erythrocytes (Fig. 20) and anemia (309–320). Other manifestations include neurologic abnormalities, fever, and renal dysfunction. Schistocyte formation may occur because the tumors in question demonstrate extensive vascular micrometastasis with endothelial disruption (320a). Alternatively, PTTP may be another autoimmune condition that is induced by a host response to an underlying neoplasm. In the idiopathic form of thrombotic thrombocytopenic purpura, autoantibody inhibitors of the ADAMTS13 metalloprotease are present (321). The latter enzyme is responsible for cleaving von Willebrand factor in nascent thrombi; accordingly, ADAMTS13 deficiency allows microthrombosis to proceed unchecked (322). It then causes microangiopathic hemolysis, thrombocytopenia, and multifocal tissue microinfarction.

Treatment is predicated on therapy for the underlying malignancy (322a), as well as administration of corticosteroid or rituximab (an anti-B-lymphocyte antibody) and serial plasma exchange (323–325). The last of these interventions is probably effective because it reduces the level of circulating anti-ADAMTS13 and replenishes the corresponding protease (325). Platelet transfusions should be avoided because they contribute to worsened microthrombosis in PTTP.

Another cause of schistocytic anemia in patients with MCUO is the presence of chronic compensated disseminated intravascular coagulation (DIC).

Leukocytosis and Leukemoid Reactions

Leukemoid reactions (LRs) represent reactive forms of leukocytosis in which >50,000 white cells/µL are present in circulation, with or without immature forms (Fig. 21) (326). They may be related to infection, systemic inflammatory disorders, or the use of therapeutic growth factors. Uncommonly, LRs also can be paraneoplastic in nature, in association with carcinomas, sarcomas, melanomas, or lymphomas (327–331). With specific reference to MCUO, leukocyte counts above 10,000/µL have been found in 15% of patients with pulmonary carcinomas, and other tumors, such as RCC, cholangiocarcinoma, pancreatic carcinoma, squamous carcinoma of the uterine cervix or head and neck, urothelial carcinomas, and nasopharyngeal carcinoma, may likewise produce such a finding (328). In some cases, concurrent hypercalcemia is also observed, especially with squamous cancers of the

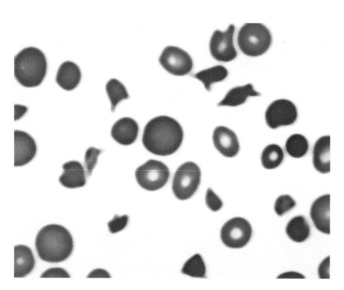

FIGURE 20 Numerous schistocytes are seen in this peripheral blood smear in a 51-year-old woman with metastatic breast carcinoma and clinical thrombotic thrombocytopenic purpura.

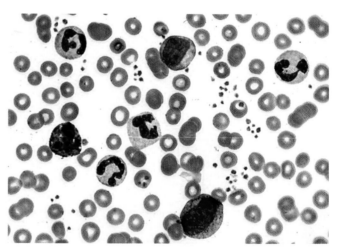

FIGURE 21 A "leukemoid" reaction is seen in this peripheral blood smear, including immature leukocytes and leukocytosis. The patient was a 65-year-old woman with ovarian serous adenocarcinoma.

oropharynx/larynx or lung. LRs are believed to be caused by tumoral synthesis or induction of granulocyte colony-stimulating factor, whereas associated elevations in calcium relate to neoplastic synthesis of PTHrP.

Extreme leukocytosis in the context of MCUO may be problematic with regard to an alternative diagnostic consideration of acute leukemia. The leukocyte alkaline phosphatase score is effective in excluding the latter possibility, inasmuch as it is high in LR and low in leukemia (332). Another difficulty concerns leukocytosis as a possible marker of sepsis, and this eventuality can only be eliminated by clinical correlation and procurement of blood cultures.

Generally speaking, patients with LR are asymptomatic in reference to that problem. However, if the white blood-cell count is extremely high (>25,000/μL), symptoms and signs of circulatory hyperviscosity may appear. These include neurologic impairments, priapism, and ischemic changes in the peripheral extremities in patients with preexisting vascular disease (333, 334). In these circumstances, cytoreductive leukapheresis may be necessary as a therapy (335); otherwise, treatment of the underlying tumor is the principal focus of management.

Thrombocytosis and Erythrocytosis

Elevations in the circulating platelet count at a level >400,000/μL fulfill the criterion for a diagnosis of thrombocytosis (336). In similarity to LRs, underlying carcinomas may be associated with this problem as well. In particular, malignant epithelial tumors of the liver, kidney, lung, and urothelial tract are best represented in this context (336, 337). Mesotheliomas also have been associated with thrombocytosis in as many as 70% of cases in some series (338). Clinical issues attending elevations in the platelet count are comparable to those discussed in reference to LRs; specifically, hyperviscosity and intravascular thrombosis are the principal concerns. Ectopic tumor-related production of thrombopoietin or IL6, or both, is felt to be the responsible mechanism in paraneoplastic thrombocytosis (339).

Therapeutic thrombopheresis may be required to reduce the platelet count. Interestingly, in patients with thrombocytosis and RCC, Blay et al. also found that daily treatment with an anti-IL6 antibody was effective in normalizing the number of circulating platelets (340).

Erythrocytosis (polycythemia) is defined by the presence of an elevated hematocrit in patients with normal blood volumes and in the absence of heavy tobacco use. It is an uncommon PS, being principally linked to RCC and hepatocellular carcinoma (340a, 340b). Both neoplasms have the potential to synthesize erythropoietin (340b, 340c), driving an increased production of erythrocytes by the bone marrow. Rarely, other tumors, such as gastric adenocarcinoma, pancreatic islet cell carcinoma, and ovarian adenocarcinomas (340d–340f), also have been associated with paraneoplastic erythrocytosis.

Treatment of this condition is necessary only if the red cell mass becomes so dense that circulation is compromised. Periodic phlebotomy is the simplest intervention.

Eosinophilia and Basophilia

Eosinophils and basophils normally account for only a small minority of circulating granulocytic leukocytes (5%). In association with some carcinomas, however, the numbers of these cellular elements are increased in the peripheral blood. Paraneoplastic eosinophilia has been linked principally to carcinomas of the lung, liver, stomach, and thyroid (341–351). Tissue infiltration of other organs by eosinophils may be present in this setting (342, 352). It appears that tumor production of interleukin-5 (IL5) may be the main causal element in paraneoplastic eosinophilia (341, 345).

Paraneoplastic basophilia seems to be associated narrowly with lung carcinomas, among all epithelial malignancies (353). The pathogenetic underpinning of this finding is unclear.

Tumor-related eosinophilia and basophilia may produce secondary symptoms and signs that simulate atopy. Urticaria, eczema, bronchospasm, and diarrhea can be seen (354). Treatment of these conditions centers on ablation of the underlying tumors, but may also include administration of antihistamines, cromolyn, and antibodies to IL5.

Immune Thrombocytopenia

Immune thrombocytopenia (ITP), with the appearance of spontaneous cutaneous petechiae and purpura (Fig. 22), is a well-known complication of malignant lymphoreticular disease, especially being connected to chronic lymphocytic leukemia/small-lymphocytic lymphoma and lymphoplasmacytic lymphoma (355). However, it has been observed in association with carcinomas as well, most often originating in the ovaries, lungs, breasts, or kidneys (356–363). Bellucci et al. have described a case in which ITP was also associated with Graves' disease and ovarian carcinoma (364). As mentioned above in connection with AIHA, the truly paraneoplastic nature of ITP linked to epithelial tumors is uncertain, as opposed to the alternate explanation that the two conditions are coincidental. Treatment for cancer-related ITP is the same as in cases of idiopathic ITP, being predicated on corticosteroids and possibly splenectomy for patients who are refractory to medical management (365). Tsoussis et al. (358) also found low-dose interferons to be an effective therapy in this setting.

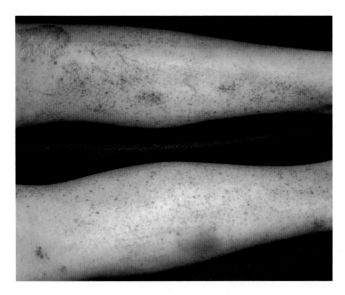

FIGURE 22 Numerous petechiae are present in the skin of the legs in this 49-year-old man with gastric adenocarcinoma. Antibodies to platelet-related proteins were present in laboratory tests.

Hypercoagulability (Trousseau's Syndrome)

One of the best known of the paraneoplasias associated with carcinomas is hypercoagulability (366), potentially leading to a variety of adverse thrombotic–embolic events. These include deep venous thrombosis with pulmonary thromboembolism (Fig. 23), marantic endocarditis with secondary arterial embolism, phlegmasia cerulea dolens (Fig. 24), phlegmasia alba dolens, and superficial migratory thrombophlebitis (367–381). Together, these problems are usually considered under the rubric of Trousseau's syndrome (TS) (366), and application of the Bradford-Hill guidelines for causation has affirmed the validity of this practice (382).

The relationship between specific malignancies and TS was examined by Ogren et al. by logistic regression in a postmortem study (383). The overall prevalence of pulmonary embolism was 23% among those autopsies; they represented 84% of all hospital deaths in Sweden during a 12-year period. The tumors that were most strongly associated with TS included carcinomas of the pancreas, gallbladder, stomach, colon, and lung. However, virtually any primary tumor type may be responsible. Adenocarcinomas had a stronger linkage with hypercoagulability than did squamous carcinomas. Similar results were obtained in another analysis by Naschitz et al. (382).

It has been suggested that the causation of TS relates to the release of tissue factor (a trigger of the extrinsic coagulation cascade) by neoplastic cells, in microvesicular form or associated with tumoral mucin production (384–387). Thrombotic or embolic events may occur months or even years before the underlying malignancy becomes clinically evident (388).

Treatment of paraneoplastic hypercoagulability relies on therapy for the underlying tumor, together with the continuous use of anticoagulant medications. These include low-molecular-weight heparin and lepirudin (389–392); coumadin is generally not effective in this specific setting and is not recommended (387, 391).

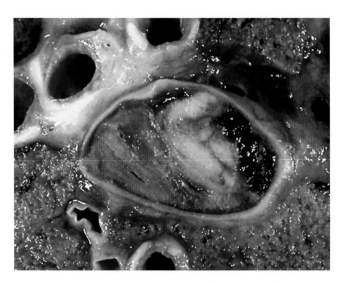

FIGURE 23 A large central laminated pulmonary thromboembolism is seen at autopsy in this 81-year-old man with pancreatic adenocarcinoma and Trousseau's syndrome.

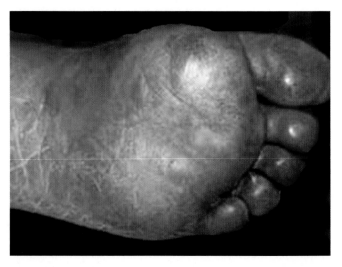

FIGURE 24 Phlegmasia cerulea dolens of the left foot in a 62-year-old woman with squamous lung carcinoma and Trousseau's syndrome. The distal extremity was blue, cold, and pulseless; a thrombus was found in the left common iliac artery.

Chronic Compensated ("Smoldering") DIC

A related problem is that of chronic compensated DIC. This condition shares with TS the potential for association with a wide variety of carcinoma morphotypes. However, carcinomas of the prostate, lung, stomach, colon, and breast are most frequently seen in this context among all solid tumors (393–396). Adenocarcinomas are again overrepresented. Carcinomas may cause DIC through the disruption of endothelial surfaces by metastases, tumoral release of tissue factor, and direct activation of the prothrombinase complex (393, 394).

Systemic signs and symptoms of DIC may include fever, hypoxia, acidosis, petechiae or purpura, hypotension, and proteinuria, potentially simulating other problems such as sepsis. Ongoing visceral microthrombosis (Fig. 25) may lead to failure of various organs, culminating in renal failure, pulmonary insufficiency, and neurologic dysfunction.

Laboratory findings in DIC include thrombocytopenia, schistocytic anemia, the presence of circulating fibrin monomer, or D-dimer, or both, and prolonged prothrombin and activated partial thromboplastin times (397). Other abnormalities are represented by increased levels of thrombin–antithrombin complexes, elevated plasminogen activator inhibitor type-1 levels, and decreased factor VII–related clotting activity (398, 399).

Therapy once again should be centered on the responsible neoplasm, in addition to administration of heparin or recombinant hirudin (390). Infusions of antithrombin-III or protein C may be used but have not yet been validated systematically. Replacement of blood components is indicated only if significant bleeding is part of the clinical picture, and it should be implemented with caution.

Monoclonal Gammopathies and Amyloidosis

The association between plasmacytic myeloma or non-Hodgkin's lymphomas and paraproteinemias or systemic amyloidosis is well known (400–402). However, selected carcinomas are also linked with the latter conditions. These include RCC, which is by far the most common amyloid-related solid tumor, as well as carcinomas of the lung, stomach, bowel, and breast (403–415). Rarely, other epithelial neoplasms have been linked to amyloidosis or paraprotein production in an anecdotal fashion as well (412, 415).

The process whereby RCC and other carcinomas induce amyloid formation is still unclear. It is felt that the tumor cells in some way transmogrify precursors of AA amyloid (e.g., C-reactive protein) and cause it to be deposited throughout the body. The distribution of carcinoma-related disease is that of "secondary" amyloidosis, principally affecting the kidneys, liver, spleen, lymph nodes, gut, and adrenal glands (Figs. 26 and 27). Similarly, mechanisms linking monoclonal gammopathies, including IgG, IgA, and IgM, to underlying epithelial tumors are rather mysterious, and the possibility once again exists that

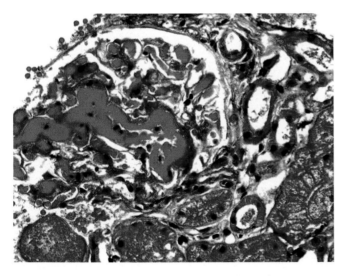

FIGURE 25 A microthrombus is present in a glomerulus in a patient with prostatic adenocarcinoma and tumor-related disseminated intravascular coagulation.

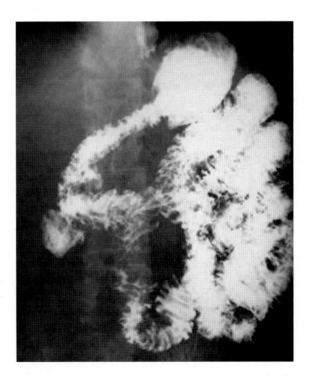

FIGURE 26 Thickened intestinal plicae are present in this barium "follow-through" study of the small bowel in a patient with malabsorption and renal cell carcinoma. Biopsy of the intestine demonstrated amyloid deposition.

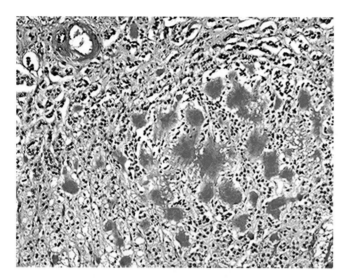

FIGURE 27 Adrenocortical deposits of amyloid are seen with the Congo red stain, in an autopsy slide taken from a 74-year-old man with renal cell carcinoma.

this relationship may be coincidental. Complications such as hyperviscosity syndromes have not been reported in this particular setting, but cryoglobulinemia has been observed in selected cases as a byproduct of paraproteinemia (Fig. 28) (416, 417).

Treatment of carcinoma-related paraproteinemias and amyloidosis is supportive. If the underlying neoplasm can be eradicated, the latter problems may cease.

Cardiovascular Paraneoplasias

Disorders of the blood vessels and heart are not uncommon in oncology patients. Many of them are the byproduct of therapeutic interventions with such agents as anthracyclines, 5-fluorouracil, trastuzumab, and interleukin-2 (418–422). In addition, carcinomatous pericarditis or metastasis to the myocardium can contribute to cardiovascular compromise in this setting (423). However, rare cases do appear to represent true paraneoplasias in association with solid tumors.

Myocarditis, particularly of the granulomatous type, and dilated cardiomyopathy have been observed as a complication of neuroendocrine, breast, and lung carcinomas (424–428). The pathogenesis of this linkage is uncertain, but it is felt to generically represent an immunologic response to antigenic determinants that are shared between the tumor cells and the myocardium. Symptoms and signs are those of cardiac insufficiency with cardiomegaly (Fig. 29), a lessened cardiac ejection fraction, pulmonary edema, peripheral edema, and elevated plasma levels of brain natriuretic peptide (BNP) and amino-terminal-proBNP (429).

Various forms of vasculitis have been reported as paraneoplastic phenomena as well. The most common of them is cutaneous leukocytoclastic vasculitis, which is considered in detail in the section in this chapter on paraneoplastic lesions of the skin. Larger-vessel lesions, such as polyarteritis nodosa, Wegener's granulomatosis, and giant cell arteritis, are additional possibilities (430–437). In paraneoplastic polyarteritis cases, the most common sites for primary carcinomas are the lung,

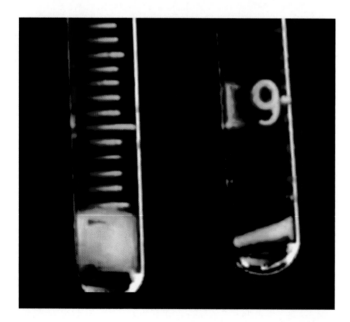

FIGURE 28 A positive "cryocrit" test (*left*) is compared with a control preparation (*right*). The specimen came from a patient with adenocarcinoma of the lung and clinical findings consistent with paraneoplastic cryoglobulinemia. The responsible paraprotein was monoclonal IgM.

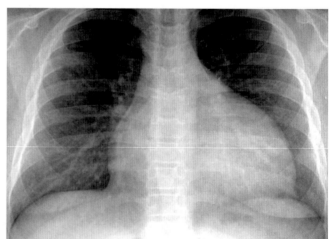

FIGURE 29 This chest radiograph was taken from a 67-year-old man with pancreatic adenocarcinoma and heart failure. Cardiomegaly is apparent. At autopsy, changes of dilated cardiomyopathy were found, with no other explanation than that of a paraneoplastic disorder.

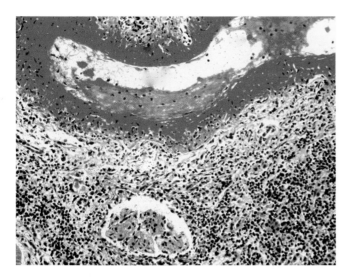

FIGURE 30 Polyarteritis nodosa is seen in a large intrarenal artery at autopsy. The patient was a 63-year-old woman with metastatic ductal breast carcinoma.

stomach, bile ducts, kidney (Fig. 30), and oropharynx–hypopharynx. Tumor-related Wegener's granulomatosis has been linked principally to carcinomas of the lungs and stomach. The diagnosis of vasculitis antedates that of malignancy in most cases. Symptoms and signs are related to the particular visceral organ sites for the vasculitic lesions. There are no laboratory markers for polyarteritis, but Wegener's granulomatosis is accompanied by autoantibodies to neutrophil cytoplasmic antigens in a high proportion of cases (430–432).

In addition to treatment of the responsible neoplasms, the therapy for cardiac and vasculitic complications of MCUO is comparable to that for the idiopathic versions of these disorders. It includes the use of corticosteroids or alkylating agents (438) and, when necessary, inotropic medications, diuretics, and inhibitors of angiotensin-converting enzyme (439).

■ REFERENCES

1. Lortholary A, Cossee M, Gamelin E, Larra F. Paraneoplastic syndromes. *Bull Cancer* 1993; 80:280–93.
2. DeLellis RA, Xia L. Paraneoplastic endocrine syndromes. *Endocr Pathol* 2003; 14:303–17.
3. Thomas L, Kwok Y, Edelman MJ. Management of paraneoplastic syndromes in lung cancer. *Curr Treat Options Oncol* 2004; 5:51–62.
4. Mitnick HJ. Paraneoplastic rheumatic syndromes. *Curr Rheumatol Rep* 2000; 2:163–70.
5. Kodousek R, Tichy T. Pathology of paraneoplastic syndromes. *Cesk Patol* 2000; 36:116–22.
6. Posner JB, Dalmau JO. Paraneoplastic syndromes of the nervous system. *Clin Chem Lab Med* 2000; 38:117–22.
7. Thomas CR, Wright CD, Loehrer PJ Jr. Thymoma: state of the art. *J Clin Oncol* 1999; 17:2280–9.
8. Zumsteg MM, Casperson DS. Paraneoplastic syndromes in metastatic disease. *Semin Oncol Nurs* 1998; 14:220–9.
9. Dropcho EJ. Principles of paraneoplastic syndromes. *Ann NY Acad Sci* 1998; 841:246–61.
10. Staszewski H. Hematological paraneoplastic syndromes. *Semin Oncol* 1997; 24:329–33.
11. Odell WD. Endocrine/metabolic syndromes of cancer. *Semin Oncol* 1997; 24:299–317.
12. Itin PH, Buchner SA, Pittelkow MR. Mucocutaneous paraneoplastic disorders. *Dev Ophthalmol* 1997; 28:73–85.
13. Kavanaugh DY, Carbone DP. Immunologic dysfunction in cancer. *Hematol Oncol Clin North Am* 1996; 10:927–51.
14. Agarwala SS. Paraneoplastic syndromes. *Med Clin North Am* 1996; 80:173–84.
15. Anderson NE. The immunobiology and clinical features of paraneoplastic syndromes. *Curr Opin Neurol* 1995; 8:424–9.
16. Szekanecz E, Andras C, Sandor Z, et al. Malignancies and soluble tumor antigens in rheumatic diseases. *Autoimmun Rev* 2006; 6:42–7.
17. Minotti AM, Kountakis SE, Stiernberg, CM. Paraneoplastic syndromes in patients with head and neck cancer. *Am J Otolaryngol* 1994; 15:336–43.
18. Aniszewski JP, Young WF Jr, Thompson GB, Grant CS, van Heerden JA. Cushing syndrome due to ectopic adrenocorticotropic hormone secretion. *World J Surg* 2001; 25:934–40.
19. Ogilvie GK. Paraneoplastic syndromes. *Vet Clin North Am Equine Pract* 1998; 14:439–49.
20. Turek MM. Cutaneous paraneoplastic syndromes in dogs and cats: a review of the literature. *Vet Dermatol* 2003; 14:279–96.
21. Finora K. Common paraneoplastic syndromes. *Clin Tech Small Anim Pract* 2003; 18:123–6.
22. Ruslander D, Page R. Perioperative management of paraneoplastic syndromes. *Vet Clin North Am Small Anim Pract* 1995; 25:47–62.
23. Feldman BF, Ruehl WW. Laboratory aspects of cancer. *Mod Vet Pract* 1984; 65:771–3.
24. Aronsohn MG, Schunk KL, Carpenter JL, King NW. Clinical and pathologic features of thymoma in 15 dogs. *J Am Vet Med Assoc* 1984; 184:1355–62.
25. Morrison WB. Paraneoplastic syndromes of the dog. *J Am Vet Med Assoc* 1979; 175:559–61.
26. Zini E, Glaus TM, Minuto F, et al. Paraneoplastic hypoglycemia due to an insulin-like growth factor type-II secreting hepatocellular carcinoma in a dog. *J Vet Intern Med* 2007; 21:193–5.
27. Battaglia L, Petterino C, Zappulli V, Castagnaro M. Hypoglycemia as a paraneoplastic syndrome associated with renal adenocarcinoma in a dog. *Vet Res Commun* 2005; 29:671–5.
28. Swain JM, Pirie RS, Hudson NP, et al. Insulin-like growth factors and recurrent hypoglycemia associated with renal cell carcinoma in a horse. *J Vet Intern Med* 2005; 19:613–6.
29. Moore AS, Nelson RW, Henry CJ, et al. Streptozotocin for treatment of pancreatic islet cell tumors in dogs: 17 cases (1989–1999). *J Am Vet Med Assoc* 2002; 15:811–8.
30. Bertazzolo W, Comazzi S, Roccabianca P, Caniatti M. Hypercalcemia associated with a retroperitoneal apocrine gland adenocarcinoma in a dog. *J Small Anim Pract* 2003; 44:221–4.
31. Anderson TE, Legendre AM, McEntee MM. Probable hypercalcemia of malignancy in a cat with bronchogenic adenocarcinoma. *J Am Anim Hosp Assoc* 2000; 36:52–5.
32. Dole RS, MacPhail CM, Lappin MR. Paraneoplastic leukocytosis with mature neutrophilia in a cat with pulmonary squamous cell carcinoma. *J Feline Med Surg* 2004; 6:391–5.

33. Peeters D, Clercx C, Thiry A, et al. Resolution of paraneoplastic leukocytosis and hypertrophic osteopathy after resection of a renal transitional cell carcinoma producing granulocyte-macrophage colony-stimulating factor in a young Bull terrier. *J Vet Intern Med* 2001; 15:407–11.

34. Hogan DF, Dhaliwal RS, Sisson DD, Kitchell BE. Paraneoplastic thrombocytosis-induced systemic thromboembolism in a cat. *J Am Anim Hosp Assoc* 1999; 35:483–6.

35. Lennox TJ, Wilson JH, Hayden DW, et al. Hepatoblastoma with erythrocytosis in a young female horse. *J Am Vet Med Assoc* 2000; 216:718–21.

36. Zini E, Bovero A, Nigrisoli E, et al. Sarcomatoid renal cell carcinoma with osteogenic differentiation and paraneoplastic hepatopathy in a dog, possibly related to human Stauffer's syndrome. *J Comp Pathol* 2003; 129:303–7.

37. Knockaert DC, Vanneste LJ, Vanneste SB, et al. Fever of unknown origin in the 1980s: an update of the diagnostic spectrum. *Arch Intern Med* 1992; 152:51–5.

38. Dinarello CA, Bunn PA Jr. Fever. *Semin Oncol* 1997; 24: 288–98.

39. Drenth JP, de Kleijn EH, de Mulder Ph, van der Meer JW. Metastatic breast cancer presenting as fever, rash, and arthritis. *Cancer* 1995; 75:1608–11.

40. Schmid HP, Szabo J. Renal cell carcinoma—a current review. *Schweiz Rundsch Med Prax* 1997; 86:837–43.

41. Stratey S. A paraneoplastic syndrome in patients with carcinoma of the upper urinary tract. *Khirurgiia* 1997; 50:10–1.

42. Gold PJ, Fefer A, Thompson JA. Paraneoplastic manifestations of renal cell carcinoma. *Semin Urol Oncol* 1996; 14:216–22.

43. Talcott JA, Siegel RD, Finberg R, et al. Risk assessment in cancer patients with fever and neutropenia: a prospective, two-center validation of a prediction rule. *J Clin Oncol* 1992; 10: 316–22.

44. Tsavaris N, Zinelis A, Tsoutsos H, Kosmidis P. The response of paraneoplastic fever of lymphomas and solid tumors to the administration of naproxen. *J Intern Med* 1991; 230:549–50.

45. Zell JA, Chang JC. Neoplastic fever: a neglected paraneoplastic syndrome. *Support Care Cancer* 2005; 13:870–7.

46. Penel N, Fournier C, Clisant S, N'Guyen M. Causes of fever and value of C-reactive protein and procalcitonin in differentiating infections from paraneoplastic fever. *Support Care Cancer* 2004; 12:593–8.

47. Penel N, Fournier C, Degardin M, Kouto H, N'Guyen M. Fever and solid tumor: diagnostic value of procalcitonin and C-reactive protein. *Rev Med Interne* 2001; 22:706–14.

48. Kettaneh A, Fain O, Stirnemann J, Thomas M. Taste disorders. *Rev Med Interne* 2002; 23:622–31.

49. Nakazato Y, Abe T, Tamura N, Shimazu K. Sweetness dysgeusia in a case of SIADH caused by lung carcinoma. *Riinsho Shinkeigaku (Clin Neurol)* 2006; 46:418–20.

50. Panayiotou H, Small SC, Hunter JH, Culpepper RM. Sweet taste (dysgeusia): the first symptom of hyponatremia in small cell carcinoma of the lung. *Arch Intern Med* 1995; 155: 1325–8.

51. Croghan CL, Salik RM. Undiagnosed lung cancer presenting with dysgeusia. *Am J Emerg Med* 2003; 21:604–5.

52. Duncan WC, Fenske NA. Cutaneous signs of internal disease in the elderly. *Geriatrics* 1990; 45:24–30.

53. Stadie V, Marsch WC. Itching attacks with generalized hyperhidrosis as initial symptoms of Hodgkin's disease. *J Eur Acad Dermatol Venereol* 2003; 17:559–61.

54. Kleyn CE, Lai-Cheong JE, Bell HK. Cutaneous manifestations of internal malignancy: diagnosis and management. *Am J Clin Dermatol* 2006; 7:71–84.

55. Giannakos G, Papanicolaou X, Trafalis D, et al. Stauffer's syndrome variant associated with renal cell carcinoma. *Int J Urol* 2005; 12:757–9.

56. Bernstein JE, Whitney DH, Soitani K. Inhibition of histamine-induced pruritus by topical tricyclic antidepressants. *J Am Acad Dermatol* 1981; 5:582–5.

57. Rivard J, Lim HW. Ultraviolet phototherapy for pruritus. *Dermatol Ther* 2005; 18:344–54.

58. Ottery FD. Cancer cachexia: prevention, early diagnosis, and management. *Cancer Pract* 1994; 2:123–31.

59. Richardson GE, Johnson BE. Paraneoplastic syndromes in lung cancer. *Curr Opin Oncol* 1992; 4:323–33.

60. van Eys J. Nutrition and cancer: physiological interrelationships. *Annu Rev Nutr* 1985; 5:435–61.

61. Hernandez-Hernandez JL, Matorras-Galan P, Riancho-Moral JA, Gonzalez-Macias J. Etiologic spectrum of solitary constitutional syndrome. *Rev Clin Esp* 2002; 202:367–74.

62. Palapattu GS, Kristo B, Rajfer J. Paraneoplastic syndromes in urologic malignancy: the many faces of renal cell carcinoma. *Rev Urol* 2002; 4:163–70.

63. Inui A. Cancer anorexia-cachexia syndrome: current issues in research and management. *CA Cancer J Clin* 2002; 52:72–91.

64. Bruera E. Anorexia, cachexia, and nutrition. *Br Med J* 1997; 315: 1219–22.

65. Woods SC, Seeley RJ, Porte D Jr, et al. Signals that regulate food intake and energy homeostasis. *Science* 1998; 280:1378–83.

66. Schwartz JW, Woods SC, Porte D Jr, et al. Central nervous system control of food intake. *Nature* 2000; 404:661–71.

67. Kalra SP, Dube MG, Pu S, et al. Interacting appetite-regulating pathways in the hypothalamic regulation of body weight. *Endocrinol Rev* 1999; 20:68–100.

68. Marks DL, Ling N, Cone RD. Role of the central melanocortin system in cachexia. *Cancer Res* 2001; 61:1432–8.

69. Lechan RM, Tatro JB. Hypothalamic melanocortin signaling in cachexia. *Endocrinology* 2001; 142:3288–91.

70. Cardona D. Pharmacological therapy of cancer anorexia-cachexia. *Nutr Hosp* 2006; 21(Suppl. 3):17–26.

71. Greaves MW. Flushing and flushing syndromes, rosacea, and perioral dermatitis. In: Champion RH, et al., eds. *Rook/Wilkinson/Ebling Textbook of Dermatology*, 6th ed. Oxford: Blackwell, 1998:2099–104.

72. Solcia E, Fiocca R, Rindi G, et al. Endocrine tumors of the small and large intestine. *Pathol Res Pract* 1995; 191:366–72.

73. de Herder WW. Tumors of the midgut (jejunum, ileum and ascending colon, including carcinoid syndrome). *Best Pract Res Clin Gastroenterol* 2005; 19:705–15.

74. Levy AD, Sobin LH. Gastrointestinal carcinoids: imaging features with clinicopathologic correlation. *Radiographics* 2007; 27:237–57.

75. Plaksin J, Landau Z, Coslovsky R. A carcinoid-like syndrome caused by a prostaglandin-secreting renal cell carcinoma. *Arch Intern Med* 1980; 140:1095–6,

76. Roberts LJ II, Hubbard WC, Bloomgarden ZT, et al. Prostaglandins: role in the humoral manifestations of medullary carcinoma of the thyroid and inhibition by somatostatin. *Trans Assoc Am Physicians* 1979; 92:286–91.

77. Dierdorf SF. Carcinoid tumor and carcinoid syndrome. *Curr Opin Anaesthesiol* 2003; 16:343–7.

78. Taal BG, Smits M. Developments in diagnosis and treatment of metastatic midgut carcinoid tumors. A review. *Minerva Gastroenterol Dietol* 2005; 51:335–44.

79. Woltering EA, Hilton RS, Zolfoghary CM, et al. Validation of serum versus plasma measurements of chromogranin a levels in patients with carcinoid tumors: lack of correlation between

absolute chromogranin A levels and symptom frequency. *Pancreas* 2006; 33:250–4.

80. Izikson L, English JC III, Zirwas MJ. The flushing patient: differential diagnosis, workup, and treatment. *J Am Acad Dermatol* 2006; 55:193–208.

81. Comaru-Schally AM, Schally AV. A clinical overview of carcinoid tumors: perspectives for improvement in treatment using peptide analogs. *Int J Oncol* 2005; 26:301–9.

82. Tan OT, Stafford TJ, Sarkany I, et al. Suppression of alcohol-induced flushing by a combination of H1 and H2 histamine antagonists. *Br J Dermatol* 1982; 107:647–52.

83. Anthony M. Serotonin antagonists. *Aust NZ J Med* 1984; 14:888–95.

84. Morandi U, Casali C, Rossi G. Bronchial typical carcinoid tumors. *Semin Thorac Cardiovasc Surg* 2006; 18:191–8.

85. Forga L, Anda E, Martinez de Esteban JP. Paraneoplastic hormonal syndromes. *An Sist Sanit Navar* 2005; 28:213–26.

86. Barbosa SL, Rodien P, Leboulleux S, et al. Ectopic adrenocorticotrophic hormone-syndrome in medullary carcinoma of the thyroid: a retrospective analysis and review of the literature. *Thyroid* 2005; 15:618–23.

87. Ilias I, Torpy DJ, Pacak K, et al. Cushing's syndrome due to ectopic corticotropin secretion: twenty years' experience at the National Institutes of Health. *J Clin Endocrinol Metab* 2005; 90:4955–62.

88. Harrison JH, Mahoney EM, Bennett AH. Tumors of the adrenal cortex. *Cancer* 1973; 32:1227–335.

89. Richie JP, Gittes RF. Carcinoma of the adrenal cortex. *Cancer* 1980; 45(Suppl. 7):1957–64.

90. Freeman DA. Steroid hormone-producing tumors in man. *Endocr Rev* 1986; 7:204–20.

91. Brown LR, Aughenbaugh GL, Wick MR, Baker BA, Salassa RM. Roentgenologic diagnosis of primary corticotropin-producing carcinoid tumors of the mediastinum. *Radiology* 1982; 142:143–8.

92. Morris DG, Grossman AB. Dynamic tests in the diagnosis and differential diagnosis of Cushing's syndrome. *J Endocrinol Invest* 2003; 26(Suppl. 7):64–73.

93. von Werder K, Muller OA. The role of corticotrophin-releasing factor in the investigation of endocrine diseases. *Ciba Found Symp* 1993; 172:317–33.

94. Tsagarakis S, Vassiliadi D, Kaskarelis IS, et al. The application of combined CRH plus desmopressin stimulation during petrosal sinus sampling is both sensitive and specific in differentiating patients with Cushing's disease from patients with the occult ectopic ACTH syndrome. *J Clin Endocrinol Metab* 2007; March 13 (E-pub).

95. Machado MC, de Sa SV, Domenice S, et al. The role of desmopressin in bilateral and simultaneous inferior petrosal sinus sampling for differential diagnosis of ACTH-dependent Cushing's syndrome. *Clin Endocrinol* 2007; 66:136–42.

96. Moncet D, Morando DJ, Pitoia F, et al. Ketoconazole therapy: an efficacious alternative to achieve eucortisolism in patients with Cushing's syndrome. *Medicina* 2007; 67:26–31.

97. Morris D, Grossman A. The medical management of Cushing's syndrome. *Ann NY Acad Sci* 2002; 970:119–33.

98. Dimopoulos MA, Fernandez JF, Samaan NA, et al. Paraneoplastic Cushing's syndrome as an adverse prognostic factor in patients who die early with small cell lung cancer. *Cancer* 1992; 69:66–71.

99. van Ditzhuijsen CI, van de Weijer R, Haak HR. Adrenocortical carcinoma. *Neth J Med* 2007; 65:55–60.

100. Hainsworth JD, Workman R, Greco FA. Management of the syndrome of inappropriate antidiuretic hormone secretion in small cell lung cancer. *Cancer* 1983; 51:161–5.

101. Tai P, Yu E, Jones K, et al. Syndrome of inappropriate antidiuretic hormone secretion (SIADH) in patients with limited stage small cell lung cancer. *Lung Cancer* 2006; 53:211–5.

102. Tho LM, Ferry DR. Is the paraneoplastic syndrome of inappropriate antidiuretic hormone secretion in lung cancer always attributable to the small-cell variety? *Postgrad Med J* 2005; 81:e17.

103. Danielides V, Miliones HJ, Karavasilis V, Briasoulis E, Elisaf MS. Syndrome of inappropriate antidiuretic hormone secretion due to recurrent oral cancer. *B-ENT* 2005; 1:151–3.

104. Maxwell EL, Witterick IJ. Syndrome of inappropriate antidiuretic hormone in a patient with metastatic supraglottic cancer. *J Otolaryngol* 2004; 33:308–9.

105. Thompson M, Adlam DM. Syndrome of inappropriate antidiuretic hormone secretion associated with oral squamous cell carcinoma. *Br J Oral Maxillofac Surg* 2002; 40:216–9.

106. Garzotto M, Beer TM. Syndrome of inappropriate antidiuretic hormone secretion: a rare complication of prostate cancer. *J Urol* 2001; 166:1386.

107. Mineta H, Miura K, Takebayashi S, et al. Immunohistochemical analysis of small cell carcinoma of the head and neck: a report of four patients and a review of sixteen patients in the literature with ectopic hormone production. *Ann Otol Rhinol Laryngol* 2001; 110:76–82.

108. Yalcin S, Erman M, Takuzman G, Ruacan S. Syndrome of inappropriate antidiuretic hormone (SIADH) associated with prostatic carcinoma. *Am J Clin Oncol* 2000; 23:384–5.

109. Ferlito A, Rinaldo A, Devaney KO. Syndrome of inappropriate antidiuretic hormone secretion associated with head and neck cancers: review of the literature. *Ann Otol Rhinol Laryngol* 1997; 106:878–83.

110. List AF, Hainsworth JD, Davis BW, et al. The syndrome of inappropriate secretion of antidiuretic hormone (SIADH) in small-cell lung cancer. *J Clin Oncol* 1986; 4:1191–8.

111. Perks WH, Crow JC, Green M. Mesothelioma associated with the syndrome of inappropriate secretion of antidiuretic hormone. *Am Rev Respir Dis* 1978; 117:789–94.

112. Mussig K, Horger M, Haring HU, Wehrmann M. Syndrome of inappropriate antidiuretic hormone secretion and ectopic ACTH production in small cell lung carcinoma. *Lung Cancer* 2007; April (E-pub).

113. Alfa-wali M, Clark GW, Bowrey DJ. A case of gastric carcinoma and the syndrome of inappropriate antidiuretic hormone secretion (SIADH). *Surgeon* 2007; 5:58–9.

114. Willis RE. Ectopic ADH production before clinical recognition of small cell carcinoma of the lung. *South Med J* 1980; 73:1415–6.

115. Giovanis P, Garna A, Marcante M, Mascanzoni A, Giusto M. Exacerbation of paraneoplastic syndrome of inappropriate antidiuretic hormone by parenteral nutrition in a patient affected by large-cell neuroendocrine pancreatic cancer. *J Pain Symptom Manage* 2006; 32:395–6.

116. Saintigny P, Chouahnia K, Cohen R, et al. Tumor lysis associated with sudden onset of syndrome of inappropriate antidiuretic hormone secretion. *Clin Lung Cancer* 2007; 8:282–4.

117. Miyagawa CI. The pharmacologic management of the syndrome of inappropriate secretion of antidiuretic hormone. *Drug Intell Clin Pharm* 1986; 20:527–31.

118. Higdon ML, Higdon JA. Treatment of oncologic emergencies. *Am Fam Physician* 2006; 74:1873–80.

119. Van Poznak C. Hypercalcemia of malignancy remains a clinically-relevant problem. *Cancer J* 2006; 12:21–3.

120. Richard V, Rosol TJ, Foley J. PTHrP gene expression in cancer: do all paths lead to Ets? *Crit Rev Eukaryot Gene Expr* 2005; 15:115–32.

121. Tanimoto M, Harada M. Hypercalcemia-leukocytosis syndrome associated with lung cancer. *Lung Cancer* 2004; 43:301–7.

122. Steffens MG, de Mulder PH, Mulders PF. Paraneoplastic syndromes in three patients with renal cell carcinoma. *Ned Tijdschr Geneeskd* 2004; 148:487–92.

123. Thomas L, Kwok Y, Edelman MJ. Management of paraneoplastic syndromes in lung cancer. *Curr Treat Options Oncol* 2004; 5: 51–62.

124. Hurtado J, Esbrit P. Treatment of malignant hypercalcemia. *Expert Opin Pharmacother* 2002; 3:521–7.

125. Gerber RB, Mazzone P, Arroliga AC. Paraneoplastic syndromes associated with bronchogenic carcinoma. *Clin Chest Med* 2002; 23:257–64.

126. Turalic H, Deamant FD, Reese JH. Paraneoplastic production of granulocyte colony-stimulating factor in a bladder carcinoma. *Scand J Urol Nephrol* 2006; 40:429–32.

127. Ijaz A, Mehmood T, Qureshi AH, et al. Estimation of ionized calcium, total calcium, and albumin corrected calcium for the diagnosis of hypercalcemia of malignancy. *J Coll Physicians Surg Pak* 2006; 16:49–52.

128. Galasko CS. Mechanisms of lytic and blastic metastatic disease of bone. *Clin Orthop Relat Res* 1982; 169:20–7.

129. Liapis H, Crouch EC, Grosso LE, Kitazawa S, Wick MR. Expression of parathyroid-like protein in normal, proliferative, and neoplastic human breast tissues. *Am J Pathol* 1993; 143: 1169–78.

130. Body JJ. Hypercalcemia of malignancy. *Semin Nephrol* 2004; 24: 48–54.

131. Sato K, Onuma E, Yocum RC, Ogata E. Treatment of malignancy-associated hypercalcemia and cachexia with humanized anti-parathyroid hormone-related protein antibody. *Semin Oncol* 2003; 30(Suppl):167–73.

132. Fernando HS, Hawkyard SJ, Poon P, Musa M. Renal cell carcinoma with non-islet cell tumor hypoglycemia. *Int J Urol* 2006; 13:985–6.

133. Fukuda I, Hizuka N, Ishikawa Y, et al. Clinical features of insulin-like growth factor-II producing non-islet cell tumor hypoglycemia. *Growth Horm IGF Res* 2006; 16:211–6.

134. Berman J, Harland S. Hypoglycemia caused by secretion of insulin-like growth factor 2 in a primary renal cell carcinoma. *Clin Oncol* 2001; 13:367–9.

135. Korn E, Van Hoff J, Buckley P, Daughaday WH, Carpenter TO. Secretion of a large molecular-weight form of insulin-like growth factor by a primary renal tumor. *Med Pediatr Oncol* 1995; 24: 392–6.

136. Nauck MA, Reinecke M, Perren A, et al. Hypoglycemia due to paraneoplastic secretion of insulin-like growth factor-I in a patient with metastasizing large-cell carcinoma of the lung. *J Clin Endocrinol Metab* 2007; Feb. (E-pub).

137. Javaprasad N, Anees T, Bijin T, Madhusoodanan S. Severe hypoglycemia due to poorly-differentiated hepatocellular carcinoma. *J Assoc Physicians India* 2006; 54:413–5.

138. Nikeghbalian S, Bananzadeh A, Yarmohammadi H. Hypoglycemia, the first presenting sign of hepatocellular carcinoma. *Saudi Med J* 2006; 27:387–8.

139. Fitzpatrick DR, Peroni DJ, Bielefeldt-Ohmann H. The role of growth factors and cytokines in the tumorigenesis and immunobiology of malignant mesothelioma. *Am J Respir Cell Mol Biol* 1995; 12:455–60.

140. Muntz HG, Brown E. Lactic acidosis and hypoglycemia: a metabolic complication of advanced gynecologic malignancy. *Int J Gynecol Cancer* 1992; 2:163–7.

141. Daughaday WH, Deuel TF. Tumor secretion of growth factors. *Endocrinol Metab Clin North Am* 1991; 20:539–63.

142. de Herder WW. Biochemistry of neuroendocrine tumors. *Best Pract Res Clin Endocrinol Metab* 2007; 21:33–41.

143. Eguchi T, Tokuyama A, Tanaka Y, et al. Hypoglycemia associated with the production of insulin-like growth factor II in adrenocortical carcinoma. *Intern Med* 2001; 40:759–63.

144. Teo SK, Ee CH. Hypoglycemia in the elderly. *Singapore Med J* 1997; 38:432–4.

145. Gutelius BJ, Korytkowski MT, Carty SE, Hamad GG. Diagnosis and minimally invasive resection of an insulinoma: report of an unusual case and review of the literature. *Am Surg* 2007; 73: 520–4.

146. Solomon CG, Dluhy RG. Paraneoplastic endocrine syndromes. *Curr Ther Endocrinol Metab* 1994; 5:537–42.

147. Frizelle FA, Pfiefer MV. Paraneoplastic hypoglycemia treated with somatostatin analogue SMS 201–995. *Eur J Surg Oncol* 1996; 22:546–7.

148. Doherty GM. Rare endocrine tumors of the gastrointestinal tract. *Best Pract Res Clin Gastroenterol* 2005; 19:807–17.

149. Brentjens R, Saltz L. Islet cell tumors of the pancreas: the medical oncologist's perspective. *Surg Clin North Am* 2001; 81: 527–42.

150. Warner RR. Enteroendocrine tumors other than carcinoid: a review of clinically-significant advances. *Gastroenterology* 2005; 128:1668–84.

151. van der Lely AJ, de Herder WW. Carcinoid syndrome: diagnosis and medical management. *Arq Bras Endocrinol Metabol* 2005; 49:850–60.

152. Diaz-Montes TP, Rosenthal LE, Bristow RE, Grumbine FC. Primary insular carcinoid of the ovary. *Gynecol Oncol* 2006; 101:175–8.

153. Hage R, de la Riviere AB, Seldenrijk CA, van den Bosch JM. Update in pulmonary carcinoid tumors: a review article. *Ann Surg Oncol* 2003; 10:697–704.

154. Nuttall KS, Pingree SS. The incidence of elevations in urine 5-hydroxyindoleacetic acid. *Ann Clin Lab Sci* 1998; 28:167–74.

155. Ruffini V, Calcagni ML, Baum RP. Imaging of neuroendocrine tumors. *Semin Nucl Med* 2006; 36:228–47.

156. Uggeri G, Arcidiaco M, Rumi A, Quarone M, Laboranti F. A rare clinical manifestation of intestinal carcinoid causing mesenteric vascular insufficiency. *Chir Ital* 1981; 33:316–24.

157. Bourgault C, Bergeron S, Bogaty P, Poirier P. A most unusual acute coronary syndrome. *Can J Cardiol* 2006; 22:429–32.

158. Connolly HM, Pellikka PA. Carcinoid heart disease. *Curr Cardiol Rep* 2006; 8:96–101.

159. de Diego C, Marcos-Alberca P, Cabrera JA, et al. Pathognomonic echocardiographic features of carcinoid syndrome. *Clin Cardiol* 2006; 29:134.

160. Moller JE, Pellikka PA, Bernheim AM, et al. Prognosis of carcinoid heart disease: analysis of 200 cases over two decades. *Circulation* 2005; 112:3320–7.

161. Raut CP, Kulke MH, Glickman JN, Swanson RS, Ashley SW. Carcinoid tumors. *Curr Probl Surg* 2006; 43:383–450.

162. Nikou GC, Toubanakis C, Nikolaou P, et al. VIPomas: an update in diagnosis and management in a series of 11 patients. *Hepato-gastroenterology* 2005; 52:1259–65.

163. Pratz KW, Ma C, Aubry MC, Vrtiska TJ, Erlichman C. Large-cell carcinoma with caltinonin and vasoactive intestinal polypeptide-associated Verner-Morrison syndrome. *Mayo Clin Proc* 2005; 80: 116–20.

164. Moody TW. Peptides and growth factors in non-small-cell lung cancer. *Peptides* 1996; 17:545–55.

165. Grier JF. WDHA (watery diarrhea, hypokalemia, achlorhydria) syndrome: clinical features, diagnosis, and treatment. *South Med J* 1995; 88:22–4.

166. de Asis DN Jr, Samaan NA. Feminizing adrenocortical carcinoma with Cushing's syndrome and pseudohyperparathyroidism. *Arch Intern Med* 1978; 138:301–3.

167. Greenwood RH, Prunty FT, Brooks RV. Selective feminization due to an adrenal carcinoma. *Proc R Soc Med* 1974; 67:671–2.

168. Masiakos PT, Flynn CE, Donahoe PK. Masculinizing and feminizing syndromes caused by functioning tumors. *Semin Pediatr Surg* 1997; 6:147–55.

169. Young RH, Scully RE. Metastatic tumors in the ovary: a problem-oriented approach and review of the recent literature. *Semin Diagn Pathol* 1991; 8:250–76.

170. Kiyokawa T, Young RH, Scully RE. Krukenberg tumors of the ovary: a clinicopathologic analysis of 120 cases with emphasis on their variable pathologic manifestations. *Am J Surg Pathol* 2006; 30:277–99.

171. Masiakos PT, Flynn CE, Donahoe PK. Masculinizing and feminizing syndromes caused by functioning tumors. *Semin Pediatr Surg* 1997; 6:147–55.

172. Mantero F, Masini AM, Opocher G, Giovagnetti M, Arnaldi G. Adrenal incidentaloma: an overview of hormonal data from the National Italian Study Group. *Horm Res* 1997; 47:284–9.

173. Schteingart DE. Conventional and novel strategies in the treatment of adrenocortical cancer. *Braz J Med Biol Res* 2000; 33:1197–200.

174. Fukai N, Hirono Y, Yoshimoto T, et al. A case of estrogen-secreting adrenocortical carcinoma with subclinical Cushing's syndrome. *Endocr J* 2006; 53:237–45.

175. Moran CA, Suster S. Primary mediastinal choriocarcinomas: a clinicopathologic and immunohistochemical study of eight cases. *Am J Surg Pathol* 1997; 21:1007–12.

176. Yaturu S, Harrara E, Nopajaroonsri C, Singal R, Gill S. Gynecomastia attributable to human chorionic gonadotropin-secreting giant cell carcinoma of lung. *Endocr Pract* 2003; 9:233–5.

177. Forst T, Beyer J, Cordes U, et al. Gynecomastia in a patient with a hCG-producing giant cell carcinoma of the lung. *Exp Clin Endocrinol Diabetes* 1995; 103:28–32.

178. Vlasveld LT, van Hulsteyn LH. Ectopic HCG production in a patient with metastatic bladder carcinoma. *Ned Tijdschr Geneeskd* 1984; 128:2092–5.

179. Caron P, Averous S, Combelles JL, Louvet JP, Sarramon JP. Gynecomastia and cancer of the bladder: an ectopic secretion of chorionic gonadotropin hormone. *Ann Urol* 1984; 18:42–4.

180. Skrabanek P, Kirrane J, Powell D. A unifying concept of chorionic gonadotrophin-production in malignancy. *Invest Cell Pathol* 1979; 2:75–85.

181. Uei Y, Koketsu H, Konda C, Kimura K. Cytodiagnosis of HCG-secreting choriocarcinoma of the stomach: report of a case. *Acta Cytol* 1973; 17:431–4.

182. Agha-Farrell L, Downey P, Keeling P, Leen E, Sreenan S. Acromegaly secondary to growth hormone releasing hormone secretion. *Ir J Med Sci* 2004; 173:215–6.

183. Osella G, Orlandi F, Caraci P, et al. Acromegaly due to ectopic secretion of GHRH by bronchial carcinoid in a patient with empty sella. *J Endocrinol Invest* 2003; 26:163–9.

184. Bhansali A, Rana SS, Bhattacharya S, et al. Acromegaly: a rare manifestation of bronchial carcinoid. *Asian Cardiovasc Thorac Ann* 2002; 10:273–4.

185. Charzistamou I, Schally AV, Pafiti A, Kiaris H, Koutselini H. Expression of growth hormone-releasing hormone in human primary endometrial carcinomas. *Eur J Endocrinol* 2002; 147:381–6.

186. Boix E, Pico A, Pinedo R, Aranda I, Kovacs K. Ectopic growth hormone-releasing hormone secretion by thymic carcinoid tumor. *Clin Endocrinol* 2002; 57:131–4.

187. Othman NH, Ezzat S, Kovacs K, et al. Growth hormone-releasing hormone (GHRH) and GHRH receptor (GHRH-R) isoform expression in ectopic acromegaly. *Clin Endocrinol* 2001; 55:135–40.

188. Mito K, Maruyama R, Uenishi Y, et al. Hypertrophic pulmonary osteoarthropathy associated with non-small-cell lung cancer demonstrating growth hormone-releasing hormone by immuno-histochemical analysis. *Intern Med* 2001; 40:532–5.

189. Losa M, von Werder K. Pathophysiology and clinical aspects of the ectopic GH-releasing hormone syndrome. *Clin Endocrinol* 1997; 47:123–35.

190. Platts JK, Child DF, Meadows P, Harvey JN. Ectopic acromegaly. *Postgrad Med J* 1997; 73:349–51.

191. Ezzat S, Ezrin C, Yamashita, Melmed S. Recurrent acromegaly resulting from ectopic growth hormone gene expression by a metastatic pancreatic tumor. *Cancer* 1993; 71:66–70.

192. Schersten T. Aspects on diagnosis and treatment of the foregut carcinoid syndrome. *Scand J Gastroenterol* 1992; 27:459–71.

193. Sorerson GD, Petterngill OS, Brinck-Johnsen T, Cate CC, Maurer LH. Hormone production by cultures of small-cell carcinoma of the lung. *Cancer* 1981; 47:1289–96.

194. Scheuer A, Grun R, Lehmann FG. Peptide hormones in liver cirrhosis and hepatocellular carcinoma. *Oncodev Biol Med* 1981; 2:1–10.

195. Lombardi G, Galdiero M, Auriermma RS, Pivonello R, Colao A. Acromegaly and the cardiovascular system. *Neuroendocrinology* 2006; 83:211–7.

196. Brooke AM, Drake WM. Serum IGF-I levels in the diagnosis and monitoring of acromegaly. *Pituitary* 2007; 10:173–9.

197. Kellett J, Friesen HG. Bromocriptine and pituitary disorders. *Ann Intern Med* 1979; 90:980–2.

198. Faglia G, Arosio M, Bazzoni N. Bromocriptine and pituitary disorders. *Ann Intern Med* 1979; 90:980–2.

199. Seccia TM, Fassina A, Nussdorfer GG, Pessina AC, Rossi GP. Aldosterone-producing adrenocortical carcinoma: an unusual cause of Conn's syndrome with an ominous clinical course. *Endocr Relat Cancer* 2005; 12:149–59.

200. Steffens J, Bock R, Braedel HU, et al. Renin-producing renal cell carcinomas—clinical and experimental investigations on a special form of renal hypertension. *Urol Res* 1992; 20:111–5.

201. Pratt JH, Ganguly A, Parkinson CA, Weinberger MH. Stimulation of aldosterone secretion by metoclopramide in humans: apparent independence of renal and pituitary mediation. *Metabolism* 1981; 30:129–34.

202. Racz K, Varga I, Kiss R, Glaz E. ACTH sensitivity of isolated human pathological adrenocortical cells: variability of responses in aldosterone, corticosterone, deoxycorticosterone and cortisol production. *J Steroid Biochem* 1984; 20:1187–94.

203. Krum H, Gilbert RE. Novel therapies blocking the renin-angiotensin-aldosterone system in the management of hypertension and related disorders. *J Hypertens* 2007; 25:25–35.

204. Togawa A, Yamamoto T, Suzuki H, et al. Membranous glomerulonephritis associated with renal cell carcinoma: failure to detect a nephritogenic tumor antigen. *Nephron* 2002; 90:219–21.

205. Porush JG. Membranous nephropathy and prostatic carcinoma. *Nephron* 2000; 86:536.

206. Matsuura H, Sakurai M, Arima K. Nephrotic syndrome due to membranous nephropathy associated with metastatic prostate cancer: rapid remission after initial endocrine therapy. *Nephron* 2000; 84:75–8.

207. Shikata Y, Hayashi Y, Yamazaki H, Shikata K, Makino H. Effectiveness of radiation therapy in nephrotic syndrome associated with advanced lung cancer. *Nephron* 1999; 83:160–4.

208. Helin K, Honkanen E, Metsaniitty J, Tornroth T. A case of membranous glomerulonephritis associated with adenocarcinoma of the pancreas. *Nephrol Dial Transplant* 1998; 13:1049–50.

209. Ahmed M, Solangi K, Abbi R, Adler S. Nephrotic syndrome, renal failure, and renal malignancy: an unusual tumor-associated glomerulonephritis. *J Am Soc Nephrol* 1997; 8:848–52.

210. Yedidag A, Zikos D, Spargo B, MacEntee P, Berkelhammer C. Esophageal carcinoma presenting with nephrotic syndrome: association with anti-neutrophil cytoplasmic antibody. *Am J Gastroenterol* 1997; 92:326–8.

211. Wagrowska-Danilewicz M, Danilewicz M. Glomerulonephritis associated with malignant diseases of non-renal origin: a report of three cases and a review of the literature. *Pol J Pathol* 1995; 46:195–8.

212. Boon ES, Vrij AA, Nieuwhof C, van Noord JA, Zeppenfeldt E. Small cell lung cancer with paraneoplastic nephrotic syndrome. *Eur Respir J* 1994; 7:1192–3.

213. Morel-Maroger-Striker L, Striker GE. Glomerular lesions in malignancies. *Contrib Nephrol* 1985; 48:111–24.

214. Papper S. Nephrotic syndrome and neoplasms: the findings to date, with practical implications. *Postgrad Med* 1984; 76:153–8.

215. Pascal RR, Slovin SF. Tumor-directed antibody and carcinoembryonic antigen in the glomeruli of a patient with gastric carcinoma. *Hum Pathol* 1980; 11:679–82.

216. Barton CH, Vaziri ND, Spear GS. Nephrotic syndrome associated with adenocarcinoma of the breast. *Am J Med* 1980; 68:308–12.

217. Yamauchi H, Linsey MS, Biava CG, Hopper J Jr. Cure of membranous nephropathy after resection of carcinoma. *Arch Intern Med* 1985; 145:2061–3.

218. Mevdanli MM, Erguvan R, Altinok MT, Ataoglu O, Kafkasli A. Rare case of neuroendocrine small cell carcinoma of the endometrium with paraneoplastic membranous glomerulonephritis. *Tumori* 2003; 89:213–7.

219. Yamagata T, Akamatsu K, Kuroda M, et al. Squamous cell lung cancer with minimal-change nephrotic syndrome. *Nihon Kokyuki Gakkai Zasshi (J Jpn Resp Soc)* 1998; 36:1032–7.

220. Usalan C, Emri S. Membranoproliferative glomerulonephritis associated with small cell lung carcinoma. *Int Urol Nephrol* 1998; 30:209–13.

221. Gandini E, Allaria P, Castiglioni A, et al. Minimal change nephrotic syndrome with cecum adenocarcinoma. *Clin Nephrol* 1996; 45:268–70.

222. Westhoff TH, Schmidt S, Zidek W, Beige J, ven der Giet M. Tacrolimus in steroid-resistant and steroid-dependent nephrotic syndrome. *Clin Nephrol* 2006; 65:393–400.

223. Esnault VL, Moreau A, Testa A, Besnier D. Crescentic glomerulonephritis. *Nephrol Ther* 2006; 2:446–60.

224. Levine SM. Cancer and myositis: new insights into an old association. *Curr Opin Rheumatol* 2006; 18:620–4.

225. Leandro MJ, Isenberg DA. Rheumatic diseases and malignancy—is there an association? *Scand J Rheumatol* 2001; 30:185–8.

226. Gabrilovich M, Raza M, Dolan S, Raza T. Paraneoplastic polymyositis associated with squamous cell carcinoma of the lung. *Chest* 2006; 129:1721–3.

227. Yamac D, Gunel N, Goker B, et al. Polymyositis and hepatitis concurrent with breast cancer. *Med Princ Pract* 2004; 13:171–5.

228. Lingor P, von Boetticher D, Bahr M, Fassbender K. Paraneoplastic polymyositis in recurring adrenal gland carcinoma. *Lancet Neurol* 2003; 2:435–6.

229. Buchbinder R, Hill CL. Malignancy in patients with inflammatory myopathy. *Curr Rheumatol Rep* 2002; 4:415–26.

230. Klausner AP, Ost MC, Waterhouse RL Jr, Savage SJ. Occult renal cell carcinoma in a patient with polymyositis. *Urology* 2002; 59:773.

231. Tanabe S, Mitomi H, Sada M, et al. Parathyroid hormone-related protein production by adenocarcinoma in Barrett's esophagus in a patient with dermatomyositis. *Dig Dis Sci* 2001; 46:1584–8.

232. Chen YJ, Wu CY, Shen JL. Predicting factors of malignancy in dermatomyositis and polymyositis: a case-control study. *Br J Dermatol* 2001; 144:825–31.

233. Fam AG. Paraneoplastic rheumatic syndromes. *Baillieres Best Pract Res Clin Rheumatol* 2000; 14:515–33.

234. Levrat E, Waeber G. Systemic sclerosis and cancer. *Schweiz Rundsch Med Prax* 2006; 95:983–8.

235. Pectasides D, Koumpou M, Gaglia A, et al. Dermatomyositis associated with breast cancer. *Anticancer Res* 2006; 26(3B):2329–31.

236. Yano S, Kobayashi K, Kato K. Progressive overlap syndrome due to small cell lung cancer as a paraneoplastic syndrome. *Respiration* 2006; March 9 (E-pub).

237. Launay D, Le Berre R, Hatron PY, et al. Association between systemic sclerosis and breast cancer: eight new cases and review of the literature. *Clin Rheumatol* 2004; 23:516–22.

238. Marmur R, Kagen L. Cancer-associated neuromusculoskeletal syndromes: recognizing the rheumatic-neoplastic connection. *Postgrad Med* 2002; 111:95–102.

239. Wenzel J. Scleroderma and malignancy: mechanisms of interrelationship. *Eru J Dermatol* 2002; 12:296–300.

240. Booton R, Jeffrey R, Prabhu PN. Systemic sclerosis and scleroderma renal crisis in association with carcinoma of the breast. *Am J Kidney Dis* 1999; 34:937–41.

241. Naschitz JE, Rosner I, Rozenbaum M, Zuckerman E, Yeshurun D. Rheumatic syndromes: clues to occult neoplasia. *Semin Arthritis Rheum* 1999; 29:43–55.

242. Loche F, Schwarze HP, Durieu C, Bazex J. A case of systemic lupus erythematosus associated with cancer of the lung: a paraneoplastic association? *Br J Dermatol* 2000; 143:210–1.

243. Blanche P, Beuzeboc P, Vincens AL, et al. Systemic lupus erythematosus paraneoplastic syndrome. *Clin Exp Rheumatol* 1997; 15:581–2.

244. Caldwell DS, McCallum RM. Rheumatologic manifestations of cancer. *Med Clin North Am* 1986; 70:385–417.

245. Kraus A, Garza-Elizondo MA, Diaz-Jouanen E. A multi-systemic disease (lupus-like) preceding bronchioloalveolar carcinoma. *Clin Rheumatol* 1985; 4:192–5.

246. Ferrer I. Pathology of paraneoplastic syndromes of the central and peripheral nervous systems and muscle. *Rev Neurol* 2000; 31:1228–36.

247. Benedek TG. Neoplastic associations of rheumatic diseases and rheumatic manifestations of cancer. *Clin Geriatr Med* 1988; 4:333–55.

248. Chinoy H, Fertig N, Oddis CV, Ollier WE, Cooper RG. The diagnostic utility of myositis autoantibody testing for predicting the risk of cancer-associated myositis. *Ann Rheum Dis* 2007; Mar 28 [Epub].

249. De Beukelaar JW, Sillevis Smitt JA. Managing paraneoplastic neurological disorders. *Oncologist* 2006; 11:292–305.

250. Rouers A, Radermecker MA, Duysinx B, Kaschten B, Limet R. Pierre-Marie-Bamberger syndrome. *Rev Med Liege* 2006; 61:142–4.

251. Campanella N, Moraca A, Pergolini M, et al. Paraneoplastic syndromes in 68 cases of respectable non-small-cell lung carcinoma: can they help in early detection? *Med Oncol* 1999; 16:129–33.

252. Baughman RP, Gunther KL, Buchsbaum JA, Lower EE. Prevalence of digital clubbing in bronchogenic carcinoma by a new digital index. *Clin Exp Rheumatol* 1998; 16:21–6.

253. Liam CK. Clubbing of the fingers in patients with primary lung cancer. *Med J Malaysia* 1997; 52:186–7.

254. Brooks PM. Rheumatic manifestations of neoplasia. *Curr Opin Rheumatol* 1992; 4:90–3.

255. Chen YC, Tiu CM, Bai LY, Liu JH. Hypertrophic pulmonary osteoarthropathy associated with disease progression in renal cell carcinoma. *J Chin Med Assoc* 2003; 66:63–6.

256. Vico P, Delcorde A, Rahier I, et al. Hypertrophic osteoarthropathy and thyroid cancer. *J Rheumatol* 1992; 19:1153–6.

256a. Sridhar KS, Lobo CF, Altman RD. Digital clubbing and lung cancer. *Chest* 1998; 114:1535–7.

256b. Dickinson CJ. The aetiology of clubbing and hypertrophic osteoarthropathy. *Eur J Clin Invest* 1993; 23:330–8.

257. Olan F, Portela M, Navarro C, et al. Circulating vascular endothelial growth factor concentrations in a case of pulmonary hypertrophic osteoarthropathy. *Correlation with disease activity.* *J Rheumatol* 2004; 31:614–6.

258. Urist MR, DeLange RJ, Finerman GA. Bone cell differentiation and growth factors. *Science* 1983; 220:680–6.

259. Fietz T, Schneider P, Knauf WU, Thiel E. Clubbed fingers and arthralgia as a reversible paraneoplastic syndrome (Pierre-Marie-Bamberger syndrome) in non-small-cell bronchial carcinoma. *Dtsch Med Wochenschr* 1998; 123:1507–11.

260. Albrecht S, Keller A. Postchemotherapeutic reversibility of hypertrophic osteoarthropathy in a patient with bronchogenic adenocarcinoma. *Clin Nucl Med* 2003; 28:463–6.

261. Giannakopoulos CHK, Kyriakidou GK, Toufexi GE. Palmar fasciitis and polyarthritis associated with secondary ovarian carcinoma: case report. *Eur J Gynaecol Oncol* 2005; 26: 339–41.

262. Denschlag D, Riener E, Vaith P, Tempfer C, Keck C. Palmar fasciitis and polyarthritis as a paraneoplastic syndrome associated with tubal carcinoma: a case report. *Ann Rheum Dis* 2004; 63: 1177–8.

263. Martorell EA, Murray PM, Peterson JJ, Menke DM, Calamia KT. Palmar fasciitis and arthritis syndrome associated with metastatic ovarian carcinoma: a report of four cases. *J Hand Surg [Am]* 2004; 29:654–60.

264. Docquier CH, Majois F, Mitine C. Palmar fasciitis and arthritis: association with endometrial adenocarcinoma. *Clin Rheumatol* 2002; 21:63–5.

265. Saxman SB, Seitz D. Breast cancer associated with palmar fasciitis and arthritis. *J Clin Oncol* 1997; 15:3515–6.

266. Enomoto M, Takemura H, Suzuki M, et al. Palmar fasciitis and polyarthritis associated with gastric carcinoma: complete resolution after total gastrectomy. *Intern Med* 2000; 39:754–7.

267. Shiel WC Jr, Prete PE, Jason M, Andrews BS. Palmar fasciitis and arthritis with ovarian and non-ovarian carcinomas: new syndrome. *Am J Med* 1985; 79:640–4.

268. Valverde-Garcia J, Juanola-Roura X, Ruiz-Martin JM, et al. Paraneoplastic palmar fasciitis-polyarthritis syndrome associated with breast cancer. *J Rheumatol* 1987; 14:1207–9.

269. Eekhoff EM, van der Lubbe PA, Breedveld FC. Flexion contractures associated with a malignant neoplasm: a paraneoplastic syndrome. *Clin Rheumatol* 1998; 17:157–9.

270. Fernandez-Guerra J, Barrot-Cortes E, Soto-Campos JG. Polymyalgia rheumatica presenting with pulmonary epidermoid carcinoma. *Aarch Bronconeumol* 1996; 32:155.

271. Bachmann LM, Vetter W. Pitfalls in the diagnosis of polymyalgia rheumatica-temporal arteritis. *Schweiz Rundsch Med Prax* 2000; 89:879–84.

272. Liozon E, Lousaud V, Fauchais AL, et al. Concurrent temporal (giant-cell) arteritis and malignancy: report of 20 patients with review of the literature. *J Rheumatol* 2006; 33:1606–14.

273. Okamoto T, Gotoh M, Masuya D, et al. Clinical analysis of interstitial pneumonia after surgery for lung cancer. *Jpn J Thorac Cardiovasc Surg* 2004; 52:323–9.

274. Yamadori I, Sato T, Fujita J, et al. A case of nonspecific interstitial pneumonia associated with primary lung cancer: possible role of antibodies to lung cancer cells in the pathogenesis of nonspecific interstitial pneumonia. *Respir Med* 1999; 93: 754–6.

275. Miyamoto Y, Tsubota N, Yoshimura M, Murotani A, Matoba Y. Postoperative interstitial pneumonia in primary lung cancer patients—its causes and management. *Nippon Kyobu Geka Gakkai Zasshi* 1995; 43:452–7.

276. Haddad L, Amsterdam A, Chi DS. Celiac disease presenting as a paraneoplastic syndrome in a patient with synchronous endometrial and ovarian cancers. *Gynecol Oncol* 2005; 97:704–6.

277. Green PH. The many faces of celiac disease: clinical presentation of celiac disease in the adult population. *Gastroenterology* 2005; 128(Suppl):S74–8.

278. Schwertz E, Kahlenberg F, Sack U, et al. Serologic assay based on gliadin-related nonapeptides as a highly sensitive and specific diagnostic aid in celiac disease. *Clin Chem* 2004; 50:2370–5.

279. Pare P, Douville P, Caron D, Lagace R. Adult celiac sprue: changes in the pattern of clinical recognition. *J Clin Gastroenterol* 1988; 10:395–400.

280. Bartholomew LG, Schutt AJ. Systemic syndromes associated with neoplastic disease including cancer of the colon. *Cancer* 1971; 28: 170–4.

281. Iida F, Sato A, Koike Y, Matsuda K. Surgical and pathologic aspects of protein-losing enteropathy. *Surg Gynecol Obstet* 1978; 147:33–7.

282. Mangla JC, Taylor E, Cristo C. Primary duodenal carcinoma with protein-losing enteropathy. *Am J Gastroenterol* 1977; 67: 73–6.

283. Waldmann TA, Broder S, Strober W. Protein-losing enteropathies in malignancy. *Ann NY Acad Sci* 1974; 230:306–17.

284. Hundegger K, Karbach U. Alpha 1-antitrypsin as an endogenous marker for the detection of intestinal protein excretion—problems and controversies in dealing with a new method. *Z Gastroenterol* 1992; 30:204–6.

285. Dahl PR, Su WPD, Cullimore KC, Dicken CH. Pancreatic panniculitis. *J Am Acad Dermatol* 1995; 33:413–7.

286. Hughes SH, Apisarnthanarax P, Mullins F. Subcutaneous fat necrosis associated with pancreatic disease. *Arch Dermatol* 1975; 111:506–10.

287. Bhatnagar A, Wig J, Vaiphei K, Majumdar S. Intracellular cytokines in cells of necrotic tissue from patients with acute pancreatitis. *Eur J Surg* 2001; 167:510–7.

288. Freeman HJ, Berean KW. Resolution of paraneoplastic collagenous enterocolitis after resection of colon cancer. *Can J Gastroenterol* 2006; 20:357–60.

289. Gardiner GW, Goldberg R, Currie D, Murray D. Colonic carcinoma associated with an abnormal collagen table: collagenous colitis. *Cancer* 1984; 54:2973–7.

290. Lazenby AJ. Collagenous and lymphocytic colitis. *Semin Diagn Pathol* 2005; 22:295–300.

291. Taha Y, Raab Y, Carlson M, et al. Vascular endothelial growth factor (VEGF)—a possible mediator of inflammation and mucosal permeability in patients with collagenous colitis. *Dig Dis Sci* 2004; 49:109–15.

292. Goff JS, Barnett JL, Pelke T, Appleman HD. Collagenous colitis: histopathology and clinical course. *Am J Gastroenterol* 1997; 92: 57–60.

293. Stauffer MH. Nephrogenic hepatosplenomegaly. *Gastroenterology* 1961; 40:694.

294. Boxer RJ, Weisman J, Leiber MM, et al. Nonmetastatic hepatic dysfunction syndrome associated with renal cell carcinoma. *J Urol* 1978; 119:468–71.

295. Walsh PN, Kissane JM. Nonmetastatic hypernephroma with reversible hepatic dysfunction. *Arch Intern Med* 1968; 122:214–22.

296. Lemmon WT Jr, Holland PV, Holand JM. The hepatopathy of hypernephroma. *Am J Surg* 1965; 110:487–91.

297. Karakolios A, Kasapis C, Kallinikidis T, Kalpidis P, Grigoriadis N. Cholestatic jaundice as a paraneoplastic manifestation of prostate adenocarcinoma. *Clin Gastroenterol Hepatol* 2003; 1: 480–3.

298. Blay JY, Rossi JF, Wijdenes J, et al. Role of interleukin-6 in the paraneoplastic inflammatory syndrome associated with renal cell carcinoma. *Int J Cancer* 1997; 72:424–30.

299. Koistinen P, Kinnula V, Timonen T. Aplastic anemia as a paraneoplastic syndrome in lung cancer. *Eur J Cancer* 1990; 26:651.

300. Saito H. Paraneoplastic syndromes: hematologic abnormalities. *Gan To Kagaku Ryoho (Cancer Chemother)* 1991; 18:337–42.

301. Johnson RA, Roodman GD. Hematologic manifestations of malignancy. *Dis Mon* 1989; 35:721–68.

302. Sans-Sabrafen J, Buxo J, Woessner S, et al. Acquired refractory anemia and neoplasms: study of 11 cases. *Med Clin* 1984; 83: 489–91.

303. Dincol G, Aktan M, Diz-Kucukkaya R, et al. Treatment of acquired severe aplastic anemia with antilymphocyte globulin, cyclosporin A, methyprednisolone, and granulocyte colony-stimulating factor. *Am J Hematol* 2007; May 15: [Epub ahead of print].

304. Sallah S, Sigounas G, Vos P, Wan JY, Nguyen NP. Autoimmune hemolytic anemia in patients with non-Hodgkin's lymphoma: characteristics and significance. *Ann Oncol* 2000; 11:1571–7.

305. Honan W, Balazs J, Jariwalla AG. Autoimmune hemolytic anemia (AHA) and lung carcinoma. *Br J Clin Pract* 1986; 40:35–6.

306. Selleslag DL, Geraghty RJ, Ganesan TS, et al. Autoimmune hemolytic anemia associated with malignant peritoneal mesothelioma. *Acta Clin Belg* 1989; 44:199–201.

307. Sokol RJ, Booker DJ, Stamps R. Erythrocyte autoantibodies, autoimmune hemolysis, and carcinoma. *J Clin Pathol* 1994; 47:340–3.

308. Philippe P. Autoimmune hemolytic anemia: diagnosis and management. *Presse Med* 2007; May 2: [Epub ahead of print].

309. Tomsova M, Zak P. Microangiopathic hemolytic anemia and thrombocytopenia (cancer-related thrombotic thrombocytopenic purpura) in a patient with diffuse gastric adenocarcinoma. *Cesk Patol* 2003; 39:26–30.

310. Teichmann J, Sieber G, Ludwig WD, Ruhl H. Thrombotic thrombocytopenic purpura within the scope of disseminated tumor disease. *Internist* 1987; 28:388–92.

311. Majhail NS, Hix JK, Almahameed A. Carcinoma of the colon in a patient presenting with thrombotic thrombocytopenic purpura-hemolytic uremic syndrome. *Mayo Clin Proc* 2002; 77:873.

312. Gonzalez N, Rios E, Martin-Nova A, Rodriguez JM. Thrombotic thrombocytopenic purpura and bone marrow necrosis as a complication of a gastric neoplasm. *Haematologica* 2002; 87: ECR01.

313. von Bubnoff N, Sandherr M, Schneller F, Peschel C. Thrombotic thrombocytopenic purpura in metastatic carcinoma of the breast. *Am J Clin Oncol* 2000; 23:74–7.

314. Gordon LI, Kwaan HC. Thrombotic microangiopathy manifesting as thrombotic thrombocytopenic purpura/hemolytic uremic syndrome in the cancer patient. *Semin Thromb Hemost* 1999; 25: 217–21.

315. Robson MG, Abbs IC. Thrombotic thrombocytopenic purpura following hemicolectomy for colonic carcinoma. *Nephrol Dial Transplant* 1997; 12:198–9.

316. Lesesne JB, Rothschild N, Erickson B, et al. Cancer-associated hemolytic-uremic syndrome: analysis of 85 cases from a national registry. *J Clin Oncol* 1989; 7:781–9.

317. Riley MG, Stead NW. Thrombotic thrombocytopenic purpura associated with small cell lung carcinoma. *J Med Assoc GA* 1985; 74:498–501.

318. Kressel BR, Ryan KP, Duong AT, Berenberg J, Schein PS. Microangiopathic hemolytic anemia, thrombocytopenia, and renal failure in patients treated for adenocarcinoma. *Cancer* 1981; 48: 1738–45.

319. Joseph RR, Day HJ, Sherwin RM, Schwartz HG. Microangiopathic hemolytic anemia associated with consumption coagulopathy in a patient with disseminated carcinoma. *Scand J Haematol* 1967; 4:271–82.

320. Knottenbelt E, Lloyd A, Jacobs P. Microangiopathic hemolytic anemia and an unusual lactate dehydrogenase isoenzyme pattern in metastatic adenocarcinoma: a case report. *S Afr Med J* 1985; 68:611–2.

320a. Forman RB, Benkel SA, Novik Y, Tsai HM. Presence of ADAMTS13 activity in a patient with metastatic cancer and thrombotic microangiopathy. *Acta Haematol* 2003; 109:150–2.

321. Sadler JE. Thrombotic thrombocytopenic purpura: a moving target. *Hematology Am Soc Hematol Educ Program* 2006; 1: 415–20.

322. Blot E, Decaudin D, Veyradier A, et al. Cancer-related thrombotic microangiopathy secondary to von Willebrand factor-cleaving protease deficiency. *Thromb Res* 2002; 106:127–30.

320a. Marcoullis G, Abebe L, Jain D, et al. Microangiopathic hemolysis refractory to plasmapheresis responding to docetaxel and cisplatin: a case report. *Med Oncol* 2002; 19:189–92.

323. Darabi K, Berg AH. Rituximab can be combined with daily plasma exchange to achieve effective B-cell depletion and clinical improvement in acute autoimmune thrombotic thrombocytopenic purpura. *Am J Clin Pathol* 2006; 125:592–7.

324. Nand S, Molokie R. Therapeutic plasmapheresis and protein A immunoadsorption in malignancy: a brief review. *J Clin Apher* 1990; 5:206–12.

325. Hwang WYK, Chai LYA, Ng HJ, Goh YT, Tan PHC. Therapeutic plasmapheresis for the treatment of the thrombotic thrombocytopenic purpura-hemolytic uremic syndromes. *Singapore Med J* 2004; 45:219–23.

326. Mukhopadhyay S, Mukhopadhyay S, Banki K, Mahajan S. Leukemoid reaction: a diagnostic clue in metastatic carcinoma mimicking classic Hodgkin lymphoma. *Arch Pathol Lab Med* 2004; 128:1445–7.

327. Kasuga I, Makino S, Kiyokawa H, et al. Tumor-related leukocytosis is linked with poor prognosis in patients with lung carcinoma. *Cancer* 2001; 92:2399–405.

328. McKee LC Jr. Excess leukocytosis (leukemoid reactions) associated with malignant diseases. *South Med J* 1985; 78: 1475–82.

329. Fahey RJ. Unusual leukocyte responses in primary carcinoma of the lung. *Cancer* 1951; 4:930–5.

328. Saussez S, Heimann P, Vandevelde L, et al. Undifferentiated carcinoma of the nasopharynx and leukemoid reaction: report of a case with literature review. *J Laryngol Otol* 1997; 111:66–9.

329. Uematsu T, Tsuchie K, Ukai K, et al. Granulocyte-colony-stimulating factor produced by pancreatic carcinoma. *Int J Pancreatol* 1996; 19:135–9.

331. Dotti G, Garratini E, Borleri G, et al. Leucocyte alkaline phosphatase identifies terminally differentiated normal neutrophils and its lack in chronic myelogenous leukaemia is not dependent on p210 tyrosine kinase activity. *Br J Haematol* 1999; 105: 163–72.

333. Rodriguez-Alonso A, Romero-Picos E, Suarez-Pascual G, et al. Priapism following paraneoplastic leukemoid reaction in a patient with bladder cancer. *Actas Urol Esp* 2004; 28:539–43.

334. Hebbar S, Thomas GA. Digital ischemia associated with squamous cell carcinoma of the esophagus. *Dig Dis Sci* 2005; 50: 691–3.

335. Blum W, Porcu P. Therapeutic apheresis in hyperleukocytosis and hyperviscosity syndromes. *Semin Thromb Hemost* 2007; 33: 350–4.

336. Hwang SJ, Luo JC, Li CP, et al. Thrombocytosis: a paraneoplastic syndrome in patients with hepatocellular carcinoma. *World J Gastroenterol* 2004; 10:2472–7.

337. Blay JY, Favrot M, Rossi JF, Wijdenes J. Role of interleukin-6 in paraneoplastic thrombocytosis. *Blood* 1993; 82:2261–2.

338. de Pangher-Manzini V. Malignant peritoneal mesothelioma. *Tumori* 2005; 91:1–5.

339. Higishihara M, Miyazaki K. Thrombopoietin-producing tumor. *Intern Med* 2003; 42:632–3.

340. Blay JY, Rossi JF, Wijdenes J, et al. Role of interleukin-6 in the paraneoplastic inflammatory syndrome associated with renal-cell carcinoma. *Int J Cancer* 1997; 72:424–30.

340a. Luo JC, Hwang SJ, Wu JC, et al. Clinical characteristics and prognosis of hepatocellular carcinoma patients with paraneoplastic syndromes. *Hepatogastroenterology* 2002; 49:1315–9.

340b. Clark D, Kersting R, Rojiani AM. Erythropoietin immunolocalization in renal cell carcinoma. *Mod Pathol* 1998; 11:24–8.

340c. Kew MC, Fisher JW. Serum erythropoietin concentrations in patients with hepatocellular carcinoma. *Cancer* 1986; 58:2485–8.

340d. Matsuo M, Koga S, Kanetake H, et al. Erythropoietin-producing gastric carcinoma in a hemodialysis patient. *Am J Kidney Dis* 2003; 42:E3–E4.

340e. Samyn I, Fontaine C, Van Tussenbroek F, Pipeleers-Marichal M, De Greve J. Paraneoplastic syndromes in cancer: polycythemia as a result of ectopic erythropoietin production in metastatic pancreatic carcinoid tumor. *J Clin Oncol* 2004; 22: 2240–2.

340f. Burchacki J, Klyszejko C. Paraneoplastic erythrocytosis in ovarian carcinoma. *Wiad Lek* 1977; 30:1477–99.

341. Pandit R, Scholnik A, Wulfekuhler L, Dimitrov N. Non-small-cell lung cancer associated with excessive eosinophilia and secretion of interleukin-5 as a paraneoplastic syndrome. *Am J Hematol* 2007; 82:234–7.

342. Saliba WR, Dharan M, Bisharat N, Elias M. Eosinophilic pancreatic infiltration as a manifestation of lung carcinoma. *Am J Med Sci* 2006; 331:274–6.

343. Niamut SM, de Vries PA, van Putten JW, de Jong RS. Eosinophilia caused by solid malignancy. *Ned Tijdschr Geneeskd* 2004; 148:1883–6.

344. Bonaventure C, Etienne-Mastroianni B, Alessio A, et al. Paraneoplastic hypereosinophilia associated with hepatocellular carcinoma. *Gastroenterol Clin Biol* 2003; 27:1167–9.

345. Balian A, Bonte E, Naveau S, et al. Intratumoral production of interleukin-5 leading to paraneoplastic peripheral eosinophilia in hepatocellular carcinoma. *J Hepatol* 2001; 34:355–6.

346. Teoh SC, Siow WY, Tan HT. Severe eosinophilia in disseminated gastric carcinoma. *Singapore Med J* 2000; 41:232–4.

347. Chang WC, Liaw CC, Wang PN, Tsai YH, Hsueh S. Tumor-associated hypereosinophilia: report of four cases. *Changgeung Yi Xue Za Zhi (Chang Gung Med J)* 1996; 19:66–70.

348. Balducci L, Chapman SW, Little DD, Hardy CL. Paraneoplastic eosinophilia: report of a case with in vitro studies of hemopoiesis. *Cancer* 1989; 64:2250–3.

349. Vassilatou E, Fisfis M, Morphopoulos G, et al. Papillary thyroid carcinoma producing granulocyte-macrophage colony-stimulating factor is associated with neutrophilia and eosinophilia. *Hormones* 2006; 5:303–9.

350. Diot P, Guimard Y, Besnier JM, et al. Pulmonary solitary mass with "a crescent sign" and blood eosinophilia. *Eur J Med* 1992; 1: 58–9.

351. Salame M, Rickaert F, Deprez C, Van Gossum A, Cremer M. Hepatocarcinoma and hypereosinophilia. *Acta Gastroenterol Belg* 1988; 51:169–72.

352. Stefanini GF, Addolorato G, Marsigli L, et al. Eosinophilic gastroenteritis in a patient with large-cell anaplastic lung carcinoma: a paraneoplastic syndrome? *Ital J Gastroenterol* 1994; 26: 354–6.

353. May ME, Waddell CC. Basophils in peripheral blood and bone marrow: a retrospective review. *Am J Med* 1984; 76: 509–11.

354. Amalich F, Lahoz C, Larrocha C, et al. Incidence and clinical significance of peripheral and bone marrow basophilia. *J Med* 1987; 18:293–303.

355. Amaral BW. Immune thrombocytopenic purpura: an overview. *Postgrad Med* 1977; 61:197–202.

356. Bir A, Bshara W, George M, Fakih MG. Idiopathic thrombocytopenic purpura in a newly diagnosed pancreatic adenocarcinoma. *JOP* 2006; 7:647–50.

357. Wakata N, Kiyozuka T, Konno S, et al. Autoimmune thrombocytopenic purpura, autoimmune hemolytic anemia, and gastric cancer in a patient with myasthenia gravis. *Intern Med* 2006; 45: 479–81.

358. Tsoussis S, Ekonomidou F, Vourliotaki E, Karalis I, Dermitzakis A. Successful treatment of idiopathic thrombocytopenic purpura-like syndrome in a cancer patient with low-dose interferon: case report and review of the literature. *Am J Hematol* 2004; 76: 353–9.

359. Chehal A, Taher A, Seoud M, Shamseddine A. Idiopathic thrombocytopenic purpura and ovarian cancer. *Eur J Gynaecol Oncol* 2003; 24:539–40.

360. Wong AS, Hon-Yoon K. Paraneoplastic Raynaud phenomenon and idiopathic thrombocytopenic purpura in non-small-cell lung cancer. *Am J Clin Oncol* 2003; 26:26–9.

361. Wahid FS, Fun LC, Keng CS, Ismail F. Breast carcinoma presenting as immune thrombocytopenic purpura. *Int J Hematol* 2001; 73:399–400.

362. Porrata LF, Alberts S, Hook C, Hanson CA. Idiopathic thrombocytopenic purpura associated with breast cancer: a case report and review of the current literature. *Am J Clin Oncol* 1999; 22: 411–3.

363. Tarraza HM, Carroll R, De Cain M, Jones M. Recurrent ovarian carcinoma: presentation as idiopathic thrombocytopenic purpura and a splenic mass. *Eur J Gynaecol Oncol* 1991; 12: 439–43.

363a. Klimberg I, Drylie DM. Renal cell carcinoma and idiopathic thrombocytopenic purpura. *Urology* 1984; 23:293–6.

363b. Garcia-Ruiz F, Martinez de Antonio E, Alonso-Navas F. Syndrome of idiopathic thrombocytopenic purpura secondary to carcinoma of the lung: report of a case. *Med Clin* 1980; 75: 435–7.

363c. Kim HD, Boggs DR. A syndrome resembling idiopathic thrombocytopenic purpura in 10 patients with diverse forms of cancer. *Am J Med* 1979; 67:371–7.

364. Bellucci S, Dosquet C, Boval B, Wautier JL, Caen J. Association of autoimmune thrombocytopenic purpura (AITP), Graves' disease, and ovarian carcinoma. *Nouv Rev Fr Hematol* 1991; 33: 307–9.

365. Bromberg ME. Immune thrombocytopenic purpura—the changing therapeutic landscape. *N Engl J Med* 2006; 355:1643–5.

366. Lin JT. Thromboembolic events in the cancer patient. *J Womens Health* 2003; 12:541–51.

367. Denko NC, Giaccia AJ. Tumor hypoxia: the physiological link between Trousseau's syndrome (carcinoma-induced coagulopathy) and metastasis. *Cancer Res* 2001; 61:795–8.

368. Rigdon EE. Trousseau's syndrome and acute arterial thrombosis. *Cardiovasc Surg* 2000; 8:214–8.

369. Lal G, Brennan TV, Hambleton J, Clark OH. Coagulopathy, marantic endocarditis, and cerebrovascular accidents as paraneoplastic features in medullary thyroid cancer—case report and review of the literature. *Thyroid* 2003; 13:601–5.

370. Fanale MA, Zeldenrust SR, Moynihan TJ. Some unusual complications of malignancies: marantic endocarditis in advanced cancer. *J Clin Oncol* 2002; 20:4111–4.

371. Chisholm JC Jr, Ireland CS, Scott RN. Bronchogenic carcinoma, leukemoid reaction, marantic endocarditis, and consumptive thrombocytopathy. *J Natl Med Assoc* 1982; 74:447–54.

372. Kooiker JC, MacLean JM, Sumi SM. Cerebral embolism, marantic endocarditis, and cancer. *Arch Neurol* 1976; 33:260–4.

373. Neufeld HN, Cadman NL, Miller AW, Edwards JE. Embolism from marantic endocarditis as a manifestation of occult carcinoma. *Mayo Clin Proc* 1960; 25:292–9.

374. Muller PH, Gmur J. Metastasizing pancreatic carcinoma with cryoproteinemia, thrombophlebitis saltans, pulmonary embolism, and phlegmasia cerulean dolens. *Schweiz Med Wochenschr* 1969; 99:682–4.

375. Vandeweghe M, Comhaire F. Phlegmasia cerulean dolens. *Acta Clin Belg* 1968; 23:394–409.

376. Howard EJ. Phlegmasia cerulea dolens secondary to carcinoma of the pancreas. *Angiology* 1960; 11:319–22.

377. Donati MB. Cancer and thrombosis: from phlegmasia alba dolens to transgenic mice. *Thromb Haemost* 1995; 74:278–81.

378. Mahorner H. Diagnosis and treatment of phlegmasia alba dolens and phlegmasia cerulea dolens. *Am Surg* 1968; 34:210–2.

379. Tasi SH, Juan CJ, Dai MS, Kao WY. Trousseau's syndrome related to adenocarcinoma of the colon and cholangiocarcinoma. *Eur J Neurol* 2004; 11:493–6.

380. Lesher JL Jr. Superficial migratory thrombophlebitis. *Cutis* 1991; 47:177–80.

381. Pinzon R, Drewinko B, Trujillo JM, Guinee V, Giacco G. Pancreatic carcinoma and Trousseau's syndrome: experience at a large cancer center. *J Clin Oncol* 1986; 4:509–14.

382. Naschitz JE, Kovaleva J, Shviv N, Rennert G, Yeshurun D. Vascular disorders preceding diagnosis of cancer: distinguishing the causal relationship based on Bradford-Hill guidelines. *Angiology* 2003; 54:11–7.

383. Ogren M, Bergqvist D, Wahlander K, Eriksson H, Sternby NH. Trousseau's syndrome—what is the evidence? A population-based autopsy study. *Thromb Haemost* 2006; 95:541–5.

384. Sato T, Tsujino I, Ikeda D, Ieko M, Nishimura M. Trousseau's syndrome associated with tissue factor produced by pulmonary adenocarcinoma. *Thorax* 2006; 61:1009–10.

385. Lisk R, O'Mahony PG. Paraneoplastic vasculitis and coexistent Trousseau's syndrome secondary to pancreatic carcinoma. *J Am Geriatr Soc* 2006; 54:1468–9.

386. Del Conde I, Bharwani LD, Dietzen DJ, et al. Microvesicle-associated tissue factor and Trousseau's syndrome. *J Thromb Haemost* 2007; 5:70–4.

387. Wahrenbrock M, Borsig L, Le D, Varki N, Varki A. Selectin-mucin interactions as a probable molecular explanation for the association of Trousseau syndrome with mucinous adenocarcinomas. *J Clin Invest* 2003; 112:853–62.

388. Sack GH Jr, Levin J, Bell WR. Trousseau's syndrome and other manifestations of chronic disseminated coagulopathy in patients with neoplasms: clinical, pathophysiologic, and therapeutic features. *Medicine* 1977; 56:1–37.

389. Andreescu AC, Cushman M, Hammond JM, Wood ME. Trousseau's syndrome treated with long-term subcutaneous lepirudin—case report and review of the literature. *J Thromb Thrombolysis* 2001; 11:33–7.

390. Baker WF Jr, Bick RL. Treatment of hereditary and acquired thrombophilic disorders. *Semin Thromb Hemost* 1999; 25: 387–406.

391. Zuger M, Demarmels-Biasiutti F, Wuillemin WA, Furlan M, Lammle B. Subcutaneous low-molecular-weight heparin for treatment of Trousseau's syndrome. *Ann Hematol* 1997; 75: 165–7.

392. Green D. Current trends in the use of heparins in thromboprophylaxis. *Semin Thromb Hemost* 1999; 25(Suppl):29–35.

393. de la Fouchardiere C, Flechon A, Droz JP. Coagulopathy in prostate cancer. *Neth J Med* 2003; 612:347–54.

394. Brechot JM, Conard J, Samama M. Coagulation and bronchopulmonary cancers: from clinical aspects to biology. *Rev Mal Respir* 1992; 9:375–84.

395. Tokar M, Bobilev D, Ariad S, Geffen DB. Disseminated intravascular coagulation at presentation of advanced gastric cancer. *Isr Med Assoc J* 2006; 8:853–5.

396. Pasquini E, Gianni L, Aitini E, et al. Acute disseminated intravascular coagulation syndrome in cancer patients. *Oncology* 1995; 52:505–8.

397. Siegman-Igra Y, Flatau E, Deligdish L. Chronic diffuse intravascular coagulation (DIC) in nonmetastatic ovarian cancer: report of a case and review of the literature. *Gynecol Oncol* 1977; 5: 92–100.

398. Kario K, Matsuo T, Kodama K, et al. Imbalance between thrombin and plasmin activity in disseminated intravascular coagulation. Assessment by the thrombin-antithrombin-III complex/plasmin-alpha-2-antiplasmin complex ratio. *Haemostasis* 1992; 22:179–86.

399. Warr TA, Rao LV, Rapaport SI. Human plasma extrinsic pathway inhibitor activity: II. Plasma levels in disseminated intravascular coagulation and hepatocellular disease. *Blood* 1989; 74: 994–8.

400. Lin P, Medeiros LJ. Lymphoplasmacytic lymphoma/Waldenstrom macroglobulinemia: an evolving concept. *Adv Anat Pathol* 2005; 12:246–55.

401. Cook L, MacDonald DH. Management of paraproteinemia. *Postgrad Med J* 2007; 83:217–23.

402. Jacobs P, Ruff P, Wood L, Moodley D, Mansvelt E. Amyloidosis: a changing clinical perspective. *Hematology* 2007; 12:163–7.

403. Enia G, Maringhini S, L'Abbate A, Zoccali C, Maggiore O. Light-chain nephropathy in patients with renal carcinoma. *Br Med J (Clin Res Ed)* 1981; 283:339–40.

404. Chen HP, Carroll JA. Monoclonal gammopathy in carcinoma of the colon. *Am J Clin Pathol* 1980; 73:607–10.

405. Burnier E, Zwahlen A, Cruchaud A. Nonmalignant monoclonal immunoglobulinemia, pernicious anemia, and gastric carcinoma: a model of immunologic dysfunction—report of two cases and review of the literature. *Am J Med* 1976; 60:1019–25.

406. Fenoglio C, Ferenczy A, Isobe T, Osserman EE. Hepatoma associated with marked plasmacytosis and polyclonal hypergammaglobulinemia. *Am J Med* 1973; 55:111–5.

407. Spencer D. Secondary amyloidosis in relation to carcinoma of the kidney. *Postgrad Med J* 1971; 47:820–2.

408. Penman HG, Thomson KJ. Amyloidosis and renal adenocarcinoma: a post-mortem study. *J Pathol* 1972; 107:45–7.

409. Lender M. Amyloidosis associated with neoplastic diseases. *S Afr Med J* 1974; 48:1944–6.

410. Svane S. Hypernephroma and systemic amyloidosis: a report on 3 cases. *Acta Chir Scand* 1970; 136:68–76.

411. Pras M, Franklin EC, Shibolet S, Frangione B. Amyloidosis associated with renal cell carcinoma of the AA type. *Am J Med* 1982; 73:426–8.

412. Lynch WJ, Joske RA. The occurrence of abnormal serum proteins in patients with epithelial neoplasms. *J Clin Pathol* 1966; 19:461–3.

413. Vanatta PR, Silva FG, Taylor WE, Costa JC. Renal cell carcinoma and systemic amyloidosis: demonstration of AA protein and review of the literature. *Hum Pathol* 1983; 14:195–201.

414. Brownstein MH, Helwig EB. Secondary systemic amyloidosis: analysis of underlying disorders. *South Med J* 1971; 64:491–6.

415. Azzopardi JG, Lehner T. Systemic amyloidosis and malignant disease. *J Clin Pathol* 1966; 19:539–48.

416. Mautner G, Roth JS, Grossman ME. Leukocytoclastic vasculitis in association with cryoglobulinemia and renal cell carcinoma. *Nephron* 1993; 63:356–7.

417. Miyachi H, Akizuki M, Yamagata H, et al. Hypertrophic osteoarthropathy, cutaneous vasculitis, and mixed-type cryoglobulinemia in a patient with nasopharyngeal carcinoma. *Arthritis Rheum* 1987; 30:825–9.

418. Schoen FJ, Berger BM, Guerina NG. Cardiac effects of noncardiac neoplasms. *Cardiol Clin* 1984; 2:657–70.

419. Eisner RM, Husain A, Clark JI. IL-2-induced myocarditis. *Cancer Invest* 2004; 22:401–4.

420. Goel M, Flaherty L, Lavine S, Redman BG. Reversible cardiomyopathy after high-does interleukin-2 therapy. *J Immunother* 1992; 11:225–9.

421. Kragel AH, Travis WD, Steis RG, Rosenberg SA, Roberts WC. Myocarditis or acute myocardial infarction associated with interleukin-2 therapy for cancer. *Cancer* 1990; 66:1513–6.

422. Antonelli D, Beker B, Barzilay J. Early cardiotoxicity of 5-fluorouracil. *G Ital Cardiol* 1981; 11:1758–61.

423. Valdes E. Metastatic and paraneoplastic cardiomyopathy. *Jpn Heart J* 1973; 14:548–53.

424. Mousa AR, Al-Din AN. Neurological and cardiac complications of carcinoma of the breast: case report. *Acta Neurol Scand* 1985; 72:518–21.

425. Fernando-Valdes E. Paraneoplastic myocardiopathies. *Rev Clin Esp* 1971; 120:247–50.

426. Agosti SJ, Espinoza CG, Ramirez G. Granulomatous myocarditis with unusual histologic features. *South Med J* 1989; 82:1180–3.

427. Benisch BM, Josephson M. Subacute (giant-cell) thyroiditis and giant-cell myocarditis in patients with carcinoma of the lung. *Chest* 1973; 64:764–5.

428. Williams JO, Pollitzer RS, Green HD. Acute interstitial myocarditis associated with carcinoma of the body of the pancreas: report of a case. *NC Med J* 1952; 13:147–50.

429. Burke MA, Cotts WG. Interpretation of B-type natriuretic peptide in cardiac disease and other comorbid conditions. *Heart Fail Rev* 2007; 12:23–36.

430. Diez-Porres L, Rios-Blanco JJ, Robles-Marhuenda A, et al. ANCA-associated vasculitis as paraneoplastic syndrome with colon cancer: a case report. *Lupus* 2005; 14:632–4.

431. Watz H, Hammerl P, Matter C, et al. Bronchioloalveolar carcinoma of the lung associated with a highly-positive pANCA titer and clinical signs of microscopic polyangiitis. *Pneumologie* 2004; 58:493–8.

432. Hutson TE, Hoffman GS. Temporal concurrence of vasculitis and cancer: a report of 12 cases. *Arthritis Care Res* 2000; 13:417–23.

433. Okada M, Suzuki K, Hidaka T, et al. Polyarteritis associated with hypopharyngeal carcinoma. *Intern Med* 2002; 41:892–5.

434. Mita T, Nakanishi Y, Ochiai A, et al. Paraneoplastic vasculitis associated with esophageal carcinoma. *Pathol Int* 1999; 49: 643–7.

435. Fortin PR. Vasculitides associated with malignancy. *Curr Opin Rheumatol* 1996; 8:30–3.

436. Navarro JF, Quereda C, Rivera M, Navarro JF, Ortuno J. Antineurtrophil cytoplasmic antibody-associated paraneoplastic vasculitis. *Postgrad Med J* 1994; 70:373–5.

437. Liozon E, Loustaud V, Fauchais AL, et al. Concurrent temporal (giant-cell) arteritis and malignancy: report of 20 patients with review of the literature. *J Rheumatol* 2006; 33:1606–14.

438. Mubashir E, Ahmed MM, Hayat S, et al. Wegener granulomatosis: a case report and update. *South Med J* 2006; 99:977–88.

439. Corey EC. Improving congestive heart failure care: a new algorithm for prehospital treatment. *JEMS* 2007; 32:68–74.

3

Histology and Cytopathology

MARK R. WICK

LISA A. CERILLI

■ INTRODUCTION

Metastatic malignancy of unknown origin (MMUO) represents a clinical and pathological challenge that is encountered in approximately 10% of cancer cases. The major goal in such instances is to identify treatable disease while minimizing unnecessary and futile therapy and iatrogenic patient morbidity. Extensive radiologic examination and evaluation of serum tumor markers generally prove to be unsatisfactory in the identification of an origin for metastases from an occult source. Indeed, detailed pathological assessment at the histological and cytological levels probably is the best means for effective characterization of MMUO. The focus of this review is to clarify some of the anatomic, histopathologic, and cytological features that help distinguish one malignant neoplasm from another. The discussion centers on "solid" tumors, and hematopoietic lesions are considered only in the context of differential diagnosis. This is because lymphomas and leukemias are not generally regarded as "metastasizing" tumors, but rather they are potentially systemic proliferations ab initio.

■ ANATOMIC CONSIDERATIONS IN EVALUATIONS OF METASTATIC CARCINOMA

Once an MMUO has proven to be carcinomatous after pathologic examination, an important, but sometimes ignored, clue regarding its origin involves the anatomic pattern of tumor distribution. Although there are certainly some exceptions, cancers arising in particular organs pursue a predictable "life history" and show definite predilections to involve predefined secondary sites. Visceral sites that are associated with particular epithelial malignancies are shown in Figure 1, and lymph node groups that are preferentially involved by selected carcinomas are depicted in Figure 2 (1).

For example, one may encounter a woman with axillary lymphadenopathy in whom a biopsy of the involved nodes demonstrates adenocarcinoma. Additional evaluation for possible metastases may show tumor deposits in the bones and liver. In assessing the most probable sources for metastases in all of those sites, one would direct principal attention to the breasts and the lungs, with the former being the more likely source. Similarly, a 32-year-old man with left supraclavicular lymphadenopathy (Virchow's node) (2) and a nodal biopsy showing poorly differentiated carcinoma, would most likely have a gonadal or gastric primary neoplasm. The prediction would be quite different if the involved lymph nodes were in the *right* supraclavicular group.

Hence, by integrating patient age, gender, and anatomic site(s) of tumor presentation, a likelihood table can be assembled of the probable sites of origin for the metastatic lesions. Pathologists use this information in a fundamental fashion, and it has substantial weight, together with nuances of morphology and other studies, in predicting the organ of origin for carcinomatous MMUOs.

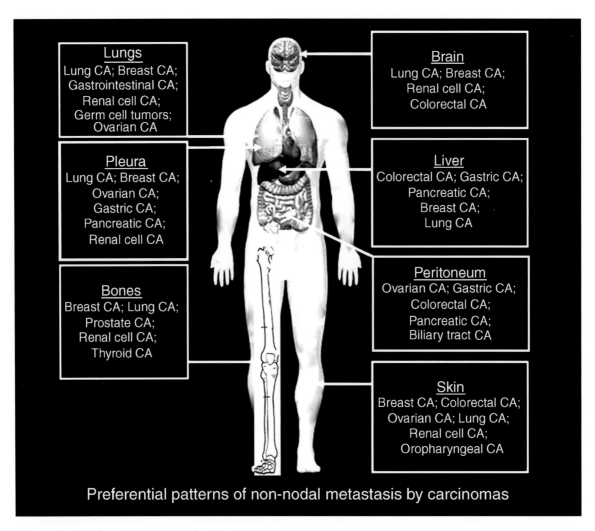

FIGURE 1 Diagram of preferential visceral sites for metastatic carcinomas.

■ SPECIAL MORPHOLOGICAL CATEGORIES OF METASTATIC TUMORS

Metastatic tumors that appear as nondescript large cell undifferentiated malignancies or "banal" adenocarcinomas are the most troublesome in regard to prediction of their sites of origin, based on conventional morphologic features alone. Indeed, one must usually rely on the age of the patient, the anatomic distribution of disease, ultrastructural or immunophenotypic findings, and results of other adjunctive studies in such cases. These ancillary evaluations are discussed in other sections of this chapter; this particular discussion focuses on morphological and histochemical "triage" of the tumors under consideration. The following sections present information on metastatic lesions that exhibit distinctive microscopic appearances that can be used to determe their possible anatomic sources.

Malignant Small Round Cell Tumors

The term *small round cell tumor* (SRCT) has traditionally been used in reference to a heterogeneous group of neoplasms that occur primarily in the soft tissue in childhood and adolescence. These lesions share the histologic image of a densely cellular proliferation with a primitive, undifferentiated appearance, and each of them may present with distant metastases to lymph nodes or viscera. SRCT is a descriptive rather than a specific diagnostic designation, and there are important therapeutic and prognostic differences attached to the different entities that comprise this group. Adjunctive techniques, especially immunohistochemical studies, cytogenetics, and electron microscopy, are critical in refining pathological interpretation and should be regarded as a routine part of the evaluation of such tumors. The application of these methods has been well described (3–8). However, the

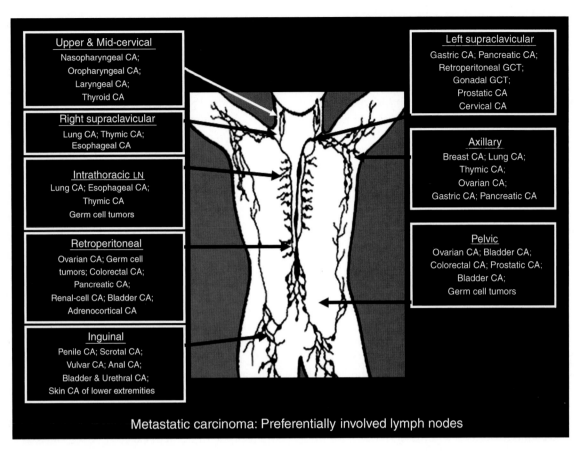

FIGURE 2 Diagram of preferential lymph node sites for metastatic carcinomas.

subsequent focus here will be on the morphological characteristics that are observed in the different tumors in this category.

These principally include Ewing sarcoma (ES) and primitive neuroectodermal tumor (PNET), both of which are considered to be part of the same neoplastic disease spectrum; juvenile-type rhabdomyosarcoma (RMS); neuroblastoma (NB); and small cell carcinomas. Only the last of those lesions is specifically germane to the topic of this monograph, but the other small cell neoplasms just listed will be considered for the sake of comparison with small cell carcinoma.

Histologically, both PNET and ES are composed of relatively monomorphic cells with round-to-oval nuclei and scant cytoplasm (3). True rosettes and pseudorosettes are potentially seen in this spectrum of neoplasms (Fig. 3). The chromatin pattern is somewhat variable, ranging from fine and homogeneous to irregularly clumped, usually with relatively indistinct nucleoli. The presence of rosettes correlates with primitive neural differentiation (i.e., the PNET portion of the tumor spectrum), but frequently these structures are absent. Surprisingly, few mitotic figures are typically visible,

given the high-grade biological nature of ES/PNET, and a prominent fibrovascular stroma—often with small "blood lakes"—is common (9).

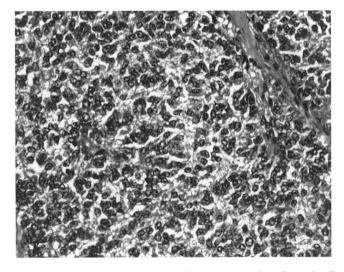

FIGURE 3 Primitive neuroectodermal—a prototypical small round cell malignancy—showing the presence of intercellular pseudorosettes.

Cytological aspirates of ES/PNET typically are highly cellular and are composed of a distinctly dimorphic cell population. Large cells demonstrating "blastic" chromatin usually predominate, and these are intermingled with smaller cells, showing dense, condensed chromatin and resembling mature lymphocytes (10). It should be noted that a dimorphic population is not diagnostic of ES/PNET in an SRCT, because degenerative changes or pyknosis may simulate this finding. When they are present, cytoplasmic vacuoles in ES/PNET are coarse and "punched out" in Romanowsky-stained preparations; finely vacuolated cytoplasm also may be encountered (11). The cytologic presence of wispy cytoplasmic extensions (or neurites) is another possibility in this group of lesions. Diffuse histochemical positivity with the periodic acid-Schiff (PAS) re-agent is typical of ES-PNET (12), and, in particular, it would not be expected in a small cell carcinoma (13).

Other tumor types may assume partial or global histological images that simulate those of ES/PNET, especially in limited biopsy specimens. For example, primary or metastatic small cell (undifferentiated) synovial sarcoma has been documented objectively, as confirmed by the presence of *SYT/SSX* fusion transcripts, which is seen in association with the characteristic t(X;18) chromosomal translocation of synovial sarcoma, and a lack of *EWS/FLI1* transcripts, which is associated with the t(11;22) chromosomal translocation of ES/PNET (14). Lymphoblastic lymphoma also may present as a localized mass that clinically, histologically, and (to some extent) immunophenotypically imitates ES/PNET. However, lymphoblastic lymphoma demonstrates more nuclear irregularity, apoptotic cellular dropout, and mitotic activity, and also may show lymphoglandular bodies in cytologic preparations (15).

RMS of the solid-alveolar variety (16) has a subtype that may manifest itself with extensive involvement of lymph nodes, and potentially of the bone marrow as well, in the absence of an obvious primary lesion in the soft tissue. This form of the tumor is known as lymphadenopathic RMS (LRMS) (17). The neoplastic cells in LRMS demonstrate a somewhat greater degree of nuclear pleomorphism than that seen in other SRCTs, occasionally with interspersed large cells possessing relatively generous amounts of eosinophilic cytoplasm. Nuclei are not dissimilar in appearance to those of ES/PNET, and LRMS also shares potential PAS positivity with neuro-ectodermal tumors. If foci suggesting an "alveolar" (dyshesive) growth pattern are observed in a PAS-reactive SRCT, the diagnosis of RMS should be favored (10, 15).

A large percentage of NB cases also have metastases to bone, liver, lymph nodes, or skin, with or without elevated levels of catecholamines or their metabolites in the urine. The primary tumors may reside in the adrenal medulla or the remainder of the sympathetic nervous system (18, 19).

Histologically, metastatic NB may be extremely difficult to distinguish from ES/PNET or other SRCT, particularly in small biopsy specimens that frequently are distorted by crush artifacts. NB is composed of primitive round-to-angulated cells with scant cytoplasm. Well-formed true rosettes and pseudorosettes, neuropil formation, and dystrophic calcification may aid in the diagnosis of this lesion (20, 21). A careful search is also worthwhile for primitive or mature ganglionic elements, represented by nucleolated cells with eccentric, relatively abundant eosinophilic cytoplasm (22).

Small cell neuroendocrine carcinomas (SCNCs) are the most important small cell malignancies that may present as an MMUO (23–25), because of their much greater frequency than all other SRCTs. The histological appearance of such tumors is that of a variably organoid proliferation of extensively apoptotic small neoplastic cells with brisk mitotic and apoptotic activity, often demonstrating prominent crush artifacts (Fig. 4) (26). Cytologically, these tumors are composed of small cells with high nuclear-to-cytoplasmic ratios, nuclear "smearing," nuclear molding, powdery chromatin, usually inconspicuous nucleoli, scant cytoplasm, and a tendency for loose cohesion and cellular dispersion (Fig. 5) (15, 27–29). Staining with Romanowsky methods may reveal fine metachromatic cytoplasmic granules. Reactivity with argyrophilic histochemical techniques, such as the Sevier-Munger, Grimelius, or Churukian-Schenk procedures, is helpful in recognizing that small cell carcinomas have neuroendocrine features (Fig. 6) (30,31). This is best appreciated in specimens that are fixed in Bouin's re-agent. In some locations, such as the skin, it may be problematic

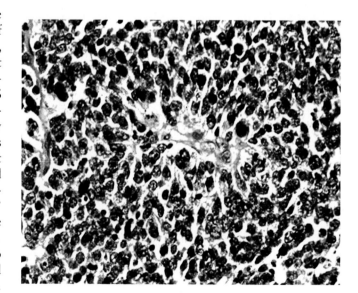

FIGURE 4 "Crush" artifact in small cell neuroendocrine carcinoma is a reflection of the fragility of the tumor cells.

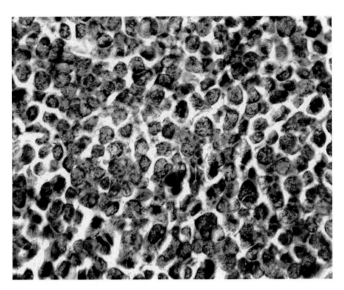

FIGURE 5 Cytological appearance of small cell neuroendocrine carcinoma, featuring the presence of nuclear "molding," in which the nuclei of adjacent tumor cells push into one another.

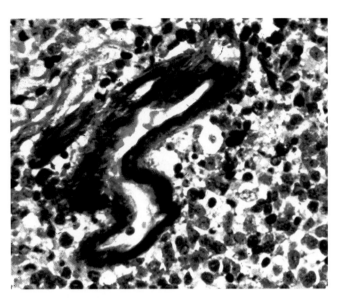

FIGURE 7 The Azzopardi phenomenon in small cell neuroendocrine carcinoma is caused by encrustation of intratumoral blood vessels by nucleic acid. It reflects the high proliferative rate of this neoplasm.

pathologically to determine whether an SCNC has arisen at that site, or, alternatively, has involved it secondarily. In that narrow context, the presence of the Azzopardi phenomenon, represented by the encrustation of intratumoral blood vessels with basophilic nucleic acid (Fig. 7) (32, 33), argues strongly for a secondary deposit.

Once metastatic SCNCs are identified, there are few other nuances of morphology or biochemistry that can be used with certainty to predict their sources. In particular, cellular peptide and amine products are broadly shared among this group of neoplasms, regardless of their topographic origins (34). Hence, anatomic patterns of

metastasis, as discussed above, and the relative frequency of SCNC in various organ systems must be used as the principal data in determining the likely source.

Malignant Oncocytoid Tumors

Cells showing intense cytoplasmic acidophilia (eosinophilia) have been referred to using a variety of terms, including oncocyte, oxyphil, Hurthle cell, Ashkenazy cell, and others (35). Although oncocytoid change reflects an abundance of mitochondria, a similar cytologic image may relate to the presence of abundant cytoplasmic organelles such as lysosomes, neuroendocrine granules, cytofilaments, and smooth endoplasmic reticulum. Detailed cytologic evaluation of the precise character of cellular eosinophilia often reveals subtle variations, such as fibrillary, globular, diffuse (homogeneous), or granular cytoplasmic patterns.

Over the past several decades, awareness has increased regarding tumors that are composed predominantly or exclusively of oncocytoid cells. Furthermore, a concept has emerged that oncocytic metaplasia may occur in lesions that are not typically associated with that feature. Oncocytic neoplasms can be encountered in virtually any organ, but they arise most often in the salivary glands, thyroid, kidneys, liver, and parathyroid glands (36–40). Those that are biologically malignant and may present with distant metastasis are listed in Table 1. They are further considered according to the detailed nature of their oncocytoid changes in the following discussion.

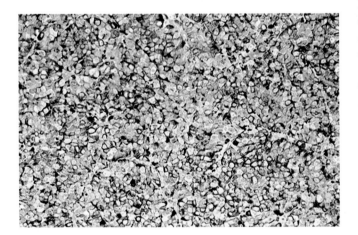

FIGURE 6 Positive Sevier-Munger (argyrophil) stain in high-grade neuroendocrine carcinoma.

Table 1 Tumors with metastatic potential and oncocytic or clear cell features

Oncocytic Neoplasms	Clear Cell Neoplasms
Carcinoid tumor	Renal cell carcinoma
Renal cell carcinoma	Mucoepidermoid carcinoma
Medullary thyroid carcinoma	Paraganglioma
Fibrolamellar hepatocellular carcinoma	Seminoma/dysgerminom
Pancreatic endocrine carcinomas	Malignant melanoma
Salivary gland carcinomas	
Hepatoid yolk-sac tumor	
Pancreatic acinar cell carcinoma	

Table 2 Cytologic findings in hepatocellular carcinoma and metastatic adenocarcinoma

	Hepatocellular Carcinoma	Metastatic Adenocarcinoma
Cellularity	High	High
Cellular arrangement	Sinusoidal capillaries	Clusters and single cells
	Endothelial cells around cell clusters	
	Trabecular structures	
Bile	Sometimes present	Absent
Nuclei	Marked anisonucleosis	Mild-to-marked nuclear pleomorphism
	Centrally placed nuclei	Central or eccentrically placed nuclei
	± Multinucleation	
	Prominent nucleoli	± Nucleolar prominence
Cytoplasm	Granular	± Cytoplasmic vacuoles
Mucin	Almost always absent	Commonly present
Necrosis	Uncommon	Common

Malignant Neoplasms with Granular Cytoplasmic Eosinophilia

Metastatic malignancies that demonstrate granular cytoplasmic acidophilia are varied in their origins and lineage of differentiation. For example, low-grade neuroendocrine carcinomas of the lung, gut, and pancreas, medullary (neuroendocrine) carcinoma of the thyroid, and metastatic ductal breast carcinomas not infrequently appear as secondary intrahepatic nodules, with the primary lesion having eluded clinical detection until that point (Figs. 8 and 9) (37, 39–41).

Histologically, in such cases, variably organoid arrays of large cells can be observed with round nuclei, inconstant mitotic activity, dispersed chromatin, and indistinct nucleoli. Cytologically, these tumors manifest as flat sheets, loose groups, cords, and singly dispersed polygonal cells, usually with a strikingly monotonous appearance. The polyhedral cells may be intermingled with spindled forms. The presence of neurosecretory granules, represented by fine red cytoplasmic granules, is highly suggestive of neuroendocrine differentiation and may be detected in Romanowsky stains. Capillaries cuffed with tumor cells are a characteristic finding, and true papillae or psammoma bodies can be seen. The presence of metachromatic amorphous stroma points to the possible presence of amyloid, and appropriate histochemical stains for amyloid (e.g., Congo red, Lieb's, Pagoda red, and thioflavine-T) (42) can then be applied to investigate this eventuality. It should be remembered that the amyloid matrix is not pathognomonic of medullary thyroid carcinoma, inasmuch as it can be present in neuroendocrine carcinomas of the lung, thymus, pancreas, and other sites as well (43–46).

Both exocrine and endocrine carcinomas of the pancreas also may show oncocytoid features, though such tumors are rare in the "pure" form (39). Most exocrine pancreatic lesions containing groups of granular eosinophilic cells demonstrate an admixture of other histologic patterns; the most common is "conventional" ductal adenocarcinoma. Acinar carcinomas of the pancreas are typified by coarsely granular cytoplasm because of the presence of cytoplasmic zymogen (proenzyme) granules (Fig. 10) (47).

Finally, hepatocellular carcinomas (HCCs) often exhibit granular cytoplasmic eosinophilia caused by the presence of lipofuscin granules and abundant endoplasmic

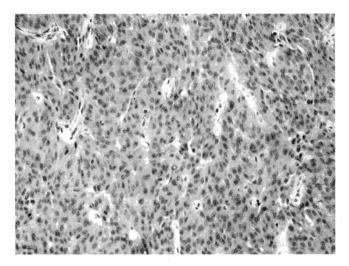

FIGURE 8 Oncocytoid metastatic neuroendocrine carcinoma, showing a composition by monomorphous tumor cells with eosinophilic cytoplasm.

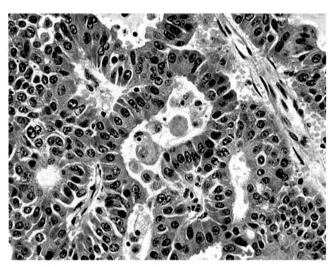

FIGURE 10 Acinar cell carcinoma of the pancreas, showing cytoplasmic eosinophilia.

reticulum (Fig. 11) (39). Up to 15% of HCCs show globular intracytoplasmic PAS-negative oxyphilic inclusions, which, when present, are useful diagnostic clues (48). In fine-needle aspiration biopsy specimens, the tumor cells may be seen singly, in sheets, or in compact cords. Intranuclear cytoplasmic invaginations, intracellular cytoplasmic globules, or bile pigment (highlighted with the Fouchet stain) (Fig. 12) may also be observed (49, 50).

Malignant Neoplasms with Globular Cytoplasmic Eosinophilia

When strictly defined by the presence of an inclusion-like mass of densely eosinophilic cytoplasm that displaces the nucleus, globular cytoplasmic eosinophilia characterizes a distinct group of heterogeneous neoplasms that are designated as "rhabdoid" (35). In the authors' opinion, malignant rhabdoid tumors demonstrate heterogeneous differentiation but have uniformly aggressive biological behavior (51). Hence, rhabdoid cells in metastatic lesions

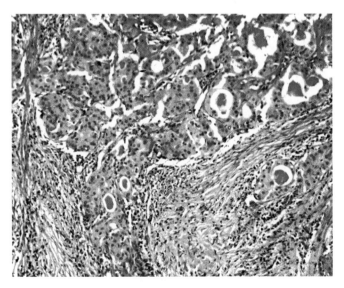

FIGURE 9 Oncocytoid invasive ductal breast carcinoma, demonstrating the presence of generous eosinophilic cytoplasm in the tumor cells.

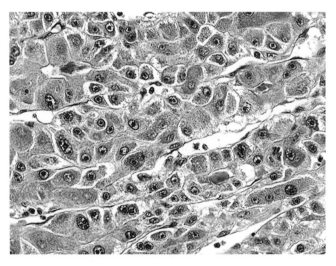

FIGURE 11 "Conventional" hepatocellular carcinoma, demonstrating oncocytoid eosinophilic cytoplasm and the presence of intercellular bile production.

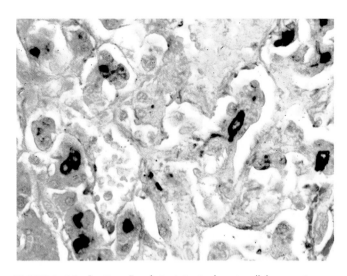

FIGURE 12 Positive Fouchet stain in hepatocellular carcinoma, labeling intratumoral deposits of bile bright green.

may be part of tumors that can arise in virtually any anatomic site. The neoplastic cells should be further scrutinized for the presence of cross striations and melanin, because RMS and malignant melanoma are potentially included in the morphologic grouping under discussion here (51, 52).

Cytologically, all forms of malignant rhabdoid tumor, regardless of whether they are carcinomatous, melanomatous, or sarcomatous, show dispersed cells with moderate nuclear pleomorphism, anisocytosis, and few other distinguishing features (Fig. 13). Therefore, special stains or ultrastructural studies again are essential in the definitive characterization of such lesions.

Malignant rhabdoid tumors often metastasize simultaneously to several anatomic sites. This fact, along with the inconstant morphologic features of this concatenation of lesions, may make it impossible to identify the origin of such neoplasms. From a practical perspective, metastatic malignant rhabdoid tumors are, as a group, generally poorly responsive to treatment (51), and localization of their primary sites or determination of their precise lineages is of academic interest only.

Malignant Neoplasms with Diffuse Cytoplasmic Eosinophilia

Complicated diagnostic problems are attached to the group of neoplasms that show diffuse cytoplasmic eosinophilia with no other discriminating features. This constellation of tumors includes high-grade carcinomas arising in several locations, melanomas, anaplastic large cell ("Ki-1;" CD30+) non-Hodgkin's lymphomas, and sarcomas with epithelioid features. In reference to MMUO, only the first two of these four possibilities are directly relevant to this discussion. Renal cell carcinoma (RCC), adrenocortical carcinoma, and large cell undifferentiated pulmonary carcinoma (Fig. 14) are the tumors that most commonly assume a large cell oncocytoid appearance with no other distinguishing features (35, 53). Such epithelial malignancies are virtually superimposable on one another morphologically, and adjunctive pathologic analyses are mandatory in discriminating between them. Likewise, amelanotic oncocytoid melanomas require similar adjunctive assessments for confident diagnostic recognition (54), especially if the Fontana-Masson stain is negative.

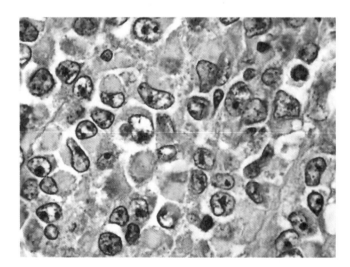

FIGURE 13 Malignant rhabdoid tumor, with abundant and hyaline eosinophilic cytoplasm that displaces nuclei with the neoplastic cells.

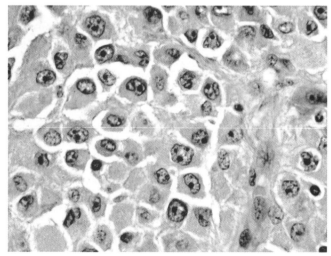

FIGURE 14 Large cell undifferentiated carcinoma of the lung, with oncocytoid eosinophilic cytoplasm.

Malignant Clear Cell Tumors

Malignant tumors with a potential for clear cell change and presentation as MMUO are also diversified. As was true of neoplasms in the preceding section, they include epithelial, mesenchymal, and melanocytic lesions (Table 1) (55). In addition, several matters complicate the evaluation of metastatic tumors in this category. The secondary lesions may undergo tumor progression to acquire clear cell change that reflects clonal evolution. As such, they could then appear dissimilar to the parent neoplasms from which they emanated. Second, selected clear cell malignancies, especially RCC (56), have the capacity to metastasize to organs in which primary clear cell neoplasms are potentially encountered. Such troublesome secondary sites include the ovaries, thyroid (Fig. 15), lungs, liver, oral mucosa, salivary glands, bones, and brain (57, 58). Third, clear cell change may reflect the presence of artifactual degenerative change from processing or fixation deficiencies (59). The following discussion is limited to the most common clear cell tumors, and to those in which clear cell change is a global rather than a focal feature.

Malignant Clear Cell Tumors with a Nested Architecture

Among all clear cell carcinomas, those arising in the kidney are the best recognized and the most frequently seen (55). These tumors may secondarily involve anatomic sites that are usually spared by other metastatic lesions (57), and it is no exaggeration to state that RCC should be entertained in the differential diagnosis of virtually any clear cell malignancy in any location. Nevertheless, the more frequent scenarios are those in which the lung, bones, liver, or brain serve as the foci for metastatic RCCs (Fig. 16). The most reliable pathologic means to address whether the kidney is indeed the source of such neoplasms is to catalog their histological nuances. In particular, if such tumors show hemorrhage into their stroma or within tubular epithelial profiles (Fig. 17), a renal origin is likely (60). Cytologically, the cytoplasm may be optically clear or granular. Cytoplasmic clearing is related to fat or glycogen accumulation, as recognized respectively using Oil-Red-O (Fig. 18) and PAS staining. Fortunately, current radiological imaging studies are sensitive for the detection of even small renal masses (61), and they should be obtained if the observed pathologic features are as cited above.

An uncommon variant of gastric carcinoma, having a tubulopapillary clear cell appearance, can simulate an RCC (62). Conversely, the latter tumor entity may secondarily involve the stomach and thereby cause diagnostic confusion (63). However, the hypervascularity that is so common in RCC is not encountered in clear cell gastric carcinoma. PAS stains are positive in many clear cell carcinomas, but intracytoplasmic diastase resistance and mucicarmine reactivity are limited to primary gastric neoplasms (64). The colloidal iron method will also label clear cell cancers of the stomach.

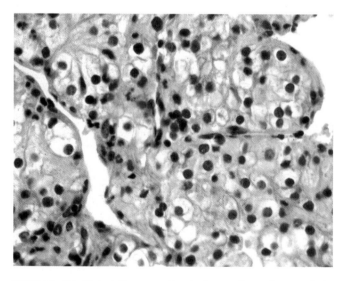

FIGURE 15 Metastatic conventional clear cell carcinoma of the kidney, presenting with metastasis to the brain.

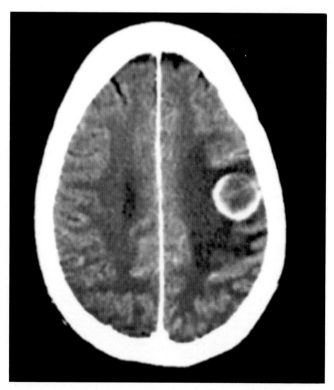

FIGURE 16 Computed tomogram of the brain, demonstrating a solitary "seminal" metastasis of renal cell carcinoma.

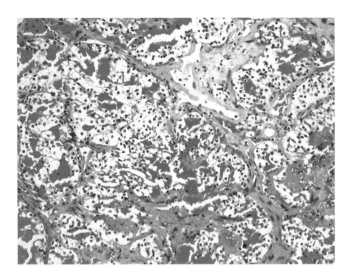

FIGURE 17 Intratumoral hemorrhage in metastatic renal cell carcinoma is a characteristic finding in this tumor.

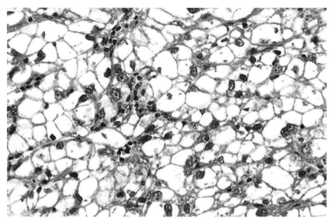

FIGURE 19 The clear cell variant of hepatocellular carcinoma can be confused pathologically with metastatic carcinomas of renal, thyroid, pulmonary, and other origins.

The clear cell form of HCC (Fig. 19) is an uncommon variant that can easily be confused with metastatic tumors, most commonly those of renal, ovarian, or adrenal origin (65, 66). Clear cell change in all of these tumors results from accumulation of intracytoplasmic fat, or glycogen, or both, making histochemical staining rather unfruitful as a differential diagnostic tool. Hence, electron microscopic evaluations are more helpful in resolving problems of identity (see Chapter 4) (66). Cytologically, smears of each of the lesions in this group are generally hypercellular; they consist of loosely cohesive groups and individually scattered malignant cells with anisonucleosis, nuclear hyperchromasia, irregular prominent nucleoli, and abundant finely vacuolated to clear cytoplasm (67).

Clear cell thyroid carcinomas of both the papillary and follicular types have been reported (68). Although clear cell change may be found focally in many thyroid lesions, both benign and malignant, the authors have limited this discussion to those in which clear cells are the predominant or exclusive cell phenotype (Fig. 20). Again, the ability of RCC to selectively involve the thyroid accounts for the fact that metastatic RCC is the principal differential diagnostic alternative to primary clear cell carcinomas within the thyroid capsule (69, 70).

In extrathyroidal sites such as lymph nodes and bone, metastatic clear cell thyroid cancers share many histological features with other clear cell malignancies.

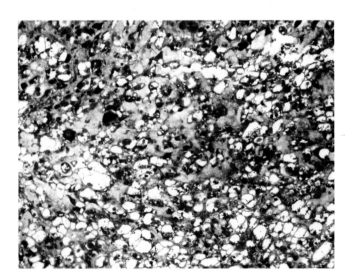

FIGURE 18 Positive Oil-Red-O stain in metastatic renal cell carcinoma.

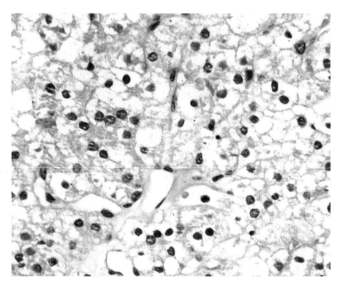

FIGURE 20 The clear cell subtype of follicular thyroid carcinoma is particularly difficult to separate diagnostically from metastatic renal cell carcinoma.

Cytological findings in clear cell papillary thyroid carcinoma (CCPTC) include the presence of nuclear pseudoinclusions and grooves, as seen in conventional papillary tumors (71). Unfortunately, these are not specific and can be observed in metastatic renal tumors as well (71). In addition, multinucleated tumor cells may be seen in CCPTC, and these are particularly helpful because they are not a part of the cytologic spectrum of other clear cell carcinomas (72). Follicular formations containing colloid-like material are likewise supportive of clear cell follicular thyroid carcinoma or CCPTC.

Sclerosing Clear Cell Malignancies

Clear cell carcinomas with a sclerotic stroma are almost entirely restricted in distribution to the salivary glands, and metastatic behavior in these tumors is distinctly unusual. Hence, they are included here principally for the sake of completeness. Hyalinizing clear cell carcinoma is a rare, recently described entity that arises in minor salivary glands and is usually confined to them (73, 74). It is characterized by solid sheets and cords of large clear cells separated by hyalinized collagen with focal myxoid degeneration. Clear cells are also seen in acinic cell carcinoma in approximately 6% of cases (Fig. 21) (74), and even fewer demonstrate intratumoral fibrosis. The vast majority of such tumors show cells with more typical amphophilic or basophilic granular cytoplasm. Acinic cell carcinomas do uncommonly involve the cervical lymph nodes metastatically, but more distant spread is exceedingly rare. Most pertinently to this discussion, such salivary gland masses may be confused with clear cell metastases from other organs, particularly the kidneys.

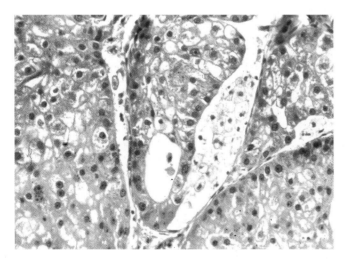

FIGURE 21 Acinic cell carcinoma of the salivary glands may be composed of clear cells, as shown here, but it rarely if ever presents with metastatic disease in the absence of a known primary tumor.

Salivary glandular clear cell carcinomas that show sclerosis can generally be regarded as primary lesions, because metastatic involvement of the salivary gland apparatus from other anatomic sources, with this particular histologic feature, is highly unlikely (73). Nevertheless, as just mentioned above, some metastatic clear cell (balloon cell) melanomas (75) may simulate the images of sclerosing clear cell carcinomas, as may selected large cell non-Hodgkin's lymphomas, both inside and outside the salivary glands (55). Hence, PAS and Fontana-Masson stains should be performed routinely in these cases; reactivity in either of these two methods militates strongly against a diagnosis of lymphoma, and Fontana-Masson positivity is diagnostic of melanoma in this particular setting. Obviously, immunohistologic evaluations and electron microscopy are also important additions.

Clear Cell Tumors Lacking Consistent Architectural Patterns

Clear cell malignancies in general are, as stated earlier, weighted toward epithelial lesions. Clear cell carcinomas with medullary growth or mixed architectural features may originate in the salivary glands, prostate ("hypernephroid" adenocarcinoma), male and female genital tracts, kidneys, adrenal glands, skin, or lungs, among other sites (55).

Other carcinomas that potentially assume a clear cell image and lack a consistent growth pattern are represented by both adenocarcinomas and "hydropic" squamous carcinomas (59). The organs of origin for such lesions are diverse and include virtually any site in which a glandular or squamous carcinoma may arise. Other than anatomic patterns of spread and histochemical or ultrastructural features in such lesions, there are no reliable architectural or cytological features that can be used to predict the topographic sources of these lesions. Fortunately, the immunophenotypes of primary clear cell prostatic, pulmonary, renal, salivary, and cutaneous tumors demonstrate many points of dissimilarity, making such profiles valuable in differential diagnosis (55) (see Chapter 5).

Classic seminoma/germinoma represents a straightforward diagnosis when the tumor arises in the gonads; however, this lesion is often misinterpreted when it presents as a metastatic lesion or as a primary extragonadal mass. A diffuse arrangement of clear tumor cells is typical of this neoplasm, sometimes with irregular separation or compartmentalization by fibrous stroma (Fig. 22) (76). The latter can be highlighted with the use of Snook's stain, showing broad investment by reticulin of neoplastic cell groups. Other common cytomorphologic features of seminoma/germinoma include well-defined cell borders, evenly spaced nuclei, and single prominent central nucleoli (77). When they are present, multinucleated

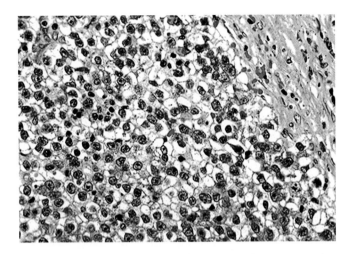

FIGURE 22 Seminoma is another tumor type that demonstrates a clear cell constituency.

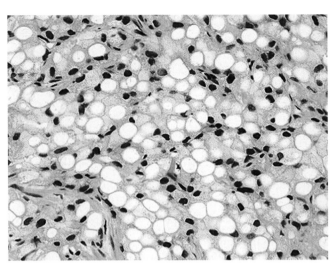

FIGURE 24 Signet-ring cell adenocarcinomas comprise neoplastic cells with intracytoplasmic vacuoles that displace the nucleus.

syncytiotrophoblastic cells, epithelioid granulomas, and a mature stromal lymphocytic infiltrate are also helpful interpretatively. Abundant intracytoplasmic glycogen is evident on PAS staining (Fig. 23).

Finally, a distinctive subset of tumors in this group are those that have a clear cell appearance because of their composition by "signet-ring" cells. These elements have an intracytoplasmic vacuole that displaces the nucleus to the periphery of the cell, yielding a configuration like that of a signet ring (Fig. 24). Signet-ring cell tumors are usually carcinomas, originating especially in the breasts or the alimentary tract (78). However, lymphomas,

melanomas, neuroendocrine tumors, and some mesenchymal malignancies (e.g., gastrointestinal stromal tumors) also can have a partial or global signet-ring cell constituency (79–82). The vacuoles in signet-ring cell adenocarcinomas typically are labeled with the PAS procedure and the colloidal iron technique (Fig. 25) (83).

Malignant Spindle Cell and Pleomorphic Tumors

Metastatic carcinomas from various organ sites may occasionally have such overwhelming spindle cell components that they virtually perfectly reproduce the appearance

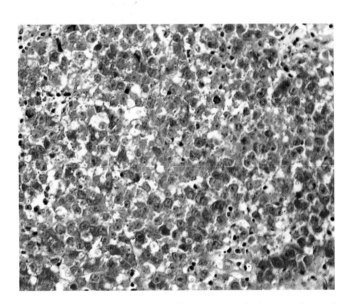

FIGURE 23 Seminoma is typically reactive with the periodic acid-Schiff (PAS) stain, as shown here.

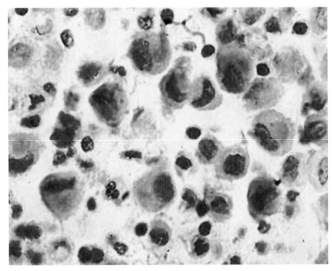

FIGURE 25 Colloidal iron positivity (for mucin) in signet-ring cell adenocarcinoma.

of sarcomas (84). For example, a relatively common setting is that of a bone lesion composed of spindle cells for which a primary osseous origin cannot be excluded on radiographic studies or conventional pathologic assessment (Fig. 26). A significant proportion of these cases represent metastatic sarcomatoid renal cell or lung carcinomas, and additional imaging reveals a mass in the kidney or thorax (85, 86). In such instances, the primary tumors may be entirely sarcomatoid (Fig. 27) or represent a preponderance of epithelioid cells with only focal spindle cell differentiation. Morphologically, similar primary sarcoma-like carcinomas may also be encountered in the urinary tract, female genital tract, alimentary tract and pancreas, thyroid, upper airway mucosa, and other locations (84). Thus, malignant spindle cell tumors in potential secondary sites such as the lymph nodes, bones, lungs, brain, and liver should be subjected to a careful search for foci of clustered polyhedral cells, which, if found, would argue strongly for a diagnosis of carcinoma.

Cytologically, the image of sarcomatoid carcinoma (SC) is much more suggestive of true sarcoma than of an epithelial neoplasm. Cellular dyshesion, anisocytosis, nuclear pleomorphism, unremarkable cytoplasmic details, and nondescript stroma are their usual features (Fig. 28) (87). Obviously, the level of suspicion for SC must be high in these circumstances, and adjunctive studies are

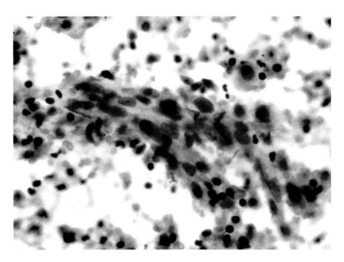

FIGURE 28 Fine-needle aspiration biopsy of sarcomatoid carcinoma, showing dyshesive and obviously atypical tumor cells. This image would also be expected in sarcomas.

mandatory to establish a firm objective diagnosis. Similar comments apply to spindle cell and pleomorphic melanomas, which likewise may present with metastatic disease and a lack of melanin pigment (88).

With regard to true spindle cell sarcomas, it should be remembered that these neoplasms only exceptionally manifest themselves initially with metastatic disease in the absence of a known primary tumor. Malignant fibrous

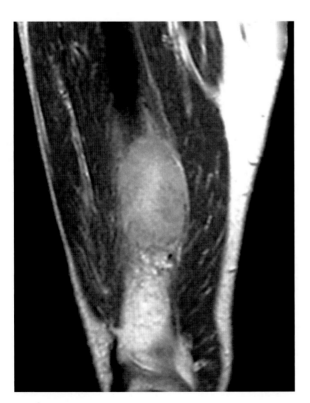

FIGURE 26 MRI showing metastatic clear cell renal cell carcinoma presenting with unifocal osseous metastasis.

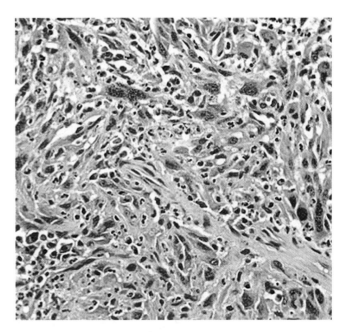

FIGURE 27 Metastatic sarcomatoid carcinomas comprise fusiform and pleomorphic cells, closely simulating the histological appearance of primary sarcomas.

histiocytomas in various locations and leiomyosarcomas of the deep soft tissue or myometrium occasionally may do so, but generally speaking, metastatic sarcomas are not associated with occult topographic origins.

■ REFERENCES

1. Lawrence W, Lenhard RE, Murphy GP, eds. American Cancer Society Textbook of Clinical Oncology, 2nd Ed. *American Cancer Society*, New York, 1995.

2. Ludwig J. Virchow-Troisier's lymph node. *J Clin Gastroenterol* 1991; 13:720–1.

3. Hicks J, Mierau GW. The spectrum of pediatric tumors in infancy, childhood, and adolescence: a comprehensive review with emphasis on special techniques in diagnosis. *Ultrastruct Pathol* 2005; 29:175–202.

4. Hill DA, O'Sullivan MJ, Zhu X, et al. Practical application of molecular genetic testing as an aid to the surgical pathologic diagnosis of sarcomas: a prospective study. *Am J Surg Pathol* 2002; 26:965–77.

5. Panani AD, Roussos C. Cytogenetic and molecular aspects of lung cancer. *Cancer Lett* 2006; 239:1–9.

6. Welborn J, Jenks H, Taplett J, Walling P. High-grade neuroendocrine carcinomas display unique cytogenetic aberrations. *Cancer Genet Cytogenet* 2004; 155:33–41.

7. Peydro-Olaya A, Llombart-Bosch A, Carda-Batalla C, Lopez-Guerrero JA. Electron microscopy and other ancillary techniques in the diagnosis of small round-cell tumors. *Semin Diagn Pathol* 2003; 20:25–45.

8. Devoe K, Weidner N. Immunohistochemistry of small round-cell tumors. *Semin Diagn Pathol* 2000; 17:216–24.

9. Dehner LP. Primitive neuroectodermal tumor and Ewing's sarcoma. *Am J Surg Pathol* 1993; 17:1–13.

10. Wakely PE Jr, Frable WJ, Kornstein MJ. Role of intraoperative cytopathology in pediatric surgical pathology. *Hum Pathol* 1993; 24:311–5.

11. Farinola MA, Weir EG, Ali SZ. CD56 expression of neuroendocrine neoplasms on immunophenotyping by flow cytometry: a novel diagnostic approach to fine needle aspiration biopsy. *Cancer* 2003; 99:240–6.

12. Sahu K, Pai RR, Khadilkar UN. Fine needle aspiration cytology of the Ewing's sarcoma family of tumors. *Acta Cytol* 2000; 44:332–6.

13. Wick MR, Scheithauer BW. Primary neuroendocrine carcinoma of the skin. In: Wick MR, ed. *Pathology of Unusual Malignant Cutaneous Tumors*. New York: Marcel-Dekker, 1985:107–80.

14. Lewis TB, Coffin CM, Bernard PS. Differentiating Ewing's sarcoma from other round blue-cell tumors: a RT-PCR translocation panel on formalin-fixed, paraffin-embedded tissues. *Mod Pathol* 2007; 20:397–404.

15. Das DK. Fine needle aspiration (FNA) cytology diagnosis of small round-cell tumors: value and limitations. *Indian J Pathol Microbiol* 2004; 47:309–18.

16. Passmore LM, Myers P, Gilbert-Barness E. Solid-variant alveolar rhabdomyosarcoma of the orbit. *Fetal Pediatr Pathol* 2006; 25:51–7.

17. Chen L, Shah HO, Lin JH. Alveolar rhabdomyosarcoma with concurrent metastasis to bone marrow and lymph nodes, simulating acute hematologic malignancy. *J Pediatr Hematol Oncol* 2004; 26:696–7.

18. Conte M, Parodi S, DeBenardi B, et al. Neuroblastoma in adolescents: the Italian experience. *Cancer* 2006; 106:1409–17.

19. Franks LM, Bollen A, Seseger RC, Stram DO, Matthay KK. Neuroblastoma in adults and adolescents. *Cancer* 1997; 79:2028–35.

20. Askin FB, Perlman EJ. Neuroblastoma and primitive neuroectodermal tumors. *Am J Clin Pathol* 1998; 109(Suppl. 4):S23–30.

21. Triche TJ, Askin FB. Neuroblastoma and the differential diagnosis of small round blue-cell tumors. *Hum Pathol* 1983; 14:569–95.

22. Shimada H, Ambros IM, Dehner LP, et al. The International Neuroblastoma Pathology Classification (the Shimada system). *Cancer* 1999; 86:364–72.

23. Lobins R, Floyd J. Small-cell carcinoma of unknown primary. *Semin Oncol* 2007; 34:39–42.

24. Galanis E, Frytak S, Lloyd RV. Extrapulmonary small cell carcinoma. *Cancer* 1997; 79:1729–36.

25. Hainsworth JD, Johnson DH, Greco FA. Poorly-differentiated neuroendocrine carcinoma of unknown primary site: a newly-recognized clinicopathologic entity. *Ann Intern Med* 1988; 109:364–71.

26. Wick MR, Ritter JH. Neuroendocrine neoplasms: evolving concepts and terminology. *Curr Diagn Pathol* 2002; 8:102–12.

27. Renshaw AA, Voytek TM, Haja J, et al. Distinguishing small cell carcinoma from non-small cell carcinoma of the lung: correlating cytologic features and performance in the College of American Pathologists' non-gynecologic cytology program. *Arch Pathol Lab Med* 2005; 129:619–23.

28. Paulose RR, Shee CD, Abdelhadi IA, Khan MR. Accuracy of touch-imprint cytology in diagnosing lung cancer. *Cytopathology* 2004; 15:109–12.

29. Nicholson SA, Ryan MR. A review of cytologic findings in neuroendocrine carcinomas including carcinoid tumors, with histologic correlation. *Cancer* 2000; 90:148–61.

30. Mosca L, Ceresoli A, Anzanello E, et al. Neuroendocrine structures in normal and diseased human lung. *Appl Pathol* 1986; 4:147–61.

31. Tateishi R, Horai T, Hattori S. Demonstration of argyrophil granules in small cell carcinoma of the lung. *Virchows Arch A Pathol Anat Histol* 1978; 377:203–10.

32. Pritt BS, Cooper K. The Azzopardi phenomenon. *Arch Pathol Lab Med* 2003; 127:1231.

33. Azzopardi JG. Oat-cell carcinoma of the bronchus. *J Pathol Bacteriol* 1959; 78:513–9.

34. Wick MR. Immunohistology of neuroendocrine and neuroectodermal tumors. *Semin Diagn Pathol* 2000; 17:194–203.

35. Nappi O, Ferrara G, Wick MR. Neoplasms composed of eosinophilic polygonal cells: an overview with consideration of different cytomorphologic patterns. *Semin Diagn Pathol* 1999; 16:82–90.

36. Paulino AF, Huvos AG. Oncocytic and oncocytoid tumors of the salivary glands. *Semin Diagn Pathol* 1999; 16:98–104.

37. Fonseca E, Soares P, Cardoso-Oliveira M, Sobrinho-Simoes M. Diagnostic criteria in well-differentiated thyroid carcinomas. *Endocr Pathol* 2006; 17:109–17.

38. Reuter VE. Renal tumors exhibiting granular cytoplasm. *Semin Diagn Pathol* 1999; 16:135–45.

39. Papotti M, Cassoni P, Taraglio S, Bussolati G. Oncocytic and oncocytoid tumors of the exocrine pancreas, liver, and gastrointestinal tract. *Semin Diagn Pathol* 1999; 16:125–34.

40. Baloch ZW, LiVolsi VA. Oncocytic lesions of the neuroendocrine system. *Semin Diagn Pathol* 1999; 16:190–9.

41. Damiani S, Dina R, Eusebi V. Eosinophilic and granular cell tumors of the breast. *Semin Diagn Pathol* 1999; 16:117–25.

42. Cooper JH. Selective amyloid staining as a function of amyloid composition and structure. *Lab Invest* 1974; 31:232–8.

43. Raikhlin NT, Smirnova EA, Satylganov IZ. Histological variants of thyroid medullary carcinoma. *Arkh Pathol* 2001; 63:10–4.

44. Steiner H. Tumors with endocrine activity producing amyloid: a morphological study of insulinomas and in calcitoninoma. *Virchows Arch A Pathol Anat* 1969; 348:170–80.

45. Marchevsky AM, Dikman SH. Mediastinal carcinoid with an incomplete Sipple's syndrome. *Cancer* 1979; 43:2497–501.

46. Abe Y, Utsunomiya H, Tsutsumi Y. Atypical carcinoid tumor of the lung with amyloid stroma. *Acta Pathol Jpn* 1992; 42:286–92.

47. Klimstra DS, Heffess CS, Oertel JE, Rosai J. Acinar cell carcinoma of the pancreas: a clinicopathologic study of 28 cases. *Am J Surg Pathol* 1992; 16:815–37.

48. Muretto P, Piantelli M, Tison V. Hepatocellular carcinoma with intracytoplasmic hyaline globules. *Tumori* 1979; 65:767–75.

49. Gondos B, Forouhar F. Fine needle aspiration cytology of liver tumors. *Ann Clin Lab Sci* 1984; 14:155–8.

50. Nguyen GK. Fine needle aspiration biopsy cytology of hepatic tumors in adults. *Pathol Annu* 1986; 21(Part 1):321–49.

51. Wick MR, Ritter JH, Dehner LP. Malignant rhabdoid tumors: a clinicopathologic review and conceptual discussion. *Semin Diagn Pathol* 1995; 12:233–48.

52. Chang ES, Wick MR, Swanson PE, Dehner LP. Metastatic malignant melanoma with "rhabdoid" features. *Am J Clin Pathol* 1994; 102:426–31.

53. Azar H, Espinoza CG, Richman AV, Saba Sr, Wang T. "Undifferentiated" large cell malignancies: an ultrastructural and immunocytochemical study. *Hum Pathol* 1982; 13:323–33.

54. Suster S. Tumors of the skin composed of large cells with abundant eosinophilic cytoplasm. *Semin Diagn Pathol* 1999; 16:162–77.

55. Nappi O, Mills SE, Swanson PE, Wick MR. Clear cell tumors of unknown nature and origin: a systematic approach to diagnosis. *Semin Diagn Pathol* 1997; 14:164–74.

56. Stenzl A, DeKernion JB. Pathology, biology, and clinical staging of renal cell carcinoma. *Semin Oncol* 1989; 16(Suppl. 1):3–11.

57. Boaziz C. Metastasis of renal cancer. *Ann Urol* 1991; 25:275–82.

58. Tongaonkar HB, Kulkami JN, Kamat MR. Solitary metastases from renal cell carcinoma: a review. *J Surg Oncol* 1992; 49:45–8.

59. Kuo TT. Clear cell carcinoma of the skin: a variant of squamous cell carcinoma that simulates sebaceous carcinoma. *Am J Surg Pathol* 1980; 4:573–83.

60. Jinzaki M, Tanimoto A, Mukai M, et al. Double-phase helical computed tomography of small renal parenchymal neoplasms: correlation with pathologic findings and tumor angiogenesis. *J Comput Assist Tomogr* 2000; 24:835–42.

61. Kim JK, Kim TK, Ahn HJ, et al. Differentiation of subtypes of renal cell carcinoma on helical CT scans. *Am J Roentgenol* 2002; 178:1499–506.

62. Govender D, Ramdial PK, Clarke B, Chetty R. Clear cell (glycogen-rich) gastric adenocarcinoma. *Ann Diagn Pathol* 2004; 8:69–73.

63. Saidi RF, Remine SG. Isolated gastric metastasis from renal cell carcinoma 10 years after radical nephrectomy. *J Gastroenterol Hepatol* 2007; 22:143–4.

64. Nesvetov AM. Gastric biopsy in the diagnosis of stomach diseases. *Arkh Patol* 1975; 37:37–41.

65. Lai CL, Wu PC, Lam KC, Todd D. Histologic-prognostic indicators in hepatocellular carcinoma. *Cancer* 1979; 44:1677–83.

66. Wu PC, Lai CL, Lam KC, Lak AS, Lin HJ. Clear cell carcinoma of the liver: an ultrastructural study. *Cancer* 1983; 552:504–7.

67. Yazdi HM. Cytopathology of clear cell hepatocellular carcinoma in ascitic fluid. *Acta Cytol* 1985; 29:911–3.

68. Carcangiu ML, Sibley RK, Rosai J. Clear cell change in primary thyroid tumors: a study of 38 cases. *Am J Surg Pathol* 1985; 9:705–22.

69. Iesalnieks I, Woenckhaus M, Glockzin G, Schlitt HJ, Agha A. Renal cell carcinoma metastases to the thyroid gland: report of 3 cases and review of the literature. *Zentralbl Chir* 2006; 131:235–9.

70. Dequanter D, Lothaire P, Larsimont D, et al. Intrathyroid metastasis: 11 cases. *Ann Endocrinol* 2004; 65:205–8.

71. Domagala W, Lasota J, Wolska H, et al. Diagnosis of metastatic renal-cell and thyroid carcinomas by intermediate filament typing and cytology of tumor cells in fine needle aspirations. *Acta Cytol* 1988; 32:415–21.

72. Shabb NS, Tawil A, Gergeos F, Saleh M, Azar S. Multinucleated giant cells in fine needle aspiration of thyroid nodules: their diagnostic significance. *Diagn Cytopathol* 1999; 21:307–12.

73. Rinaldo A, McLaren KM, Boccato P, Maran AG. Hyalinizing clear cell carcinoma of the oral cavity and the parotid gland. *J Otorhinolaryngol Relat Spec* 1999; 61:48–51.

74. Mairorano E, Altini M, Favia G. Clear cell tumors of the salivary glands, jaws, and oral mucosa. *Semin Diagn Pathol* 1997; 14:203–12.

75. Kao GF, Helwig EB, Graham JH. Balloon cell malignant melanoma of the skin. *Cancer* 1992; 69:2942–52.

76. Moran CA, Suster S, Przygodski RM, Koss MN. Primary germ cell tumors of the mediastinum. II. Mediastinal seminomas—a clinicopathologic and immunohistochemical study of 120 cases. *Cancer* 1997; 80:691–8.

77. Caraway NP, Fanning CV, Amato RJ, Sneige N. Fine needle aspiration cytology of seminoma: a review of 16 cases. *Diagn Cytopathol* 1995; 12:327–33.

78. Goldstein NS, Long A, Kuan SF, Hart J. Colon signet ring-cell adenocarcinoma: immunohistochemical characterization and comparison with gastric and typical colon adenocarcinomas. *Appl Immunohistochem Molec Morphol* 2000; 8:183–8.

79. Golouh R, Us-Krasovec M, Auersperq M, et al. Amphicrine-composite calcitonin and mucin-producing carcinoma of the thyroid. *Ultrastruct Pathol* 1985; 8:197–206.

80. Nagasaki A, Oshiro A, Miyagi T, et al. Signet ring-cell lymphoma. *Intern Med* 2003; 42:1055–6.

81. Sheibani K, Battifora H. Signet-ring-cell melanoma: a rare morphologic variant of malignant melanoma. *Am J Surg Pathol* 1988; 12:28–34.

82. Suster S, Fletcher CDM. Gastrointestinal stromal tumors with prominent signet-ring-cell features. *Mod Pathol* 1996; 9:609–13.

83. Fadare O. Pleomorphic lobular carcinoma in-situ of the breast composed almost entirely of signet ring cells. *Pathol Int* 2006; 56:683–7.

84. Wick MR, Swanson PE. "Carcinosarcomas:" current perspectives and an historical review of nosological concepts. *Semin Diagn Pathol* 1993; 10:118–27.

85. Reuter VE. Sarcomatoid lesions of the urogenital tract. *Semin Diagn Pathol* 1993; 10:188–201.

86. Nappi O, Wick MR. Sarcomatoid neoplasms of the respiratory tract. *Semin Diagn Pathol* 1993; 10:137–47.

87. Silverman JF, Dabbs DJ, Finley JL, Geisinger KR. Fine needle aspiration biopsy of pleomorphic (giant-cell) carcinoma of the pancreas. *Am J Clin Pathol* 1988; 89:714–20.

88. Wick MR, Fitzgibbon JF, Swanson PE. Cutaneous sarcomas and sarcomatoid neoplasms of the skin. *Semin Diagn Pathol* 1993; 10:148–58.

4

Electron Microscopy

MARK R. WICK

carcinoma or a prostatic adenocarcinoma, or separating a malignant epithelioid mesothelioma from adenocarcinoma involving the serosal surfaces.

Some poorly differentiated tumors have sufficiently distinctive histological features that they can be reliably identified on conventional microscopy. However, these lesions are generally few in number, and widely divergent opinions may therefore be expected in evaluating high-grade malignancies by examination of routinely stained tissue sections. The latter statement is true regardless of the amount of interpretative experience that various observers have accrued. For this reason, adjunctive morphological methods now have an important role in the evaluation of histologically indeterminate or anaplastic malignancies. This section addresses the application of electron microscopy in the previously mentioned settings, and considers the strengths and the limitations of this procedure.

■ INTRODUCTION

Rather commonly, pathologists are faced with the need to determine the characteristics of an obviously epithelial malignancy, with respect to its primary or secondary nature, or, if it is clearly metastatic, its anatomic site of origin. Examples of these situations include small cell "undifferentiated" carcinomas in many locations, adenocarcinomas presenting with lymph nodal or visceral metastasis, and cases in which histologically similar tumors are seen synchronously in two organ sites such as the lung and liver, the breast and lung, or the lung and adrenal gland. Another related problem is "regional" differential diagnosis of high-grade carcinomas or other histologically similar tumors. In this setting one may be interested in distinguishing a renal neoplasm from an adrenocortical lesion when analyzing a large mass that encompasses both the kidney and adrenal gland, distinguishing between hepatocellular carcinoma and cholangiocarcinoma in the liver, determining whether a tumor straddling the bladder and prostate is a transitional-cell

■ GENERAL ULTRASTRUCTURAL APPROACH TO MORPHOLOGICALLY INDETERMINATE TUMORS

When one is faced with a histologically undifferentiated or indeterminate malignant neoplasm, the first task in diagnosis is to determine the general lineage of the lesion. Is the tumor a sarcoma, a lymphoma, a melanoma, or a carcinoma? Indeed, this question still drives the principal application of electron microscopy in surgical pathology (1).

In the sarcomatous group of neoplasms, several have distinguishing ultrastructural characteristics that allow for a definitive diagnosis. For example, rhabdomyosarcomas contain actin and myosin filaments in register with one another, recapitulating, in a primitive way, normal sarcomeric structure (Fig. 1) (2–5). Leiomyosarcomas contain skeins of thin filaments that are punctuated by dense bodies, and cell membranes demonstrate the presence of dense plaques and pinocytotic vesicles

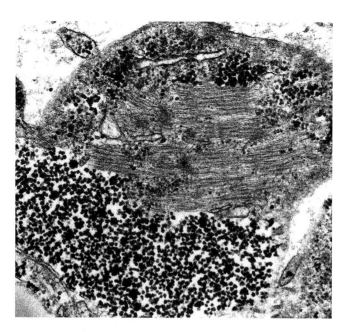

FIGURE 1 Electron photomicrograph of embryonal rhabdomyosarcoma, showing abundant intracellular glycogen and primitive sarcomeric arrays comprising thin and thick filaments.

(Fig. 2) (6). Peripheral nerve sheath sarcomas exhibit elongated, overlapping, and attenuated cellular processes, which are invested by the basal lamina and may embrace

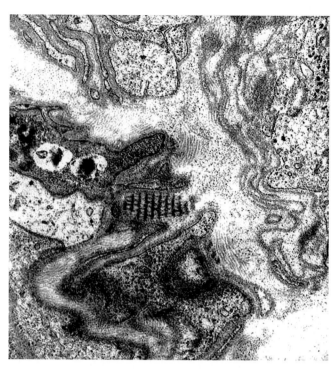

FIGURE 3 A Schwann cell, peripheral-nerve sheath tumor is shown here, with overlapping cell processes, pericellular basal lamina, and "long-spaced" collagen (*center of figure*).

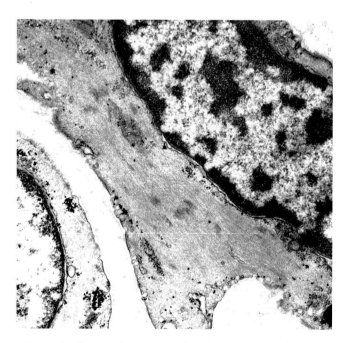

FIGURE 2 Electron photomicrograph of leiomyosarcoma, demonstrating parallel arrays of intermediate filaments that are punctuated by dense bodies. Subplasmalemmal dense patches and pinocytotic vesicles are also present.

long-spaced collagen in the intercellular spaces (Fig. 3) (7). On the other hand, the electron microscopic image of Ewing's sarcoma-primitive neuroectodermal tumor (PNET) represents a possible diagnostic pitfall in that it can be mistaken for an epithelial neoplasm. This is because PNET often shows small intercellular junctional complexes and may contain abundant cytoplasmic glycogen (Fig. 4) (5, 8, 9), features that one usually associates with carcinomas. Paradoxically, it is notable that small cell carcinomas, with which PNET can be confused histologically, are only very glycogen-rich in rare cases (10).

Melanomas are typified ultrastructurally by their content of premelanosomes. These cytoplasmic inclusions are ovoid or rounded structures of medium- or high-electron density, and they contain internal striations (Fig. 5) (11–14). The detection of premelanosomes may require a diligent search of several electron microscopic sections, because amelanotic melanomas contain very few of them (13). This is an important caveat, because the overall ultrastructural image of melanoma cells may otherwise be quite similar to those of undifferentiated carcinomas (11, 15).

Regardless of the particular subtype of lymphoma under study, the basic ultrastructural composition of this tumor group is similar (16–20). Only the most basic

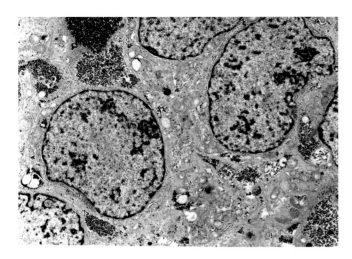

FIGURE 4 A primitive neuroectodermal tumor (PNET) is shown in this electron photomicrograph. Tumor cells are constitutively primitive, except for their content of abundant intracytoplasmic glycogen.

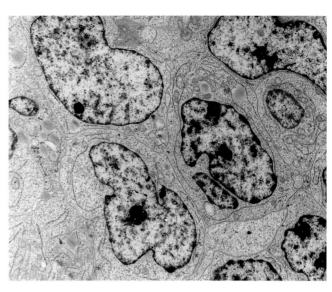

FIGURE 6 Large cell lymphoma is ultrastructurally nondescript. It does not manifest the presence of intercellular junctional complexes, and cytoplasmic organelles are "basic."

cytoplasmic organelles, such as endoplasmic reticulum, mitochondria, lysosomes, and Golgi apparatus, are present. Lymphomas do not manifest intercellular junctions, skeins of microfilaments, neurosecretory granules (NSGs), or any other distinctive cytoplasmic inclusions (Fig. 6) (20). Thus, it should be no surprise that electron microscopy is not particularly definitive in identifying lymphoid lesions. From a diagnostic perspective, the lack of salient ultrastructural findings is never as helpful as their presence.

Finally, carcinomas are, first and foremost, characterized by their formation of well-defined intercellular junctional attachments. These vary in complexity—from

macular to complex and elongated—but their general structure includes well-defined densities in apposing and adjacent cell membranes, with an intervening zone of dense matrix (Fig. 7) (1, 15, 21–24). In addition, most

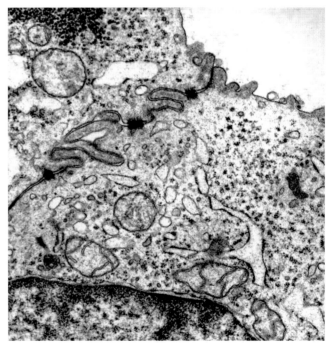

FIGURE 7 Well-formed intercellular junctional complexes, as typically seen in epithelial cells, demonstrate appositional plasmalemmal plaques and an intervening zone of extracellular density.

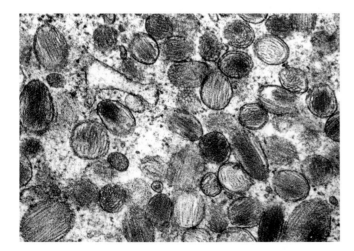

FIGURE 5 Melanomas contain variable numbers of premelanosomes, as shown here. They are cytoplasmic structures that resemble lysosomes, except for the presence of internal striations.

carcinomas (even "undifferentiated" ones) contain identifiable skeins of cytoplasmic intermediate filaments, which often insert into junctional intercellular attachments (Fig. 8) (21, 22).

Further definition of squamous cell carcinoma or transitional cell carcinoma is possible when one observes densely aggregated intermediate filaments forming tonofibrils (also called tonofilaments) (Fig. 9). These very commonly are attached to intercellular junctional complexes (25–28). In comparison, adenocarcinomas are generically recognized by their formation of glandular lumina, which may either be intercellular or intracellular (Fig. 10) (27–32). The latter possibility is especially true of signet-ring cell adenocarcinomas (29, 33). The luminal spaces may contain amorphous secretory material or poorly electron-dense mucin. Tonofibrils are not observed.

Neuroendocrine carcinomas (NECs) are described in a subsequent section of this chapter.

■ ELECTRON MICROSCOPY OF SELECTED EPITHELIAL MALIGNANCIES

Once a metastatic lesion is defined as a carcinoma, further details of its electron microscopic phenotype should be studied for further classification. Because the ultrastructural features of all epithelial neoplasms cannot be covered

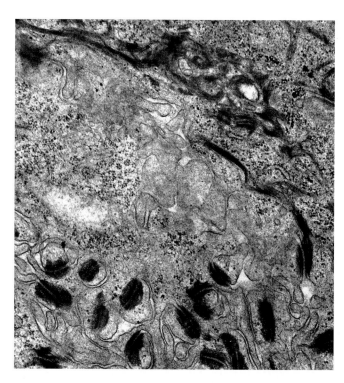

FIGURE 9 Tonofibrils (aggregated bundles of intermediate filaments) often insert into well-formed intercellular junctions in squamous carcinomas.

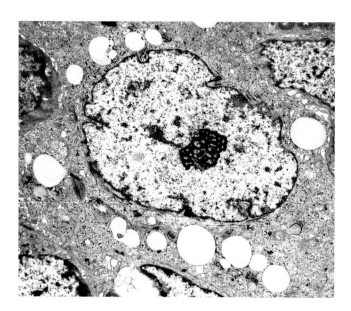

FIGURE 8 Even poorly differentiated carcinoma, including the lymphoepithelioma-like carcinoma shown here, contain intercellular junctional complexes and at least some definable cytoplasmic intermediate filament bundles.

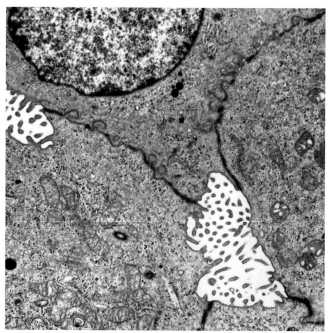

FIGURE 10 This metastatic adenocarcinoma shows the formation of intercellular lumina that are bound by junctional complexes. Plasmalemmal microvilli project into the spaces.

in this chapter, only selected tumor entities in which electron microscopic findings are in some way distinctive are considered here. There are few epithelial tumors the ultrastructural features of which are so singular that they allow for a conclusive diagnosis to be made. Indeed, only epithelioid malignant mesotheliomas and NECs truly fall into this category.

Malignant Epithelioid Mesotheliomas

In mesotheliomas, a constellation of findings that includes abundant skeins of cytoplasmic intermediate filaments (with focal formation of tonofibrils), elongated and complex intercellular junctional complexes, an absence of mucin droplets, and the presence of branched microvilli with a length-to-diameter ratio (LDR) of 10:1 or more is virtually pathognomonic (Figs. 11 and 12) (31, 34–38). Relatively few neoplasms show all of these characteristics (39), but most mesothelial proliferations demonstrate enough of them so as to make their recognition possible. In contrast, adenocarcinomas of various anatomic origins—which represent the principal diagnostic alternative to malignant mesothelioma—exhibit short truncated microvilli and an absence of tonofibrils, and rather commonly also show intracytoplasmic mucin granules (Figs. 13 and 14) (26, 30–32, 40–42).

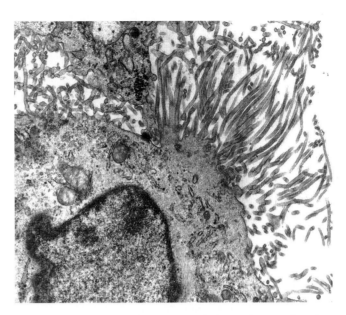

FIGURE 12 The microvilli in mesothelioma have a length-to-diameter ratio of at least 1:10, as opposed to a lower denominator in adenocarcinomas.

Illustrative Case 1: Pseudomesotheliomatous Adenocarcinoma of the Lung

A 59-year-old man presented with a three-month history of cough, right-sided chest pain, and progressive shortness of breath. He had a 40-pack-year cigarette smoking history. Chest radiographs and computed tomograms showed a large right pleural effusion, as well as diffuse thickening of the right pleura by a soft tissue mass. There were no discrete intrapulmonary tumors. Videoscopic

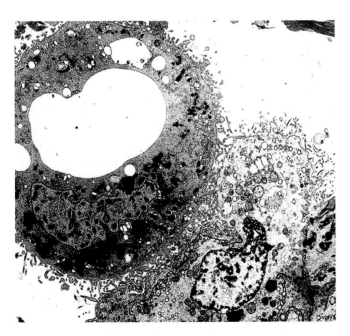

FIGURE 11 Epithelioid mesothelioma, shown here, is characterized by elongated and often-branching microvilli on the surfaces of the tumor cells.

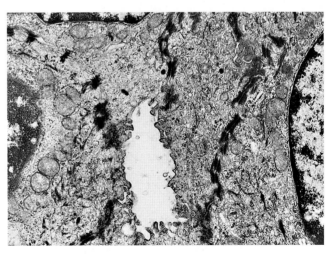

FIGURE 13 The microvilli in this metastatic adenocarcinoma have a length-to-diameter ratio of 1:4 or 1:5.

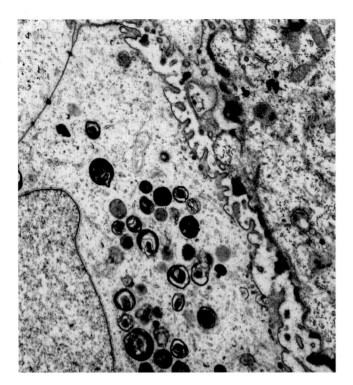

FIGURE 14 This metastatic adenocarcinoma exhibits "stubby" cell-surface microvilli and also the presence of cytoplasmic mucin granules.

thoracoscopy showed that the right pleura was markedly indurated, and that the right lung was encased by a dense "rind" of tissue. A biopsy of the latter was obtained and is represented by the neoplasm shown in Figure 15.

Because a diagnostic decision between epithelioid mesothelioma and "pseudomesotheliomatous" adenocarcinoma of the lung could not be reached on the basis of conventional histology alone, electron microscopy was performed on glutaraldehyde-fixed tissue. This procedure showed the presence of an epithelial neoplasm with nonbranching surface microvilli having an LDR of 1:6 (Fig. 16), in addition to occasional cytoplasmic mucin granules. No tonofibrils or complicated intercellular junctions were apparent. These characteristics indicated a diagnosis of adenocarcinoma, which was felt to be a primary pleurotropic ("pseudomesotheliomatous") pulmonary lesion.

Neuroendocrine Carcinomas

NECs have comparable electron microscopic attributes regardless of their sites of anatomic origin. They feature the presence of small, macular, intercellular junctional complexes, a relative prominence of Golgi apparatus and rough endoplasmic reticulum, and dispersed NSGs. The latter inclusions are round, dense-core structures with a peripheral zone of lucency, varying from 50 to 450 nm in diameter (Figs. 17 and 18) (43). Their intracellular numbers vary inversely with the grade of the tumor; in other words, well-differentiated NECs contain numerous NSGs, whereas high-grade small cell or large cell NECs show only scattered cytoplasmic inclusions of this type (44). Many NECs also show a paranuclear aggregation of intermediate (7–10 nm) filaments, in which dense-core granules may be enmeshed (Fig. 19) (22, 43, 45).

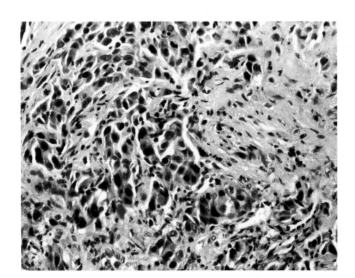

FIGURE 15 Pleural biopsy in illustrative case 1, showing the presence of a malignant, poorly differentiated, epithelioid neoplasm, the differential diagnosis for which is adenocarcinoma versus mesothelioma.

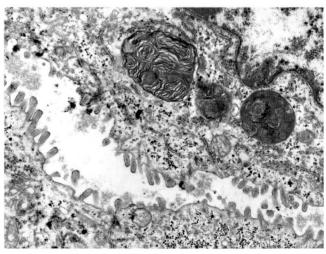

FIGURE 16 Electron photomicrograph from illustrative case 1, showing short cell surface microvilli with a length-to-diameter ratio of 1:6. The final diagnosis was that of "pseudomesotheliomatous" (pleurotropic) adenocarcinoma of the lung.

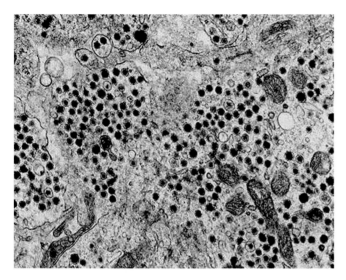

FIGURE 17 Neuroendocrine carcinomas contain variable numbers of cytoplasmic neurosecretory granules. These structures have a dense core, a peripheral "halo" beneath a limiting membrane, and a size ranging from 50 to 450 nm in diameter.

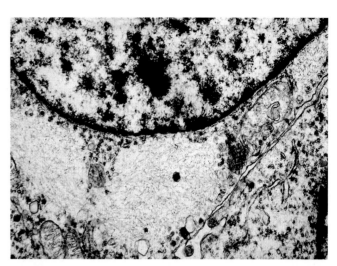

FIGURE 19 In some neuroendocrine carcinomas, particularly those with a small cell appearance, neurosecretory granules may be enmeshed in paranuclear whorls of intermediate filaments.

Otherwise, the organelles seen in NECs are relatively nondescript, including mitochondria, rough endoplasmic reticulum, and scattered lysosomes. The latter may sometimes be difficult to distinguish from neurosecretory inclusions, necessitating such techniques as the uranaffin reaction (which is selective for NSGs) (46). Exceptions to this ultrastructural profile are NECs with brisk secretory activity, e.g., those that synthesize high levels of neuropeptides such as ACTH. They have a much expanded rough endoplasmic reticulum and prominent Golgi bodies (47). Tonofibrils, intracellular lumina, and intercellular lumina are not seen in "pure" NECs, but they may be demonstrable in neoplasms with mixed attributes, e.g., mixed small cell NEC squamous cell carcinoma, or carcinomas that do have a neuroendocrine phenotype on light microscopy but show "occult" neuroendocrine differentiation (48) (see Chapter 1). Lastly, there are no reliable electron microscopic features of NECs that allow for prediction of a primary site, when they present as metastatic malignancy of unknown origin.

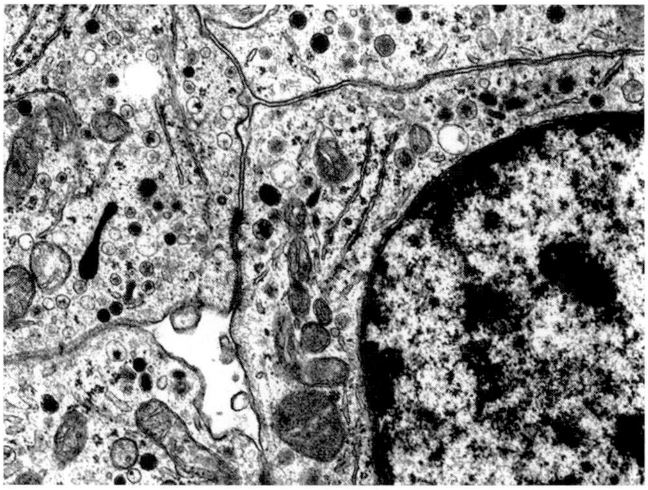

Illustrative Case 2: Metastatic Large Cell NEC

A 61-year-old male smoker presented with abrupt onset of grand-mal seizures. Radiographic studies of the brain demonstrated a single 3-cm lesion in the frontal lobe, with a peripheral rim of edema (Fig. 20). Additional imaging of the chest, thorax, and pelvis failed to reveal another mass. Craniotomy and resection of the tumor demonstrated a large cell neoplasm with numerous mitoses and "geographic" zones of necrosis on histological examination (Fig. 21). The tumor cells were arranged in broad clusters and sheets, and focal nuclear molding was observed (Fig. 22). There were no glandular lumina or foci of keratinization.

Electron microscopy showed the presence of well-defined macular intercellular junctional complexes. Only dispersed intermediate filaments were present in the cytoplasm, but a moderate number of NSGs were apparent, together with relatively prominent Golgi bodies

FIGURE 18 The number of neurosecretory granules in neuroendocrine carcinoma is inversely related to the grade of the tumor. Figure 17 was taken from a low-grade lesion, whereas this electron photomicrograph depicts a grade 2 neoplasm.

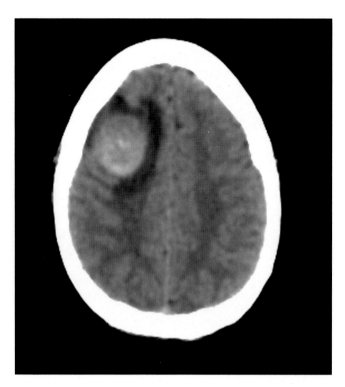

FIGURE 20 CT of the head in illustrative case 2, showing a nodular mass in the right frontal lobe with a zone of perilesional edema. This appearance is consistent with that of a metastasis.

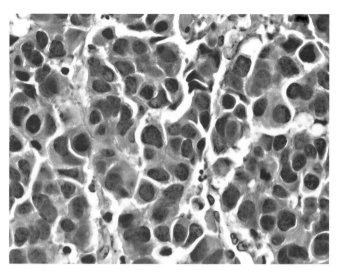

FIGURE 22 High-power photomicrograph of the lesion shown in Figure 20, showing the presence of relatively monomorphic large tumor cells with dispersed chromatin and nuclear molding.

In light of this information, and with the mode of tumor presentation in mind, a high-resolution CT of the thorax was taken. It demonstrated a small peripheral mass in the right lung (Fig. 24), and fine-needle aspiration of the lesion confirmed the diagnosis of primary lung carcinoma.

(Fig. 23). No tonofibrils or glandular lumina were evident. When taken together with the histopathological attributes of the lesion, the ultrastructural findings were felt to be diagnostic of large cell, poorly differentiated NEC.

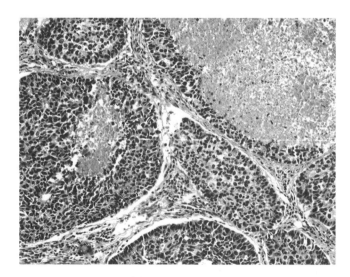

FIGURE 21 Excision of the mass shown in Figure 20 demonstrated a largely necrotic carcinoma.

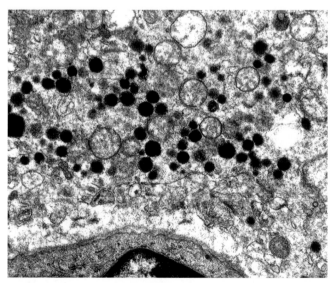

FIGURE 23 This electron photomicrograph of the tumor shown in Figures 20 and 21 reveals the presence of cytoplasmic neurosecretory granules. Together with the histological features of the lesion, this finding establishes the diagnosis of metastatic large cell neuroendocrine carcinoma. The most likely organ of origin was thought to be the lung.

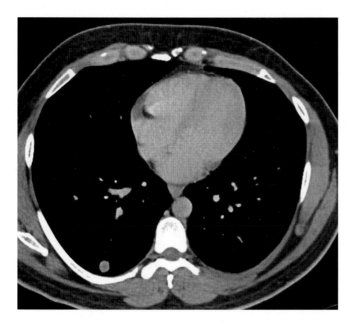

FIGURE 24 Subsequent CT of the chest in illustrative case 2, showing a small peripheral mass in the right lung field. Fine-needle aspiration biopsy of the nodule confirmed the diagnosis of large cell, neuroendocrine carcinoma.

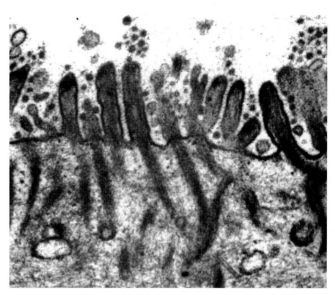

FIGURE 25 Enteric-type adenocarcinomas are characterized by the presence of a "terminal web" of intermediate filaments, which insert into the cores of plasmalemmal microvilli ("core rootlets").

GROUPS OF CARCINOMAS WITH SPECIAL ULTRASTRUCTURAL FEATURES

Aside from the neoplasms just described, there are really no individual malignant epithelial lesions that have truly unique electron microscopic features. Nonetheless, one may still gain useful information from ultrastructural studies of several other carcinomatous morphotypes, in the sense that extensive differential diagnostic considerations may be abridged using the observations that are made. In this context, there are four major groups of epithelial malignancies that can be considered as units on the basis of their fine structural attributes.

Carcinomas with Specialized Cell-Surface Structures

Some normal epithelia and related tumors show distinctive alterations of the cellular surfaces. In particular, enteric lining cells demonstrate two specific features, a terminal subplasmalemmal "web" and glycocalyceal bodies, which set them apart from other epithelia (49–51). The first of these structures is a network of filaments that extends into the centers of surface microvilli, as well as forming a perpendicular connection of the latter "core rootlets" (Fig. 25) (52). On one hand, terminal webs are most typical of intestinal epithelial tumors, but they also have been reported in pulmonary adenocarcinomas with enteric features (53). On the other hand, glycocalyceal bodies are membrane-bound vesicular

structures that are located in the apices of epithelial cells that surround luminal spaces (Fig. 26) (49). They are variously thought to be formed by "budding" of the plasmalemma or exocytosis of cytoplasmic vesicles, and they contain relatively uniformly electron-dense, granular, amorphous material (54). As distinguished from other endocytotic vesicles, glycocalyceal bodies are another

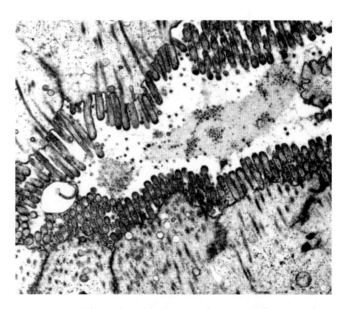

FIGURE 26 Glycocalyceal bodies are also typical of enteric adenocarcinomas. These structures are round, with a thin external zone of density, and they are found in lumina formed by adjacent tumor cells.

marker of enteric epithelial differentiation. Like terminal webs, they are observed in most gastrointestinal tumors and selected pulmonary neoplasms (53, 54).

Illustrative Case 3: Metastatic Colonic Adenocarcinoma

A 49-year-old man consulted his physician with a four-month history of progressive right upper abdominal pain, which was unassociated with oral intake and noncolicky in character. Hepatic ultrasonography showed no abnormalities of the gallbladder, but it did demonstrate several hypoechoic lesions of the hepatic parenchyma, which were confirmed by CT (Fig. 27). Laparoscopic biopsy yielded the specimen represented in Figure 28, showing the presence of a metastatic adenocarcinoma. This tumor was thought to have enteric characteristics on conventional microscopy, but electron microscopy was pursued to confirm this impression. The latter evaluation demonstrated the presence of a terminal web in the neoplastic cells (Fig. 29), objectifying the light microscopic interpretation. Subsequent colonoscopy revealed a cecal adenocarcinoma and numerous adenomatous polyps of the large intestine.

Carcinomas with Distinctive Intracytoplasmic Inclusions

Certain adenocarcinomas display intracellular structures in the tumor cells, which may permit one to restrict attention to just a few possible primary sites for metastatic lesions. For example, the finding of intracytoplasmic lumina (Fig. 30) would suggest that a secondary glandular tumor may have arisen in the breasts or the gastrointestinal tract (29, 33). Similarly, large cytoplasmic mucin granules (Fig. 31) suggest a potential origin in the

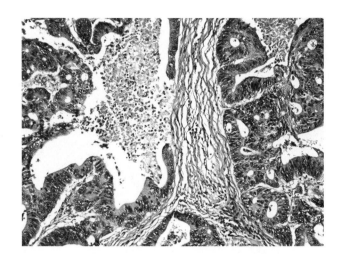

FIGURE 28 A liver biopsy in illustrative case 3 revealed the presence of metastatic adenocarcinoma.

gastrointestinal tract, endocervix, ovary, or lung (40, 41, 52, 55). Two forms of adenocarcinoma exhibit the presence of intracellular inclusions that are sufficiently unusual that they allow the observer to localize one site of origin for metastatic deposits in lymph nodes or other sites. These are pulmonary tumors with at least some features of bronchioloalveolar carcinoma (BAC), in which small dense mucin granules and lamellated "myelinoid" inclusions are seen in the cytoplasm (27, 30, 41, 51), and selected examples of prostatic adenocarcinoma that

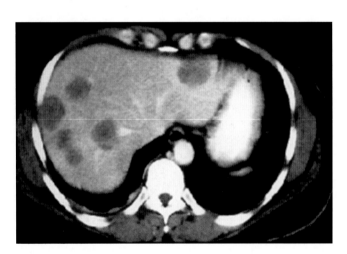

FIGURE 27 CT of the abdomen in illustrative case 3, showing the presence of numerous nodular hypodense lesions throughout the liver.

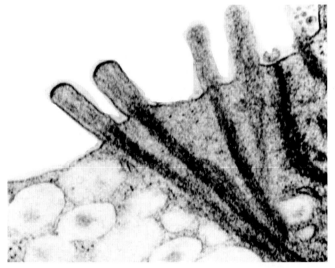

FIGURE 29 Electron microscopy of the lesion shown in Figure 28, demonstrating a terminal web in the neoplastic cells. This finding indicated a probable gastrointestinal origin for the tumor, which was subsequently confirmed at colonoscopy.

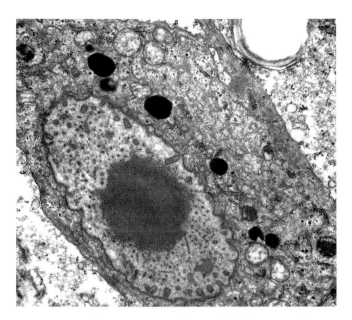

FIGURE 30 Adenocarcinomas with intracellular lumina, as shown in this electron photomicrograph, usually originate in the breasts or the gastrointestinal tract.

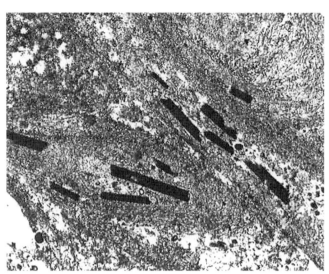

FIGURE 32 Rarely, adenocarcinomas are associated with the formation of elongated intercellular crystalloids, as seen by electron microscopy. This finding is virtually pathognomonic of a prostatic origin.

display the presence of intercellular or intracytoplasmic crystalloids at an ultrastructural level (Fig. 32) (56, 57). Very rarely, the latter inclusions also may be evident in metastases by light microscopy (58).

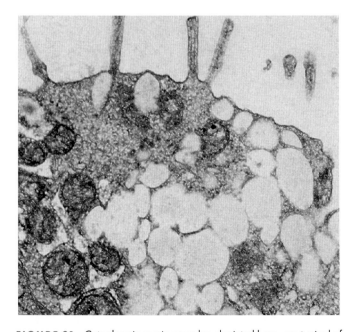

FIGURE 31 Cytoplasmic mucin granules, depicted here, are typical of adenocarcinomas arising in the lungs, pancreas, or gastrointestinal tract.

Illustrative Case 4: Metastatic Pulmonary Micropapillary Adenocarcinoma

A 57-year-old man experienced progressive weight loss and fatigue over the course of six months. He had not altered his diet or other personal habits during that time. Social habits included smoking (two packs per day for 40 years) as well as periodic alcohol abuse; the patient was employed as a laborer in a foundry. Physical examination showed to be a thin individual with signs of chronic obstructive pulmonary disease. In addition, an enlarged right supraclavicular lymph node was palpable, measuring 3 cm in greatest dimension. Chest radiographs showed consolidation of the right middle lobe, which was felt to be a focus of probable bronchopneumonia. An excisional supraclavicular lymph node biopsy was obtained, revealing metastatic adenocarcinoma with micropapillary features (Fig. 33). Ultrastructural examination of the tumor showed the presence of scattered cytoplasmic "myelinoid" surfactant-like bodies (Fig. 34), which were thought to be typical of those seen in BAC. Subsequent sputum cytology specimens were indeed found to contain malignant glandular epithelial cells.

Carcinomas with Distinctive Constellations of Organelles

Three forms of adenocarcinoma are typified by their aggregate cytoplasmic contents, in the sense that one or more of the "usual" metabolic organelles assume an unusual prominence that may permit the observer to localize the anatomic source of the tumor. The lesions in this category include renal cell carcinoma and its variants

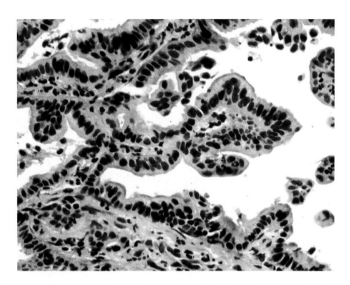

FIGURE 33 A right supraclavicular lymph node biopsy in illustrative case 4 showed metastatic adenocarcinoma with micropapillary features.

(59–61), hepatocellular carcinoma (62, 63), and adrenocortical carcinoma (64, 65). Dominant organelles that these tumors may contain are used in combination (and with attention to their semiquantitative nature) to bias the investigator toward one or the other of the specified neoplasms. Renal cell carcinomas typically contain a mixture of cytoplasmic glycogen and lipid deposits that are visible ultrastructurally. They may show small cell

surface microvilli and pericellular basal lamina as well, and mitochondrial structure is usually banal (Fig. 35) (61). In contrast, adrenocortical carcinomas do not often show cytoplasmic glycogen pools, although they certainly do contain lipid deposits; their mitochondria have an unusual internal configuration featuring "tubulovesicular" cristae (Fig. 36), and basal lamina formation is not common (65). Hepatocellular carcinomas demonstrate a potential mixture of all of these features, but in addition, they may contain intracellular or intercellular bile droplets (63).

It should be readily apparent that the above-cited features are sometimes less than definitive. However, an example in which an intrapulmonary deposit of carcinoma shows abundant basal lamina together with numerous glycogen granules, well-developed cell junctions, and an absence of cytoplasmic bile droplets would certainly skew the probable diagnosis toward that of metastatic renal cell carcinoma (60).

Carcinomas with Sarcomatoid Features

In general, neoplasms with the histological characteristics of sarcomas, but which arise in the mucosae or visceral organs, are best considered as sarcomatoid carcinomas until proven otherwise. Tumors with such features have

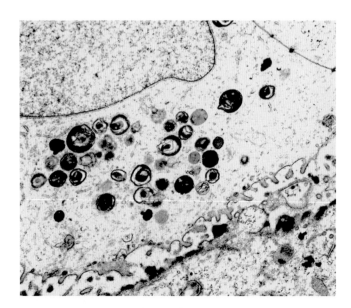

FIGURE 34 Ultrastructural study of the tumor seen in Figure 33 showed cytoplasmic "myelinoid" figures, representing surfactant-related inclusions. This feature indicated a probable pulmonary origin for the metastatic nodal lesion.

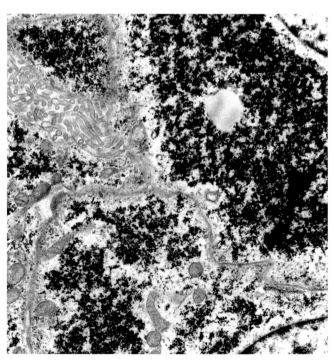

FIGURE 35 Renal cell carcinomas are typified ultrastructurally by abundant glycogen content, with or without cytoplasmic lipid as well. Formation of short microvilli is also relatively common.

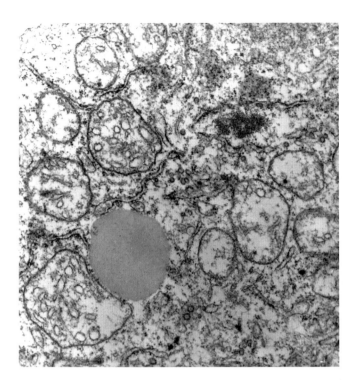

FIGURE 36 This electron photomicrograph shows an adrenocortical carcinoma, with "tubulovesicular" mitochondrial cristae. These structures correlate with steroid-hormone production by the neoplastic cells.

been reported in a wide variety of anatomic locations and under several nosologic designations, but they are most common in the kidney, lungs, and upper aerodigestive tract mucosa (66). Although it is true that these peculiar forms of poorly differentiated squamous carcinomas, adenocarcinomas, or transitional cell carcinomas commonly lose many of the expected ultrastructural attributes of epithelial differentiation, electron microscopy is still potentially valuable in establishing their nonsarcomatous nature (67–69). In the author's experience, approximately 50% of sarcomatoid carcinomas demonstrate retention of at least some epithelial characteristics, such as identifiable intercellular junctional complexes, cytoplasmic tonofibrils, intracellular or intercellular lumen formation, and elaboration of basal laminar material (60, 70). Tissue sampling is a critical issue in this context, as many sarcomatoid carcinomas may exhibit "divergent" differentiation into specialized mesenchymal-like elements that closely simulate striated muscle, cartilage, or bone (in so-called "carcinosarcomas") (66). Hence, unless several tissue blocks are examined in such cases, an erroneous diagnosis of a true sarcoma may be made. It should also be remembered that immunohistologic analysis is, in most instances, more effective than electron microscopy for the elucidation of epithelial differentiation in sarcomatoid carcinomas (70).

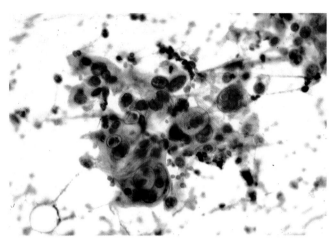

FIGURE 37 Urine cytology specimen in illustrative case 4, showing a loosely cohesive group of bluntly fusiform malignant cells.

Illustrative Case 5: Sarcomatoid Transitional Cell Carcinoma of Urinary Bladder

A 76-year-old man presented to his physician with a four-month history of progressively worsening but painless gross hematuria. An involuntary 10-pound weight loss had also been experienced during the same time period. Cytological examination of the urine showed the presence of malignant cells with spindled and pleomorphic shapes (Fig. 37), and cystoscopy demonstrated the presence of a large, ulcerated, polypoid tumor mass in the posterior wall of the bladder. A biopsy of the latter lesion showed

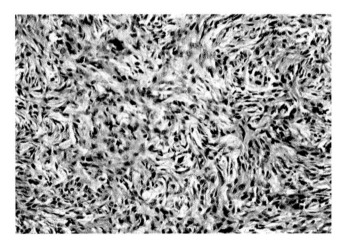

FIGURE 38 Cytoscopy in illustrative case 4 showed a large, ulcerated, polypoid tumor in the bladder, a biopsy of which is shown here. The appearance is that of a malignant lesion with the histological features of a sarcoma.

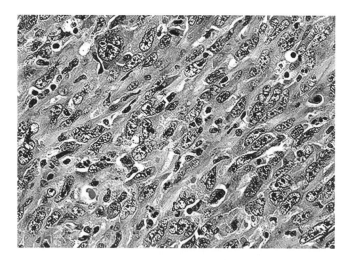

FIGURE 39 Cytoscopy in illustrative case 4 showed a large, ulcerated, polypoid tumor in the bladder, a biopsy of which is shown here. The appearance is that of a malignant lesion with the histological features of a sarcoma.

a tumor with the apparent histological features of malignant fibrous histiocytoma (Figs. 38 and 39), but electron microscopy of the mass revealed intercellular junctions between the neoplastic cells as well as rare cytoplasmic tonofibrils (Fig. 40). In light of these findings, a diagnosis of sarcomatoid transitional cell carcinoma was made and a total cystectomy was performed.

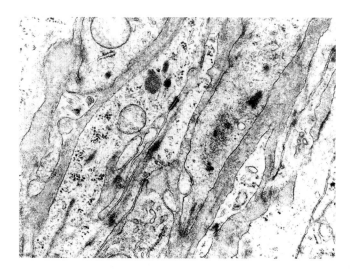

FIGURE 40 Despite the microscopic attributes seen in Figures 38 and 39, electron microscopy of the tumor demonstrated the focal presence of intercellular junctional complexes into which intermediate filaments inserted. The final diagnosis was that of sarcomatoid urothelial carcinoma.

■ REFERENCES

1. Azar HA, Espinoza CG, Richman AV, Saba SR, Wang T. "Undifferentiated" large cell malignancies: an ultrastructural and immunocytochemical study. *Hum Pathol* 1982; 13:323–33.
2. Parham DM, Ellison DA. Rhabdomyosarcomas in adults and children: an update. *Arch Pathol Lab Med* 2006; 130:1454–65.
3. Franchi A, Massi D, Santucci M. The comparative role of immunohistochemistry and electron microscopy in the identification of myogenic differentiation in soft tissue pleomorphic sarcomas. *Ultrastruct Pathol* 2005; 29:295–304.
4. Kindblom LG, Widehn S, Meis-Kindblom JM. The role of electron microscopy in the diagnosis of pleomorphic sarcomas of soft tissue. *Semin Diagn Pathol* 2003; 20:72–81.
5. Peydro-Olaya A, Llombart-Bosch A, Carda-Batalla C, Lopez-Guerrero JA. Electron microscopy and other ancillary techniques in the diagnosis of small-round-cell tumors. *Semin Diagn Pathol* 2003; 20:25–45.
6. Suo Z, Nesland JM. Electron microscopy in the diagnosis of spindle-cell tumors. *Semin Diagn Pathol* 2003; 20:5–12.
7. Mackay B, Bruner JM, Ordonez NG. Soft tissue sarcoma with neural differentiation. *Ultrastruct Pathol* 1985; 9:181–8.
8. Carvajal R, Meyers P. Ewing's sarcoma and primitive neuroectodermal tumor family of tumors. *Hematol Oncol Clin North Am* 2005; 19:501–25.
9. Suh CH, Ordonez NG, Hicks J, Mackay B. Ultrastructure of the Ewing's sarcoma family of tumors. *Ultrastruct Pathol* 2002; 26:67–76.
10. Wick MR, Scheithauer BW. Primary neuroendocrine carcinoma of the skin. In: Wick MR, ed. *Pathology of Unusual Malignant Cutaneous Tumors*. New York: Marcel Dekker, 1985:107–70.
11. Mazur MT, Katzenstein AL. Metastatic melanoma: the spectrum of ultrastructural morphology. *Ultrastruct Pathol* 1980; 1:337–56.
12. Bhuta S. Electron microscopy in the evaluation of melanocytic tumors. *Semin Diagn Pathol* 1993; 10:92–101.
13. Gibson LE, Goeller JR. Amelanotic melanoma: cases studied by Fontana stain, S100 immunostain, and ultrastructural examination. *Mayo Clin Proc* 1988; 63:777–82.
14. Turbat-Herrera EA, Herrera GA. Electron microscopy renders the diagnostic capabilities of cytopathology more precise: an approach to everyday practice. *Ultrastruct Pathol* 2005; 29:475–82.
15. Herrera GA, Alexander CB, Jones JM. Ultrastructural characteristics of pulmonary neoplasms. II. The role of electron microscopy in the characterization of uncommon epithelial pulmonary neoplasms, metastatic neoplasms to and from lung, and other tumors, including mesenchymal neoplasms. *Surv Synth Pathol Res* 1985; 4:163–84.
16. Goedhals J, Benkes CA, Cooper J. The ultrastructural features of plasmablastic lymphoma. *Ultrastruct Pathol* 2006; 30:427–33.
17. Said JW, Hargreaves HK, Pinkus GS. Non-Hodgkin's lymphomas: an ultrastructural study correlating morphology and immunologic cell type. *Cancer* 1979; 44:504–28.
18. Denti S, Pittaluga S, Bosincu L, Tanda F, Costanzi G. Ultrastructural studies in the differential diagnosis of some non-Hodgkin's lymphatic neoplasms. *Pathologica* 1979; 71:495–510.
19. Kelenyi G. Non-Hodgkin's lymphomas of high-grade malignancy: pathologic and differential diagnosis. *Arch Geschwulstforsch* 1979; 49:648–61.
20. Gillespie JJ. The ultrastructural diagnosis of diffuse large cell ("histiocytic") lymphoma: fine structural study of 30 cases. *Am J Surg Pathol* 1978; 2:9–20.
21. Michaels L, Hyams VJ. Undifferentiated carcinoma of the nasopharynx: light and electron microscopical study. *Clin Otolaryngol Allied Sci* 1977; 2:105–14.

22. Battifora H, Applebaum EL. Electron microscopy in the diagnosis of head and neck tumors. *Head Neck Surg* 1979; 1:202–12.

23. Ordonez NG, Mackay B. Electron microscopy in tumor diagnosis: indications for its use in the immunohistochemical era. *Hum Pathol* 1998; 29:1403–11.

24. Mackay B, Ordonez NG. Pathological evaluation of neoplasms with unknown primary tumor site. *Semin Oncol* 1993; 20:206–28.

25. Banks ER, Frierson HF Jr, Mills SE, et al. Basaloid squamous cell carcinoma of the head and neck: a clinicopathologic and immunohistochemical study of 40 cases. *Am J Surg Pathol* 16:939–46.

26. Chen HP, Berardi RS. A light and electron microscopic study of lung cancers: clinical implications. *Int Surg* 1993; 78:124–6.

27. Leong ASY. The relevance of ultrastructural examination in the classification of primary neoplasms of the lung. *Pathology* 1982; 14:37–46.

28. Sidhu GS. The ultrastructure of malignant epithelial neoplasms of the lung. *Pathol Annu* 1982; 17(Part 1):235–66.

29. Battifora H. Intracytoplasmic lumina in breast carcinoma. *Arch Pathol Lab Med* 1975; 99:614–7.

30. Hammar SP. Adenocarcinoma and large cell carcinoma of the lung. *Ultrastruct Pathol* 1987; 11:263–91.

31. Warhol M, Corson JM. An ultrastructural comparison of mesotheliomas with adenocarcinomas of the lung and breast. *Hum Pathol* 1985; 16:50–5.

32. Wick MR, Loy TS, Mills SE, et al. Malignant epithelioid pleural mesothelioma versus peripheral pulmonary adenocarcinoma: a histochemical, ultrastructural, and immunohistologic study of 103 cases. *Hum Pathol* 1990; 21:759–66.

33. Yamashiro K, Suzuki H, Nagayo T. Electron microscopic study of signet ring cells in diffuse carcinoma of the human stomach. *Virchows Arch A Pathol Anat Histol* 1977; 374:275–84.

34. Suzuki Y, Kannerstein M. Ultrastructure of human malignant diffuse mesothelioma. *Am J Pathol* 1976; 85:241–62.

35. Stoebner P, Brambilla E. Ultrastructural diagnosis of pleural tumors. *Pathol Res Pract* 1982; 173:402–16.

36. Burns TR, Johnson EH, Cartwright JJ, Greenberg SD. Desmosomes of epithelial malignant mesotheliomas. *Ultrastruct Pathol* 1988; 12:385–8.

37. Leong ASY, Stevens MW, Mukherjee TM. Malignant mesothelioma: cytologic diagnosis with histologic, immunohistochemical, and ultrastructural correlation. *Semin Diagn Pathol* 1992; 9: 141–50.

38. Weidner N. Malignant mesothelioma of peritoneum. *Ultrastruct Pathol* 1991; 15:515–20.

39. Dardick I, Jabi M, McCaughey WT. Diffuse epithelial mesothelioma: a review of the ultrastructural spectrum. *Ultrastruct Pathol* 1987; 11:503–33.

40. Ferenczy A. Diagnostic electron microscopy in gynecologic pathology. *Pathol Annu* 1979; 14(Part 1):353–81.

41. McGregor DH, Dixon AY, McGregor DK. Adenocarcinoma of the lung: a comparative diagnostic study using light and electron microscopy. *Hum Pathol* 1988; 19:901–13.

42. Oury TD, Hammar SP, Roggli VL. Ultrastructural features of diffuse malignant mesotheliomas. *Hum Pathol* 1998; 29:1382–92.

43. Hammond EH, Yowell RL, Flinner RL. Neuroendocrine carcinomas: role of immunocytochemistry and electron microscopy. *Hum Pathol* 1998; 29:1367–71.

44. Linnoila RI. Spectrum of neuroendocrine differentiation in lung cancer cell lines featured by cytomorphology, markers, and their corresponding tumors. *J Cell Biochem Suppl* 1996; 24: 92–106.

45. Wenig BM, Hyams VJ, Haffner DK. Moderately-differentiated neuroendocrine carcinoma of the larynx: a clinicopathologic study of 54 cases. *Cancer* 1988; 62:2658–76.

46. Payne CM, Nagle RB, Borduin V. An ultrastructural cytochemical stain specific for neuroendocrine neoplasms. *Lab Invest* 1984; 51:350–65.

47. Wick MR, Scheithauer BW. Thymic carcinoid. *A histologic, immunohistochemical, and ultrastructural study of 12 cases.* *Cancer* 1984; 53:475–84.

48. Cerilli LA, Ritter JH, Mills SE, Wick MR. Neuroendocrine neoplasms of the lung. *Am J Clin Pathol* 2001; 116(Suppl):S65–96.

49. Marcus PB, Martin JH, Green RH, Krouse MA. Glycocalyceal bodies and microvillous core rootlets. *Arch Pathol Lab Med* 1979; 103:89–92.

50. Seiler MW, Reilova-Velez J, Hickey W, Bono L. Ultrastructural markers of large bowel cancer. *Prog Cancer Res Ther* 1984; 29: 51–65.

51. Hammar SP. Metastatic adenocarcinoma of unknown primary origin. *Hum Pathol* 1998; 29:1393–402.

52. Hickey WF, Seiler MW. Ultrastructural markers of colonic adenocarcinoma. *Cancer* 1981; 47:140–5.

53. Weidner N. Pulmonary adenocarcinoma with intestinal-type differentiation. *Ultrastruct Pathol* 1992; 16:7–10.

54. Marcus PB. Glycocalyceal bodies and their role in tumor typing. *J Submicr Cytol* 1981; 13:483–500.

55. Nevalainen TV, Jarvi OH. Ultrastructure of intestinal and diffuse type gastric carcinoma. *J Pathol* 1977; 122:129–36.

56. Ro JY, Ayala AG, Ordonez NG. Intraluminal crystalloids in prostatic adenocarcinoma: immunohistochemical, electron microscopic, and X-ray microanalytic studies. *Cancer* 1986; 55: 2397–407.

57. Ohtsuki Y, Fuihata M, Inoue K. Immunohistochemical and ultrastructural studies of intraluminal crystalloids in human prostatic carcinomas. *Virchows Arch* 1992; 421:421–5.

58. Molberg KH, Mikhail A, Vuitch F. Crystalloids in metastatic prostatic adenocarcinoma. *Am J Clin Pathol* 1994; 101:266–8.

59. Tannenbaum M. Ultrastructural pathology of human renal cell tumors. *Pathol Annu* 1971; 6:249–77.

60. Mackay B, Ordonez NG, Khoursand J, Bennington JL. The ultrastructure and immunocytochemistry of renal cell carcinoma. *Ultrastruct Pathol* 1987; 11:483–502.

61. Sun CN, Bissada NK, White HJ, Redman JF. Spectrum of ultrastructural patterns of renal cell adenocarcinoma. *Urology* 1977; 9:195–200.

62. Toker C, Trevino N. Ultrastructure of human primary hepatic carcinoma. *Cancer* 1966; 19:1594–606.

63. Ordonez NG, Mackay B. Ultrastructure of liver-cell and bile-duct carcinoma. *Ultrastruct Pathol* 1983; 5:201–41.

64. Silva EG, Mackay B, Samaan NA, Hickey RC. Adrenal cortical carcinomas: an ultrastructural study of 22 cases. *Ultrastruct Pathol* 1982; 3:1–7.

65. Mackay B, El-Naggar A, Ordonez NG. Ultrastructure of adrenal cortical carcinoma. *Ultrastruct Pathol* 1994; 18:181–90.

66. Wick MR, Swanson PE. Carcinosarcomas: current perspectives and an historical review of nosological concepts. *Semin Diagn Pathol* 1993; 10:118–27.

67. Battifora H. Spindle-cell carcinoma: ultrastructural evidence of squamous origin and collagen production by the tumor cells. *Cancer* 1976; 37:2275–82.

68. Morikawa Y, Tohya K, Kusuyama Y. Sarcomatoid renal cell carcinoma: an immunohistochemical and ultrastructural study. *Int J Urol Nephrol* 1993; 25:51–8.

69. Winfield HL, Rosenberg AS, Antonescu CR, Weil M, Wang AR. Monophasic sarcomatoid carcinoma of the scalp. *J Cutan Pathol* 2003; 30:393–400.

70. Nappi O, Wick MR. Sarcomatoid neoplasms of the respiratory tract. *Semin Diagn Pathol* 1993; 10:137–47.

5 Immunohistology

ROHIT BHARGAVA

MARK R. WICK

DAVID J. DABBS

■ INTRODUCTION

A malignancy is labeled as a metastatic cancer of unknown primary site (CUP) when meticulous clinical and radiographic examination and tissue evaluation fails to accurately identify the primary source of growth. However, a tumor diagnosed as CUP two decades ago might not be classified as such today, because the technological advancement in radiographic techniques and immunohistologic/molecular evaluation of tumor tissue can predict the site of origin to a degree of certainty that was never before possible. Even with currently available techniques, approximately 5% of all malignancies are still finally classified as CUP (1, 2).

Although the term *carcinoma of unknown primary site* is often used interchangeably with *cancer* of unknown origin, not all such malignancies are epithelial in nature. This chapter reviews the pathological triage and evaluation of all types of malignant neoplasms that may present with metastasis with the main focus on carcinomas, which comprise the predominant category (approximately 90–95%) of CUP cases (2–4).

A general surgical pathologist encounters most examples of CUP in core biopsies or incisional or excisional biopsies of a clinically accessible lesion. The amount of tissue provided is generally small, which sometimes significantly limits definitive evaluation of the lesion. Whenever possible, the pathologist should ask for a reasonably generous sample if CUP is the suspected clinical diagnosis. It is also advisable to request that fresh tissue be submitted, which can then be used for cytogenetic studies, electron microscopy (EM), flow cytometry, and molecular analysis. Recent advances in molecular pathology have, to some extent, obviated the need for some of these techniques. If not enough tissue is available, the recommendation is to freeze at least some of the sample after triaging a portion for morphological analysis, because frozen tissue is the most desirable for molecular assessment (5).

After a biopsy is obtained in a suspected CUP case, the responsibility falls on the surgical pathologist to make a definitive diagnosis and, if possible, to determine the site of origin for the tumor in question. CUP cases are among the most challenging ones seen by pathologists. Clinical history is crucial, as obtained from clinicians or from electronic medical records. In particular, the past surgical history occasionally may provide a critical clue to the source of CUP. For example, a small cell tumor in the pelvis may represent a recurrent endometrial stromal sarcoma that was not recognized in a previous hysterectomy specimen. The pathologist therefore should review any surgical specimen that might be pertinent.

■ TRIAGE IN ANATOMIC PATHOLOGY

The first step in the pathological evaluation of CUP is histological evaluation with conventional hematoxylin and eosin stains. This process allows for confident recognition in a good number of cases of carcinoma morphotypes, sarcomas, melanomas, lymphomas, and germ cell tumors (6). When a tumor presents as CUP, however, it may sometimes be so poorly differentiated that additional evaluations are needed for diagnostic characterization. One procedure used to that end is EM, as considered in Chapter 4. In addition, many antibodies have now been developed for diagnostic use that are active in formalin-fixed and paraffin-embedded (FFPE) tissues. Indeed, immunohistochemical evaluation is often the second step in the triage of CUP cases (6–11).

"Screening" Immunohistochemistry

An abbreviated initial panel to address the lineage of differentiation in CUP comprises epithelial markers (pan-keratins, MOC-31, E-cadherin), mesenchymal markers (vimentin, N-cadherin), hematolymphoid determinants [e.g., CD45 (leukocyte common antigen)], and melanocytic markers (S100 protein, melan-A). Vimentin is considered to be a pan-mesenchymal intermediate filament protein (12), but it may be expressed in many poorly differentiated carcinomas and melanomas as well (13). With this specific exception, the other markers just listed are helpful in pointing to a likely lineage for the tumor in question.

Lymphoid Lesions

The preliminary panel generally is followed by a more extensive immunohistological evaluation. For example, CD45-positive tumors are studied with antibodies to CD20, CD79a, PAX5, CD3, CD5, CD43, and other lymphoid-subset markers (14, 15). If granulocytic sarcoma is judged to be a possibility, myeloid markers may be employed (16–18). These stains include myeloperoxidase, lysozyme, and CD117 (19–21). CD43 and CD68 are also potentially positive in granulocytic sarcomas (17, 22, 23).

Melanocytic Lesions

Diffuse and strong nucleocytoplasmic staining for S100 protein in the absence of keratin or CD45, constitutes good evidence that the tumor is a melanoma (Fig. 1) (24–26). This conclusion can be confirmed by additional melanocyte-related markers such as HMB-45, melan-A (MART-1), tyrosinase, or PNL2 (Fig. 1). S100 protein may also be expressed by selected carcinomas (27, 28) and sarcomas (liposarcoma; chondrosarcoma; malignant peripheral nerve sheath tumors) (29, 30). An additional pitfall is that rare melanomas may show reactivity with heteroantisera to carcinoembryonic antigen (CEA) and antibodies to keratins 8 and 18 (31–33).

Sarcomas

Strong vimentin expression in a nonmelanocytic, non-lymphoid neoplasm is generally an indication of sarcoma. Most, but not all, mesenchymal malignancies are negative for epithelial markers; however, epithelioid sarcoma, as its name suggests, reproducibly shows epithelial differentiation, and synovial sarcoma does so as well (34–37). Nonetheless, mesenchymal neoplasms

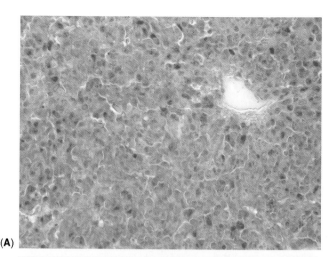

(A)

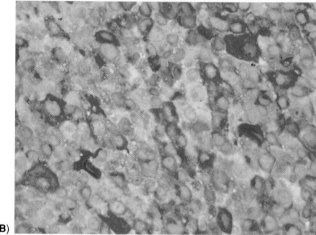

(B)

FIGURE 1 Typical diffuse nucleocytoplasmic S100 expression in a melanoma (**A**). Contrast this with cytoplasmic Melan-A staining in another case of melanoma (**B**). Fast red was used as chromogen.

that are usually considered in CUP cases are those that have a more indeterminate morphological image than those of epithelioid or synovial sarcoma, for example, Ewing's sarcoma/primitive neuroectodermal tumor (PNET), desmoplastic small round cell tumor, rhabdomyosarcoma, clear cell sarcoma, and "solid" angiosarcoma. In some cases, many immunostains must be obtained in order to render a diagnosis of a specific sarcoma morphotype (38), and, in CUP cases, one must have a high index of suspicion that the lesion is, in fact, not epithelial but mesenchymal (Fig. 2).

Immunohistochemistry (IHC) is valuable in this context (39, 40). For example, a small round-cell tumor that expresses CD99 in a young adult may be a PNET. At a molecular level, the EWS-FLI1 fusion transcript is expected in this entity, and, currently, reverse transcriptase–polymerase chain reaction assays can be done on FFPE tissue to detect it (41, 42). Triage for sarcomas in general is outlined in Table 1.

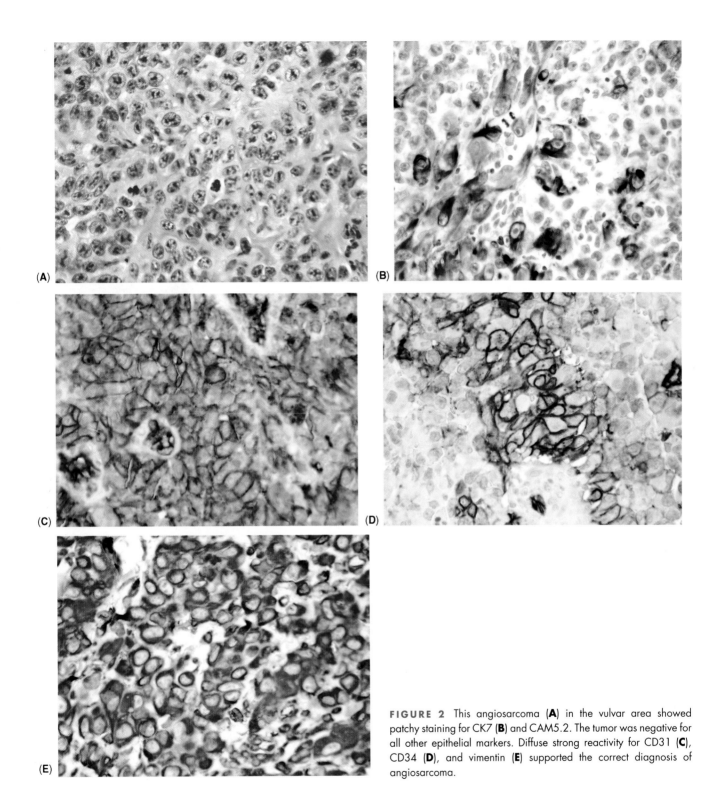

FIGURE 2 This angiosarcoma (**A**) in the vulvar area showed patchy staining for CK7 (**B**) and CAM5.2. The tumor was negative for all other epithelial markers. Diffuse strong reactivity for CD31 (**C**), CD34 (**D**), and vimentin (**E**) supported the correct diagnosis of angiosarcoma.

■ **Table 1** Sarcomas that can present as CUP

Sarcoma Type	Age/Site	Morphology	Special Stains/IHC	Ancillary Techniques for Confirmation of Diagnosis
Ewings sarcoma/ PNET	Usually <30 yr. Chest wall, extremities, retroperitoneum, pelvis. Metastases to lungs and bone	Small round blue cell tumor	PAS+, CD99+, FLI1+	RT-PCR for EWS-FLI1, EWS-ERG, EWS-ETV1, EWS-E1AF, EWS-FEV. EWS translocation can also be shown by FISH with EWS break-apart probe
Rhabdomyosarcoma (RMS)-alveolar (A), embryonal (E), and pleomorphic (P)	A-RMS: 10–20 yrs. Extremities and perineum E-RMS: 3–10 yrs. Prostate, paratesticular, orbit, nasal cavity P-RMS: 50+ yrs. Abdomen, retroperitoneum, chest wall, testes, and extremities	Small round blue cells with alveolar growth pattern in alveolar RMS; round and spindle cells in embryonal; round, spindle and pleomorphic cells in pleomorphic RMS	Muscle-specific actin (MSA)+, desmin+, myoglobin+, myogenin (most specific)+, myoD1+	RT-PCR for PAX3-FKHR and PAX7-FKHR in alveolar RMS only
Desmoplastic, small round cell tumor	Young adults, often adolescent boys. Abdomen and pelvis, peritoneal implants	Round/oval cells in desmoplastic stroma in classic cases, other cases with variable morphology	Vimentin+, cytokeratin+, EMA+, desmin+, WT1+	RT-PCR for EWS-WT1
Synovial sarcoma	Young adults. Extremities around large joints. Now described in various locations including lung and pleura	Spindle cell or biphasic glandular and spindle cell pattern. Small round cells in poorly differentiated tumor	EMA+, keratin+ (biphasic tumors), CD99+, bcl2+. Recently TLE1+	RT-PCR for SYT-SSX1 and SYT-SSX2
Clear cell sarcoma (melanoma of soft parts)	Young adults. Deep soft tissue with nodal and lung metastases	Mixed epithelioid and spindle cells in nested growth pattern	S100+, HMB45+, melanA+	RT-PCR for EWS-ATF1 (not seen in cutaneous melanoma)
Alveolar soft part sarcoma	Young adults, often females. Deep soft tissue. Lung metastases common	Large polygonal cells, granular cytoplasm, prominent nucleoli, rare mitoses	PASD+, TFE3+	Membrane-bound rhomboidal crystals by electron microscopy (EM). RT-PCR for ASPL-TFE3
PEComas	40–50 yr, usually females. Various visceral organs and soft tissue	Epithelioid and spindle cells with perivascular arrangement, clear to granular cytoplasm	HMB45+, melanA+, but S100 negative	EM: glycogen, pre-melanosomes, occasional dense bodies
Epithelioid sarcoma	Young adults. Deep soft tissue of extremities. Metastases to lung, lymph node, and skin	Epithelioid tumor cells, granuloma-like growth pattern	Keratin+, EMA+, vimentin+, CD34+, CK5/6-, p63-	Nothing specific. EM may be helpful

(Continued)

| Table 1 | Sarcomas that can present as CUP (Continued) | | | |
Sarcoma Type	Age/Site	Morphology	Special Stains/IHC	Ancillary Techniques for Confirmation of Diagnosis
Vascular tumors	Adults. Soft tissue and various visceral organs	Angiosarcoma: epithelioid and spindle cell tumor, vasoformative areas. Epithelioid in hemangioendothelioma	FVIII+, CD31+, CD34+, FLI1+, thrombomodulin+, patchy keratin+	EM to identify endothelial cells is rarely required
Leiomyosarcoma	Adults. Abdomen, pelvis and various other locations	Spindle or epithelioid cells with areas of smooth muscle differentiation	SMA+, HHF35+, desmin+, caldesmon+, patchy keratin+	EM: smooth muscle differentiation
Malignant peripheral nerve sheath tumor	Adults. NF1 patients (50%). Deep soft tissue in association with major nerve	Spindle cells with neural differentiation, abundant mitosis, necrosis+/−. Rarely epithelioid	S100+ (weak, patchy), CD56+, CD57+, PGP9.5+, CD99+. Negative for melanoma and vascular markers	Negative for SYT-SSX1 and SYT-SSX2 EM: neural differentiation
Chordoma	Adults, usually males. Sacrococcygeal, thoracolumbar spine	Physaliferous cells, vacuolated cytoplasm, mucoid stroma	S100+, keratin+, but CK7 /CK20−, EMA+	EM rarely required
Extraskeletal myxoid chondrosarcoma	Adults. Deep soft tissues of extremities. Metastases may be confused with myoepithelial type carcinomas	Cords of spindle and epithelioid cells in myxoid stroma	S100+, NSE+, synaptophysin+/−, keratin-, chromogranin-	RT-PCR for EWS-CHN and TAF2N-CHN
Endometrial stromal sarcoma	Adult females. Abdominopelvic region. Distant metastases to lungs	Oval/round to spindle cells. Vague resemblance to proliferative pattern endometrial stroma	CD10+, ER+, bcl2−, CD34−, SMA and desmin positivity with smooth muscle differentiation	FISH for 7p15 translocation better than RT-PCR for JAZF1-JJAZ fusion
Gastrointestinal stromal tumor	Adults. GI tract. Abdominopelvic region. Metastases often to the liver	Spindle or epithelioid cells	CD117+, CD34+, often negative for S100, actin and desmin	KIT activating mutations

Abbreviations: CUP, carcinoma of unknown primary site; EMA, epithelial membrane antigen; IHC, immunohistochemistry; PNET, primitive neuroectodermal tumor.

Epithelial Neoplasms

Cytokeratin stains are reliable epithelial markers, as seen in carcinomas and mesotheliomas (43). However, selected uncommon examples of keratin positivity have also been described in other tumor types (44–51). In spite of this, intense and diffuse pankeratin reactivity points to a diagnosis of carcinoma in the context of CUP. The next step, which is the main focus in cases of metastatic carcinoma of unknown origin, is to assess the possible site of tumor origin by looking for other specific epithelial determinants. Knowledge of the primary site improves therapeutic choices in such circumstances (52–55).

■ METASTATIC CUP

The majority (approximately 70%) of CUPs are adeno-carcinomas (56). The poorly differentiated carcinoma [not further specified (NFS)] group comprises approximately 15% to 20% of cases, with the remainder being constituted by squamous cell carcinomas (SCCs) (5%) and neuroendocrine carcinomas (5%). Determinations of the site of origin of metastatic squamous cell or neuro-endocrine carcinomas are more dependent on clinical presentation than on the results of immunostains.

SCC of Unknown Primary Site

If upper and mid cervical lymph nodes are involved by carcinomatous metastases, the primary tumor is likely located in the head and neck (57–60), where SCCs are predominant. Although the latter tumors are readily identified in conventionally stained sections, immunos-taining for CK5/6 and p63 may be advisable for securing the diagnosis of SCC in selected cases (Fig. 3) (61, 62). If nasopharyngeal carcinoma is suspected, in situ hybrid-ization for Epstein–Barr virus-encoded RNA may be useful in confirming the diagnosis (63–65). Metastatic SCC involving low cervical lymph nodes is suspicious for a pulmonary or lower esophageal origin (66, 67). There are no specific markers for SCCs in these sites. Antibodies to thyroid transcription factor (TTF-1), a protein seen in lung and thyroid adenocarcinomas, very infrequently label pulmonary SCCs (68–70).

Most patients with SCC involving the inguinal nodes have primary tumors in the anogenital region (71), including the vulva, vagina, uterine cervix, and anus. However, there are no immunohistologic markers that specifically delineate an origin in such sites.

Neuroendocrine Tumor of Unknown Primary Site

The neuroendocrine tumors that may present as CUP include low-grade neuroendocrine carcinoma ("classical carcinoid"), small cell neuroendocrine carcinoma, and large cell neuroendocrine carcinoma (high-grade neuro-endocrine carcinoma, large cell type). Carcinoids and small cell carcinomas have typical morphological images that are readily recognizable, but immunostains for endocrine markers are often required for a definite diagnosis of large cell neuroendocrine carcinoma. These include chromogranin-A, synaptophysin, CD56, and CD57 (72–76).

Carcinoid tumors show diffuse positivity for virtually all of the determinants, but high-grade neuroendocrine carcinomas of both small cell and large cell types generally do not. Some studies have suggested that immunostains are useful in distinguishing carcinoids arising in the gut

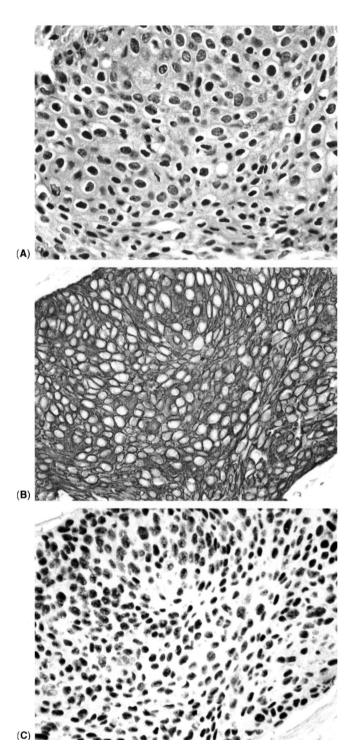

FIGURE 3 Poorly differentiated carcinoma involving bladder wall (**A**). The tumor cells were strongly positive for CK5/6 (**B**) and p63 (**C**), confirming recurrence of a known squamous cell carcinoma.

from those of other origins (77, 78). One analysis showed that midgut carcinoids were often CDX2-positive, but those originating in the foregut and hindgut were usually CDX2-negative (79).

Widely metastatic small cell neuroendocrine carcinomas usually have a pulmonary origin, but such tumors may also arise in salivary glands, esophagus, urinary bladder, prostate, ovary, uterine cervix, breast, and other locations. TTF-1 labeling in a small cell carcinoma does not necessarily indicate a pulmonary source for the lesion, because it has also been identified in a variety of primary extrapulmonary small cell carcinomas (80). Similarly, high-grade large cell neuroendocrine carcinomas lack site-specific immunostaining features.

It may be more important to prove the presence of neuroendocrine differentiation in these cases than it is to localize the anatomic origin of the tumor. This is because similar chemotherapy, irrespective of site or origin, is generally used for neuroendocrine carcinomas, grade for grade (81).

Adenocarcinoma and Poorly Differentiated Carcinoma of Unknown Primary Site

The largest and the most significant group of CUP is that of metastatic adenocarcinomas. Although it is important to note the clinical presentation and morphology of such lesions, a more definitive diagnosis requires immunohistological analysis. Determining sites of origin for adenocarcinoma of unknown primary site is complex, and can be more easily understood when broken down into three steps: selection of immunostains that are useful in this differential diagnosis, delineation of the immunoprofiles of site-specific adenocarcinomas, and an algorithmic approach to this topic. The following discussion includes poorly differentiated carcinoma, NFS, and malignant germ cell tumors.

Step 1: Markers that are Useful in Determining Anatomic Site of Origin

CYTOKERATIN 7 AND CYTOKERATIN 20 (CK7 AND CK20). There are roughly 20 well-defined subclasses of keratin that have been identified on the basis of their molecular weights and isoelectric points (82). Several of these proteins have relatively tissue-selective distributions, and combinations of them can be exploited to determine sites of tumor origin in CUP cases (83). Common keratin antibodies that are often used in this process are those directed against CK7 and CK20 (84–86). CK7+/CK20– adenocarcinomas include those in the breasts, lungs, gynecological tract, thyroid, and salivary glands. Mesotheliomas also have a similar keratin profile. The majority of CK7–CK20+ tumors are of intestinal origin, but similar expressions are seen in a third of gastric adenocarcinomas and almost all Merkel cell carcinomas of the skin. Dual positivity (CK7+/CK20+) is present in adenocarcinomas of the pancreas, bile ducts, and urothelial tract, and in one-third of gastric adenocarcinomas. CK7–/CK20– tumors originate in the adrenal cortex, liver, prostate, and kidneys, although some CK7+ renal carcinomas do exist. Germ cell tumors also show a CK7–/CK20– profile, except that embryonal carcinoma manifests CK7 reactivity in up to 50% of cases (84, 87, 88).

WILMS' TUMOR PROTEIN (WT1). The WT1 gene encodes a zinc finger DNA-binding protein that acts as a transcriptional activator or repressor depending on the cellular or chromosomal context (89). WT1 protein is required for the normal development of genitourinary epithelium and mesothelium (90). In the context of neoplasia, nuclear WT1 expression is seen in Wilms' tumor, mesothelioma, and müllerian carcinomas (especially of the ovarian serous type) (91, 92). The literature regarding WT1 in endometrial serous adenocarcinomas is contradictory, but it appears that nuclear expression (Fig. 4) can be seen in approximately one-third of these tumors (93–98).

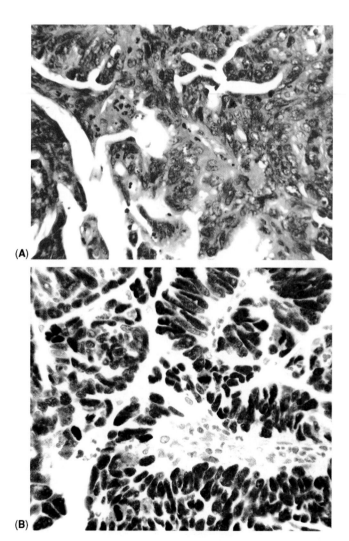

(A)

(B)

FIGURE 4 An endometrial serous carcinoma (**A**), showing unequivocal positivity for Wilms' tumor protein (**B**).

CDX2. This protein is also known as caudal-type homeobox transcription factor-2. The corresponding gene encodes a transcription factor that plays a role in the proliferation and differentiation of intestinal epithelial cells. CDX2 polypeptide is highly expressed in the intestinal mucosa (Fig. 5) and in carcinomas that demonstrate enteric differentiation (99). Virtually all colorectal adenocarcinomas are CDX2+ (100).

THYROID TRANSCRIPTION FACTOR-1. TTF-1 is a 38-kD nuclear protein that mediates thyroid-specific gene transcription (101) and shows nuclear labeling by IHC (Fig. 6). TTF-1 activates thyroglobulin and thyroperoxidase gene transcription in thyroid adenocarcinomas and transcription of human surfactant protein B in the lung. This marker is seen in almost all thyroid carcinomas (except anaplastic tumors) and the majority (~80%) of pulmonary adenocarcinomas (102–105). Squamous tumors of the lung are infrequently positive, and other pulmonary tumors (neuroendocrine and undifferentiated carcinomas) are variably TTF-1-reactive. Merkel cell carcinoma is reproducibly negative for this determinant (80, 106).

THYROGLOBULIN. Thyroglobulin is a glycoproteinaceous precursor of thyroid hormones. It is a specific marker of thyroid epithelial differentiation and is potentially expressed by all thyroid malignancies except anaplastic carcinoma (107).

GROSS CYSTIC DISEASE FLUID PROTEIN-15 (GCDFP-15). GCDFP-15 is also known as prolactin-inducible protein (108). This hormonally responsive polypeptide is expressed by a benign and malignant mammary

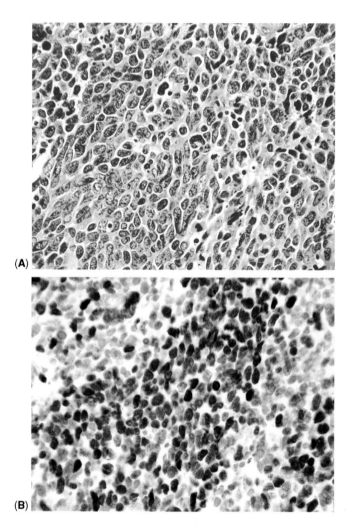

FIGURE 6 A small cell neuroendocrine carcinoma (**A**), showing diffuse strong nuclear reactivity for thyroid transcription factor-1 (**B**).

epithelium. It is a marker for apocrine differentiation; therefore, GCDFP-15 labeling is stronger in those carcinomas that manifest "decapitation secretion" in tumor glands (109). This protein is considered to be highly selective for breast carcinomas, but immunoreactivity for it can also be seen in selected tumors of sweat glands, salivary glands, bronchial glands, and lacrimal glands (110). Staining for GCDFP-15 in breast carcinomas is often patchy (Fig. 7), and its sensitivity is lessened in small core biopsies. Overall, 50% to 70% of breast carcinomas of all types (except medullary carcinoma) are GCDFP-15-positive in excision specimens.

MAMMAGLOBIN (MGB). MGB is a secretory protein with a predicted molecular mass of 10.5 kD. It shares a high degree of homology with rat prostatic steroid-binding protein subunit C3 (rPSC3), human Clara cell 10 kD protein, and rabbit uteroglobin (111–113).

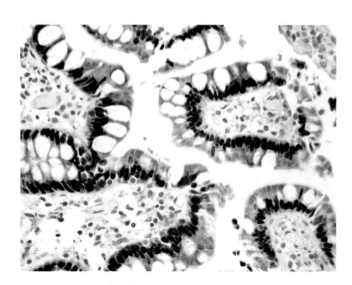

FIGURE 5 Typical nuclear staining of colonic epithelium for CDX2.

Immunohistological studies on FFPE tissues have demonstrated diffuse MGB expression in breast and endometrioid adenocarcinomas (114–117). MGB is also potentially observed in sweat gland and salivary gland adenocarcinomas. With respect to mammary carcinomas, MGB is a more sensitive but less specific marker as compared with GCDFP-15 (Fig. 7).

BER-EP4, BG8, AND MOC31. Ber-EP4, Bg8, and MOC31 are generic markers of epithelial differentiation. They are most often used to distinguish adenocarcinomas from mesotheliomas (118–120). Ber-EP4 and MOC31 antibodies are directed against glycoproteins that are present on the surfaces of glandular epithelial cells of endodermal derivation. Squamous carcinoma virtually never is Ber-EP4-positive (121). Characteristic staining with Ber-EP4 and MOC31 is cell-membrane based. Bg8 antibody is directed against the Lewis Y antigen and shows cytoplasmic labeling in adenocarcinomas and some SCCs. When Ber-EP4, Bg8, and MOC31 are combined with calretinin, podoplanin, and WT1, one can achieve a high level of sensitivity and specificity for the diagnostic separation of metastatic serosal adenocarcinoma and epithelioid mesothelioma (122).

CALRETININ. Calretinin is a 29-kD calcium-binding protein that is one of the most sensitive markers of mesothelial differentiation (Fig. 8) (123). Nevertheless, because of its potential expression in various carcinomas, sarcomas, ovarian stromal tumors, and other neoplasms, calretinin must be combined with other stains in a diagnostic setting (124–127).

MUCIN IMMUNOSTAINS. Mucin or MUC immunostains label a heterogeneous group of glycoproteins that are expressed by various glandular epithelia. The three most common MUC stains that have been applied to human tumors include MUC1 (also known as epithelial

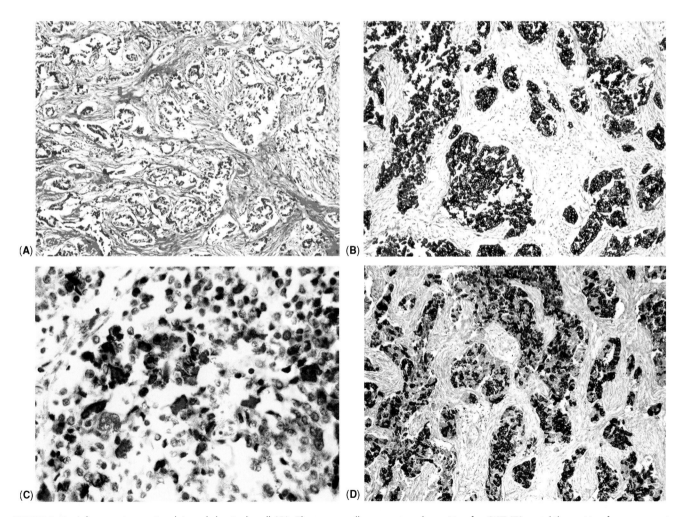

FIGURE 7 Adenocarcinoma involving abdominal wall (A). The tumor cells were strongly positive for CK7 (B), patchily positive for gross cystic disease fluid protein-15 (C), and diffusely reactive for mammaglobin (D). This profile was consistent with a known history of breast carcinoma.

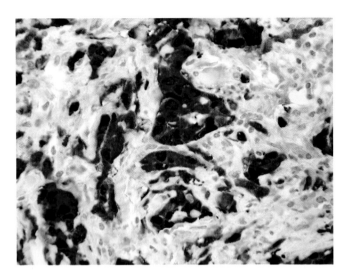

FIGURE 8 Characteristic nuclear and cytoplasmic reactivity for calretinin in a case of mesothelioma.

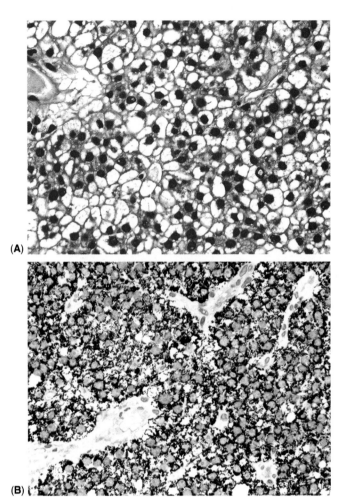

FIGURE 9 Hepatocellular carcinoma with clear cell features (**A**), showing granular cytoplasmic positivity for Hep-Par1 (**B**).

membrane antigen or EMA), MUC2, and MUC5AC. It is well known that adenocarcinomas from many sites express EMA. MUC2 is seen in gastrointestinal (GI) carcinomas and colloid carcinomas in various locations (128–130). MUC5AC has a more limited distribution, being present principally in GI neoplasms. It is often seen in tumors of pancreaticobiliary origin and also endocervical adenocarcinomas (131–133). The expression of MUC5AC may be related to the type of mucin that is produced, rather than the site of tumor origin. Nevertheless, the differential expression of these three MUC moieties may be helpful in selected differential diagnoses (134). None of them is present in adrenocortical carcinoma (ACC) and only rarely in hepatocellular carcinomas (HCCs). Thus, a panel of MUC1/MUC2/MUC5AC could be used to distinguish HCC (negative for all three markers or occasionally MUC1+) from cholangiocarcinoma (MUC1+/MUC2−/MUC5AC+); renal cell carcinoma (MUC1+/MUC2−/MUC5AC−); and ACC (negative for all three).

HEPATOCYTE MARKER FOR PARAFFIN-1 (HEP-PAR1). Hep-Par1 is a sensitive and relatively selective marker of hepatocytic differentiation, and it was specifically designed for use with paraffin-embedded tissue. The antibody is directed against a mitochondrial antigen in hepatocytes (Fig. 9). However, Hep-Par1 labeling is also observed in selected other tumors as well (135–137).

CYTOKERATIN 5/6 (CK5/6). Keratins 5 and 6 are basic polypeptides that are expressed in nonkeratinizing stratified squamous epithelia. Therefore, antibodies to CK5/6 are potential markers for squamous differentiation in carcinomas. CK5/6 is also expressed in mesotheliomas,

metaplastic and basal-like breast carcinomas, urothelial carcinomas, selected salivary gland and sweat gland tumors, and thymomas. In cases of poorly differentiated carcinomas, positivity for CK5/6 and p63 can be useful in establishing a squamous lineage (138).

UROPLAKIN III. The ultrastructure of urothelium demonstrates an asymmetrical unit membrane that is believed to involve strengthening and stabilizing of the urothelial apical surface, thus preventing the cells from rupturing during bladder distention. The asymmetric unit membrane is composed of "uroplakins," including uroplakin III. The latter protein is a specific marker of urothelial differentiation, but is present in only ~50% of transitional cell carcinomas (139, 140). So far, uroplakin III has not been reported in any nonurothelial tumors.

THROMBOMODULIN. In contrast to uroplakin III, thrombomodulin is a highly sensitive but nonspecific marker for urothelial differentiation. Thrombomodulin is a cell-surface glycoprotein on endothelia, which forms a complex with thrombin. It is expressed in vascular neoplasms (141, 142), but is also observed in SCCs and transitional cell carcinomas (143). Moreover, thrombomodulin is a sensitive marker for mesotheliomas but is absent in most adenocarcinomas (144).

ESTROGEN AND PROGESTERONE RECEPTOR PROTEINS (ERP AND PRP). Steroid hormone receptors, particularly ERP, can be useful in the evaluation of CUP. Although some degree of staining for ERP and PRP has been described in several carcinoma morphotypes, diffuse nuclear labeling for these markers is predominantly seen in malignancies of the breast and gynecological tract (145, 146). Immunoreactivity for PRP in the absence of ERP should be interpreted with more caution with regard to determinations of tumor origin (45, 147).

PROSTATE-SPECIFIC ANTIGEN (PSA). PSA is a kallikrein-like protease that is present in seminal fluid (148). It is a specific marker of prostatic adenocarcinoma, more so than prostatic acid phosphatase (PAP). However, the specificity of PSA is not absolute, and it has been rarely detected in nonprostatic carcinomas as well (149, 150).

DELETED IN PANCREATIC CARCINOMA, LOCUS-4 GENE (DPC4). DPC4 is a tumor-suppressor gene (151), the expression of which is lost in approximately 45% to 50% of pancreatic adenocarcinomas. DPC4 protein expression is retained in many other malignancies that enter into differential diagnosis with pancreatic carcinoma (152). Because DPC4 stains are meaningful when they are *negative*, they must be interpreted with caution.

MELAN-A/MART-1. The melan-A gene encodes an antigen in premelanosomes that is recognized by cytotoxic T cells. Antibodies against this marker not only label melanomas, but also stain steroid-hormone–producing tumors such as ACC (153). If other immunostaining results exclude melanoma and ovarian sex cord tumors (154), melan-A-positivity supports the presence of adrenocortical differentiation in CUP cases.

CD10. CD10 (common acute lymphoblastic leukemia antigen) is a marker of early lymphoid progenitors and normal germinal center cells in lymph nodes. However, in the sphere of nonhematopoietic tumors, CD10 is present mainly in renal cell carcinomas, HCCs, and endometrial stromal sarcomas. This protein may also be seen in transitional cell carcinomas, prostatic adenocarcinomas, schwannomas, melanomas, rhabdomyosarcomas, leiomyosarcomas, hemangiopericytomas, solitary fibrous tumors, fibrous histiocytomas, and mesotheliomas (155).

RENAL CELL CARCINOMA ANTIGEN (RCC-AG). RCC-Ag is a 200-kD glycoprotein that is seen in the renal proximal tubules, mammary epithelium, epididymis, parathyroid glands, and thyroid. Positive staining for CD10 and RCC-Ag in a clear cell CUP constitutes strong evidence for a renal origin. Other rarer tumors of the kidney (chromophobe carcinoma; collecting duct carcinoma) are usually negative for RCC-Ag. Other carcinomas that can show RCC-Ag positivity may arise in the breasts, gonads (embryonal carcinoma), and parathyroids (156).

GERM CELL TUMOR MARKERS. Determinants that are often present in malignant germ cell tumors include placental alkaline phosphatase (PLAP), OCT3/4, CD117, CD57, CD30, alpha-fetoprotein (AFP), and beta-human chorionic gonadotropin (HCG). PLAP, CD117, and CD57 mark stem cells and are most often seen in seminomas and dysgerminomas. OCT3/4 is an octameric binding transcription factor involved in the regulation of pluripotency. It is also present in seminomas (Fig. 10) as well

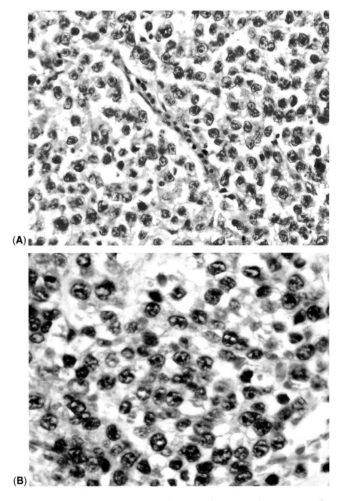

FIGURE 10 A seminoma (**A**), showing distinct nuclear staining for OCT3/4 (**B**).

as embryonal carcinomas, but yolk sac tumors, teratomas, and choriocarcinomas are consistently OCT3/4 negative (157, 158). CD30 labels embryonal carcinomas, AFP is present in ~50% of yolk sac tumors, and HCG is positive in choriocarcinomas. None of these determinants is entirely specific for malignant germ cell tumors (159–162). In particular, HCG-positive tumor cells have been reported in several somatic carcinomas in various anatomic locations (162).

It should be noted that other carcinoma-related immunostains such as CA125 and CA19-9 have not been discussed here. This is true simply as a reflection of the authors' approach to this topic, and other pathologists may well elect to employ these markers in cases of CUP.

Step 2: Immunohistological Profiles of Carcinomas That Can Present as CUP

SALIVARY GLAND TUMORS. Malignant tumors of the major and minor salivary glands include carcinoma *ex* pleomorphic adenoma, basal cell adenocarcinoma (basaloid carcinoma), myoepithelial carcinoma, epithelial–myoepithelial carcinoma, hyalinizing clear cell carcinoma, mucoepidermoid carcinoma, adenoid cystic carcinoma, acinic cell carcinoma, and salivary duct carcinoma. Most of them have distinctive histological features, IHC typically shows a CK7+/CK20– profile (163) and myoepithelial differentiation may be seen. Some specific markers, such as CD117, are overrepresented in adenoid cystic carcinoma, but histologically identical lesions in other organs are also CD117 positive (164, 165). The most common sites of metastases from salivary gland tumors include the regional lymph nodes and lungs. Immunostains are generally not helpful in differential diagnosis with other histologically similar neoplasms, with the possible exception of clear cell carcinomas. Those in the salivary glands lack RCC-Ag, as opposed to metastatic renal cell carcinomas (166). Another important point to remember is that salivary *duct* carcinomas are morphologically analogous to mammary ductal adenocarcinomas. Statistical differences in the incidence of ERP expression do exist between those tumor types, but they are not reliable in a case-specific setting. Both salivary glandular and breast tumors may also be reactive for androgen-receptor protein (167), as well as PSA-like moieties and PAP (168, 169).

UPPER RESPIRATORY TRACT CARCINOMAS. The only tumor of the upper respiratory tract that is relevant to this discussion is sinonasal adenocarcinoma. This lesion can be broadly classified into intestinal and nonintestinal types. Intestinal type sinonasal adenocarcinoma (ITAC) is extremely difficult to separate from colorectal adenocarcinomas that metastasize to the nose. The number of immunostained cases of ITAC is rather limited, but most of them have been positive for CK7, CK20, CDX2, villin, and MUC2 (170–172). Variable reactivity has been seen for neuroendocrine markers, MUC5AC, and CEA. Therefore, tumors with a CK7+, CK20+, MUC2+, and CDX2+ immunophenotype are likely to be primary sinonasal lesions, whereas others with a CK7–, CK20+, MUC2+, and CDX2+ profile suggest the possibility of metastasis from the GI tract.

THYROID GLAND TUMORS. The major subtypes of thyroid carcinomas are papillary, follicular, Hurthle-cell, poorly differentiated (insular), anaplastic, and medullary. All of these tumors are positive for pankeratin, but anaplastic tumors demonstrate only spotty immunolabeling for this protein. The usual profile of the other lesions in this category is CK7+/CK20–. The two stains that are most helpful in determining a thyroid origin for CUP are thyroglobulin and TTF-1 (173). All carcinoma subtypes are potentially positive for TTF-1 and thyroglobulin except for anaplastic tumors. Because medullary carcinomas are neuroendocrine tumors, they also express chromogranin-A, CD56, synaptophysin, and the specific product of C cells, calcitonin. Another important feature of medullary carcinoma is its consistent positivity for CEA.

With regard to anaplastic thyroid carcinoma (ATC), it is difficult not only to prove the site of origin for this lesion, but also to show that it is a carcinoma and not a sarcoma. Vimentin positivity is more diffusely seen than is keratin in the neoplastic cells of ATC; however, EMA (MUC1) reactivity may be identified as well, particularly in squamoid components (174).

The most common sites of metastases for thyroid carcinomas are the regional cervical lymph nodes (especially with papillary tumors) and the lungs. Much less commonly, the bones and central nervous system may be involved at presentation.

MEDIASTINUM. Primary mediastinal tumors that may be confused with CUP include thymic neoplasms (atypical thymoma, thymic carcinoid, and thymic carcinoma), ectopic thyroid tumors (discussed above), lymphomas, paragangliomas, and malignant germ cell tumors. The following discussion is limited to thymic epithelial neoplasms and germ cell tumors. Thymomas are generally recognized in a straightforward way because of a characteristic admixture of neoplastic thymic epithelial cells with nonneoplastic lymphocytes. The epithelial elements are positive for keratin (175) and also may exhibit CEA and EMA (176, 177). Thymic lymphocytes are of T-cell derivation but do not stain for markers of mature T cells. Instead, they are positive for terminal

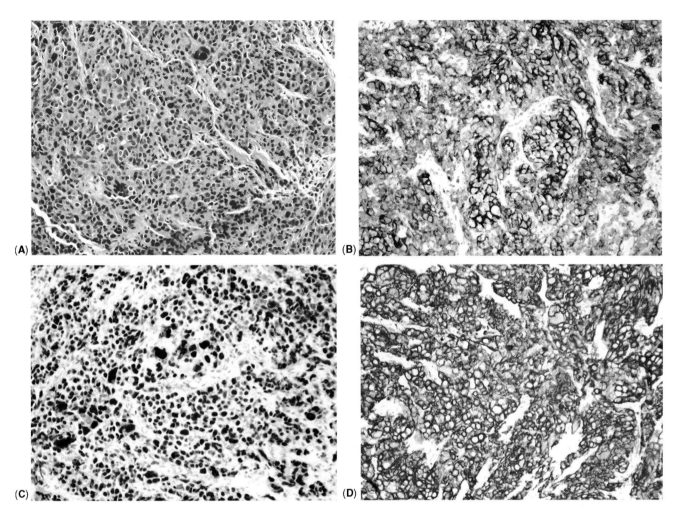

FIGURE 11 A pleural biopsy showing metastatic ovarian adenocarcinoma (**A**), positive for BER-EP4 (**B**), WT1 (**C**), and CK7 (**D**). The tumor cells were negative for calretinin and CK20 (not shown).

deoxynucleotidyl transferase, CD1a, and CD99 (178, 179). Thymic carcinomas are usually distinctive morphologically and do not resemble thymoma; rather, they are similar to carcinoma morphotypes in other organs. Therefore, their identification as primary lesions of the thymus is difficult or sometimes impossible. The two immunostains that have been claimed to be specific to thymic carcinoma are CD5 and CD70. Of these, more experience has been accrued with CD5; it is present in ~70% of thymic carcinomas but is consistently absent in thymoma and carcinomas of nonthymic origin (180–182). CD70 has not yet been assessed sufficiently in nonthymic tumors (183); for example, renal cell carcinomas may express this determinant (184–186).

Mediastinal germ cell tumors are often primary in the thorax, and this is especially likely if there is a single lesion in the chest with no evidence of retroperitoneal involvement. All types of germ cell tumors are potentially encountered in the mediastinum (187).

Their immunohistochemical profiles are generally similar to those of their gonadal counterparts (188). Seminoma is often reactive for PLAP, OCT3/4, CD117, podoplanin, and CD57, and it generally lacks keratin (189–191). In contrast, embryonal carcinoma is keratin positive; it also labels for CD30 and often for OCT3/4 and PLAP as well (192, 193). Yolk sac tumors are positive for AFP, and choriocarcinomas demonstrate HCG staining (194). However, the latter two determinants are nonspecific and have been reported in many somatic carcinomas as well. In this respect, EMA (MUC1) becomes an important discriminant, because it is generally lacking in germ cell neoplasms and present in somatic epithelial malignancies.

Another important feature of all germ cell tumors is the presence of isochromosome 12p [i$(12p)$] in the tumor cells (195). This aberration results in a net gain of 12p, which can be identified by in situ hybridization using FFPE samples (196).

PULMONARY TUMORS. As mentioned earlier, TTF-1 is seen in approximately 80% of pulmonary adenocarcinomas, regardless of morphological subtype [e.g., enteric, clear cell, goblet cell, mucinous (colloid), and acinar (conventional)] or grade (197, 198). However, the mucinous subtype of bronchioloalveolar carcinoma (BAC) is usually TTF-1 negative (199). The general keratin profile for lung adenocarcinoma is CK7+/CK20−, except again for mucinous BAC; it is usually reactive for CK20. In view of its immunoprofile, mucinous BAC may be difficult to distinguish from metastatic tumors from the alimentary tract or pancreas. However, mucinous BACs are CDX2 negative, a finding that promotes their diagnostic separation (200).

PLEURAL TUMORS. Pleural involvement by metastatic malignancies, in the absence of a known primary lesion, always raises the differential diagnostic possibility of mesothelioma. Most immunohistochemical studies on this topic have dealt with the comparative immunophenotypes of pleural mesothelioma and pulmonary adenocarcinoma. The immunohistochemical approach applied to this distinction could be used in reference to nonpulmonary adenocarcinomas as well, but with some caveats.

The selected panel of antibodies in this setting should include at least two markers for carcinomas (Bg8, BER-EP4, TAG72.3, CD15, CEA, MOC-31, TTF-1) and at least two markers for mesothelioma (calretinin, WT1, thrombomodulin, CK5/6, podoplanin). Pankeratin stains are also recommended to assure the antigenic integrity of the tissue sample being studied. No single stain is wholly specific in the latter group of reagents (188, 201). For example, metastatic serous papillary carcinoma would label for generic epithelial markers and WT1 and possibly for calretinin as well, and no staining for TTF-1 would be expected (Fig. 11). Similarly, poorly differentiated metastatic urothelial carcinoma often demonstrates labeling for CK5/6 and thrombomodulin. In such instances, the lesions may be misdiagnosed as mesotheliomas if a sufficient number of other appropriately discriminatory stains is not employed.

In spite of these pitfalls, the great majority of serosal epithelioid malignancies can be reliably identified as mesothelioma or adenocarcinoma with IHC. EM is still a useful technique in this setting, and it is particularly helpful in resolving immunophenotypically equivocal cases (202) (see Chapter 4).

UPPER GI TRACT. Empirically, it is known that the majority of upper GI adenocarcinomas (i.e., esophageal, gastric, and duodenal) that present as CUP originate in the stomach. The keratin profiles of such lesions are variable.

Most gastric and esophageal adenocarcinomas are CK7+, and CK20 positivity is seen in approximately 30% of stomach tumors (203). CDX2 reactivity is present predominantly in *intestinal*-type carcinomas, and this fact limits its use in identifying signet-ring cell carcinomas as enteric in origin (204). Currently, there are no specific markers for upper GI carcinomas, and their diagnosis is based on an exclusionary process.

COLORECTAL AND ANAL CARCINOMAS. Colorectal adenocarcinomas are characteristically CK7− and CK20+, and the majority express CDX2 and villin as well (205, 206). Although CEA reactivity is present in many nonenteric tumors, the *lack* of this marker in a CUP makes a colorectal origin highly improbable (207). Differential mucin expression may sometimes be helpful

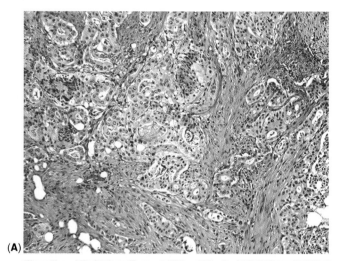

(A)

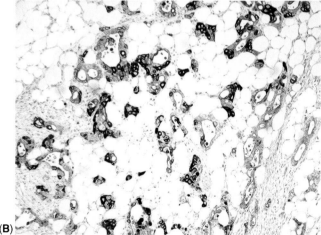

(B)

FIGURE 12 An adenocarcinoma with extensive desmoplasia and focal mucin production involving the omentum (**A**). The tumor cells show CK17 positivity (**B**). The morphology and immunoprofile supported a pancreatic primary lesion.

in distinguishing colorectal tumors from pancreaticobiliary carcinomas. Colorectal neoplasms infrequently show MUC5AC expression, and this fact separates them from most carcinomas of the pancreas and biliary tree.

The majority of anal canal carcinomas are of the keratinizing squamous cell type, but approximately 20% show a basaloid, nonkeratinizing squamous morphotype (the so-called cloacogenic tumors). The latter tumors also may have a confusing immunophenotype; they may be labeled for "squamoid" markers (e.g., CK5/6, p63) but also show expression of CK7. CK20 and CEA are typically absent in basaloid squamous carcinomas (208).

LIVER, GALLBLADDER, AND BILE DUCT TUMORS. HCCs can manifest several growth patterns and thereby simulate metastatic adenocarcinoma in the liver. Immunohistochemically, HCCs are generally negative for both CK7 and CK20 (209), with the exception of CK7+ "fibrolamellar" variants (210). HCCs are also negative with the AE1 keratin antibody (as opposed to cholangiocarcinoma), but they are immunoreactive with the CAM5.2 antibody. In our experience, the most helpful stains in recognizing HCC are Hep-Par1 and AFP (135). This neoplasm is consistently negative for MOC-31 and CEA (as detected with monoclonal antibodies), further distinguishing them from bile duct tumors and metastatic adenocarcinomas (211). EMA is generally absent or only focally seen in HCC, but other carcinomas in the differential diagnosis are typically diffusely positive for this marker. Another useful tool for establishing hepatic origin in CUP cases is the demonstration of albumin mRNA by in situ hybridization (212, 213).

In contrast to HCC, no specific stains exist for cholangiocarcinoma or gallbladder carcinomas. They are usually CK7+/CK20+, except that *intrahepatic* cholangiocarcinomas often lack CK20–(214, 215).

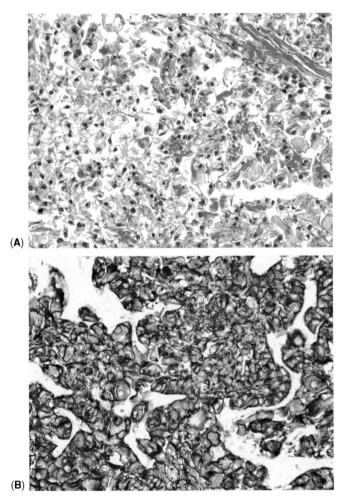

FIGURE 13 A renal tumor with mixed features of clear cell and chromophobe type carcinoma (**A**), demonstrating diffuse cytoplasmic and membranous reactivity for CD10 (**B**).

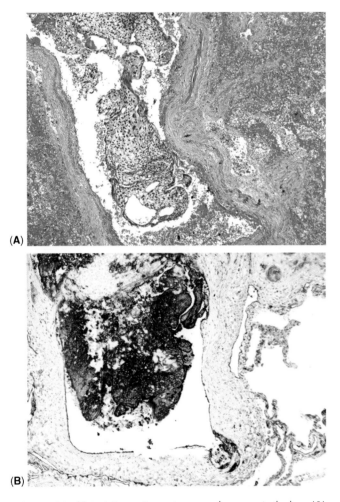

FIGURE 14 Metastatic carcinoma in a vascular space in the lung (**A**). The tumor cells were strongly positive for thrombomodulin (**B**), and showed focal staining for uroplakin III (not shown), confirming the presence of urothelial differentiation in the tumor cells.

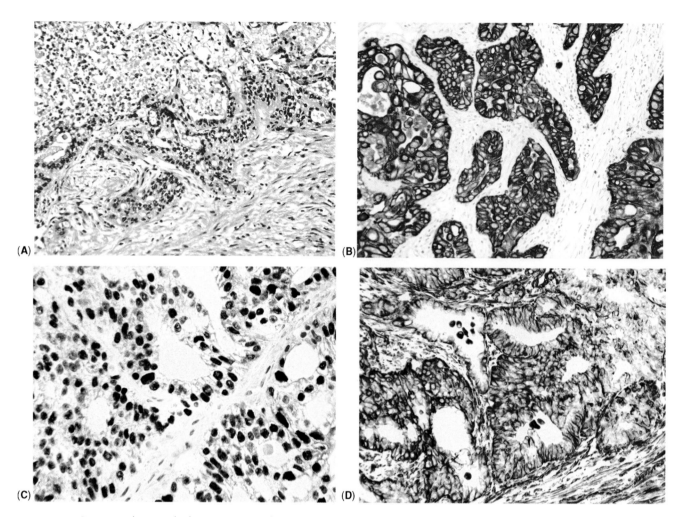

FIGURE 15 Ovarian endometrioid adenocarcinoma with necrosis (**A**), showing positivity for CK7 (**B**), estrogen receptor proteins (**C**), and vimentin (**D**). The tumor cells were negative for CK20 and CDX2. The patient had had colonic carcinoma in the past.

PANCREATIC AND DUODENAL TUMORS. The majority of pancreatic carcinomas are of the ductal type, with expression of CK7+. CK20 labeling is much less frequent, but it may be observed in primary ampullary (duodenal) adenocarcinomas. Diffuse CK17 expression has also been described in pancreaticobiliary tumors and may be helpful in distinguishing them from primary carcinomas of other sites (Fig. 12) (216). CK5/6 is infrequently present in pancreatic or ampullary neoplasms, unless partial squamous differentiation is apparent morphologically (217).

An important subtype of these lesions is mucinous (colloid) adenocarcinoma. When it presents with metastases in the abdominal cavity ("pseudomyxoma peritonei"), the differential diagnosis includes metastatic carcinoma from the appendix, colon and rectum, stomach, endometrium, or ovary. These cases are extremely difficult to resolve, and immunohistochemical stains have limited value. A lack of DPC4 expression may be helpful in suggesting a pancreatic tumor, but some nonpancreatic primary carcinomas (in the duodenal ampulla, small intestine, and gallbladder) have also been shown DPC4 deletion (218–220). On the other hand, the DPC4 gene is inactivated in only 50% of pancreatic malignancies.

ADRENOCORTICAL CARCINOMA. In similarity to hepatocellular and renal neoplasms, ACCs are among the few tumors that are nonreactive for both CK7 and CK20 (221). Occasional labeling for low molecular-weight keratins may be seen in adrenal carcinomas, but most are entirely keratin negative in FFPE specimens. Moreover, they are negative for EMA, MOC31, TAG-72, CEA, CD10, and B72.3. Hence, it may be immunohistologically difficult to prove that the lesion is a carcinoma at all. The most useful stains for ACC are inhibin and melan-A, for which most lesions show diffuse positivity (153, 222). ACCs typically are positive for vimentin, and some can show focal labeling for synaptophysin, but all of these tumors are negative for chromogranin-A (223).

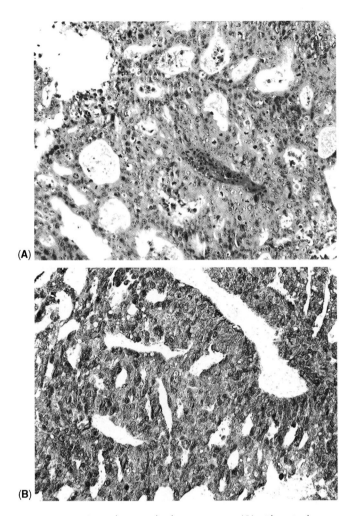

FIGURE 16 An endocervical adenocarcinoma (**A**) with typical strong staining of all tumor cells for p16 (**B**).

Any case of CUP that is negative for both CK7 and CK20 should be further analyzed for a possible adrenocortical, hepatocellular, or renal origin. In contrast to ACC, metastatic nonrenal carcinomas in the adrenal gland usually are CK7+ and MOC31+ or EMA+; renal cell carcinoma is CD10+; and metastatic melanoma is reactive for S100 protein, tyrosinase, and PNL2.

RENAL TUMORS. The form of renal cell carcinoma that most often presents as CUP is the conventional clear cell type (224), which may metastasize to virtually any site in the body (225, 226). To reiterate, renal cell carcinomas are negative for both CK7 and CK20. They coexpress keratin and vimentin and are also positive for EMA (227). Two supportive stains to establish a renal origin for clear cell carcinomas are RCC-Ag and CD10 (Fig. 13) (228). Another recently described "renal cell" stain is PAX2, but it has not been extensively tested to date (229–231).

BLADDER AND URETHRAL TUMORS. The majority of malignant bladder and urethral tumors are urothelial carcinomas, with rare examples of clear cell, enteric, and enteric adenocarcinoma or squamous and neuroendocrine carcinoma. Urothelial carcinomas classically have a CK7+/CK20+ immunoprofile. As mentioned earlier, "urothelial" markers include thrombomodulin and uroplakin III, neither of which is both sensitive and specific (140). Because of their individual drawbacks, these two stains should be used together as a means of assessing a potential urothelial origin for CUP (Fig. 14). Adenocarcinomas, squamous carcinomas, and neuroendocrine carcinomas of the bladder and urethra lack specific markers to suggest that they have arisen in the urinary tract (232, 233).

PROSTATIC CARCINOMA. All but the most undifferentiated prostatic adenocarcinomas are positive for PSA and PAP (234). Prostatic tumors rarely stain for CK20, a feature that helps to distinguish them from urothelial carcinomas (235). However, they are positive for low molecular weight cytokeratins and EMA.

MÜLLERIAN ADENOCARCINOMAS. The major histological subtypes of "müllerian" carcinomas are endometrioid, serous, clear cell, and mucinous adenocarcinomas. Their sites of potential origin include the ovary, endometrium, cervix, fallopian tubes, and peritoneal surfaces. Adenocarcinomas of müllerian origin usually have a CK7+/CK20− immunoprofile. On the other hand, primary ovarian mucinous carcinomas may show CK20 reactivity, and up to 40% may be CDX2+ (236, 237). Ovarian serous adenocarcinomas often show diffuse WT1 expression, as do primary peritoneal ("surface") serous carcinomas (93, 238). Up to one-third of primary uterine serous carcinomas are also WT1+. Hormonal receptors (ERP or PRP) are usually diffusely present in endometrioid müllerian carcinomas regardless of anatomic origin (239), and serous carcinomas often express them as well, albeit in a patchy fashion.

Endometrioid carcinomas label for vimentin but not for CEA, potentially helping to distinguish them from colorectal or cervical adenocarcinomas (Fig. 15) (240). The "usual" cervical adenocarcinomas are typically nonreactive for vimentin, ERP, and PRP, but they are CEA positive (241). Nonetheless, *endometrioid* lesions of the cervix are indistinguishable immunophenotypically from primary endometrial carcinoma (242).

Recently, diffuse p16 (INK4A) expression (Fig. 16) has been proposed as a distinctive marker of cervical adenocarcinoma (243). Although other tumor types can be p16 positive as well (244, 245), if this marker is seen in a mucinous tumor of the ovary or omentum it is highly suggestive of a cervical primary lesion (246). In situ hybridization or polymerase chain reaction assays for human papillomavirus nucleic acid in the tumor cells would be even more definitive in this regard. Müllerian clear cell tumors do not have a specific immunoprofile, but they need to be distinguished from clear cell carcinomas arising in other organ systems.

PERITONEAL CARCINOMATOSIS. In women who have diffuse peritoneal involvement by serous papillary adenocarcinoma, in the absence of an apparent lesion of the ovaries, fallopian tubes, or endometrium, the diagnosis of primary peritoneal serous carcinoma (PPSC) is usually assigned. The immunophenotype of PPSC is identical to that of ovarian serous tumors.

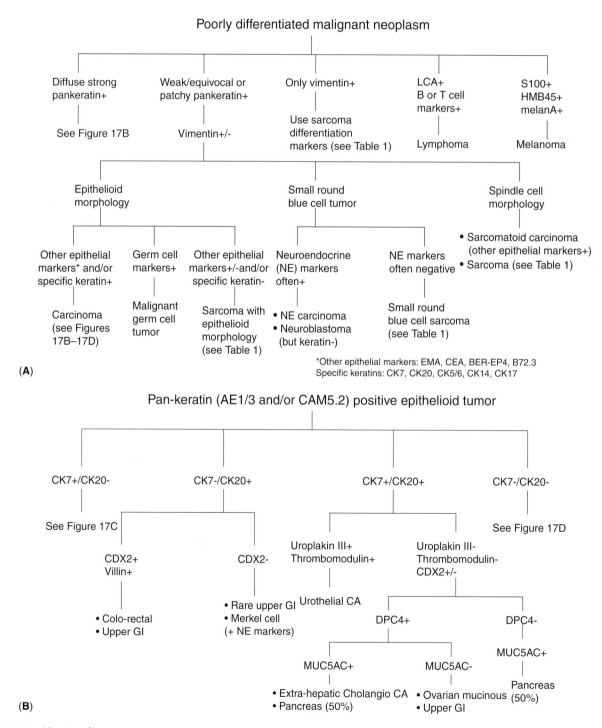

FIGURE 17 *(Continued on next page.)*

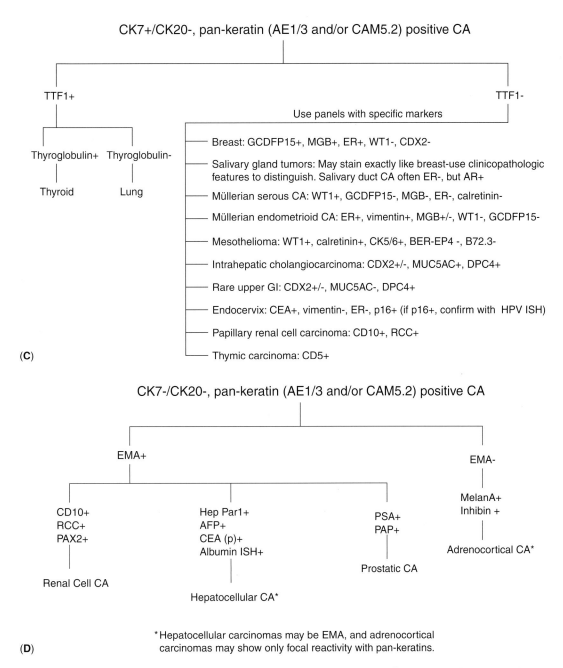

FIGURE 17 **(A)** Algorithmic approach to determining a line of differentiation in a poorly differentiated malignant neoplasm. **(B)** Algorithmic approach to determine site of origin in an adenocarcinoma or a poorly differentiated carcinoma. Further workup of a CK7+/CK20– **(C)** and CK7/CK20– **(D)** tumor. *Abbreviations*: EMA, epithelial membrane antigen; CEA, carcinoembryonic antigen; MUC, mucin; TTF, thyroid transcription factor; GCDFP-15, gross cystic disease fluid protein-15; MGB, mammaglobin; RCC, renal cell carcinoma; AFP, alpha-fetoprotein; DPC, deleted in pancreatic carcinoma; PAP, prostatic acid phosphatase; GI, gastrointestinal; PSA, prostate specific antigen.

The differential diagnosis is more challenging when the tumor shows a mucinous morphology, as discussed above (247). A combination of stains for CK7, CK20, CDX2, DPC4, several MUC determinants, p16, and vimentin is recommended as an approach to this problem (248). Metastatic ovarian stromal tumors occasionally enter this differential diagnosis as well. They may show

keratin positivity, but are almost always negative for EMA and positive for inhibin, calretinin, and CD99 (154, 249, 250).

BREAST CARCINOMAS. Breast carcinomas are broadly classified as ductal or lobular adenocarcinomas, although several other special morphological variants do exist. Ductal and lobular tumors show differential immunoreactivity for E-cadherin and p120; the ductal lesions manifest membranous expression of both, whereas lobular carcinomas are negative for E-cadherin and show diffuse *cytoplasmic* reactivity for p120. The latter p120 pattern is also shared by gastric signet-ring cell carcinomas and signet-ring cell colorectal carcinomas (251). Irrespective of morphotypes, breast carcinomas are usually CK7+/CK20–(252). The most specific immunostain for breast carcinoma is GCDFP-15, but it has a suboptimal sensitivity of approximately 50% to 60% (253). MGB is more sensitive, but it is also present in a significant number of endometrioid müllerian carcinomas. Approximately 70% of breast carcinomas are convincingly positive for ERP or PRP or both, in similarity to endometrial carcinomas and ovarian tumors (146, 254–256).

Step 3: Algorithms to Determine the Site of Origin for CUP

The availability of many disparate antibodies, and potentially confusing information in the literature on immunohistology, may occasionally lead to misinterpretation or worse, a mistaken diagnosis. This unwanted outcome can be minimized by using an algorithmic approach to IHC. Algorithms may vary by generic morphological categorization, such as those pertaining to small cell, large cell, epithelioid, and spindle cell neoplasms. The algorithms described herein apply to poorly differentiated malignant neoplasms in general. After an initial screening approach, more specific markers are used in a panel format to arrive at a detailed diagnosis (Fig. 17).

Although such algorithms provide a useful guide for the evaluation of CUP, it is important to remember that they are guidelines and not rules. The algorithms have been devised to include the most common immunoprofiles of the most common histological types of carcinoma in a particular anatomic site. *Exceptions do occur and if an immunophenotype is discordant with the morphological image, caution is advised and the use of additional analyses (e.g., EM) is suggested.*

There are several preanalytical, analytical, and postanalytical factors that can affect immunostaining results. Recently, standards have been proposed to control these elements (257). However, in spite of such efforts, discordant staining continues to happen because of variations in tumor biology. Therefore, a prediction of site of origin for CUP should not be entirely based on the immunoprofile, but must always incorporate clinical, morphological, immunohistologic (ultrastructural), and molecular data to arrive at the final determination.

■ REFERENCES

1. Shaw PH, Adams R, Jordan C, Crosby TD. A clinical review of the investigation and management of carcinoma of unknown primary in a single cancer network. *Clin Oncol (R Coll Radiol)* 2007; 19:87–95.
2. Yakushiji S, Ando M, Yonemori K, et al. Cancer of unknown primary site: review of consecutive cases at the National Cancer Center Hospital of Japan. *Int J Clin Oncol* 2006; 11:421–5.
3. Blaszyk H, Hartmann A, Bjornsson J. Cancer of unknown primary: clinicopathologic correlations. *Apmis* 2003; 111:1089–94.
4. Greco FA, Burris HA 3rd, Erland JB, et al. Carcinoma of unknown primary site. *Cancer* 2000; 89:2655–60.
5. Frayling IM. Methods of molecular analysis: mutation detection in solid tumours. *Mol Pathol* 2002; 55:73–9.
6. Armstrong AC, Blackhall FH. Management of cancer from an unknown primary. *Expert Opin Pharmacother* 2007; 8:445–55.
7. Chan JK. Advances in immunohistochemistry: impact on surgical pathology practice. *Semin Diagn Pathol* 2000; 17:170–7.
8. Dennis JL, Hvidsten TR, Wit EC, et al. Markers of adenocarcinoma characteristic of the site of origin: development of a diagnostic algorithm. *Clin Cancer Res* 2005; 11:3766–72.
9. Hainsworth JD, Wright EP, Johnson DH, Davis BW, Greco FA. Poorly differentiated carcinoma of unknown primary site: clinical usefulness of immunoperoxidase staining. *J Clin Oncol* 1991; 9: 1931–8.
10. Jaffer S, Bleiweiss IJ. Beyond hematoxylin and eosin–the role of immunohistochemistry in surgical pathology. *Cancer Invest* 2004; 22:445–65.
11. van der Gaast A, Verwij J, Planting AS, Stoter G, Henzen-Logmans SC. The value of immunohistochemistry in patients with poorly differentiated adenocarcinomas and undifferentiated carcinomas of unknown primary. *J Cancer Res Clin Oncol* 1996; 122:181–5.
12. Leader M, Collins M, Patel J, Henry K. Vimentin: an evaluation of its role as a tumour marker. *Histopathology* 1987; 11:63–72.
13. Azumi N, Battifora H. The distribution of vimentin and keratin in epithelial and nonepithelial neoplasms. A comprehensive immunohistochemical study on formalin- and alcohol-fixed tumors. *Am J Clin Pathol* 1987; 88:286–96.
14. Kurtin PJ, Pinkus GS. Leukocyte common antigen—a diagnostic discriminant between hematopoietic and nonhematopoietic neoplasms in paraffin sections using monoclonal antibodies: correlation with immunologic studies and ultrastructural localization. *Hum Pathol* 1985; 16:353–65.
15. Ries S, Barr R, LeBoit P, McCalmont T, Waldman J. Cutaneous sarcomatoid B-cell lymphoma. *Am J Dermatopathol* 2007; 29: 96–98.
16. Colella G, Tirelli A, Capone R, Rubini C, Guastafierro S. Myeloid sarcoma occurring in the maxillary gingiva: a case without leukemic manifestations. *Int J Hematol* 2005; 81: 138–41.
17. Menasce LP, Banerjee SS, Beckett E, Harris M. Extra-medullary myeloid tumour (granulocytic sarcoma) is often misdiagnosed: a study of 26 cases. *Histopathology* 1999; 34:391–8.
18. Sadahira Y, Sugihara T, Yawata Y, Manabe T. Cutaneous granulocytic sarcoma mimicking immunoblastic large cell lymphoma. *Pathol Int* 1999; 49:347–53.
19. Chen J, Yanuck RR 3rd, Abbondanzo SL, Chu WS, Aguilera NS. c-Kit (CD117) reactivity in extramedullary myeloid tumor/granulocytic sarcoma. *Arch Pathol Lab Med* 2001; 125:1448–52.
20. Palomino-Portilla EA, Valbuena JR, Quinones-Avila Mdel P, Medeiros LJ. Myeloid sarcoma of appendix mimicking acute appendicitis. *Arch Pathol Lab Med* 2005; 129:1027–31.

21. Roth MJ, Medeiros LJ, Elenitoba-Johnson K, et al. Extramedullary myeloid cell tumors. An immunohistochemical study of 29 cases using routinely fixed and processed paraffin-embedded tissue sections. *Arch Pathol Lab Med* 1995; 119: 790–8.

22. Hudock J, Chatten J, Miettinen M. Immunohistochemical evaluation of myeloid leukemia infiltrates (granulocytic sarcomas) in formaldehyde-fixed, paraffin-embedded tissue. *Am J Clin Pathol* 1994; 102:55–60.

23. Traweek ST, Arber DA, Rappaport H, Brynes RK. Extramedullary myeloid cell tumors. An immunohistochemical and morphologic study of 28 cases. *Am J Surg Pathol* 1993; 17: 1011–9.

24. Blessing K, Sanders DS, Grant JJ. Comparison of immunohistochemical staining of the novel antibody melan-A with S100 protein and HMB-45 in malignant melanoma and melanoma variants. *Histopathology* 1998; 32:139–46.

25. DeYoung BR, Wick MR. Immunohistologic evaluation of metastatic carcinomas of unknown origin: an algorithmic approach. *Semin Diagn Pathol* 2000; 17:184–93.

26. Drlicek M, Bodenteich A, Urbanits S, Grisold W. Immunohistochemical panel of antibodies in the diagnosis of brain metastases of the unknown primary. *Pathol Res Pract* 2004; 200:727–34.

27. Drier JK, Swanson PE, Cherwitz DL, Wick MR. S100 protein immunoreactivity in poorly differentiated carcinomas. Immunohistochemical comparison with malignant melanoma. *Arch Pathol Lab Med* 1987; 111:447–52.

28. Stroup RM, Pinkus GS. S-100 immunoreactivity in primary and metastatic carcinoma of the breast: a potential source of error in immunodiagnosis. *Hum Pathol* 1988; 19:949–53.

29. Hashimoto H, Daimaru Y, Enjoji M. S-100 protein distribution in liposarcoma. An immunoperoxidase study with special reference to the distinction of liposarcoma from myxoid malignant fibrous histiocytoma. *Virchows Arch A Pathol Anat Histopathol* 1984; 405:1–10.

30. Nakajima T, Watanabe S, Sato Y, et al. An immunoperoxidase study of S-100 protein distribution in normal and neoplastic tissues. *Am J Surg Pathol* 1982; 6:715–27.

31. Miettinen M, Franssila K. Immunohistochemical spectrum of malignant melanoma. The common presence of keratins. *Lab Invest* 1989; 61:623–8.

32. Selby WL, Nance KV, Park HK. CEA immunoreactivity in metastatic malignant melanoma. *Mod Pathol* 1992; 5:415–9.

33. Zarbo RJ, Gown AM, Nagle RB, Visscher DW, Crissman JD. Anomalous cytokeratin expression in malignant melanoma: one- and two-dimensional western blot analysis and immunohistochemical survey of 100 melanomas. *Mod Pathol* 1990; 3: 494–501.

34. Laskin WB, Miettinen M. Epithelioid sarcoma: new insights based on an extended immunohistochemical analysis. *Arch Pathol Lab Med* 2003; 127:1161–8.

35. Machen SK, Fisher C, Gautam RS, Tubbs RR, Goldblum JR. Utility of cytokeratin subsets for distinguishing poorly differentiated synovial sarcoma from peripheral primitive neuroectodermal tumour. *Histopathology* 1998; 33:501–7.

36. Olsen SH, Thomas DG, Lucas DR. Cluster analysis of immunohistochemical profiles in synovial sarcoma, malignant peripheral nerve sheath tumor, and Ewing sarcoma. *Mod Pathol* 2006; 19: 659–68.

37. Ordonez NG, Mahfouz SM, Mackay B. Synovial sarcoma: an immunohistochemical and ultrastructural study. *Hum Pathol* 1990; 21:733–49.

38. Sebire NJ, Gibson S, Rampling D, et al. Immunohistochemical findings in embryonal small round cell tumors with molecular diagnostic confirmation. *Appl Immunohistochem Mol Morphol* 2005; 13:1–5.

39. Folpe AL, Goldblum JR, Rubin BP, et al. Morphologic and immunophenotypic diversity in Ewing family tumors: a study of 66 genetically confirmed cases. *Am J Surg Pathol* 2005; 29: 1025–33.

40. Lazar A, Abruzzo LV, Pollock RE, Lee S, Czerniak B. Molecular diagnosis of sarcomas: chromosomal translocations in sarcomas. *Arch Pathol Lab Med* 2006; 130:1199–207.

41. Fritsch MK, Bridge JA, Schuster AE, Perlman EJ, Argani P. Performance characteristics of a reverse transcriptase-polymerase chain reaction assay for the detection of tumor-specific fusion transcripts from archival tissue. *Pediatr Dev Pathol* 2003; 6:43–53.

42. Scicchitano MS, Dalmas DA, Bertiaux MA, et al. Preliminary comparison of quantity, quality, and microarray performance of RNA extracted from formalin-fixed, paraffin-embedded, and unfixed frozen tissue samples. *J Histochem Cytochem* 2006; 54: 1229–37.

43. Spagnolo DV, Michie SA, Crabtree GS, Warnke RA, Rouse RV. Monoclonal anti-keratin (AE1) reactivity in routinely processed tissue from 166 human neoplasms. *Am J Clin Pathol* 1985; 84: 697–704.

44. Al-Abbadi MA, Almasri NM, Al-Quran S, Wilkinson EJ. Cytokeratin and epithelial membrane antigen expression in angiosarcomas: an immunohistochemical study of 33 cases. *Arch Pathol Lab Med* 2007; 131:288–92.

45. Bhargava R, Shia J, Hummer AJ, et al. Distinction of endometrial stromal sarcomas from "hemangiopericytomatous" tumors using a panel of immunohistochemical stains. *Mod Pathol* 2005; 18: 40–7.

46. Fuchs U, Kivela T, Summanen P, Immonen I, Tarkkanen A. An immunohistochemical and prognostic analysis of cytokeratin expression in malignant uveal melanoma. *Am J Pathol* 1992; 141: 169–81.

47. Gustmann C, Altmannsberger M, Osborn M, Griesser H, Feller AC. Cytokeratin expression and vimentin content in large cell anaplastic lymphomas and other non-Hodgkin's lymphomas. *Am J Pathol* 1991; 138:1413–22.

48. Korabiowska M, Fischer G, Steinacker A, et al. Cytokeratin positivity in paraffin-embedded malignant melanomas: comparative study of KL1, A4 and Lu5 antibodies. *Anticancer Res* 2004; 24:3203–7.

49. Srivastava A, Rosenberg AE, Selig M, Rubin BP, Nielsen GP. Keratin-positive Ewing's sarcoma: an ultrastructural study of 12 cases. *Int J Surg Pathol* 2005; 13:43–50.

50. Traweek ST, Liu J, Battifora H. Keratin gene expression in nonepithelial tissues. Detection with polymerase chain reaction. *Am J Pathol* 1993; 142:1111–8.

51. Vakar-Lopez F, Ayala AG, Raymond AK, Czerniak B. Epithelial Phenotype in Ewing's Sarcoma/Primitive Neuroectodermal Tumor. *Int J Surg Pathol* 2000; 8:59–65.

52. Abbruzzese JL, Abbruzzese MC, Lenzi R, Hess KR, Raber MN. Analysis of a diagnostic strategy for patients with suspected tumors of unknown origin. *J Clin Oncol* 1995; 13:2094–103.

53. Bartsch R, Wenzel C, Zielinski CC, Steger GG. HER-2-Positive Breast Cancer: Hope Beyond Trastuzumab. *BioDrugs* 2007; 21: 69–77.

54. Molina JR, Adjei AA, Jett JR. Advances in chemotherapy of non-small cell lung cancer. *Chest* 2006; 130:1211–9.

55. Ramalingam S, Belani CP. Recent advances in targeted therapy for non-small cell lung cancer. *Expert Opin Ther Targets* 2007; 11:245–57.

56. Hammar SP. Metastatic adenocarcinoma of unknown primary origin. *Hum Pathol* 1998; 29:1393–402.

57. Conessa C, Clement P, Foehrenbach H, Poncet JL. [Positron emission tomography in head and neck squamous cell carcinomas]. *Ann Otolaryngol Chir Cervicofac* 2006; 123:227–39.

58. Schmalbach CE, Miller FR. Occult primary head and neck carcinoma. *Curr Oncol Rep* 2007; 9:139–46.

59. Silva P, Hulse P, Sykes AJ, et al. Should FDG-PET scanning be routinely used for patients with an unknown head and neck squamous primary? *J Laryngol Otol* 2007; 121:149–53.

60. Gluckman JL, Robbins KT, Fried MP. Cervical metastatic squamous carcinoma of unknown or occult primary source. *Head Neck* 1990; 12:440–3.

61. Dotto JE, Glusac EJ. p63 is a useful marker for cutaneous spindle cell squamous cell carcinoma. *J Cutan Pathol* 2006; 33:413–7.

62. Kaufmann O, Fietze E, Mengs J, Dietel M. Value of p63 and cytokeratin 5/6 as immunohistochemical markers for the differential diagnosis of poorly differentiated and undifferentiated carcinomas. *Am J Clin Pathol* 2001; 116:823–30.

63. Chao TY, Chow KC, Chang JY, et al. Expression of Epstein-Barr virus-encoded RNAs as a marker for metastatic undifferentiated nasopharyngeal carcinoma. *Cancer* 1996; 78:24–9.

64. Gulley ML, Amin MB, Nicholls JM, et al. Epstein-Barr virus is detected in undifferentiated nasopharyngeal carcinoma but not in lymphoepithelioma-like carcinoma of the urinary bladder. *Hum Pathol* 1995; 26:1207–14.

65. Pathmanathan R, Prasad U, Chandrika G, et al. Undifferentiated, nonkeratinizing, and squamous cell carcinoma of the nasopharynx. Variants of Epstein-Barr virus-infected neoplasia. *Am J Pathol* 1995; 146:1355–67.

66. Jereczek-Fossa BA, Jassem J, Orecchia R. Cervical lymph node metastases of squamous cell carcinoma from an unknown primary. *Cancer Treat Rev* 2004; 30:153–64.

67. Calabrese L, Jereczek-Fossa BA, Jassem J, et al. Diagnosis and management of neck metastases from an unknown primary. *Acta Otorhinolaryngol Ital* 2005; 25:2–12.

68. Chang YL, Lee YC, Liao WY, Wu CT. The utility and limitation of thyroid transcription factor-1 protein in primary and metastatic pulmonary neoplasms. *Lung Cancer* 2004; 44:149–57.

69. Jerome Marson V, Mazieres J, Groussard O, et al. Expression of TTF-1 and cytokeratins in primary and secondary epithelial lung tumours: correlation with histological type and grade. *Histopathology* 2004; 45:125–34.

70. Tan D, Li Q, Deeb G, et al. Thyroid transcription factor-1 expression prevalence and its clinical implications in non-small cell lung cancer: a high-throughput tissue microarray and immunohistochemistry study. *Hum Pathol* 2003; 34:597–604.

71. Zaren HA, Copeland EM 3rd. Inguinal node metastases. *Cancer* 1978; 41:919–23.

72. Chejfec G, Falkmer S, Grimelius L, et al. Synaptophysin. A new marker for pancreatic neuroendocrine tumors. *Am J Surg Pathol* 1987; 11:241–7.

73. Gosney JR, Gosney MA, Lye M, Butt SA. Reliability of commercially available immunocytochemical markers for identification of neuroendocrine differentiation in bronchoscopic biopsies of bronchial carcinoma. *Thorax* 1995; 50:116–20.

74. O'Connor DT, Burton D, Deftos LJ. Chromogranin A: immunohistology reveals its universal occurrence in normal polypeptide hormone producing endocrine glands. *Life Sci* 1983; 33: 1657–63.

75. Pahlman S, Esscher T, Nilsson K. Expression of gamma-subunit of enolase, neuron-specific enolase, in human non-neuroendocrine tumors and derived cell lines. *Lab Invest* 1986; 54:554–60.

76. Schurmann G, Betzler M, Buhr HJ. Chromogranin A, neuron-specific enolase and synaptophysin as neuroendocrine cell

77. markers in the diagnosis of tumours of the gastro-entero-pancreatic system. *Eur J Surg Oncol* 1990; 16:298–303.

77. Cai YC, Banner B, Glickman J, Odze RD. Cytokeratin 7 and 20 and thyroid transcription factor 1 can help distinguish pulmonary from gastrointestinal carcinoid and pancreatic endocrine tumors. *Hum Pathol* 2001; 32:1087–93.

78. Saqi A, Alexis D, Remotti F, Bhagat G. Usefulness of CDX2 and TTF-1 in differentiating gastrointestinal from pulmonary carcinoids. *Am J Clin Pathol* 2005; 123:394–404.

79. Jaffee IM, Rahmani M, Singhal MG, Younes M. Expression of the intestinal transcription factor CDX2 in carcinoid tumors is a marker of midgut origin. *Arch Pathol Lab Med* 2006; 130: 1522–6.

80. Kaufmann O, Dietel M. Expression of thyroid transcription factor-1 in pulmonary and extrapulmonary small cell carcinomas and other neuroendocrine carcinomas of various primary sites. *Histopathology* 2000; 36:415–20.

81. Galanis E, Frytak S, Lloyd RV. Extrapulmonary small cell carcinoma. *Cancer* 1997; 79:1729–36.

82. Moll R, Franke WW, Schiller DL, Geiger B, Krepler R. The catalog of human cytokeratins: patterns of expression in normal epithelia, tumors and cultured cells. *Cell* 1982; 31:11–24.

83. Moll R. Molecular diversity of cytokeratins: significance for cell and tumor differentiation. *Acta Histochem Suppl* 1991; 41:117–27.

84. Chu P, Wu E, Weiss LM. Cytokeratin 7 and cytokeratin 20 expression in epithelial neoplasms: a survey of 435 cases. *Mod Pathol* 2000; 13:962–72.

85. Rubin BP, Skarin AT, Pisick E, Rizk M, Salgia R. Use of cytokeratins 7 and 20 in determining the origin of metastatic carcinoma of unknown primary, with special emphasis on lung cancer. *Eur J Cancer Prev* 2001; 10:77–82.

86. Tot T. Adenocarcinomas metastatic to the liver: the value of cytokeratins 20 and 7 in the search for unknown primary tumors. *Cancer* 1999; 85:171–7.

87. Cheville JC, Rao S, Iczkowski KA, Lohse CM, Pankratz VS. Cytokeratin expression in seminoma of the human testis. *Am J Clin Pathol* 2000; 113:583–8.

88. Ramalingam P, Malpica A, Silva EG, et al. The use of cytokeratin 7 and EMA in differentiating ovarian yolk sac tumors from endometrioid and clear cell carcinomas. *Am J Surg Pathol* 2004; 28:1499–505.

89. Call KM, Glaser T, Ito CY, et al. Isolation and characterization of a zinc finger polypeptide gene at the human chromosome 11 Wilms' tumor locus. *Cell* 1990; 60:509–20.

90. Little M, Wells C. A clinical overview of WT1 gene mutations. *Hum Mutat* 1997; 9:209–25.

91. Shimizu M, Toki T, Takagi Y, Konishi I, Fujii S. Immunohistochemical detection of the Wilms' tumor gene (WT1) in epithelial ovarian tumors. *Int J Gynecol Pathol* 2000; 19:158–63.

92. Waldstrom M, Grove A. Immunohistochemical expression of wilms tumor gene protein in different histologic subtypes of ovarian carcinomas. *Arch Pathol Lab Med* 2005; 129:85–8.

93. Acs G, Pasha T, Zhang PJ. WT1 is differentially expressed in serous, endometrioid, clear cell, and mucinous carcinomas of the peritoneum, fallopian tube, ovary, and endometrium. *Int J Gynecol Pathol* 2004; 23:110–8.

94. Al-Hussaini M, Stockman A, Foster H, McCluggage WG. WT-1 assists in distinguishing ovarian from uterine serous carcinoma and in distinguishing between serous and endometrioid ovarian carcinoma. *Histopathology* 2004; 44:109–15.

95. Dupont J, Wang X, Marshall DS, et al. Wilms Tumor Gene (WT1) and p53 expression in endometrial carcinomas: a study of 130 cases using a tissue microarray. *Gynecol Oncol* 2004; 94:449–55.

96. Egan JA, Ionescu MC, Eapen E, Jones JG, Marshall DS. Differential expression of WT1 and p53 in serous and endometrioid carcinomas of the endometrium. *Int J Gynecol Pathol* 2004; 23:119–22.

97. Goldstein NS, Uzieblo A. WT1 immunoreactivity in uterine papillary serous carcinomas is different from ovarian serous carcinomas. *Am J Clin Pathol* 2002; 117:541–5.

98. Hashi A, Yuminamochi T, Murata S, et al. Wilms tumor gene immunoreactivity in primary serous carcinomas of the fallopian tube, ovary, endometrium, and peritoneum. *Int J Gynecol Pathol* 2003; 22:374–7.

99. Moskaluk CA, Zhang H, Powell SM, et al. Cdx2 protein expression in normal and malignant human tissues: an immunohistochemical survey using tissue microarrays. *Mod Pathol* 2003; 16:913–9.

100. Kaimaktchiev V, Terracciano L, Tornillo L, et al. The homeobox intestinal differentiation factor CDX2 is selectively expressed in gastrointestinal adenocarcinomas. *Mod Pathol* 2004; 17: 1392–9.

101. Guazzi S, Price M, De Felice M, et al. Thyroid nuclear factor 1 (TTF-1) contains a homeodomain and displays a novel DNA binding specificity. *Embo J* 1990; 9:3631–9.

102. Fabbro D, Di Loreto C, Beltrami CA, et al. Expression of thyroid-specific transcription factors TTF-1 and PAX-8 in human thyroid neoplasms. *Cancer Res* 1994; 54:4744–9.

103. Nakamura N, Miyagi E, Murata S, Kawaoi A, Katoh R. Expression of thyroid transcription factor-1 in normal and neoplastic lung tissues. *Mod Pathol* 2002; 15:1058–67.

104. Reis-Filho JS, Carrilho C, Valenti C, et al. Is TTF1 a good immunohistochemical marker to distinguish primary from metastatic lung adenocarcinomas? *Pathol Res Pract* 2000; 196: 835–40.

105. Yatabe Y, Mitsudomi T, Takahashi T. TTF-1 expression in pulmonary adenocarcinomas. *Am J Surg Pathol* 2002; 26: 767–73.

106. Agoff SN, Lamps LW, Philip AT, et al. Thyroid transcription factor-1 is expressed in extrapulmonary small cell carcinomas but not in other extrapulmonary neuroendocrine tumors. *Mod Pathol* 2000; 13:238–42.

107. Stanta G, Carcangiu ML, Rosai J. The biochemical and immunohistochemical profile of thyroid neoplasia. *Pathol Annu* 1988; 23 Pt 1:129–57.

108. Myal Y, Robinson DB, Iwasiow B, et al. The prolactin-inducible protein (PIP/GCDFP-15) gene: cloning, structure and regulation. *Mol Cell Endocrinol* 1991; 80:165–75.

109. Viacava P, Naccarato AG, Bevilacqua G. Spectrum of GCDFP-15 expression in human fetal and adult normal tissues. *Virchows Arch* 1998; 432:255–60.

110. Myal Y, Gregory C, Wang H, Hamerton JL, Shiu RP. The gene for prolactin-inducible protein (PIP), uniquely expressed in exocrine organs, maps to chromosome 7. *Somat Cell Mol Genet* 1989; 15:265–70.

111. Watson MA, Darrow C, Zimonjic DB, Popescu NC, Fleming TP. Structure and transcriptional regulation of the human mammaglobin gene, a breast cancer associated member of the uteroglobin gene family localized to chromosome 11q13. *Oncogene* 1998; 16: 817–24.

112. Watson MA, Fleming TP. Mammaglobin, a mammary-specific member of the uteroglobin gene family, is overexpressed in human breast cancer. *Cancer Res* 1996; 56:860–5.

113. Zhao C, Nguyen T, Yusifov T, Glasgow BJ, Lehrer RI. Lipophilins: human peptides homologous to rat prostatein. *Biochem Biophys Res Commun* 1999; 256:147–55.

114. Bhargava R, Beriwal S, Dabbs DJ. Mammaglobin vs GCDFP-15: an immunohistologic validation survey for sensitivity and specificity. *Am J Clin Pathol* 2007; 127:103–13.

115. Ciampa A, Fanger G, Khan A, Rock KL, Xu B. Mammaglobin and CRxA-01 in pleural effusion cytology: potential utility of distinguishing metastatic breast carcinoma from other cytokeratin 7-positive/cytokeratin 20-negative carcinomas. *Cancer* 2004; 102:368–72.

116. Han JH, Kang Y, Shin HC, et al. Mammaglobin expression in lymph nodes is an important marker of metastatic breast carcinoma. *Arch Pathol Lab Med* 2003; 127:1330–4.

117. Sasaki E, Tsunoda N, Hatanaka Y, et al. Breast-specific expression of MGB1/mammaglobin: an examination of 480 tumors from various organs and clinicopathological analysis of MGB1-positive breast cancers. *Mod Pathol* 2007; 20:208–14.

118. Ordonez NG. Value of the MOC-31 monoclonal antibody in differentiating epithelial pleural mesothelioma from lung adenocarcinoma. *Hum Pathol* 1998; 29:166–9.

119. Ordonez NG. Value of the Ber-EP4 antibody in differentiating epithelial pleural mesothelioma from adenocarcinoma. The M.D. Anderson experience and a critical review of the literature. *Am J Clin Pathol* 1998; 109:85–9.

120. Riera JR, Astengo-Osuna C, Longmate JA, Battifora H. The immunohistochemical diagnostic panel for epithelial mesothelioma: a reevaluation after heat-induced epitope retrieval. *Am J Surg Pathol* 1997; 21:1409–19.

121. Rossen K, Thomsen HK. Ber-EP4 immunoreactivity depends on the germ layer origin and maturity of the squamous epithelium. *Histopathology* 2001; 39:386–9.

122. Yaziji H, Battifora H, Barry TS, et al. Evaluation of 12 antibodies for distinguishing epithelioid mesothelioma from adenocarcinoma: identification of a three-antibody immunohistochemical panel with maximal sensitivity and specificity. *Mod Pathol* 2006; 19:514–23.

123. Doglioni C, Tos AP, Laurino L, et al. Calretinin: a novel immunocytochemical marker for mesothelioma. *Am J Surg Pathol* 1996; 20:1037–46.

124. Cao QJ, Jones JG, Li M. Expression of calretinin in human ovary, testis, and ovarian sex cord-stromal tumors. *Int J Gynecol Pathol* 2001; 20:346–52.

125. Gotzos V, Wintergerst ES, Musy JP, Spichtin HP, Genton CY. Selective distribution of calretinin in adenocarcinomas of the human colon and adjacent tissues. *Am J Surg Pathol* 1999; 23:701–11.

126. Miettinen M, Limon J, Niezabitowski A, Lasota J. Calretinin and other mesothelioma markers in synovial sarcoma: analysis of antigenic similarities and differences with malignant mesothelioma. *Am J Surg Pathol* 2001; 25:610–7.

127. Miettinen M, Sarlomo-Rikala M. Expression of calretinin, thrombomodulin, keratin 5, and mesothelin in lung carcinomas of different types: an immunohistochemical analysis of 596 tumors in comparison with epithelioid mesotheliomas of the pleura. *Am J Surg Pathol* 2003; 27:150–8.

128. Adsay NV, Merati K, Nassar H, et al. Pathogenesis of colloid (pure mucinous) carcinoma of exocrine organs: coupling of gel-forming mucin (MUC2) production with altered cell polarity and abnormal cell-stroma interaction may be the key factor in the morphogenesis and indolent behavior of colloid carcinoma in the breast and pancreas. *Am J Surg Pathol* 2003; 27:571–8.

129. Matsukita S, Nomoto M, Kitajima S, et al. Expression of mucins (MUC1, MUC2, MUC5AC and MUC6) in mucinous carcinoma of the breast: comparison with invasive ductal carcinoma. *Histopathology* 2003; 42:26–36.

130. Pinto-de-Sousa J, David L, Reis CA, et al. Mucins MUC1, MUC2, MUC5AC and MUC6 expression in the evaluation of

differentiation and clinico-biological behaviour of gastric carcinoma. *Virchows Arch* 2002; 440:304–10.

131. Baker AC, Eltoum I, Curry RO, et al. Mucinous expression in benign and neoplastic glandular lesions of the uterine cervix. *Arch Pathol Lab Med* 2006; 130:1510–5.

132. Lee MJ, Lee HS, Kim WH, Choi Y, Yang M. Expression of mucins and cytokeratins in primary carcinomas of the digestive system. *Mod Pathol* 2003; 16:403–10.

133. Riethdorf L, O'Connell JT, Riethdorf S, Cviko A, Crum CP. Differential expression of MUC2 and MUC5AC in benign and malignant glandular lesions of the cervix uteri. *Virchows Arch* 2000; 437:365–71.

134. Lau SK, Weiss LM, Chu PG. Differential expression of MUC1, MUC2, and MUC5AC in carcinomas of various sites: an immunohistochemical study. *Am J Clin Pathol* 2004; 122:61–9.

135. Chu PG, Ishizawa S, Wu E, Weiss LM. Hepatocyte antigen as a marker of hepatocellular carcinoma: an immunohistochemical comparison to carcinoembryonic antigen, CD10, and alpha-fetoprotein. *Am J Surg Pathol* 2002; 26:978–88.

136. Fan Z, van de Rijn M, Montgomery K, Rouse RV. Hep par 1 antibody stain for the differential diagnosis of hepatocellular carcinoma: 676 tumors tested using tissue microarrays and conventional tissue sections. *Mod Pathol* 2003; 16:137–44.

137. Kakar S, Muir T, Murphy LM, Lloyd RV, Burgart LJ. Immunoreactivity of Hep Par 1 in hepatic and extrahepatic tumors and its correlation with albumin in situ hybridization in hepatocellular carcinoma. *Am J Clin Pathol* 2003; 119:361–6.

138. Reis-Filho JS, Simpson PT, Martins A, et al. Distribution of p63, cytokeratins 5/6 and cytokeratin 14 in 51 normal and 400 neoplastic human tissue samples using TARP-4 multi-tumor tissue microarray. *Virchows Arch* 2003; 443:122–32.

139. Moll R, Wu XR, Lin JH, Sun TT. Uroplakins, specific membrane proteins of urothelial umbrella cells, as histological markers of metastatic transitional cell carcinomas. *Am J Pathol* 1995; 147: 1383–97.

140. Parker DC, Folpe AL, Bell J, et al. Potential utility of uroplakin III, thrombomodulin, high molecular weight cytokeratin, and cytokeratin 20 in noninvasive, invasive, and metastatic urothelial (transitional cell) carcinomas. *Am J Surg Pathol* 2003; 27:1–10.

141. Appleton MA, Attanoos RL, Jasani B. Thrombomodulin as a marker of vascular and lymphatic tumours. *Histopathology* 1996; 29:153–7.

142. Yonezawa S, Maruyama I, Sakae K, et al. Thrombomodulin as a marker for vascular tumors. *Comparative study with factor VIII and Ulex europaeus I lectin. Am J Clin Pathol* 1987; 88:405–11.

143. Lager DJ, Callaghan EJ, Worth SF, Raife TJ, Lentz SR. Cellular localization of thrombomodulin in human epithelium and squamous malignancies. *Am J Pathol* 1995; 146:933–43.

144. Kushitani K, Takeshima Y, Amatya VJ, et al. Immunohistochemical marker panels for distinguishing between epithelioid mesothelioma and lung adenocarcinoma. *Pathol Int* 2007; 57: 190–9.

145. Kaufmann O, Deidesheimer T, Muehlenberg M, Deicke P, Dietel M. Immunohistochemical differentiation of metastatic breast carcinomas from metastatic adenocarcinomas of other common primary sites. *Histopathology* 1996; 29:233–40.

146. O'Connell FP, Wang HH, Odze RD. Utility of immunohistochemistry in distinguishing primary adenocarcinomas from metastatic breast carcinomas in the gastrointestinal tract. *Arch Pathol Lab Med* 2005; 129:338–47.

147. Nash JW, Morrison C, Frankel WL. The utility of estrogen receptor and progesterone receptor immunohistochemistry in the distinction of metastatic breast carcinoma from other tumors in the liver. *Arch Pathol Lab Med* 2003; 127:1591–5.

148. Diamandis EP, Yousef GM, Luo LY, Magklara A, Obiezu CV. The new human kallikrein gene family: implications in carcinogenesis. *Trends Endocrinol Metab* 2000; 11:54–60.

149. Alanen KA, Kuopio T, Koskinen PJ, Nevalainen TJ. Immunohistochemical labelling for prostate specific antigen in non-prostatic tissues. *Pathol Res Pract* 1996; 192:233–7.

150. Elgamal AA, Ectors NL, Sunardhi-Widyaputra S, et al. Detection of prostate specific antigen in pancreas and salivary glands: a potential impact on prostate cancer overestimation. *J Urol* 1996; 156:464–8.

151. Hahn SA, Schutte M, Hoque AT, et al. DPC4, a candidate tumor suppressor gene at human chromosome 18q21.1. *Science* 1996; 271:350–3.

152. Ji H, Isacson C, Seidman JD, Kurman RJ, Ronnett BM. Cytokeratins 7 and 20, Dpc4, and MUC5AC in the distinction of metastatic mucinous carcinomas in the ovary from primary ovarian mucinous tumors: Dpc4 assists in identifying metastatic pancreatic carcinomas. *Int J Gynecol Pathol* 2002; 21:391–400.

153. Busam KJ, Iversen K, Coplan KA, et al. Immunoreactivity for A103, an antibody to melan-A (Mart-1), in adrenocortical and other steroid tumors. *Am J Surg Pathol* 1998; 22:57–63.

154. McCluggage WG, Young RH. Immunohistochemistry as a diagnostic aid in the evaluation of ovarian tumors. *Semin Diagn Pathol* 2005; 22:3–32.

155. Chu P, Arber DA. Paraffin-section detection of CD10 in 505 nonhematopoietic neoplasms. Frequent expression in renal cell carcinoma and endometrial stromal sarcoma. *Am J Clin Pathol* 2000; 113:374–82.

156. McGregor DK, Khurana KK, Cao C, et al. Diagnosing primary and metastatic renal cell carcinoma: the use of the monoclonal antibody "renal cell carcinoma marker". *Am J Surg Pathol* 2001; 25:1485–92.

157. Cheng L, Sung MT, Cossu-Rocca P, et al. OCT4: biological functions and clinical applications as a marker of germ cell neoplasia. *J Pathol* 2007; 211:1–9.

158. Honecker F, Oosterhuis JW, Mayer F, et al. New insights into the pathology and molecular biology of human germ cell tumors. *World J Urol* 2004; 22:15–24.

159. Miettinen M, Lasota J. KIT (CD117): a review on expression in normal and neoplastic tissues, and mutations and their clinicopathologic correlation. *Appl Immunohistochem Mol Morphol* 2005; 13:205–20.

160. Miettinen M, Sobin LH, Sarlomo-Rikala M. Immunohistochemical spectrum of GISTs at different sites and their differential diagnosis with a reference to CD117 (KIT). *Mod Pathol* 2000; 13: 1134–42.

161. Al-Shamkhani A. The role of CD30 in the pathogenesis of haematopoietic malignancies. *Curr Opin Pharmacol* 2004; 4:355–9.

162. Grammatico D, Grignon DJ, Eberwein P, et al. Transitional cell carcinoma of the renal pelvis with choriocarcinomatous differentiation. Immunohistochemical and immunoelectron microscopic assessment of human chorionic gonadotropin production by transitional cell carcinoma of the urinary bladder. *Cancer* 1993; 71:1835–41.

163. Nikitakis NG, Tosios KI, Papanikolaou VS, et al. Immunohistochemical expression of cytokeratins 7 and 20 in malignant salivary gland tumors. *Mod Pathol* 2004; 17:407–15.

164. Andreadis D, Epivatianos A, Poulopoulos A, et al. Detection of C-KIT (CD117) molecule in benign and malignant salivary gland tumours. *Oral Oncol* 2006; 42:57–65.

165. Azoulay S, Lae M, Freneaux P, et al. KIT is highly expressed in adenoid cystic carcinoma of the breast, a basal-like carcinoma associated with a favorable outcome. *Mod Pathol* 2005; 18: 1623–31.

166. Ozolek JA, Bastacky SI, Myers EN, Hunt JL. Immunophenotypic comparison of salivary gland oncocytoma and metastatic renal cell carcinoma. *Laryngoscope* 2005; 115:1097–100.

167. Kapadia SB, Barnes L. Expression of androgen receptor, gross cystic disease fluid protein, and CD44 in salivary duct carcinoma. *Mod Pathol* 1998; 11:1033–8.

168. Fan CY, Wang J, Barnes EL. Expression of androgen receptor and prostatic specific markers in salivary duct carcinoma: an immunohistochemical analysis of 13 cases and review of the literature. *Am J Surg Pathol* 2000; 24:579–86.

169. James GK, Pudek M, Berean KW, Diamandis EP, Archibald BL. Salivary duct carcinoma secreting prostate-specific antigen. *Am J Clin Pathol* 1996; 106:242–7.

170. Franchi A, Massi D, Palomba A, Biancalani M, Santucci M. CDX-2, cytokeratin 7 and cytokeratin 20 immunohistochemical expression in the differential diagnosis of primary adenocarcinomas of the sinonasal tract. *Virchows Arch* 2004; 445:63–7.

171. Kennedy MT, Jordan RC, Berean KW, Perez-Ordonez B. Expression pattern of CK7, CK20, CDX-2, and villin in intestinal-type sinonasal adenocarcinoma. *J Clin Pathol* 2004; 57: 932–7.

172. Resto VA, Krane JF, Faquin WC, Lin DT. Immunohistochemical distinction of intestinal-type sinonasal adenocarcinoma from metastatic adenocarcinoma of intestinal origin. *Ann Otol Rhinol Laryngol* 2006; 115:59–64.

173. Bejarano PA, Nikiforov YE, Swenson ES, Biddinger PW. Thyroid transcription factor-1, thyroglobulin, cytokeratin 7, and cytokeratin 20 in thyroid neoplasms. *Appl Immunohistochem Mol Morphol* 2000; 8:189–94.

174. Ordonez NG, El-Naggar AK, Hickey RC, Samaan NA. Anaplastic thyroid carcinoma. Immunocytochemical study of 32 cases. *Am J Clin Pathol* 1991; 96:15–24.

175. Kodama T, Watanabe S, Sato Y, Shimosato Y, Miyazawa N. An immunohistochemical study of thymic epithelial tumors. I. Epithelial component. *Am J Surg Pathol* 1986; 10:26–33.

176. Fukai I, Masaoka A, Hashimoto T, et al. The distribution of epithelial membrane antigen in thymic epithelial neoplasms. *Cancer* 1992; 70:2077–81.

177. Truong LD, Mody DR, Cagle PT, et al. Thymic carcinoma. A clinicopathologic study of 13 cases. *Am J Surg Pathol* 1990; 14: 151–66.

178. Chan JK, Tsang WY, Seneviratne S, Pau MY. The MIC2 antibody 013. Practical application for the study of thymic epithelial tumors. *Am J Surg Pathol* 1995; 19:1115–23.

179. Pomplun S, Wotherspoon AC, Shah G, et al. Immunohistochemical markers in the differentiation of thymic and pulmonary neoplasms. *Histopathology* 2002; 40:152–8.

180. Dorfman DM, Shahsafaei A, Chan JK. Thymic carcinomas, but not thymomas and carcinomas of other sites, show CD5 immunoreactivity. *Am J Surg Pathol* 1997; 21:936–40.

181. Hishima T, Fukayama M, Fujisawa M, et al. CD5 expression in thymic carcinoma. *Am J Pathol* 1994; 145:268–75.

182. Kornstein MJ, Rosai J. CD5 labeling of thymic carcinomas and other nonlymphoid neoplasms. *Am J Clin Pathol* 1998; 109: 722–6.

183. Hishima T, Fukayama M, Hayashi Y, et al. CD70 expression in thymic carcinoma. *Am J Surg Pathol* 2000; 24:742–6.

184. Adam PJ, Terrett JA, Steers G, et al. CD70 (TNFSF7) is expressed at high prevalence in renal cell carcinomas and is rapidly internalised on antibody binding. *Br J Cancer* 2006; 95:298–306.

185. Diegmann J, Junker K, Gerstmayer B, et al. Identification of CD70 as a diagnostic biomarker for clear cell renal cell carcinoma by gene expression profiling, real-time RT-PCR and immunohistochemistry. *Eur J Cancer* 2005; 41:1794–801.

186. Junker K, Hindermann W, von Eggeling F, et al. CD70: a new tumor specific biomarker for renal cell carcinoma. *J Urol* 2005; 173:2150–3.

187. Weidner N. Germ-cell tumors of the mediastinum. *Semin Diagn Pathol* 1999; 16:42–50.

188. Suster S, Moran CA. Applications and limitations of immunohistochemistry in the diagnosis of malignant mesothelioma. *Adv Anat Pathol* 2006; 13:316–29.

189. Cossu-Rocca P, Jones TD, Roth LM, et al. Cytokeratin and CD30 expression in dysgerminoma. *Hum Pathol* 2006; 37: 1015–21.

190. Moran CA, Suster S, Przygodzki RM, Koss MN. Primary germ cell tumors of the mediastinum: II. Mediastinal seminomas—a clinicopathologic and immunohistochemical study of 120 cases. *Cancer* 1997; 80:691–8.

191. Ulbright TM. Germ cell tumors of the gonads: a selective review emphasizing problems in differential diagnosis, newly appreciated, and controversial issues. *Mod Pathol* 2005; 18(Suppl. 2): S61–79.

192. Cheng L. Establishing a germ cell origin for metastatic tumors using OCT4 immunohistochemistry. *Cancer* 2004; 101: 2006–10.

193. Sung MT, Jones TD, Beck SD, Foster RS, Cheng L. OCT4 is superior to CD30 in the diagnosis of metastatic embryonal carcinomas after chemotherapy. *Hum Pathol* 2006; 37:662–7.

194. Jacobsen GK, Jacobsen M. Alpha-fetoprotein (AFP) and human chorionic gonadotropin (HCG) in testicular germ cell tumours. A prospective immunohistochemical study. *Acta Pathol Microbiol Immunol Scand [A]* 1983; 91:165–76.

195. Bosl GJ, Ilson DH, Rodriguez E, et al. Clinical relevance of the i (12p) marker chromosome in germ cell tumors. *J Natl Cancer Inst* 1994; 86:349–55.

196. Kernek KM, Brunelli M, Ulbright TM, et al. Fluorescence in situ hybridization analysis of chromosome 12p in paraffin-embedded tissue is useful for establishing germ cell origin of metastatic tumors. *Mod Pathol* 2004; 17:1309–13.

197. Merchant SH, Amin MB, Tamboli P, et al. Primary signet-ring cell carcinoma of lung: immunohistochemical study and comparison with non-pulmonary signet-ring cell carcinomas. *Am J Surg Pathol* 2001; 25:1515–9.

198. Tsuta K, Ishii G, Nitadori J, et al. Comparison of the immunophenotypes of signet-ring cell carcinoma, solid adenocarcinoma with mucin production, and mucinous bronchioloalveolar carcinoma of the lung characterized by the presence of cytoplasmic mucin. *J Pathol* 2006; 209:78–87.

199. Lau SK, Desrochers MJ, Luthringer DJ. Expression of thyroid transcription factor-1, cytokeratin 7, and cytokeratin 20 in bronchioloalveolar carcinomas: an immunohistochemical evaluation of 67 cases. *Mod Pathol* 2002; 15:538–42.

200. Saad RS, Cho P, Silverman JF, Liu Y. Usefulness of Cdx2 in separating mucinous bronchioloalveolar adenocarcinoma of the lung from metastatic mucinous colorectal adenocarcinoma. *Am J Clin Pathol* 2004; 122:421–7.

201. Ordonez NG. Immunohistochemical diagnosis of epithelioid mesothelioma: an update. *Arch Pathol Lab Med* 2005; 129: 1407–14.

202. Hammar SP. Macroscopic, histologic, histochemical, immunohistochemical, and ultrastructural features of mesothelioma. *Ultrastruct Pathol* 2006; 30:3–17.

203. Gulmann C, Counihan I, Grace A, et al. Cytokeratin 7/20 and mucin expression patterns in oesophageal, cardia and distal gastric adenocarcinomas. *Histopathology* 2003; 43:453–61.

204. Mizoshita T, Inada K, Tsukamoto T, et al. Expression of the intestine-specific transcription factors, Cdx1 and Cdx2, correlates

shift to an intestinal phenotype in gastric cancer cells. *J Cancer Res Clin Oncol* 2004; 130:29–36.

205. De Lott LB, Morrison C, Suster S, Cohn DE, Frankel WL. CDX2 is a useful marker of intestinal-type differentiation: a tissue microarray-based study of 629 tumors from various sites. *Arch Pathol Lab Med* 2005; 129:1100–5.

206. Nishizuka S, Chen ST, Gwadry FG, et al. Diagnostic markers that distinguish colon and ovarian adenocarcinomas: identification by genomic, proteomic, and tissue array profiling. *Cancer Res* 2003; 63:5243–50.

207. Sheahan K, O'Brien MJ, Burke B, et al. Differential reactivities of carcinoembryonic antigen (CEA) and CEA-related monoclonal and polyclonal antibodies in common epithelial malignancies. *Am J Clin Pathol* 1990; 94:157–64.

208. Chetty R, Serra S, Hsieh E. Basaloid squamous carcinoma of the anal canal with an adenoid cystic pattern: histologic and immunohistochemical reappraisal of an unusual variant. *Am J Surg Pathol* 2005; 29:1668–72.

209. Maeda T, Kajiyama K, Adachi E, et al. The expression of cytokeratins 7, 19, and 20 in primary and metastatic carcinomas of the liver. *Mod Pathol* 1996; 9:901–9.

210. Klein WM, Molmenti EP, Colombani PM, et al. Primary liver carcinoma arising in people younger than 30 years. *Am J Clin Pathol* 2005; 124:512–8.

211. Porcell AI, De Young BR, Proca DM, Frankel WL. Immunohistochemical analysis of hepatocellular and adenocarcinoma in the liver: MOC31 compares favorably with other putative markers. *Mod Pathol* 2000; 13:773–8.

212. Oliveira AM, Erickson LA, Burgart LJ, Lloyd RV. Differentiation of primary and metastatic clear cell tumors in the liver by in situ hybridization for albumin messenger RNA. *Am J Surg Pathol* 2000; 24:177–82.

213. Varma V, Cohen C. Immunohistochemical and molecular markers in the diagnosis of hepatocellular carcinoma. *Adv Anat Pathol* 2004; 11:239–49.

214. Rullier A, Le Bail B, Fawaz R, et al. Cytokeratin 7 and 20 expression in cholangiocarcinomas varies along the biliary tract but still differs from that in colorectal carcinoma metastasis. *Am J Surg Pathol* 2000; 24:870–6.

215. Sasaki A, Kawano K, Aramaki M, et al. Immunohistochemical expression of cytokeratins in intrahepatic cholangiocarcinoma and metastatic adenocarcinoma of the liver. *J Surg Oncol* 1999; 70:103–8.

216. Chu PG, Schwarz RE, Lau SK, Yen Y, Weiss LM. Immunohistochemical staining in the diagnosis of pancreatobiliary and ampulla of Vater adenocarcinoma: application of CDX2, CK17, MUC1, and MUC2. *Am J Surg Pathol* 2005; 29:359–67.

217. Kardon DE, Thompson LD, Przygodzki RM, Heffess CS. Adenosquamous carcinoma of the pancreas: a clinicopathologic series of 25 cases. *Mod Pathol* 2001; 14:443–51.

218. McCarthy DM, Hruban RH, Argani P, et al. Role of the DPC4 tumor suppressor gene in adenocarcinoma of the ampulla of Vater: analysis of 140 cases. *Mod Pathol* 2003; 16:272–8.

219. Parwani AV, Geradts J, Caspers E, et al. Immunohistochemical and genetic analysis of non-small cell and small cell gallbladder carcinoma and their precursor lesions. *Mod Pathol* 2003; 16:299–308.

220. Svrcek M, Jourdan F, Sebbagh N, et al. Immunohistochemical analysis of adenocarcinoma of the small intestine: a tissue microarray study. *J Clin Pathol* 2003; 56:898–903.

221. Gaffey MJ, Traweek ST, Mills SE, et al. Cytokeratin expression in adrenocortical neoplasia: an immunohistochemical and biochemical study with implications for the differential diagnosis of adrenocortical, hepatocellular, and renal cell carcinoma. *Hum Pathol* 1992; 23:144–53.

222. Pan CC, Chen PC, Tsay SH, Ho DM. Differential immunoprofiles of hepatocellular carcinoma, renal cell carcinoma, and adrenocortical carcinoma: a systemic immunohistochemical survey using tissue array technique. *Appl Immunohistochem Mol Morphol* 2005; 13:347–52.

223. Miettinen M. Neuroendocrine differentiation in adrenocortical carcinoma. New immunohistochemical findings supported by electron microscopy. *Lab Invest* 1992; 66:169–74.

224. Mai KT, Landry DC, Robertson SJ, et al. A comparative study of metastatic renal cell carcinoma with correlation to subtype and primary tumor. *Pathol Res Pract* 2001; 197:671–5.

225. Pagano S, Franzoso F, Ruggeri P. Renal cell carcinoma metastases. Review of unusual clinical metastases, metastatic modes and patterns and comparison between clinical and autopsy metastatic series. *Scand J Urol Nephrol* 1996; 30:165–72.

226. Weiss L, Harlos JP, Torhorst J, et al. Metastatic patterns of renal carcinoma: an analysis of 687 necropsies. *J Cancer Res Clin Oncol* 1988; 114:605–12.

227. Waldherr R, Schwechheimer K. Co-expression of cytokeratin and vimentin intermediate-sized filaments in renal cell carcinomas. Comparative study of the intermediate-sized filament distribution in renal cell carcinomas and normal human kidney. *Virchows Arch A Pathol Anat Histopathol* 1985; 408:15–27.

228. Avery AK, Beckstead J, Renshaw AA, Corless CL. Use of antibodies to RCC and CD10 in the differential diagnosis of renal neoplasms. *Am J Surg Pathol* 2000; 24:203–10.

229. Daniel L, Lechevallier E, Giorgi R, et al. Pax-2 expression in adult renal tumors. *Hum Pathol* 2001; 32:282–7.

230. Mazal PR, Stichenwirth M, Koller A, et al. Expression of aquaporins and PAX-2 compared to CD10 and cytokeratin 7 in renal neoplasms: a tissue microarray study. *Mod Pathol* 2005; 18:535–40.

231. Memeo L, Jhang J, Assaad AM, et al. Immunohistochemical analysis for cytokeratin 7, KIT, and PAX2: value in the differential diagnosis of chromophobe cell carcinoma. *Am J Clin Pathol* 2007; 127:225–9.

232. Oliva E, Amin MB, Jimenez R, Young RH. Clear cell carcinoma of the urinary bladder: a report and comparison of four tumors of mullerian origin and nine of probable urothelial origin with discussion of histogenesis and diagnostic problems. *Am J Surg Pathol* 2002; 26:190–7.

233. Oliva E, Young RH. Clear cell adenocarcinoma of the urethra: a clinicopathologic analysis of 19 cases. *Mod Pathol* 1996; 9:513–20.

234. Hameed O, Humphrey PA. Immunohistochemistry in diagnostic surgical pathology of the prostate. *Semin Diagn Pathol* 2005; 22:88–104.

235. Mhawech P, Uchida T, Pelte MF. Immunohistochemical profile of high-grade urothelial bladder carcinoma and prostate adenocarcinoma. *Hum Pathol* 2002; 33:1136–40.

236. Vang R, Gown AM, Barry TS, et al. Cytokeratins 7 and 20 in primary and secondary mucinous tumors of the ovary: analysis of coordinate immunohistochemical expression profiles and staining distribution in 179 cases. *Am J Surg Pathol* 2006; 30:1130–9.

237. Vang R, Gown AM, Wu LS, et al. Immunohistochemical expression of CDX2 in primary ovarian mucinous tumors and metastatic mucinous carcinomas involving the ovary: comparison with CK20 and correlation with coordinate expression of CK7. *Mod Pathol* 2006; 19:1421–8.

238. Lee BH, Hecht JL, Pinkus JL, Pinkus GS. WT1, estrogen receptor, and progesterone receptor as markers for breast or ovarian

primary sites in metastatic adenocarcinoma to body fluids. *Am J Clin Pathol* 2002; 117:745–50.

239. Darvishian F, Hummer AJ, Thaler HT, et al. Serous endometrial cancers that mimic endometrioid adenocarcinomas: a clinico-pathologic and immunohistochemical study of a group of problematic cases. *Am J Surg Pathol* 2004; 28:1568–78.

240. Dabbs DJ, Sturtz K, Zaino RJ. The immunohistochemical discrimination of endometrioid adenocarcinomas. *Hum Pathol* 1996; 27:172–7.

241. McCluggage WG, Sumathi VP, McBride HA, Patterson A. A panel of immunohistochemical stains, including carcinoembryonic antigen, vimentin, and estrogen receptor, aids the distinction between primary endometrial and endocervical adenocarcinomas. *Int J Gynecol Pathol* 2002; 21:11–5.

242. Kamoi S, AlJuboury MI, Akin MR, Silverberg SG. Immunohistochemical staining in the distinction between primary endometrial and endocervical adenocarcinomas: another viewpoint. *Int J Gynecol Pathol* 2002; 21:217–23.

243. McCluggage WG, Jenkins D. p16 immunoreactivity may assist in the distinction between endometrial and endocervical adenocarcinoma. *Int J Gynecol Pathol* 2003; 22:231–5.

244. Raspollini MR, Nesi G, Baroni G, Girardi LR, Taddei GL. p16 (INK4a) expression in urinary bladder carcinoma. *Arch Ital Urol Androl* 2006; 78:97–100.

245. Reid-Nicholson M, Iyengar P, Hummer AJ, et al. Immuno-phenotypic diversity of endometrial adenocarcinomas: implications for differential diagnosis. *Mod Pathol* 2006; 19:1091–100.

246. O'Neill CJ, McCluggage WG. p16 expression in the female genital tract and its value in diagnosis. *Adv Anat Pathol* 2006; 13:8–15.

247. Elishaev E, Gilks CB, Miller D, et al. Synchronous and metachronous endocervical and ovarian neoplasms: evidence supporting interpretation of the ovarian neoplasms as metastatic endocervical adenocarcinomas simulating primary ovarian surface epithelial neoplasms. *Am J Surg Pathol* 2005; 29:281–94.

248. Nonaka D, Kusamura S, Baratti D, et al. CDX-2 expression in pseudomyxoma peritonei: a clinicopathological study of 42 cases. *Histopathology* 2006; 49:381–7.

249. Baker PM, Oliva E. Immunohistochemistry as a tool in the differential diagnosis of ovarian tumors: an update. *Int J Gynecol Pathol* 2005; 24:39–55.

250. Deavers MT, Malpica A, Liu J, Broaddus R, Silva EG. Ovarian sex cord-stromal tumors: an immunohistochemical study including a comparison of calretinin and inhibin. *Mod Pathol* 2003; 16:584–90.

251. Dabbs DJ, Bhargava R, Chivukula M. Lobular versus ductal breast neoplasms: the diagnostic utility of p120 catenin. *Am J Surg Pathol* 2007; 31:427–37.

252. Tot T. Patterns of distribution of cytokeratins 20 and 7 in special types of invasive breast carcinoma: a study of 123 cases. *Ann Diagn Pathol* 1999; 3:350–6.

253. Tornos C, Soslow R, Chen S, et al. Expression of WT1, CA 125, and GCDFP-15 as useful markers in the differential diagnosis of primary ovarian carcinomas versus metastatic breast cancer to the ovary. *Am J Surg Pathol* 2005; 29:1482–9.

254. Helin HJ, Helle MJ, Kallioniemi OP, Isola JJ. Immunohistochemical determination of estrogen and progesterone receptors in human breast carcinoma. Correlation with histopathology and DNA flow cytometry. *Cancer* 1989; 63:1761–7.

255. Lal P, Tan LK, Chen B. Correlation of HER-2 status with estrogen and progesterone receptors and histologic features in 3,655 invasive breast carcinomas. *Am J Clin Pathol* 2005; 123:541–6.

256. Nadji M, Gomez-Fernandez C, Ganjei-Azar P, Morales AR. Immunohistochemistry of estrogen and progesterone receptors reconsidered: experience with 5,993 breast cancers. *Am J Clin Pathol* 2005; 123:21–7.

257. Taylor CR. Standardization in immunohistochemistry: the role of antigen retrieval in molecular morphology. *Biotech Histochem* 2006; 81:3–12.

Serum Tumor Markers

GEORGE PENTHEROUDAKIS

NICHOLAS PAVLIDIS

■ INTRODUCTION

Tumor markers are biological molecules associated with the cellular aberrations that contribute to the development of the malignant phenotype. These substances may be proteins, nucleic acids, or lipids produced by the tumor cells or by normal tissues as a secondary effect of malignancy. Tumor markers can be evaluated in tissues, exfoliated or circulating cells, and body fluids, such as serum, urine, saliva, sputum, serosal effusions, or cerebrospinal fluid. Most often they are glycoproteins released by malignant epithelia into the bloodstream and evaluated in the serum. These biomolecules may be produced strictly by carcinomatous cells as a result of distinct genetic and epigenetic alterations, or they may be relatively overexpressed in malignant versus normal tissues.

The detection and serial determination of serum tumor markers, which is performed relatively easily, aids in the study of surrogate markers for early cancer detection and diagnosis, molecular classification of tumors, evaluation of response to treatment, assessment of prognosis, and patient follow-up (1). Bigbee and Herberman elegantly summarized the characteristics of an ideal tumor marker, the most important of which were specific production by malignant tissue at detectable levels in the serum in all patients in an organ-site-specific manner; quantitative association between serum marker levels and tumor volume; and availability of a standardized, validated assay to perform the measurements (2). Such ideal tumor markers have the potential to influence clinical decisions in screening, diagnosis, prognosis, treatment selection, monitoring of therapy, and detection of relapse in a clinically useful manner. Clinical utility dictates that knowledge of the tumor marker should contribute to a decision-making process that results in a more favorable patient outcome. Such an outcome may be defined as improved survival, improved quality of life, avoidance of ineffective or toxic treatment, and reduction in the cost of health care (3).

The serum tumor markers used today are far from ideal, because they have low sensitivity (especially in early tumor stages), unsatisfactory specificity, unrestricted organ-site expression, and an unreliable association with tumor volume changes. As a result, there are only rare clinical scenarios where tumor markers alone can impact management and prognosis. In most instances, they are used as adjuncts that are coupled with clinical assessment of the patient, tumor imaging, biopsy results, and molecular studies. The nature of tumor markers and their approved uses in oncology are summarily presented in this chapter.

Metastatic cancer of unknown primary site (CUP) comprises 3% to 5% of all new diagnoses of malignancy and ranks as the fourth to seventh most common cause of cancer-related death (4). The acronym CUP is used when metastases are present in the absence of an identifiable tumor primary site, despite a thorough, systematic diagnostic evaluation. The latter consists of history, physical examination, hemogram screening, biochemical tests, chest and abdominopelvic CT scans, pathological evaluation of biopsy material, and additional symptom- or sign-driven endoscopic and imaging studies. CUP is characterized by primary site tumor dormancy or regression, early systemic dissemination, resistance to therapy, and a poor prognosis (5). Recently, a minority of patients have been identified that belong to specific clinicopathologic CUP subsets with a more favorable prognosis (Table 1). The identification of either the primary tumor related to the CUP or the presence of a "good risk" CUP subset is believed to be clinically meaningful, because it will allow physicians to better define prognosis and administer tailored primary or CUP subset-dependent therapy. The available evidence and recommendations for the use of serum tumor markers in this setting are also considered in this chapter.

■ WIDELY USED TUMOR MARKERS AND APPROVED APPLICATIONS

The serum tumor markers most widely used in clinical practice today are carcinoembryonic antigen (CEA), CA19-9, CA15-3, CA-125, prostate-specific antigen (PSA), alpha-fetoprotein (AFP), and beta-human chorionic gonadotropin (HCG). These determinants, along with their approved and extant clinical uses, are shown in Table 2.

Carcinoembryonic Antigen

CEA was defined in 1965 as an antigen that is expressed in colonic adenocarcinoma and the fetal colon, but absent in healthy adults. It is a glycoprotein composed of one polypeptide chain of 641 amino acids, with a molecular weight of 150 to 300 KDa, depending on the extent of glycosylation. CEA is encoded by one gene in the CEA gene family of 29 genes, and its biological function is still unknown. New, highly specific CEA antibodies have demonstrated their expression in normal colonic epithelial cells, gastric mucous cells, prostatic epithelium, and squamous epithelial cells of the tongue, esophagus, and uterine cervix. In normal colonic epithelium, CEA is released from the apical surface of columnar cells into the gut lumen, whereas in the dysregulated cell growth of colon cancer, it is released into the bloodstream in greater amounts (6).

CEA monitoring is widely used in the surveillance of patients after curative surgical resection for colorectal adenocarcinoma. Serial CEA determination detects recurrent disease with 80% sensitivity and 70% specificity, providing a median lead-time of five months (3). Three meta-analyses have compared outcomes in patients with colon cancer who were followed intensively with serial CEA determinations every three months, versus controls who had only symptom-driven assessment (7–9). All of those publications showed a modest (9–20%) improvement in the five-year overall survival of patients in the first group; they had earlier detection of recurrences and a doubling of curative re-resections. Accordingly, recommendations issued by the American Society of Clinical Oncology (ASCO) and the European Group on Tumor Markers advise follow-up of patients with resected colon cancer who are eligible

Table 1 Clinicopathologic carcinoma of unknown primary site subsets	
Favorable Subsets	**Unfavorable Subsets**
Poorly differentiated carcinoma with midline distribution (extragonadal germ cell syndrome)	Adenocarcinoma metastatic to the liver or other organs
Women with papillary adenocarcinoma of peritoneal cavity	Nonpapillary malignant ascites (adenocarcinoma)
Women with adenocarcinoma involving only axillary lymph nodes	Multiple cerebral metastases (adeno or squamous carcinoma)
Squamous cell carcinoma involving cervical lymph nodes	Multiple lung/pleural metastases (adenocarcinoma)
Isolated inguinal adenopathy (squamous carcinoma)	Multiple metastatic bone (adenocarcinoma)
Poorly differentiated neuroendocrine carcinomas	
Men with blastic bone metastases and elevated prostate-specific antigen (adenocarcinoma)	
Patients with a single, small, potentially resectable tumor	

■ Table 2 Serum tumor markers and approved or widely applied clinical uses

Serum Tumor Marker	Use
CEA	Surveillance after resection of stage II and III colorectal cancer in patients suitable for liver resection Monitoring response to therapy of patients with advanced colorectal cancer
CA19-9	Monitoring response to antineoplastic therapy for patients with advanced pancreatic cancer, provided confirmation with imaging studies is sought in case of elevation
CA15-3	U.S. Food and Drug Administration–approved test for the follow-up of patients with resected breast cancer Monitoring treatment efficacy in patients with metastatic breast cancer in exceptional circumstances with disease difficult to evaluate, such as osseous metastases. When used in such a setting, the marker should be combined with clinical evaluation and imaging studies
CA-125	Screening of high-risk women in combination with pelvic ultrasound Monitoring response to therapy of patients with ovarian cancer Surveillance in ovarian cancer patients after completion of primary therapy
PSA	Screening average-risk men from the age of 50 yr and high-risk men from the age of 40 yr for prostate cancer Surveillance of prostate cancer patients after completion of primary therapy Monitoring disease course in patients with advanced prostate cancer receiving endocrine ablative therapies
HCG/AFP	Screening for hepatoma in high-risk groups, combined with liver ultrasound (AFP) Diagnosis, monitoring of response to treatment, and follow-up of patients with gestational trophoblastic neoplasia (HCG) Diagnosis, staging, monitoring of response to treatment, and follow-up of patients with germ cell tumors (HCG, AFP)

Abbreviations: AFP, alpha-fetoprotein; CEA, carcinoembryonic antigen; HCG, human chorionic gonadotropin; PSA, prostate-specific antigen.

for liver resection, using regular CEA determinations for at least two years postoperatively (10, 11). Serial CEA evaluation is also useful for monitoring the response to therapy of patients with metastatic colon carcinoma (12). CEA serum levels may also be elevated in patients with benign conditions such as proliferative breast disease, inflammatory bowel disease, cirrhosis, and chronic obstructive pulmonary disease. A wide variety of noncolonic solid epithelial tumors may synthesize this marker as well, negating its potentially organ-localizing application in CUP cases.

CEA is not recommended as a screening test. Moreover, the prognostic significance of its preoperative serum level is not strong enough to guide decisions regarding adjuvant systemic therapy (12, 13).

CA19-9

CA19-9 is a sialylated lactofucopentanose oligosaccharide that is related to the Lewis-A blood group antigen. It is present in cell-surface mucins in normal and neoplastic epithelia of the pancreas, colon, stomach, bile ducts, liver,

and esophagus (14). CA19-9 was initially defined as the target of the 1116-NS19-9 antibody, which was produced by inoculating BALB/c mice with a human colorectal carcinoma cell line (15). Although a regulatory role in cell adhesion, apoptosis, immune surveillance, and signal transduction has been proposed for mucins related to CA19-9 (heavily glycosylated proteins), its precise biological function is not known.

The use of CA19-9 is not recommended for diagnosis, follow-up, or monitoring of treatment response for patients with colorectal cancer. Serum CA19-9 levels are elevated in association with many other gastrointestinal tract tumors—especially exocrine carcinomas of the pancreas—as well as ovarian carcinomas and hepatocellular carcinomas, militating against its effectiveness in defining a specific primary site in CUP cases.

Benign conditions such as hepatobiliary disorders, pancreatitis, inflammatory bowel disease, diverticulitis, diabetes mellitus, and cystic fibrosis may also increase blood levels of CA19-9 (14). This marker also cannot be used in isolation for screening, diagnosis, or monitoring of patients with pancreatic cancer. ASCO states that serial determination of serum CA19-9 values may be employed for monitoring response to antineoplastic therapy for advanced pancreatic carcinoma, provided that confirmation of disease status is sought with imaging studies in cases showing an elevation (12).

CA15-3

CA15-3 is a breast-associated antigen defined by reactivity to two monoclonal antibodies, DF3 and 115D8, which were raised against a membrane-enriched fraction of a human breast carcinoma and human milk-fat globule membranes respectively (16). The CA15-3 epitope is a glycopeptide sequence on MUC1 mucin, a 250 to 1000 KDa transmembrane glycoprotein consisting of a large extracellular domain, a membrane-spanning domain (31 amino acids), and a cytoplasmic tail (69 amino acids). MUC1 is present in the apical surface of normal ductal breast epithelium, uterine endometrium, and gastrointestinal tract epithelium, and is glycosylated to varying extents. In malignant tumor tissue, the mucin is overexpressed as well as aberrantly glycosylated, and loses its apical polarity (16, 17).

Serum CA15-3 levels are used for monitoring patients with early or advanced breast adenocarcinoma in many medical centers worldwide. An ASCO panel recently found that 67% of 352 breast cancer patients with elevated CA15-3 values had confirmed tumor relapses. Only 8% of 1320 patients who were free of recurrence had serum CA15-3 elevations by immunoassay (10). Still, CA15-3 elevation mainly occurs in the setting of metastatic disease that is incurable, blunting its utility as a guide to early and effective therapy for recurrence. High CA15-3 values are also seen in association with benign breast diseases, hepatic disorders, endometriosis, autoimmune conditions, drug or cytokine administration, and infections. Moreover, serum CA15-3 elevations have been linked to other solid tumors apart from breast carcinoma. Therefore, it is not satisfactory as a directive marker in patients with CUP.

Because early treatment of asymptomatic individuals with relapsed breast cancer does not enhance outcome, ASCO and German "expert" panels were unable to recommend the routine use of CA15-3 in the surveillance of patients with resected breast cancer. Nonetheless, the U.S. Food and Drug Administration did approve this application of CA15-3, as well as the related marker BR 27.29 (16, 18). Data from 11 studies showed a good correlation between changes in serum CA15-3 concentrations and the response to therapy of patients with advanced breast cancer. Thus, ASCO has stated that the marker can be used for monitoring treatment efficacy in selected patients with metastatic breast cancer, such as those with osseous involvement (10). When used in such a

setting, CA15-3 cannot be used alone to define response to treatment, and additional information must always be obtained from clinical evaluation and imaging studies.

CA-125

CA-125 was initially defined by the OC125 monoclonal antibody, obtained through immunization of BALB/c mice with the ovarian serous adenocarcinoma cell line OVCA433 (19). CA-125 is a 40 KDa proteolytic fragment of the MUC16 transmembrane glycoprotein, characterized by an N-terminal region of nine sequences of 156 amino acids repeated in tandem, and a C-terminal region containing a membrane-spanning domain and a cytoplasmic tail (20). MUC16 is present in the coelomic epithelium of the ovary, peritoneum, pericardium, and pleura. It is overexpressed in serous papillary carcinoma, and, to a lesser extent, in mucinous adenocarcinoma of the ovary (21).

CA-125 levels are also elevated in benign conditions such as ovarian cysts, endometriosis, uterine leiomyomas, serosal inflammatory disorders such as peritonitis, pericarditis, and pleuritis, serosal bleeding; and pregnancy (22). Moreover, CA-125 is potentially synthesized by carcinomas of the pancreas, bile ducts, breast, lung, thyroid, distal esophagus and stomach, and liver, as well as by mesotheliomas (22, 24). This characteristic interferes with the use of this marker in attempts at primary tumor localization in examples of CUP.

Serum CA-125 testing has a relatively low sensitivity and specificity as a screen in healthy women for ovarian cancer (25). Screening of high-risk women by means of serial serum CA-125 determinations and ultrasound yields false-positive findings in 1% to 4% of cases. The latter should be considered as an experimental strategy that is still under study (25). Several trials reported that serum CA-125 concentrations show concordance with the clinical course of advanced ovarian carcinoma (22). It is now accepted that CA-125 is an accurate, convenient, and relatively cheap method for assessing response to treatment in patients with that tumor. Following surgery and initial chemotherapy, many ovarian cancer patients are monitored with serial determinations of serum CA-125 levels, based on the assumption that early administration of salvage chemotherapy could improve survival. The lead time between CA-125 elevations and clinical progression varies from 1 to 15 months, though it is not known if this fact has an impact on patient outcome or quality of life in a beneficial way (22). Until results of ongoing randomized studies become available, there is no established role for monitoring asymptomatic patients with serum CA-125 after completion of primary therapy for ovarian carcinoma (27). Once relapse occurs, serum measurements of this marker can again be used for monitoring the disease course.

Prostate-Specific Antigen

PSA belongs to the family of kallikrein proteases. It is a 30 KDa macromolecule synthesized primarily, but not exclusively, by prostatic epithelial cells. PSA is bound in serum by the endogenous protease inhibitors alpha-1-antichymotrypsin and alpha-2-microglobulin.

Although an elevated serum PSA level is potentially associated with benign prostatic hyperplasia, prostatic ischemia, prostatic intraepithelial neoplasia, and prostatitis it is currently the best available noninvasive test for prostate carcinoma screening and early diagnosis (28). Serum PSA testing at a cutoff point of 4 µg/L has a sensitivity of 71%, a specificity of 35% to 75%, a false-positive rate of 25% to 65%, and a false-negative rate of 20% to 30% (3, 29). PSA screening detects prostatic carcinomas at a median of five years in advance of clinical presentation, with the vast majority being organ confined. Nonetheless, it is not known whether earlier diagnosis and therapy enhances patient outcome. Two large prospective trials comparing survival in screened and control patient groups are currently underway in Europe and the United States (30). Despite the lack of evidence, American and European observers have recommended annual digital rectal examination and serum PSA testing in all men over 50 years of age (31, 32).

In addition to screening, serum PSA testing is widely used in clinical practice for staging and monitoring the clinical course of patients with known prostate cancer. Serum PSA has an independent predictive value vis-à-vis pathological stage as well as locoregional invasion and prognosis (33). PSA testing is useful for monitoring patients after completion of primary therapy and those with advanced disease on endocrine ablative therapies.

With respect to localizing a primary site in CUP cases, PSA is an effective and specific marker, with only a few exceptions (33a). The extraprostatic spread of prostate cancer is typically associated with marked elevations in the serum PSA level. This fact, together with the selectivity of this marker for prostatic epithelial differentiation, gives it considerable value with regard to predicting the source of metastases of unknown anatomic origin.

AFP and β-HCG

AFP and HCG are produced by trophoblastic or yolk-sac elements in germ cell tumors. These include choriocarcinoma (HCG), selected examples of seminoma (HCG), and yolk-sac tumor and polyembryoma (AFP). Regenerating or neoplastic liver cells also may synthesize AFP, and a host of somatic malignancies—including gastric carcinoma, lung cancer, and bladder carcinoma, among others (34, 35)—may show divergent germinal differentiation with corresponding synthesis of *either* AFP or HCG. As expected, this variability of tumor types may interfere with the use of AFP and HCG in CUP cases to locate a primary lesion. Nevertheless, it should be understood that their ectopic production by nongestational, nongerminal tumors is relatively rare.

HCG is a 45 KDa α/β heterodimeric glycoprotein hormone that is exclusively produced by trophoblastic cells of the placenta under normal circumstances (36). AFP is a 70 KDa, single, glycosylated polypeptide chain that is synthesized in the fetal liver, but only in low amounts during adult life (37). Several functions have been proposed for both molecules, including regulation of cellular growth, differentiation, adhesion, angiogenesis, immune function, and ligand transport.

These two biological molecules possess some of the characteristics that approximate those of ideal tumor markers. They are elevated in the serum of 80% to 100% of patients with gestational choriocarcinoma and metastatic nonseminomatous germ cell tumors (NSGCT) and are quite selective for those tumors. Serum concentrations of AFP and HCG reflect changes in the tumor burden and may be used to judge the efficacy of antineoplastic therapy. Moreover, their baseline serum levels provide useful staging and prognostic information for gestational trophoblastic neoplasms and NSGCT (2, 3).

Serum HCG testing is pivotal for the diagnosis of gestational trophoblastic neoplasia, risk classification, monitoring of treatment, and ongoing surveillance of patients after completion of therapy (38). Pretreatment serum AFP and HCG concentrations are independent prognostic factors for patients with NSGCT and were the first tumor markers to be incorporated into the AJCC/UICC staging system for those lesions (39, 40). In addition to their prognostic and monitoring functions, serial determinations of AFP/HCG are mandatory in the long-term evaluation of NSGCT patients who are believed to be cured (41). In this setting, rising marker concentrations, even in the absence of radiological or clinical evidence of disease, would suffice to reinitiate treatment.

In accordance with information presented earlier, other clinical entities must be excluded that may cause modest, spurious, or temporary elevation of serum HCG/AFP concentrations (hepatitis, cirrhosis, pregnancy, cannabis use, hepatocellular carcinoma, and other solid tumors) before concluding that a trophoblastic or germ cell tumor is present. In the majority of circumstances, appropriate physical examination, evaluation of patient demographics, and the evolution of serum-marker concentrations can distinguish nongerminal tumors from germ cell neoplasms.

Serum AFP testing is also used in conjunction with ultrasound imaging in screening high-risk patients with cirrhosis for hepatocellular carcinoma. However, no consensus exists regarding survival benefits that might be associated with this strategy (42).

■ TUMOR-MARKER EXPRESSION IN CUP

CUP cases represent a heterogeneous group of malignancies, with the common denominator of early systemic dissemination, quite often involving uncommon organ sites, in the absence of a definable primary tumor. Several hypotheses have been proposed to explain the peculiar natural history of CUP. All of them postulate the emergence of a metastasis-capable clone of malignant cells that can spread distantly and proliferate at secondary sites. At the same time, the primary tumor fails to grow, either as a result of intrinsic biochemical defects or suppressive effects of the local microenviromment. A lack of angiogenetic effectors or cell survival–growth transducers, as well as the impact of proapoptotic and metastasis-growth suppressing proteins in the milieu of the primary tumor, have been proposed as mechanisms responsible for its dormancy (43, 44). To date, no preclinical evidence has been generated to confirm or refute these hypotheses. Debate over the true nature of CUPs still revolves around the basic question of whether they simply reflect metastases from missed primary neoplasms—in which case it would represent an artificial grouping of metastatic tumors—or are they truly separate clinical entities with distinct genetic and epigenetic aberrations, characterized by a CUP-specific molecular signature? If the latter scenario proves to be true, the multigene molecular signature of a CUP would differ in regard to several key genes from that of the primary tumor (45).

As described earlier, the commonly used tumor markers for carcinomas are glycoproteins that are relatively overexpressed in malignant cells compared with their normal epithelial counterparts, with aberrant glycosylation and architectural distribution. They are released into the blood in greater amounts than normal tissues would yield. It is crucial to emphasize that these markers are not tumor *specific* (i.e., present in malignant tissues only), but are instead tumor *associated* (relatively overexpressed in cancers). Moreover, their overexpression is not restricted to a specific tumor type, but quite commonly spans a range of solid tumor sites and histological categories. Coexpression and release into the blood of more than one tumor marker is not rare in clinical practice, in reference to cancers of the breast, ovary, lung, kidney, and gastrointestinal tract (1, 3, 46).

Unfortunately, this experience with known primary tumors does not offer much help in locating a "missing" primary malignancy for reasons implicit in the foregoing discussion. Still, this is a highly desirable goal, because knowledge of the primary tumor would enable oncologists to furnish more accurate information concerning prognosis, and to choose specific primary site–dependent antineoplastic therapies. Even though it can be argued that such treatments are unlikely to alter the prognosis

substantially in the setting of widespread metastases, such knowledge would at least allow for classification of patients with CUP into favorable or high-risk clinicopathologic groups. Finally, the diagnosis of metastases of a CUP seems to generate considerable anxiety and uncertainty in both the physician and the patient regarding proper treatment and prognosis. These feelings are seemingly even more marked than those pertaining to metastasis of a *known* primary tumor, probably because of the compounded uncertainty in CUP cases.

Koch and McPherson reviewed 542 patients with metastatic tumors of known anatomic origin and reported that elevated serum CEA levels >10 ng/mL were most often associated with tumors from endodermally derived organs (i.e., gastrointestinal tract and lung), as well as the breasts, endometrium, uterine cervix, and ovaries (47). The authors then attempted to validate these observations in a cohort of 32 patients with metastases from unknown primary sites. They concluded that normal or moderately elevated plasma CEA levels (0–10 ng/mL) were not useful, because they could be seen in association with many tumor types. However, CEA plasma levels >10 ng/mL were felt to indicate that the primary lesion was in an endodermally derived organ, or the breast or ovary, thus narrowing the search for the "parent" tumor.

These preliminary data (from 1981) were not confirmed by other investigators. In another series of 147 CUP patients from the M.D. Anderson Cancer Center, reported by Varadhachary et al., 41 patients had CEA values >10 ng/mL (48). At that cutoff level, the marker concentration did not help to establish a primary site. Similarly, in a study by Fritsche, 41 patients with CUP had serum CEA values >10 ng/mL, and primary localization was not aided by the marker in that group either (49). Gupta et al. measured serum CEA and CA19-9 concentrations in patients with different malignancies, 15 of whom had liver metastases of tumors in unknown primary sites (50). CEA was elevated in 40% and CA19-9 in 27% of these patients, but there was no correlation of the markers to other specific clinicopathologic findings. It is possible that metastatic dissemination, with involvement of several organs and tissues, resulted in nonspecific overexpression of CEA and CA19-9.

Our group retrospectively evaluated six tumor markers (CEA, CA19-9, CA-125, CA15-3, β-HCG, and AFP) in 85 patients with CUP. We attempted to relate serum levels with histological features of the tumors, metastatic sites, responses to therapy, and outcome (51). More than 40% of the patients had increased serum levels of all six markers except for AFP, which was elevated in only 17% of cases. Patients with liver involvement had higher mean levels of CEA and CA19-9, as compared to those with only lymph nodal disease. High serum CA19-9 and CA15-3 concentrations showed a relationship with advanced disease. None of the markers had any predictive value for response to treatment, nor were they prognostic. We concluded that patients with CUP have a nonspecific overexpression of the specified markers, and that the routine use of these analytes does not provide any diagnostic or prognostic assistance.

Milovic et al. assessed serum concentrations of CEA, CA19-9, CA15-3, and CA-125 in 46 patients with CUP. They looked for relationships with histological findings, metastatic sites, treatment efficacy, and outcome (52). Thirty-three patients had increased serum levels of at least one marker. There was no correlation of marker values with histological tumor type, metastatic pattern, treatment response, or outcome. The authors similarly concluded that the serum tumor markers in question had little value in CUP cases.

Yonemori et al. evaluated the usefulness of tumor-marker measurements and searched for prognostic factors in 93 CUP patients who received platinum-based combination chemotherapy (53). Ninety-one of them manifested at least one abnormal serum tumor-marker concentration, with a median number of elevated markers of 5. The proportion of patients with elevated values of CEA, CA19-9, CA15-3, and CA-125 (women only) were 44%, 39%, 28%, and 64% respectively. High serum PSA (men only), β-HCG, and AFP levels were seen in 8%, 55%, and 5% of cases, respectively. The performance status, number of involved organs, and elevated serum lactate dehydrogenase (LDH) levels were the only independent prognostic factors for outcome in multivariate statistical analysis. The authors concluded that routine tumor-marker measurements were ineffective in identifying a primary tumor site. Moreover, they were not capable of predicting response to platinum-based therapy or prognosticating the survival of patients with CUP. Published clinical experience regarding serum tumor-marker use in CUP is summarized in Table 3.

■ TUMOR-MARKER USES AND ABUSES IN CASES OF CUP

Cumulative evidence supports the contention that routine measurement of CEA, CA19-9, CA15-3, and CA-125 in all patients with CUP is unsupportable as a standard practice. Loi et al. performed a cross-sectional, retrospective study of tumor-marker use in a tertiary hospital over a three-month period (54). Among 476 marker tests that were ordered, only 0.8% had any diagnostic value. Among the 106 assays with abnormal results, 45% were useful for monitoring the growth of a preexisting cancer, but only 1.9% served to localize a primary site in CUP cases. The latter group principally concerned AFP and hepatocellular carcinoma. In addition, not only do CEA and CA19-9 show poor organ specificity, but the tumors likely to be associated with those markers are, for the moment, largely resistant to available systemic therapies.

On the other hand, the potential clinical utility of serum AFP, HCG, and PSA, or that of CA15-3 and CA-125 in selected patients, is less straightforward. Although most patients with CUP will succumb to their tumors in less than one year after diagnosis, it is crucial for physicians not to miss treatable CUP subsets (4, 5). Patients with poorly differentiated carcinomas that mainly involve lymph node groups with a midline distribution may have extragonadal germ cell tumors (EGCTs). Women with disseminated papillary serous adenocarcinoma of the peritoneal cavity can have either metastatic ovarian tumors or primary peritoneal serous carcinomas. Men presenting with blastic osseous metastases likely have prostate cancer with a missed or regressed primary tumor. Finally, women with isolated axillary lymphadenopathy may harbor an occult breast carcinoma on the ipsilateral side. Patients with these clinical complexes should be treated with therapies that are tailored to the corresponding primary tumors. These include platinum-based combination chemotherapy for patients with likely EGCTs, surgical debulking and platinum–taxane regimens for papillary serous peritoneal adenocarcinomas, nodal dissection with chemotherapy and breast irradiation or surgery for women with isolated axillary adenopathy, and, finally, endocrine-ablative therapy for men with blastic bony implants of prostatic carcinoma.

A proportion of these patients will enjoy long-term disease remission after appropriate treatment. Luckily, EGCTs and occult prostatic tumors often produce relatively specific tumor markers at concentrations that are easily detectable in the serum. Accordingly, testing for those analytes increases the identification of patients with treatable CUP subsets.

Keeping in mind that the most important aim is to avoid missing a treatable malignancy, and given the restrictive nature of selected serum markers at primary sites, all male patients with CUP should have a basic panel of AFP, HCG, and PSA. The European Society of Medical Oncology has recommended this strategy in its Minimum Clinical Recommendations (55). Even though the rate of detection may be low, this practice will ensure that most men with a treatable occult malignancy are identified.

In view of the nonspecific overexpression of mucins by malignant epithelial cells, the authors do not advocate the routine measurement of serum CA15-3 and CA-125 in all female patients with CUP. These tests should be obtained in selected cases with a clinical picture that is compatible with breast or ovarian cancer. These include

■ **Table 3** Published clinical experience on use of serum tumor markers in CUP

Authors (Ref.)	Number of CUP Patients (n)	Markers Studied	Diagnostic Utility	Predictive/ Prognostic Utility
Koch and McPherson (47)	32	CEA	Yes	No
Varadhachary et al. (48)	147	CEA	No	No
Fritsche (49)	41	CEA	No	No
Gupta et al. (50)	15	CEA, CA19-9	No	No
Pavlidis et al. (51)	85	CEA, CA19-9, CA-125; CA15-3, β-HCG, AFP	No	No
Milovic et al. (52)	46	CEA, CA19-9; CA15-3, CA-125	No	No
Yonemori et al. (53)	93	CEA, CA19-9; CA15-3, CA-125; PSA, AFP, β-HCG	No	No

Abbreviations: CUP, carcinoma of unknown primary site; CEA, carcinoembryonic antigen; HCG, human chorionic gonadotropin; AFP, alpha-fetoprotein; PSA, prostate-specific antigen.

isolated involvement of axillary lymph nodes (occult breast cancer) and peritoneal deposits or involvement of pelvic and retroperitoneal lymph nodes by serous papillary or undifferentiated carcinomas (occult ovarian or primary peritoneal cancers) (56). In these circumstances, elevated serum concentrations of CA15-3 or CA-125 strengthen the case for a treatable CUP subset and guide therapy.

It is important to remember that elevation of these tumor markers alone is neither necessary nor adequate for the diagnosis of a treatable CUP subset or for reliable prognostication. Curow et al. reported 15 patients with midline nodal carcinoma who had elevated serum AFP or HCG. Only two responses to platinum-based chemotherapy were achieved in that group (57). The median survival of all patients, excluding one long-term survivor, was only 4.5 months. On the other hand, Motzer et al. reported a 75% response rate to platinum-based chemotherapy and prolonged survival among 12 CUP patients who had *no* serum AFP/HCG elevation but harbored malignancies with the isochromosome 12p (a cytogenetic marker of germ cell tumors) (58). A thorough, conjoint evaluation of marker levels with patient characteristics, clinical presentations, histological findings, adjunctive pathological studies, and results of imaging tests is mandatory in CUP cases.

■ **CONCLUSIONS AND FUTURE OPTIONS**

Metastatic carcinomas from unknown primary sites commonly overexpress several tumor markers in a non-specific fashion. Accordingly, routine serum marker testing does not furnish much useful diagnostic, predictive, or prognostic information. Serum AFP, HCG, and PSA analysis is a notable exception to this rule, because their systematic measurement will ensure that the majority of patients with treatable CUP subsets (EGCTs and occult prostatic cancers) are identified. Serum CA15-3 and CA-125 levels may be determined in selected patients whose clinical presentations suggest an occult breast carcinoma or ovarian–peritoneal tumors of Mullerian type. Those are likewise treatable CUP subsets (Table 4).

High-throughput multigene expression or multiprotein profiling with oligonucleotide or tissue protein microarrays offer promise for the identification of the primary tumor site in CUP cases, relying on tissue-specific genetic signatures. These techniques are discussed in detail in Chapter 8. Dennis et al. used 15 publicly available SAGE data libraries and performed hierarchical clustering to demonstrate that common metastatic adenocarcinomas clustered according to their site of origin (59). Su et al. employed oligonucleotide arrays to determine the expression of 12,533 genes from 11 tumor types, in a sample of 100 primary tumors

Table 4 Suggested use of tumor markers in CUP

Serum Tumor Marker	Use in CUP
Alpha-fetoprotein, human chorionic gonadotropin	Testing in all patients
Prostate-specific antigen	Testing in all men
CA-125	Testing in women with ascites/peritoneal deposits and/or inguinal nodes involved by papillary serous or poorly differentiated adenocarcinoma
CA15-3	Testing in women with axillary node involvement by adenocarcinoma
Carcinoembryonic antigen, CA19-9	Testing not recommended

Abbreviation: CUP, carcinoma of unknown primary site.

(60). A set of 110 genes (10 per tumor type), which were differentially expressed according to anatomical site, succeeded in accurately classifying a validation set of 75 tumors according to tissue and organ site of origin in 75% to 87% of cases. Bloom et al. used both oligonucleotide and spotted cDNA microarrays to profile 78 adenocarcinomas from seven common anatomic sites (61). A set of 400 genes was required for 50 metastatic tumors with known primaries to be classified according to their sites of origin with 84% accuracy. Ma et al. and Talantov et al. recently used data from gene microarrays to devise 92-gene and 10-gene real-time polymerase chain reaction assays that classified tumor validation sets as to their primary sites with accuracies of 87% and 78% (62, 63). Tothill et al. used a single cDNA microarray platform and profiled 229 primary and metastatic tumors, representing 14 tumor types, with 89% accuracy in training and validation sets (64). Use of the microarray was successful in 11 of 13 CUP cases in predicting the probable anatomic site of origin. Dennis et al. assessed the expression of 27 proteins in 352 primary adenocarcinomas from seven sites (65). A simplified diagnostic panel of 10 peptides and a decision tree were devised in that study, which were able to correctly classify 88% of primary and metastatic tumors in an independent validation set.

All of these multigene or multiprotein profiling studies have attempted to classify the genetic pattern of tumors according to their primary sites. However, none has examined the potential presence of a CUP-specific primary site–independent genetic signature. Whether such a signature does indeed exist remains to be seen. Hopefully, the cited technological platforms will provide tools for screening the expression of genes and their proteins to guide therapies tailored to the genotype of each CUP, rather than relying on comparatively nonspecific expressions of a few circulating tumor markers.

■ REFERENCES

1. Canil CM, Tannock IF. Doctor's dilemma: incorporating tumor markers into clinical decision-making. *Semin Oncol* 2002; 29: 286–93.
2. Bigbee W, Herberman RB. Tumor markers and immunodiagnosis. In: Kufe DW, Pollock RE, Weichselbaum RR, et al., eds. *Cancer Medicine*, 6th ed. Hamilton, London: BC Decker, 2003:209–20.
3. Duffy MJ. Evidence for the clinical use of tumor markers. *Ann Clin Biochem* 2004; 41:370–7.
4. Pavlidis N, Fizazi K. Cancer of unknown primary (CUP). *Crit Rev Oncol Hematol* 2005; 54:243–50.
5. Pentheroudakis G, Briasoulis E, Karavasilis V, et al. Chemotherapy for patients with two favourable subsets of unknown primary carcinoma: active, but how effective? *Acta Oncol* 2005; 44:155–60.
6. Hammarstrom S. The carcinoembryonic antigen (CEA) family. Structures, suggested functions and expression in normal and malignant tissues. *Cancer Bio* 1999; 9:67–81.
7. Bruinvels DJ, Stiggelbout AM, Kievit J, et al. Follow up of colorectal cancer: a meta-analysis. *Ann Surg* 1994; 219:174–82.
8. Rosen M, Chan L, Beart RW, Vukasin P, Anthone G. Follow up of colorectal cancer: a meta-analysis. *Dis Colon Rectum* 1998; 41:1116–26.
9. Renehan AG, Egger M, Saunders MP, O'Dwyer ST. Impact on survival of intensive follow up after curative resection for colorectal cancer: systematic review and meta-analysis of randomised trials. *BMJ* 2002; 324:813–6.
10. Anonymous. Clinical practice guidelines for use of tumor markers in breast and colorectal cancer. *J Clin Oncol* 1996; 14:2843–77.
11. Duffy MJ, van Dalen A, Haglund C. Clinical utility of biochemical markers in colorectal cancer: European Group on Tumor Markers (EGTM) guidelines. *Eur J Cancer* 2003; 39: 718–27.
12. Locker GY, Hamilton S, Harris J, et al. ASCO 2006 update of recommendations for the use of tumor markers in gastrointestinal cancer. *J Clin Oncol* 2006; 24:5313–27.
13. Fletcher RH. Carcinoembryonic antigen. *Ann Intern Med* 1996; 104:66–73.
14. Duffy MJ. CA 19-9 as a marker for gastrointestinal cancers: a review. *Ann Clin Biochem* 1998; 35:364–70.
15. Koprowski H, Steplewski Z, Mitchell K, et al. Colorectal carcinoma antigens detected by hybridoma antibodies. *Somatic Cell Genet* 1979; 5:957–72.
16. Duffy MJ. CA 15-3 and related mucins as circulating markers in breast cancer. *Ann Clin Biochem* 1999; 36:579–86.
17. Gendler SJ, Spicer AP. Epithelial mucin genes. *Ann Rev Physiol* 1995; 57:607–34.
18. Bast RC, Ravdin P, Hayes DF, et al. 2000 Update of recommendations for the use of tumor markers in breast and colorectal: clinical practice guidelines of the American Society of Clinical Oncology. *J Clin Oncol* 2001; 19:1865–78.

19. Bast RC, Freeney M, Lazarus H, et al. Reactivity of a monoclonal antibody with human ovarian carcinoma. *J Clin Invest* 1981; 68: 1331–7.

20. Yin BW, Dnistrian A, Lloyd KO. Ovarian cancer antigen CA 125 is encoded by the MUC16 mucin gene. *Int J Cancer* 2002; 98:737–40.

21. Kabawat SE, Bast RC, Bhan AK, et al. Tissue distribution of a coelomic epithelium related antigen recognised by the monoclonal antibody OC125. *Int J Gynecol Pathol* 1983; 2:275–85.

22. Tuxen MK, Soletormos G, Dombernowsky P. Tumor markers in the management of patients with ovarian cancer. *Cancer Treat Rev* 1995; 21:215–43.

23. Loy TS, Quesenberry JT, Sharp SC. Distribution of CA-125 in adenocarcinomas: an immunohistochemical study of 481 cases. *Am J Clin Pathol* 1992; 98:175–9.

24. Bollinger DJ, Wick, MR, Dehner LP, et al. Peritoneal malignant mesothelioma versus serous papillary adenocarcinoma: a histochemical and immunohistochemical comparison. *Am J Surg Pathol* 1989; 13:659–70.

25. Jacobs IJ, Skates SJ, MacDonald N, et al. Screening for ovarian cancer: a pilot randomised controlled trial. *Lancet* 1999; 353: 1207–10.

26. National Institutes of Health Consensus Development Conference Statement. Ovarian cancer: screening, treatment, and follow up. *Gynecol Oncol* 1994; 55:S4–14.

27. Guppy AE, Rustin GJS. CA 125 response: can it replace the traditional response criteria in ovarian cancer. *Oncologist* 2002; 7:437–43.

28. Polascik TJ, Oesterling JE, Partin AW. Prostate specific antigen. A decade of discovery—what we have learned and where are we going. *J Urol* 1999; 162:293–306.

29. Neal DE, Leung HY, Powell PH, et al. Unanswered questions in screening for prostate cancer. *Eur J Cancer* 2000; 36:1316–21.

30. De Koning HJ, Auvinen A, Berenguer Sanchez A, et al. Large scale randomised prostate cancer screening trials: program performances in the European randomised screening for prostate cancer trial and the prostate, lung, colorectal and ovary cancer trial. *Int J Cancer* 2002; 97:237–44.

31. Von Eschenbach A, Ho R, Murphy GP, Cunningham M, Lins N. American Cancer Society guideline for the early detection of prostate cancer, update 1997. *CA Cancer J Clin* 1997; 47:261–4.

32. Semjonow A, Albrecht W, Bialk P, et al. Tumor markers in prostate cancer: EGTM recommendations. *Anticancer Res* 1999; 19:2785–820.

33. Partin AW, Yoo J, Carter HB, et al. The use of prostate specific antigen, clinical stage and Gleason score to predict pathological stage in men with localised prostate cancer. *J Urol* 1993; 150: 110–4.

33a. Leibovici D, Spiess PE, Agarwal PK, et al. Prostate cancer progression in the presence of undetectable or low serum prostate-specific antigen levels. *Cancer* 2007; 109:198–204.

34. Iles RK. Ectopic hCG-beta expression by epithelial cancer: malignant behavior, metastasis, and inhibition of tumor cell apoptosis. *Mol Cell Endocrinol* 2007; 1:260–70.

35. Crawford SM, Lederman JA, Turkle W, et al. Is ectopic production of human chorionic gonadotrophin (hCG) or alpha-fetoprotein (AFP) by tumors a marker of chemosensitivity? *Eur J Cancer Clin Oncol* 1986; 22:1483–7.

36. Alfthan H, Stenman UH. Pathophysiological importance of various molecular forms of human choriogonadotropin. *Mol Cell Endocrinol* 1996; 125:107–20.

37. Mizejewski GJ. Apha-fetoprotein structure and function: relevance to isoforms, epitopes and conformational variants. *Exp Biol Med* 2001; 226:377–408.

38. Fisher PM, Hancock BW. Gestational trophoblastic disease and their treatment. *Cancer Treat Rev* 1997; 23:1–16.

39. Green FL, Page DL, Fleming ID, et al. *AJCC Cancer Staging Manual*, 6th ed. New York: Springler-Verlag, 2000.

40. International Germ Cell Cancer Collaborative Group. International Germ Cell Consensus Classification: a prognostic factor-based staging system for metastatic germ cell cancers. *J Clin Oncol* 1997; 15:594–603.

41. Sturgeon C. Practical guidelines for tumor marker use in the clinic. *Clin Chem* 2002; 48:1151–9.

42. Yuen MF, Cheng CC, Lauder IJ, et al. Early detection of hepatocellular carcinoma increases the chance of treatment: Hong Kong experience. *Hepatology* 2000; 31:330–5.

43. Naresh KN. Do metastatic tumors from an unknown primary reflect angiogenic incompetence of the tumor at the primary site?—A hypothesis. *Med Hypotheses* 2002; 59:357–60.

44. Van de Wouw AJ, Jansen RLH, Speel EJM, Hillen HFP. The unknown biology of the unknown primary tumor: a literature review. *Ann Oncol* 2003; 14:191–6.

45. Pentheroudakis G, Pavlidis N. Cancer of unknown primary site: missing primary or missing biology? *The Oncologist* 2007; 12:418–25.

46. Perkins GL, Slater ED, Sanders GK, Prichard JG. Serum tumor markers. *Am Fam Physician* 2003; 68:1075–82.

47. Koch M, McPherson TA. CEA levels as an indicator of the primary site in metastatic disease of unknown origin. *Cancer* 1981; 48:1242–4.

48. Varadhachary GR, Abbruzzese JL, Lenzi R. Diagnostic strategies for unknown primary cancer. *Cancer* 2004; 100:1776–85.

49. Fritsche HA. Serum tumor markers for patient monitoring: a case-oriented approach illustrated with carcinoembryonic antigen. *Clin Chem* 1993; 39:2431–4.

50. Gupta MK, Arciaga R, Bosci L, et al. Measurement of a monoclonal antibody defined antigen (CA 19-9) in the sera of patients with malignant and non-malignant diseases. Comparison with carcinoembryonic antigen. *Cancer* 1985; 15:277–83.

51. Pavlidis N, Kalef-Ezra J, Briasoulis E, et al. Evaluation of six tumor markers in patients with carcinoma of unknown primary. *Med Pediatr Oncol* 1994; 22:162–7.

52. Milovic M, Popov I, Jelic S. Tumor markers in metastatic disease from cancer of unknown primary origin. *Med Sci Monit* 2002; 8: MT25–MT30.

53. Yonemori K, Ando M, Shibata T, et al. Tumor-marker analysis and verification of prognostic models in patients with cancer of unknown primary, receiving platinum-based combination chemotherapy. *J Cancer Res Clin Oncol* 2006, Springer-Verlag, DOI 10.1007/s00432-006-0110-z.

54. Loi S, Haydon AMM, Shapiro J, Schwarz MA, Schneider HG. Towards evidence-based use of serum tumor marker requests: an audit of use in a tertiary hospital. *Intern Med J* 2004; 34: 545–50.

55. Briasoulis E, Tolis C, Bergh J, Pavlidis N. ESMO Guideline Task Force. ESMO Minimum Clinical Recommendations for diagnosis, treatment and follow-up of cancers of unknown primary site (CUP). *Ann Oncol* 2005; 16(Suppl. 1):i75-i76.

56. Greco FA, Hainsworth JD. Cancer of unknown primary site. In: DeVita VT Jr, Hellman S, Rosenberg SA, et al., eds. *Cancer, Principles and Practice of Oncology*, 6th ed. Philadelphia: Lippincott William and Wilkins, 2001:2537–60.

57. Curow DC, Findlay M, Cox K, Harnett PR. Elevated germ cell markers in carcinoma of uncertain primary site do not predict response to platinum based chemotherapy. *Eur J Cancer* 1996; 32A:2357–9.

58. Motzer RJ, Rodriguez E, Reuter VE, et al. Molecular and cytogenetic studies in the diagnosis of patients with poorly differentiated carcinomas of unknown primary site. *J Clin Oncol* 1995; 13:274–82.

59. Dennis JL, Vass K, Wit EC, Keith N, Oien KA. Identification from public data of molecular markers of adenocarcinoma characteristic of the site of origin. *Cancer Res* 2002; 62:5999–6005.

60. Su AI, Welsh JB, Sapinoso LM, et al. Molecular classification of human carcinomas by use of gene expression signatures. *Cancer Res* 2001; 61:7388–93.

61. Bloom G, Yang IV, Boulware D, et al. Multi-platform, multi-site, microarray-based human tumor classification. *Am J Pathol* 2004; 164:9–16.

62. Ma XJ, Patel R, Wang X, et al. Molecular classification of human cancers using a 92-gene real-time quantitative polymerase chain reaction assay. *Arch Pathol Lab Med* 2006; 130:465–73.

63. Talantov D, Baden J, Jatkoe T, et al. A quantitative reverse transcriptase-polymerase chain reaction assay to identify metastatic carcinoma tissue of origin. *J Mol Diagn* 2006; 8:320–9.

64. Tothill RW, Kowalczyk A, Rischin D, et al. An expression-based site of origin diagnostic method designed for clinical application to cancer of unknown origin. *Cancer Res* 2005; 65:4031–40.

65. Dennis JL, Hvidsten TR, Wit EC, et al. Markers of adenocarcinoma characteristic of the site of origin: development of a diagnostic algorithm. *Clin Cancer Res* 2005; 11:3766–72.

7 Tissue Microarrays and Gene Chips

JEFFREY S. ROSS

ABHIJIT MAZUMDER

■ INTRODUCTION

The incidence of carcinoma of unknown primary site (CUP), the clinical syndrome of metastatic carcinoma presenting without an identifiable primary tumor, is thought to pertain to 3% to 7% of newly diagnosed cancer patients (1–7). Thus, as many as 35,000 new cases of CUP occur each year in the United States alone, ranking among the more common presentations of malignancy. Less frequent than breast, prostate, lung, and colorectal cancers, CUPs are similar in frequency to carcinomas of the ovary and pancreas. CUPs represent a diverse group of tumors including many moderately to poorly differentiated adenocarcinomas that involve the liver, bone, lung, lymph nodes, pleura, and brain (8). Approximately 50% of CUPs are from well- to mode-rately differentiated adenocarcinomas, 30% are poorly differentiated adeno-carcinomas and undifferentiated carcinomas, 15% are squamous cell carcinomas, and 5% are undifferentiated malignant neoplasms (9). The prognosis for CUP is generally quite poor, with the median survival rarely reaching one year (9). However, it is generally agreed that the knowledge of the primary site of malignancy in a patient who presents with CUP can potentially improve the patient's overall outcome (3, 9).

In particular, in the era of targeted therapies for cancer, it could be possible that a more accurate determination of the primary site of origin for cases presenting as CUP could potentially yield an improvement in the survival of these patients by selecting a tumor-specific form of treatment (9). The diagnosis of CUP requires a biopsy-proven malignancy that could not have originated at the biopsy site, the absence of a confirmed primary tumor site identified after a thorough medical history or physical examination and routine medical imaging, and noncontributory laboratory test results.

■ TYPICAL EVALUATION FOR DETERMINATION OF PRIMARY TUMOR ORIGIN

In approximately 50% of the 30,000 new cases of CUP in the United States each year, the primary site of origin can be determined by clinical information including a variety of routine laboratory tests, routine imaging including CT scans, and a detailed medical history (Fig. 1). Approximately 35% of CUP cases require an immunohistochemical analysis, including a large panel of antibodies, to address the location of the primary site of the tumor. Approximately 85% of CUPs are identifiable as to their probable anatomic origins, at or near the time of presentation, using the clinical testing that is available in most diagnostic facilities. In the remaining 15% of CUP cases the sources cannot be determined by standard surgical pathological methods, and so the application of molecular technologies has been focused on those lesions (7, 9–12). In these cases of CUP, the clinical history, laboratory data, imaging results, and immunostaining pattern have not been helpful in pointing to a specific primary site of origin of the malignant process.

Using either fresh or frozen tumor tissue (when available) and/or formalin-fixed paraffin-embedded (FFPE) tumor tissues, with or without some type of tumor enrichment by microdissection, molecular techniques have generally complemented morphological information. They use extracted DNA or RNA from the samples and gene-expression profiling technologies to characterize the disease. This chapter reviews the various methods of gene-expression profiling and approaches to data analysis that

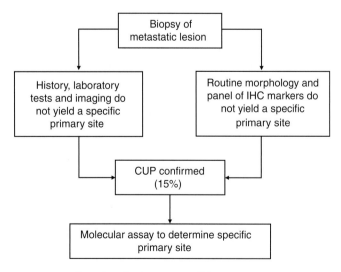

FIGURE 1 Flow chart for CUP origin. *Abbreviations:* CUP, carcinoma of unknown primary site; IHC, immunohistochemistry.

have been used to evaluate transcriptional profiling patterns. The main focus is on the competing techniques of multiplex real-time reverse transcription–polymerase chain reaction (RT-PCR) methods, as compared with gene-expression microarray technologies (cDNA and oligonucleotide). In addition, the emerging approach of profiling microRNA expression (miRNA) is considered as an approach to determining the origin of CUPs. A brief consideration of proteomic profiling using capillary electrophoresis and spectroscopic methods are also discussed.

■ TISSUE MICROARRAYS

Tissue microarrays (TMAs) have been designed to produce high-throughput testing of many characterized tumor samples, often with known clinical status and follow-up data, using a single microscopic glass slide (13–16). TMAs can facilitate the discovery of biomarkers and drug targets by allowing for rapid assessment of disease associations, as well as improvements in efficiency and productivity by conserving reagents and reducing "hands-on" testing time. Patient population studies as large as 600 cases can be assessed by in situ hybridization and immunohistology using a single microscopic slide. New hardware and software for digital image analysis has been specifically designed to facilitate TMA analysis, allowing for individual core scoring to be performed in a semiautomated manner. TMAs facilitate drug discovery and development by industrializing the assessment of mRNA and protein target expression in large numbers of clinically defined samples (17–20). TMAs are also used to validate disease-specific associations of novel tumor biomarkers as prognostic and predictive factors (21). Finally, TMAs have also been used to validate the discovery of gene sets that are designed to predict the sites of origin for CUPs.

■ TRANSCRIPTIONAL PROFILING: GENOMIC MICROARRAYS

The measurement of relative gene expression by detecting mRNA levels has evolved into a major technique in the field of oncological molecular diagnostics. The development of printed and spotted genomic microarrays has allowed for rapid screening and accumulation of new information concerning germ-line genotypes, gene mutations, and mRNA expression in human malignancies (22, 23). Transcriptional profiling done via hybridizing labeled probes, derived from cancer specimens, and arrayed oligonucleotide or cDNA libraries can provide a "snapshot" of a given tumor's transcriptome. The mRNA expression levels of well-characterized and/or novel genes from neoplastic specimens can be compared with the gene expression levels of reference samples. The latter specimens typically include cell lines, normal tissues, and precancerous clinical lesions. Biochip and microarray technologies have contributed to the industrialization of the genomic and proteomic discovery process, and they facilitate the development of "personalized medicine" and individualized therapies (24).

Table 1 lists the major types of arrays or biochips, as well as the associated fluorescent, radioisotopic, or mass-spectroscopic reporter systems that are in current

■ Table 1 Types of microarrays				
Feature	**cDNA Microarray (Spotted Arrays)**	**Oligonucleotide Microarrays**	**Comparative Genomic Hybridization—BAC/YAC Microarrays**	**Tissue Microarrays**
Target type and technology	Double-stranded cDNA Made from tumor mRNA >100 nucleotides Polymerase chain reaction products from cDNA clones Competitive hybridization	16–24 bp oligonucleotides in situ synthesis or printing Up to 240,000 oligos/chip Probe redundancy decreases false positives	DNA fragment arrays Bacterial/yeast artificial chromosomes 100 bp to 100 kb; 5000 spots 1 Mb resolution	Paraffin section arrays Frozen section arrays
Types of array surfaces	Glass slides Silicon Nylon membranes	Glass slides Silicon Nylon membranes Gels Beads		Glass slides
Signal detection systems	Fluorophores Radioisotopes Typically dual color	Fluorophores Typically single color	Fluorophores	Fluorophores Chromagens Radioisotopes
Technical limitations	Printing inaccuracies False hybridizations	Greater density, but limited by cross-hybridization errors	Limited resolution	Tumor heterogeneity Formalin-based protein and RNA degradation
Automation capability	Robot printing Laser scanning	Robot printing Laser scanning	Fluorescence microscopy Digital imaging	Image analysis
Clinical applications	Leukemia/lymphoma classification Solid tumor classification Carcinoma of unknown primary site Drug selection	Gene resequencing Single nucleotide polymorphism (SNP) discovery Tumor classification SNP prediction of toxicity Drug selection	High-resolution cytogenetics for gains and losses Tumor classification New primary tumor vs. metastasis	Currently used for research purposes only
Drug discovery and development applications	Drug target selection Pharmacogenomics discovery Biomarker discovery	Drug target selection Pharmacogenomics discovery Biomarker discovery	Drug target discovery	Drug target validation Pharmacogenomic target validation Biomarker validation

use or in development for cancer molecular diagnostics. Each of these techniques has in common the ability to generate hundreds of thousands of data points. Such a volume of information requires sophisticated and complex informational systems for accurate and useful data analysis.

cDNA Microarrays

cDNA microarrays were introduced in the mid-1990s and are now widely used for the expression profiling of human clinical samples. Using sequence-verified cDNA clones, robotic printing, fluorescent or radioisotope-based signal detection, and usually either glass-slide or nylon-membrane hybridization surfaces (Fig. 2), this technique can generate a wealth of new information in subtyping leukemia/lymphoma, solid tumor classification, pharmacogenomics, and drug and biomarker target discovery (22, 23). In addition, oligonucleotide-based cDNA microarrays, as produced by companies such as Affymetrix, Inc. and Agilent Technologies, Inc. (Santa Clara, California, U.S.A.) have been used extensively to map the human gene transcriptome.

Oligonucleotide Microarrays

Unlike most cDNA microarray platforms that compare the expression of the unknown tumor sample to reference tissue mRNA expression levels in a two-color system, oligonucleotide arrays typically feature a single-color system and do not include a reference mRNA sample that is cohybridized with the unknown material. Oligonucleotide arrays have been extensively used for transcriptional profiling and detection of single nucleotide polymorphisms (SNPs), as well as individual gene-point mutations. This method employs photolithography techniques to apply a large number of oligonucleotides to glass and nylon surfaces (22). Often, there is redundancy in the microarray so that a single gene is represented by more than 20 oligonucleotides, spanning its entire length, reducing the rate of false-negative results (22). This "single-color" approach has been employed to profile relative gene expression differences between samples of human tumors from different patients.

Oligonucleotide arrays are also highly regarded for their ability to provide automated, high-throughput genome-wide analysis of SNPs and other clinically relevant DNA polymorphisms. In addition, they have been used to classify subtypes of breast carcinoma and predict disease progression. Recently, oligonucleotide arrays have shown substantial promise in helping to select the most efficacious therapy for a particular disease.

Comparative Genomic Hybridization Microarrays

In DNA–array-based comparative genomic hybridization (array-CGH), the original CGH technique, which was applied to metaphase chromosomes, has been replaced by spots of cloned cDNA or artificial human chromosomes derived from bacteria (BAC) or yeast (YAC) (25). The resolution of array-CGH is significantly greater compared to standard metaphase CGH. The former technique can be automated to increase throughput and open the door to further discovery of specific genetic targets that may be exploited by future anticancer drugs (25, 26). Recent studies of breast cancer cell lines and clinical specimens have shown a significant correlation between DNA abnormalities discovered by array-CGH and RNA expression measured in the same samples as profiled on genomic microarrays (27).

Data Analysis and Data Display

Each DNA microarray produces tens of thousands of measurements that require significant computer-based data analysis to query biologically relevant patterns. It is critical to have systems in place that efficiently combine associative, functional, and gene expression data to assess the potential of a gene as a disease marker or drug target. Four techniques have emerged as the predominant method of DNA microarray data analysis: hierarchical clustering, self-organizing maps, multidimensional scaling, and pathway associations (27, 28).

Originally described in 1997, the arrangement of hybridization data into a cluster order based on color-coded intensities (a measure of comparative gene signals), provided clues as to which genes were signaling in groups (29–35). Typically, genes whose expression was significantly greater than that of a reference sample were depicted with increasing intensity on the "red" scale and those with less gene expression as increasing "green" signals (30). In hierarchical clustering, an algorithm groups genes in an array, based on similarities in their patterns of gene expression. Typically, those genes featuring the most similar patterns of expression are placed next to one other in the vertical axis, and patient samples with similar clinical or disease outcome features are arranged along the horizontal axis. This process yields a "heat map" (Fig. 3). The grouping of samples with similar gene expression with others that are linked to similar disease outcomes is known as a dendrogram.

Cluster analysis of genes can be performed in both a *supervised* and an *unsupervised* manner. In supervised analysis, the bioinformatics system uses machine learning after the computer is provided with an initial batch of categorized data. It features additional information

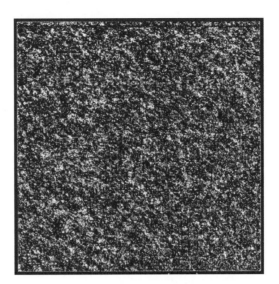

(A)

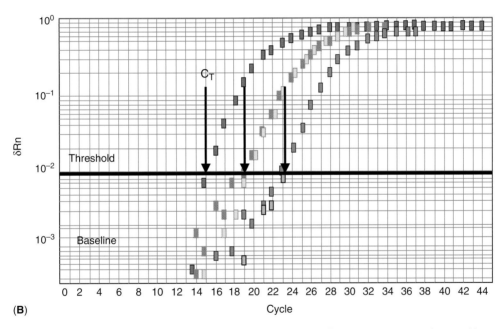

(B)

FIGURE 2 Gene expression evaluation systems. **(A)** The Affymetrix GeneChip System (Affymetrix Corp, Santa Clara, California, U.S.A.) features a single-color oligonucleotide microarray where each gene is represented by multiple probe pairs. The sequences of the probes are specific for a particular gene and the probe pairing design facilitates identification and subtraction of nonspecific hybridization and background signals. Hybridization signals are developed using immunochemistry and detected using a high-resolution scanner. **(B)** Basic principles of quantitative real-time polymerase chain reaction (RT-PCR). qRT-PCR amplification curves plot fluorescence-signal intensity (δRn) versus cycle number. The curves for three samples, run in duplicate, are shown. C_T values are indicated by arrows and represent the cycle fractions where the instrument can first reliably detect fluorescence derived from the amplification reaction. The fluorescence signal during the initial cycles of the polymerase chain reaction (PCR) is below the instrument's detection threshold and defines the baseline for the amplification plot. An increase in fluorescence above the threshold indicates the detection of accumulated PCR product. The amount of target in an unknown sample is quantified by measuring the C_T and using the standard curve to determine starting copy number.

on classification, such as tumor subtype, grade, stage, and disease outcome. This initial profiling step is known as the "learning or training set." In unsupervised analysis, the computer attempts to perform the clustering process without exposure to a set of previous training cases.

■ TRANSCRIPTIONAL PROFILING:
MULTIPLEX RT-PCR

The introduction of the real-time RT-PCR technique has allowed for rapid growth in gene expression studies, pertaining to both hematologic malignancies and solid

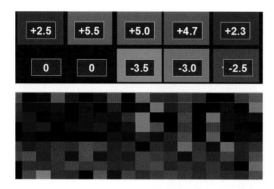

FIGURE 3 The heat map. The image demonstrates the standard data expression for gene clustering using the heat-map display system. Gene expression at levels greater than baseline are displayed in deepening red color and genes expressed below baseline are shown in deepening green color. Gene expressions equal to the reference housekeeping gene-expression level are shown in black. The patient's tumor samples are represented in the columns and the individual genes are represented in the rows. *Source:* From Ref. 97.

tumors (36). In multiplex RT-PCR, "housekeeping" and gene-specific oligonucleotide primers and dye conjugated probes are added to cDNA. The latter moiety is produced from RNA isolated from clinical samples, and a quantitative level of mRNA expression is obtained by normalizing the amplification cycle time for the target gene against that of a "housekeeping" gene (36). A variety of commercial closed-system RT-PCR technologies are used for clinical applications, predominantly represented by the TaqMan (ABI, Inc. Foster City, California, U.S.A.) and the Lightcycler (Roche Applied Science, Inc. Indianapolis, Indiana, U.S.A.) instruments. RT-PCR applications generally focus on the enhanced sensitivity that is associated with PCR-based strategies, owing to an ability to detect RNA over a 7-log range.

Leukemia and Lymphoma Diagnosis and Management

RT-PCR techniques found their first clinical applications in the field of leukemia and lymphoma management (37–40). RT-PCR can be used to detect the presence of non-Hodgkin's lymphoma in minute tissue samples (38, 40), as well as the recurrence of the disease after bone marrow transplantation (39). Although the sensitivity of PCR-based methods in detecting recurrent tumor has caused concern regarding their specificity for clinically significant [versus "molecular-only" (biologically irrelevant?)] disease relapse, most major cancer centers do employ the technique regularly to follow patients after intensive ablative treatments and/or bone marrow transplantation.

Micrometastasis Detection, Sentinel Lymph Node Evaluation, and Evaluation of Surgical Resection Margins

Recently, RT-PCR methods have been used to detect minute amounts of tumor-derived mRNA in lymph-node samples and surgical resection margin specimens, taken from patients with breast cancer (41–43) and a variety of other solid tumors (44–49). This approach has been compared with serial tissue sectioning and immunohisto-chemical assessment (50, 51), in reference to the detection of "micrometastases" in sentinel lymph-node biopsies. The methods designed to enhance the diagnosis of micrometastasis are currently controversial. It is not certain whether lymph-node samples that do not show malignant cells by routine microscopy, but contain abnormal mRNA expression as detected by RT-PCR, are clinically different from lymph nodes that are truly free of metastases by all parameters (52). Long-term clinical follow-up and treatment-specific surveillance will be needed to determine whether ultrasensitive methods, such as RT-PCR, are superior to traditional pathological evaluations in guiding therapeutic decisions and improving patient outcomes.

"Rare Event" Detection in Peripheral Blood and Body Fluids

Detection of rare circulating tumor cells in peripheral blood and body fluids by RT-PCR has been used as a method for the diagnosis of early-stage breast cancer, molecular staging of the disease, and monitoring therapeutic response (53–57).

Gene Methylation Status

RT-PCR-based measurement of "CpG" island promoter-gene hypermethylation has been extensively studied as an adjunct for the diagnosis of solid tumors (58–60). Gene silencing by methylation has also been studied in breast carcinoma (61–63). The "silencing" of important disease-related gene pathways such as those relating to estrogen receptor (ER) protein-related genes and BRCA1 have been identified in tumor cell lines and clinical samples (64–66). Methylating enzymes have recently emerged as targets in cancer therapeutics (67).

Pharmacogenomics

The RT-PCR technique has enabled the introduction of pharmacogenomics into clinical practice. In view of the fact that most human tumor samples are stored after formalin-fixation in paraffin blocks, strategies have been designed to amplify mRNA targets after extraction from paraffin. Most notable among these is Taqman RT-PCR quantitation of thymidylate synthase and dihydro-pyrimidine dehydrogenase mRNAs, extracted from paraffin-embedded tissues. These markers are felt to be predictors of response to 5-fluorouracil-based therapy for colorectal carcinomas (68).

■ COMPARISON OF GENOMIC MICROARRAY AND RT-PCR TECHNOLOGIES

As seen in Table 2, genomic microarray and RT-PCR technologies have been commercialized for the evaluation of clinical cancer samples. Microarrays have the advantage of being able to profile thousands of genes on a single chip or glass slide. This process generates enormous databases and expression signatures. RT-PCR features a broader dynamic range than microarrays can provide, and this may be critical for developing satisfactory reproducibility among testing sites. In addition, RT-PCR is more readily applied to FFPE tissue and may not require tissue microdissection for most clinical applications. The commercial assays that use these technologies are expensive, with prices exceeding $3000 per test.

■ SERIAL ANALYSIS OF GENE EXPRESSION

Serial analysis of gene expression (SAGE) is a direct and quantitative measure of expression that is based on the isolation and sequencing of unique sequence SAGE tags (69). Sequence data are analyzed to identify the presence and level of gene expression, and they are combined to form a SAGE "library." This process is similar to that of "differential display," and the SAGE method is currently applied principally for the discovery of biomarkers. By using a SAGE strategy with hierarchical clustering of publicly available data, it has been shown that adenocarcinomas and their metastases cluster according to their anatomic sites of origin (70). The strategy used was a novel bioinformatic approach, contrasting the differences between clusters and employing diverse sources. These included public expression data from analyses of SAGE and digital differential displays, as well as published microarray studies (70).

A 61-gene marker set identified from the expression-profiling databases was then converted to an 11-gene RT-PCR assay for testing on primary adenocarcinomas from a range of sites. Seven (64%) were site restricted (70).

■ TRANSCRIPTIONAL PROFILING FOR SOLID TUMOR CLASSIFICATION AND DETERMINING SITES OF ORIGIN FOR CUP

Genomic microarrays and RT-PCR techniques have also been used extensively to advance and revise the classification of malignancies (71–78). The initial "molecular

Table 2 Comparison of microarray and RT-PCR technologies

	Genomic Microarray	Multiplex Quantitative RT-PCR
Commercial providers	Affymetrix, Agilent	Roche, Applied BioScience
Maximum number of genes that reasonably can be profiled	30,000–40,000	10–100
Typical commercial assay	60–1550 genes	10–92 genes
Paraffin tissue capability	Limited	Widely accepted
Micro-dissection	May be required	Rarely required
Dynamic range	Intermediate	High
Bioinformatic data analysis systems	Highly complex	Complex; near-standardized for technique
	Not standardized for either technique or data	Not standardized for data
Reproducibility across different platforms	Limited documentation	Significant documentation
Testing platform	Predominantly centralized to commercial laboratories	Both centralized and decentralized platforms
Commercialized test cost	High (>$3000)	High (>$3000)

Abbreviation: RT-PCR, reverse-transcription polymerase chain reaction.

classification" of cancer used a DNA microarray profiling system to create an algorithm for cancer class discovery and prediction (70). This schema was then applied to classify acute leukemias, and an accuracy of 100% was achieved (70). A subsequent study from the same investigators used an algorithm for support vector machines (SVM), and a "one versus all" (OVA) classifier, in a DNA microarray-profiling study of 14 different tumor types (72). In that assessment, 78% accuracy was obtained (72). The molecular classification of breast carcinoma is also currently in use to assess the prognosis and potential selection of targeted therapies (71).

Expression profiling studies to determine the sites of origin for CUPs have used classification algorithms to determine the molecular "portrait" of human neoplasms. The gene expression profile of a test sample is compared with a reference database of known tumor profiles (79). This system uses a "nearest neighbor" identification system, generating a "k" value, which numerically estimates whether the expression profile of the unknown specimen matches that of a known tumor type (79).

Another large-scale RNA profiling study used supervised machine-learning algorithms to construct a first-generation molecular classification scheme. It was applied to carcinomas of the prostate, breast, lung, ovary, colon and rectum, kidney, liver, pancreas, bladder and ureter, stomach, and esophagus (77). The classification scheme that was developed in this study was based on identifying gene subsets. Their expression typified each cancer class; it led to a prediction of the primary site of tumor origin for 90% of 175 carcinomas, including 9 of 12 metastatic lesions (77). Predictor gene subsets include those whose expression is characteristic of various normal epithelia, as well as others that demonstrate elevated expression profiles after malignant transformation (77).

More recently, a single cDNA microarray platform was used to profile 229 primary and metastatic tumors, representing 14 tumor types with multiple histological subtypes. It generated a data set that was used for training and validation of an SVM classifier (12). This approach generated 89% accuracy using a 13-class model. Using fresh-frozen and FFPE tissues, the data set was then translated into a 5-class quantitative PCR platform using 79 gene markers, applied to a low-density microarray (12). Data generated from the microarray and quantitative PCR approaches were then used to train and validate a cross-platform SVM model. It successfully identified the site of origin in 11 of 13 cases (85%) of CUP (12).

Finally, using a simplified approach and a quantitative RT-PCR platform, a 10-gene marker set was employed to classify 205 CUP cases into one of six tumor types (80). In the validation assay for that study, a gene-based algorithm used an overall "leave-one-out" cross-validation approach. It achieved an accuracy of 78% for predicting the site of origin in 260 cases of CUP (80). The assay also produced an accuracy of 76% when tested on an independent set of 48 metastatic samples, 37 of which were from known primary tumors or CUPs for which the site of origin had been subsequently determined by other means (80).

■ PROGNOSTIC AND PREDICTIVE MOLECULAR ASSAYS IN CURRENT COMMERCIAL USE

A number of microarray-based and RT-PCR assays, designed to predict prognosis and response to specific chemotherapies, are in various stages of clinical and commercial development. Two molecular profiling tests for lymph node–negative, ER-positive breast cancer are now commercially marketed.

Oncotype Dx

Oncotype Dx (Genomic Health, Redwood City, California, U.S.A.) is a multigene RT-PCR multiplex assay. It uses a 21-gene probe set and mRNA that is extracted from paraffin blocks of stored breast carcinoma samples (81). The assay features 16 cancer-related genes and 5 reference genes that were selected based on a series of transcriptional profiling experiments. The cancer-related genes include markers of proliferation, including Ki-67; markers of apoptosis, including survivin; invasion-associated protease genes, including MMP11 and cathepsin L2; ER and HER2/neu gene family members; the glutathione-S transferase genotype M1; CD68 (a lysosomal monocytes/macrophage marker); and BAG1, a cochaperone glucocorticoid receptor that is associated with *bcl*-2 and related to apoptosis. Using a cohort of 688 lymph node-negative, ER-positive tumors, obtained from patients who were enrolled in the National Surgical Adjuvant Breast Program (NSABP) B-14 clinical trial and treated with Tamoxifen alone, the 21-gene assay produced three prognosis scores (low, intermediate, and high risk). Recurrence rates for these patients at 10-year follow-up was 7% for the low-risk, 14% for intermediate-risk, and 31% for high-risk groups. The difference between the low- and high-risk patients was highly significant ($p < 0.001$). With multivariate analysis, this assay predicted an adverse outcome independent of tumor size; it also predicted overall survival (81).

Although this assay is not currently approved by the U.S. Food and Drug Administration (FDA), interest in it has been intense, and it has significantly grown in use since its original introduction. Further studies are needed to validate the testing platform, and learn its best uses and limitations. Given the evolving approach to hormonal therapy with non-tamoxifen–related drugs and the use of adjuvant cytotoxic agents for node-negative patients, there is enthusiasm for the availability of RT-PCR-based and non-RT-PCR approaches for predicting response to antiestrogenic and other antineoplastic agents for the treatment of breast cancer (82).

Recently, the Trial Assigning IndividuaLized Options for Treatment (TAILORx) clinical trial was opened under the auspices of the U.S. National Cancer Institute. It is intended to prospectively test whether the Oncotype Dx recurrence score can guide chemotherapeutic decisions and result in improved patient outcomes (83).

MammaPrint (70-Gene Prognosis Score)

Gene expression profiles can define cellular functions, biochemical pathways, cell-proliferation activity, and regulatory mechanisms. In a cDNA microarray analysis using the Agilent Technologies system on primary breast tumors from 117 node-negative patients, a supervised system of classification was used to identify a poor-prognosis gene expression signature. Aberrant expression of genes that regulate the cell cycle, invasion, metastasis, and angiogenesis strongly predicted a short interval to the appearance of distant metastases (84). In a follow-up study, the "poor prognosis" gene profile outperformed currently used clinical parameters in predicting disease outcome. The estimated hazard ratio for distant metastases was 5.1 (95% confidence interval, 2.9–9.0; $p < 0.001$) (85).

The commercialized version of the 70-gene predictor known as MammaPrint (Agendia, Amsterdam, The Netherlands) was recently approved by the FDA in a 510k format. The Microarray In Node-negative Disease may Avoid ChemoTherapy (MINDACT) clinical trial is designed to provide evidence regarding the clinical relevance of the 70-gene prognostic signature and to assess the performance of that signature compared with that of traditional prognostic indicators in choosing therapy for node-negative breast cancer (86).

■ COMMERCIALIZED MOLECULAR ASSAYS FOR DETERMINING THE LIKELY PRIMARY SITE FOR CUP

Shortly after gene-expression profiling became available for use with human cancer samples, investigators began to apply the technology to the clinical dilemma of CUP. Over the past five years, four assays that utilize micro-array-based and RT-PCR technologies have been commercialized and are in varying stages of clinical development (Table 3).

CupPrint

This CupPrint (Agendia) assay uses FFPE tissue sections of tumor tissue. It measures the expression of 495 genes and is designed to detect 43 cancer types using the "k-nearest neighbor" bioinformatic strategy (87). CupPrint has achieved an 88% overall accuracy for determining a primary site in CUP cases. The test is commercialized and is performed at two sites, Amsterdam, the Netherlands, and Phoenix, Arizona, U.S.A., in a centralized format. It is not currently FDA approved.

MCID

MCID (AviaraDx, Carlsbad, California, U.S.A.), known as the "molecular cancer identification" test, uses an FFPE-ready RT-PCR assay to measure 92 genes; it is capable of identifying 32 tumor classes. The proprietary bioinformatic data-analysis system in MCID also uses the k-nearest neighbor strategy. It can be applied to small-needle biopsies, does not require tissue microdissection in most settings, and was associated in one study with an 87% success rate in classifying the 32 tumor classes (79). This assay is currently commercialized and is offered by U.S. national laboratories such as Quest Diagnostics, Inc. (Teterboro, New Jersey, U.S.A.) and the Laboratory Corporation of America, Inc. (Burlington, North Carolina, U.S.A.).

Pathwork Tissue of Origin Test

The Pathwork test (Pathwork Diagnostics, Sunnyvale, California, U.S.A.) uses the Affymetrix GeneChip oligo-nucleotide microarray technology to measure the expression of approximately 1550 genes in fresh or frozen tissues. The Pathchip assay, which is available from the same supplier, does not allow the use of FFPE tissues. Fifteen tumor classes are evaluated using a proprietary bioinformatic data analysis system. According to the manufacturer, the test has good reproducibility between laboratories. A sensitivity of 87% and specificity of 98% have been reported across the 15 tumor classes evaluated. In a recent report, the Pathwork Tissue of Origin Test (TOT) achieved 89% success in identifying a primary tumor site in 499 cases of CUP (88). This assay is commercial and is currently under review by the FDA.

GeneSearch

After querying a series of microarray-based profiling databases, the GeneSearch FFPE tissue-ready RT-PCR assay (Veridex, LLC, Warren, New Jersey, U.S.A.) was developed by Applied Biosystems, Inc, (Foster City, California, U.S.A.). This approach reduced the number of profiled genes to 10 and the number of tumor classes evaluated to 6. The embedded bioinformatic system is the Modern Applied Statistics with S (MASS) library function ("lda" in R language) and it uses the leave-one-out cross-validation strategy. This test produced an overall accuracy

■ Table 3 Molecular assays using gene-expression profiling for determining the primary site of carcinoma of unknown primary site

Test	CupPrint	MCID	Pathwork Tissue of Origin Test	GeneSearch
Commercial organization	Agendia	AviaraDx	Pathwork Diagnostics	Veridex, LLC
Location	Amsterdam, The Netherlands	Carlsbad, California	Sunnyvale, California	Warren, New Jersey
Platform	cDNA microarray	RT-PCR	Oligonucleotide microarray	RT-PCR
Platform source	Arcturus GE/Agilent	TaqMan Applied Biosystems	Affymetrix	TaqMan Applied Biosystems
Starting material	FFPE	FFPE	Fresh/frozen	FFPE
Number of genes profiled	495	92	>1550	10
Number of tumor classes	43	32	15	6
Bioinformatic strategy	k-nearest neighbor	Proprietary (k-nearest neighbor)	Proprietary	MASS (Venables and Ripley) library function "lda" in the R language
Overall success rate (%)	88	87	84	78
On-the-market status	Yes (centralized)	Yes (centralized)	Yes (decentralized)	In development
Food and Drug Administration approval status	No	No	In review	No

Abbreviations: MCID, molecular cancer identification test; cDNA, complementary DNA; FFPE, formalin-fixed paraffin-embedded; RT-PCR, reverse transcription-polymerase chain reaction; MASS, modern applied statistics with S.

of 79% in its initial clinical application (89) and 80% in a follow-up validation study (Table 4) (90). It is currently in development and has not been generally marketed.

■ SUMMARY OF COMMERCIALIZED MOLECULAR TESTS FOR CUP

As seen in Table 3, two of the assays discussed in the foregoing section use genomic microarrays to determine the gene expression profile of CUP specimens. The CupPrint appears to have an advantage over the Pathwork TOT because it has been customized to perform with FFPE specimens. On the other hand, the Pathwork TOT is the only one of the four assays that is in a late stage of the FDA approval process. These two microarray profiling tests evaluate the expression of more genes than the two RT-PCR assays do, but they do not automatically attempt to classify a greater number of tumor classes. The CupPrint assay includes the largest number of tumor classes (at 43), whereas the GeneSearch test includes only 6. Both the RT-PCR assays utilize FFPE tissues. The MCID RT-PCR test profiles more than >9 times the number of genes as the GeneSearch does (92 vs. 10) and attempts to place CUP specimens into 1 of 32 tumor classes. In addition, the MCID test is fully commercial and is available from national clinical laboratories. In contrast, the GeneSearch test is not, as yet, on the market. It remains to be seen whether the simpler GeneSearch test, with CUPs placed into only six tumor classes, will outperform more complex and higher-density molecular assays.

Table 4 Assay cross-validation by "leave-one-out" cross validation test on 260 formalin-fixed paraffin-embedded metastatic and primary tissue samples

Prediction	Breast	Colon	Lung	Ovary	Pancreas	Prostate	Other	Total
Breast	22	0	2	1	1	0	0	
Colon	1	27	3	2	4	0	4	
Lung	1	2	45	2	3	0	5	
Other	1	1	3	1	4	0	16	
Ovary	5	0	0	43	0	0	1	
Pancreas	0	0	3	0	31	0	6	
Prostate	0	0	0	0	0	20	0	
Total	30	30	56	49	43	20	32	260
Number correct	22	27	45	43	31	20	16	204
Accuracy (%)	73	90	80	88	72	100	50	79

Source: From Ref. 80.

MIRNA PROFILING FOR DETERMINATION OF CUP

miRNAs are small noncoding RNA sets of between 19 to 24 nucleotides, which are members of a class of small regulatory RNAs. These also include the small interfering RNAs known as siRNAs (90–92). miRNAs regulate the expression of downstream gene targets including transcription factors, oncogenes, and tumor-supressor genes. Transcriptional profiling using genomic microarrays and beads has enabled the discovery of numerous miRNAs that are differentially expressed in normal tissues as compared with tumors. These nucleic acid sequences are associated with cancer development, as well as clinical diagnosis and prognosis (90–93).

miRNA signatures can be used to detect and classify malignancies as well as predict the severity of disease. Certain profiles of miRNA expression are linked to aggressive tumors that typically demonstrate advanced disease at diagnosis (90–93). In the future, it is possible that miRNA profiling may also prove to be a more accurate method of determining the site of origin for CUP, compared with current strategies for profiling mRNA.

SERUM PROTEOMIC PROFILING OF CANCER

The proteomic profiling of human malignancies uses readily available serum samples and a variety of techniques. These include capillary electrophoresis and mass spectroscopy and show significant promise for potential clinical use in determining the primary sites for CUPs (94–96). To date, the development of cancer serum proteomics has been limited by sample procurement and bioinformatic issues, as well as a lack of standardized techniques (94–96). Whether this approach will eventually replace gene expression profiling of tumor tissues themselves, as a method of evaluating newly diagnosed CUP cases, remains to be seen.

IMMUNOHISTOCHEMISTRY AND MOLECULAR PROFILING: COMPLEMENTARY TECHNIQUES OR COMPETING PLATFORMS?

In this chapter, the molecular approaches for determining the site of origin for CUPs have been reviewed. From this information, it can be seen that the majority of CUP cases can be classified as to their probable primary sites using clinical history, physical examination, conventional laboratory testing, radiologic imaging, careful morphological assessment, and immunohistochemistry. Nonetheless, a group of approximately 15% of CUP cases remains, conceivably including 3000 to 4000 patients in the United States each year, that cannot be completely characterized by such approaches. For these patients, molecular testing, using available gene expression platforms, offers significant promise as a further level of diagnostic assessment. Given the complexity, limited in-house availability, and high cost of these gene expression profiling procedures, it is highly unlikely that they will be employed as "front line" evaluations for CUPs. However, there is increasing acceptance of the concept that improved clinical outcomes may be obtained if the site of origin for a CUP can be defined. For immunohistologically indeterminate cases, it is likely that molecular approaches will be pursued on an increasing basis toward this purpose.

■ REFERENCES

1. Abbruzzese JL, Lenzi R, Raber MN, Pathak S, Frost P. The biology of unknown primary tumors. *Semin Oncol* 1993; 20:238–43.

2. van de Wouw AJ, Janssen-Heijnen ML, Coebergh JW, Hillen HF. Epidemiology of unknown primary tumours; incidence and population-based survival of 1285 patients in Southeast Netherlands, 1984–1992. *Eur J Cancer* 2002; 38:409–13.

3. Abbruzzese JL, Abbruzzese MC, Lenzi R, Hess KR, Raber MN. Analysis of a diagnostic strategy for patients with suspected tumors of unknown origin. *J Clin Oncol* 1995; 13:2094–103.

4. Jemal A, Murray T, Samuels A, Ghafoor A, Ward E, Thun MJ. Cancer statistics, 2003. *CA Cancer J Clin* 2003; 53:5–26.

5. Bugat R, Bataillard A, Lesimple T, et al. Summary of the standards, options and recommendations for the management of patients with carcinoma of unknown primary site (2002). *Br J Cancer* 2003; 89(Suppl. 1):S59–66.

6. Dowell JE. Cancer from an unknown primary site. *Am J Med Sci* 2003; 326:35–46.

7. Varadhachary GR, Abbruzzese JL, Lenzi R. Diagnostic strategies for unknown primary cancer. *Cancer* 2004; 100:1776–85.

8. Le Chevalier T, Cvitkovic E, Caille P, et al. Early metastatic cancer of unknown primary origin at presentation: a clinical study of 302 consecutive autopsied patients. *Arch Intern Med* 1988; 148:2035–9.

9. Pavlidis N, Briasoulis E, Hainsworth J, Greco FA. Diagnostic and therapeutic management of cancer of an unknown primary. *Eur J Cancer* 2003; 39:1990–2005.

10. Dennis JL, Oien KA. Hunting the primary: novel strategies for defining the origin of tumours. *J Pathol* 2005; 205:236–47.

11. Tothill RW, Kowalczyk A, Rischin D, et al. An expression-based site of origin diagnostic method designed for clinical application to cancer of unknown origin. *Cancer Res* 2005; 65(10):4031–40.

12. Viale G, Mastropasqua MG. Diagnostic and therapeutic management of carcinoma of unknown primary: histopathological and molecular diagnosis. *Ann Oncol* 2006; 17(Suppl. 10):163–7.

13. Moch H, Kononen T, Kallioniemi OP, Sauter G. Tissue microarrays: what will they bring to molecular and anatomic pathology? *Adv Anat Pathol* 2001; 8:14–20.

14. Bubendorf L, Nocito A, Moch H, Sauter G. Tissue microarray (TMA) technology: miniaturized pathology archives for high-throughput in situ studies. *J Pathol* 2001; 195:72–9.

15. Skacel M, Skilton B, Pettay JD, Tubbs RR. Tissue microarrays: a powerful tool for high-throughput analysis of clinical specimens: a review of the method with validation data. *Appl Immunohistochem Mol Morphol* 2002; 10:1–6.

16. Kallioniemi OP, Wagner U, Kononen J, Sauter G. Tissue microarray technology for high-throughput molecular profiling of cancer. *Hum Mol Genet* 2001; 10:657–62.

17. Battifora H. The multitumor (sausage) tissue block: novel method for immunohistochemical antibody testing. *Lab Invest* 1986; 55:244–8.

18. Kononen J, Bubendorf L, Kallioniemi A, et al. Tissue microarrays for high-throughput molecular profiling of tumor specimens. *Nat Med* 1998; 4:844–7.

19. Zarrinkar PP, Mainquist JK, Zamora M, et al. Arrays of arrays for high-throughput gene expression profiling. *Genome Res* 2001; 11:1256–61.

20. Hoos A, Cordon-Cardo C. Tissue microarray profiling of cancer specimens and cell lines: opportunities and limitations. *Lab Invest* 2001; 81:1331–8.

21. Torhorst J, Bucher C, Kononen J, et al. Tissue microarrays for rapid linking of molecular changes to clinical endpoints. *Am J Pathol* 2001; 159:2249–56.

22. Harkin DP. Uncovering functionally relevant signaling pathways using microarray based expression profiling. *Oncologist* 2000; 5:501–7.

23. Polyak K, Riggins GJ. Gene discovery using the serial analysis of gene expression technique: implications for cancer research. *J Clin Oncol* 2001; 19:2948–58.

24. Kallioniemi OP. Biochip technologies in cancer research. *Ann Med* 2001; 33:142–7.

25. Monni O, Hyman E, Mousses S, Barlund M, Kallioniemi A, Kallioniemi OP. From chromosomal alterations to target genes for therapy: integrating cytogenetic and functional genomic views of the breast cancer genome. *Semin Cancer Biol* 2001; 11:395–401.

26. Monni O, Barlund M, Mousses S, et al. Comprehensive copy number and gene expression profiling of the 17q23 amplicon in human breast cancer. *Proc Natl Acad Sci USA* 2001; 98:5711–76.

27. Pollack JR, Sorlie T, Perou CM, et al. Microarray analysis reveals a major direct role of DNA copy number alteration in the transcriptional program of human breast tumors. *Proc Natl Acad Sci USA* 2002; 99:12963–68.

28. Zhang MQ. Large-scale gene expression data analysis: a new challenge to computational biologists. *Genome Res* 1999; 9:681–8.

29. Werner T. Cluster analysis and promoter modeling as bioinformatics tools for the identification of target genes from expression array data. *Pharmacogenomics* 2001; 2:25–36.

30. Scherf U, Ross DT, Waltham M, et al. A gene expression database for the molecular pharmacology of cancer. *Nat Genet* 2000; 24:236–44.

31. Johnson KF, Lin SM. Critical assessment of microarray data analysis: the 2001 challenge. *Bioinformatics* 2001; 17:857–8.

32. Goryachev AB, Macgregor PF, Edwards AM. Unfolding of microarray data. *J Comput Biol* 2001; 8:443–61.

33. Davenport RJ. Microarrays. *Data standards on the horizon.* *Science* 2001; 292:414–5.

34. Ayers M, Symmans WF, Stec J, et al. Gene expression profiles predict complete pathologic response to neoadjuvant paclitaxel and fluorouracil, doxorubicin, and cyclophosphamide chemotherapy in breast cancer. *J Clin Oncol* 2004; 22:2284–93.

35. Chang JC, Wooten EC, Tsimelzon A, et al. Gene expression profiling for the prediction of therapeutic response to docetaxel in patients with breast cancer. *Lancet* 2003; 362:362–9.

36. Jung R, Soondrum K, Neumaier M. Quantitative PCR. *Clin Chem Lab Med* 2000; 38:833–6.

37. Morgan GJ, Pratt G. Modern molecular diagnostics and the management of haematological malignancies. *Clin Lab Haematol* 1998; 20(3):135–41.

38. Gleissner B, Thiel E. Detection of immunoglobulin heavy chain gene rearrangements in hematologic malignancies. *Expert Rev Mol Diagn* 2001; 1:191–200.

39. Dolken G. Detection of minimal residual disease. *Adv Cancer Res* 2001; 82:133–85.

40. Diaz-Cano SJ, Blanes A, Wolfe HJ. PCR techniques for clonality assays. *Diagn Mol Pathol* 2001; 10:24–33.

41. Turner RR, Giuliano AE, Hoon DS, Glass EC, Krasne DL. Pathologic examination of sentinel lymph node for breast carcinoma. *World J Surg* 2001; 25:798–805.

42. Baker M, Gillanders WE, Mikhitarian K, et al. The molecular detection of micrometastatic breast cancer. *Am J Surg* 2003; 186:351–8.

43. Inokuchi M, Ninomiya I, Tsugawa K, et al. Quantitative evaluation of metastases in axillary lymph nodes of breast cancer. *Br J Cancer* 2003; 89:1750–6.

44. Raj GV, Moreno JG, Gomella LG. Utilization of polymerase chain reaction technology in the detection of solid tumors. *Cancer* 1998; 82:1419–42.

45. Pantel K, Hosch SB. Molecular profiling of micrometastatic cancer cells. *Ann Surg Oncol* 2001; 8:18S–21S.

46. von Knebel Doeberitz M, Weitz J, Koch M, Lacroix J, Schrodel A, Herfarth C. Molecular tools in the detection of micrometastatic cancer cells—technical aspects and clinical relevance. *Recent Results Cancer Res* 2001; 158:181–6.

47. Taback B, Morton DL, O'Day SJ, Nguyen DH, Nakayama T, Hoon DS. The clinical utility of multimarker RT-PCR in the detection of occult metastasis in patients with melanoma. *Recent Results Cancer Res* 2001; 158:78–92.

48. Jung R, Soondrum K, Kruger W, Neumaier M. Detection of micrometastasis through tissue-specific gene expression: its promise and problems. *Recent Results Cancer Res* 2001; 158:32–9.

49. van Diest PJ, Torrenga H, Meijer S, Meijer CJ. Pathologic analysis of sentinel lymph nodes. *Semin Surg Oncol* 2001; 20:238–45.

50. Noura S, Yamamoto H, Miyake Y, et al. Immunohistochemical assessment of localization and frequency of micrometastases in lymph nodes of colorectal cancer. *Clin Cancer Res* 2002; 8:759–67.

51. Ishida M, Kitamura K, Kinoshita J, Sasaki M, Kuwahara H, Sugimachi K. Detection of micrometastasis in the sentinel lymph nodes in breast cancer. *Surgery* 2002; 131:S211–6.

52. Hermanek P. Disseminated tumor cells versus micrometastasis: definitions and problems. *Anticancer Res* 1999; 19:2771–4.

53. Hu XC, Chow LW. Detection of circulating breast cancer cells by reverse transcriptase polymerase chain reaction (RT-PCR). *Eur J Surg Oncol* 2000; 26:530–5.

54. Shivers SC, Stall A, Goscin C, et al. Molecular staging for melanoma and breast cancer. *Surg Oncol Clin N Am* 1999; 8:515–26.

55. Baker MK, Mikhitarian K, Osta W, et al. Molecular detection of breast cancer cells in the peripheral blood of advanced-stage breast cancer patients using multimarker real-time reverse transcription-polymerase chain reaction and a novel porous barrier

56. density gradient centrifugation technology. *Clin Cancer Res* 2003; 9:4865–71.

56. Schroder CP, Ruiters MH, de Jong S, et al. Detection of micrometastatic breast cancer by means of real time quantitative RT-PCR and immunostaining in perioperative blood samples and sentinel nodes. *Int J Cancer* 2003; 106:611–8.

57. Stathopoulou A, Mavroudis D, Perraki M, et al. Molecular detection of cancer cells in the peripheral blood of patients with breast cancer: comparison of CK-19, CEA and maspin as detection markers. *Anticancer Res* 2003; 23:1883–90.

58. Herman JG, Baylin SB. Promoter-region hypermethylation and gene silencing in human cancer. *Curr Top Microbiol Immunol* 2000; 249:35–54.

59. Esteller M, Herman JG. Cancer as an epigenetic disease: DNA methylation and chromatin alterations in human tumours. *J Pathol* 2002; 196:1–7.

60. Wong IH. Methylation profiling of human cancers in blood: molecular monitoring and Prognostication. *Int J Oncol* 2001; 19:1319–24.

61. Widschwendter M, Jones PA. DNA methylation and breast carcinogenesis. *Oncogene* 2002; 21:5462–82.

62. Asch BB, Barcellos-Hoff MH. Epigenetics and breast cancer. *J Mammary Gland Biol Neoplasia* 2001; 6:151–2.

63. Yang X, Yan L, Davidson NE. DNA methylation in breast cancer. *Endocr Relat Cancer* 2001; 8:115–27.

64. Hayashi SI, Eguchi H, Tanimoto K, et al. The expression and function of estrogen receptor alpha and beta in human breast cancer and its clinical application. *Endocr Relat Cancer* 2003; 10:193–202.

65. Mueller CR, Roskelley CD. Regulation of BRCA1 expression and its relationship to sporadic breast cancer. *Breast Cancer Res* 2003; 5:45–52.

66. Esteller M, Silva JM, Dominguez G, et al. Promoter hypermethylation and BRCA1 inactivation in sporadic breast and ovarian tumors. *J Natl Cancer Inst* 2000; 92:564–9.

67. Szyf M. Towards a pharmacology of DNA methylation. *Trends Pharmacol Sci* 2001; 22:350–4.

68. Salonga D, Danenberg KD, Johnson M, et al. Colorectal tumors responding to 5-fluorouracil have low gene expression levels of dihydropyrimidine dehydrogenase, thymidylate synthase, and thymidine phosphorylase. *Clin Cancer Res* 2000; 6:1322–7.

69. Yamamoto M, Wakatsuki T, Hada A, Ryo A. Use of serial analysis of gene expression (SAGE) technology. *J Immunol Methods* 2001; 250:45–66.

70. Dennis JL, Vass JK, Wit EC, Keith WN, Oien KA. Identification from public data of molecular markers of adenocarcinoma characteristic of the site of origin. *Cancer Res* 2002; 62:5999–6005.

71. Golub TR, Slonim DK, Tamayo P, et al. Molecular classification of cancer: class discovery and class prediction by gene expression monitoring. *Science* 1999; 286:531–7.

72. Perou CM, Jeffrey SS, van de Rijn M, et al. Distinctive gene expression patterns in human mammary epithelial cells and breast cancers. *Proc Natl Acad Sci USA* 1999; 96:9212–7.

73. Ramaswamy S, Tamayo P, Rifkin R, et al. Multiclass cancer diagnosis using tumor gene expression signatures. *Proc Natl Acad Sci USA* 2001; 98:15149–54.

74. Khan J, Wei JS, Ringner M, et al. Classification and diagnostic prediction of cancers using gene expression profiling and artificial neural networks. *Nat Med* 2001; 7:673–9.

75. Su AI, Welsh JB, Sapinoso LM, et al. Molecular classification of human carcinomas by use of gene expression signatures. *Cancer Res* 2001; 61:7388–93.

76. Giordano TJ, Shedden KA, Schwartz DR, et al. Organ-specific molecular classification of primary lung, colon, and ovarian

adenocarcinomas using gene expression profiles. *Am J Pathol* 2001; 159:1231–8.

77. Shedden KA, Taylor JM, Giordano TJ, et al. Accurate molecular classification of human cancers based on gene expression using a simple classifier with a pathological tree-based framework. *Am J Pathol* 2003; 163:1985–95.

78. Bloom G, Yang IV, Boulware D, et al. Multi-platform, multi-site, microarray-based human tumor classification. *Am J Pathol* 2004; 164:9–16.

79. Ma XJ, Patel R, Wang X, et al. Molecular classification of human cancers using a 92-gene real-time quantitative polymerase chain reaction assay. *Arch Pathol Lab Med* 2006; 130:465–73.

80. Talantov D, Baden J, Jatkoe T, et al. A quantitative reverse transcriptase-polymerase chain reaction assay to identify metastatic carcinoma tissue of origin. *J Mol Diagn* 2006; 8:320.

81. Paik S, Shak S, Tang G, et al. A multigene assay to predict recurrence of tamoxifen-treated, node-negative breast cancer. *N Engl J Med* 2004; 351:2817–26.

82. Bast RC Jr, Hortobagyi GN. Individualized care for patients with cancer—a work in progress. *N Engl J Med* 2004; 351:2865–7.

83. Sparano JA. TAILORx: trial assigning individualized options for treatment (Rx). *Clin Breast Cancer* 2006; 7:347–50.

84. van't Veer LJ, Dai H, van de Vijver MJ, et al. Gene expression profiling predicts clinical outcome of breast cancer. *Nature* 2002; 415:530–6.

85. van de Vijver MJ, He YD, van't Veer LJ, et al. A gene-expression signature as a predictor of survival in breast cancer. *N Engl J Med* 2002; 347:1999–2009.

86. Bogaerts J, Cardoso F, Buyse M, et al. TRANSBIG consortium. Gene signature evaluation as a prognostic tool: challenges in the design of the MINDACT trial. *Nat Clin Pract Oncol* 2006; 3: 540–51.

87. Horlings HM, Warmoes MO, Kerst JM, Helgason H, De Jong D, Van 't Veer L. Successful classification of metastatic carcinoma of known primary using the CUPPRINT. *Proceed ASCO*, 2006: 20028.

88. Monzon FA, Dumur CI, Lyons-Weiler M, et al. Clinical validation of a gene expression microarray-based tissue of origin test applied to primary and metastatic tumors. *J Molec Diagn* 2006; 8:662.

89. Ibrahim CK, Baden J, Major C, et al. Validation of a 10 gene multiplex quantitative reverse transcriptase-polymerase chain reaction (qrt-pcr) assay to detect the primary site of metastatic carcinoma of unknown origin (CUP). *Modern Pathology* 2007; 20:350A.

90. Garzon R, Fabbri M, Cimmino A, Calin GA, Croce CM. MicroRNA expression and function in cancer. *Trends Mol Med* 2006; 12:580–7.

91. Liu CG, Calin GA, Meloon B, et al. An oligonucleotide microchip for genome-wide microRNA profiling in human and mouse tissues. *Proc Natl Acad Sci USA* 2004; 101:9740–4.

92. Volinia S, Calin GA, Liu CG, et al. A microRNA expression signature of human solid tumors defines cancer gene targets. *Proc Natl Acad Sci USA* 2006; 103:2257–61.

93. Lu J, Getz G, Miska EA, et al. MicroRNA expression profiles classify human cancers. *Nature* 2005; 435:834–8.

94. Omenn GS. Strategies for plasma proteomic profiling of cancers. *Proteomics* 2006; 6:5662–73.

95. Solassol J, Jacot W, Lhermitte L, Boulle N, Maudelonde T, Mange A. Clinical proteomics and mass spectrometry profiling for cancer detection. *Expert Rev Proteomics* 2006; 3: 311–20.

96. Wulfkuhle JD, Edmiston KH, Liotta LA, Petricoin EF 3rd. Technology insight: pharmacoproteomics for cancer—promises of patient-tailored medicine using protein microarrays. *Nat Clin Pract Oncol* 2006; 3:256.

97. Ross JS, Hortobagyi GH, eds. *The Molecular Oncology of Breast Cancer*. Sudbury, MA: Jones and Bartlett, Inc., 2005.

8 Endoscopic Evaluation of the Head and Neck

JAMES F. REIBEL

■ INTRODUCTION

Head-and-neck surgeons are routinely asked to participate in the evaluation of patients with potential neck metastases. The role of such physicians is to evaluate the upper aerodigestive tract for primary disease and stage whatever neoplasms may be found in the neck. This process includes endoscopy and biopsy to provide a diagnosis for the primary lesion and sampling of lymph nodal tissue to confirm the presence and nature of metastatic disease when no primary is identified. Tissue procurement from the neck mass is customarily deferred until a thorough head-and-neck examination is performed, because biopsy of any suspected primary tumors can establish the diagnosis and avoid unnecessary expense. Nevertheless, consultation sometimes follows fine-needle aspiration (FNA) or open biopsy by other physicians that has identified a cervical metastasis without a known primary lesion. In this instance, the otolaryngologist's primary objective is to identify the primary neoplasm, if possible, and to distinguish cases of occult primary carcinoma from true examples of metastatic carcinoma of unknown origin (MCUO).

■ CLINICAL AND RADIOGRAPHIC EVALUATIONS

Patients in the scenario just presented must undergo a standard historical review, where symptoms that would raise suspicion of a head-and-neck malignancy are noted. These include dysphagia, odynophagia, otalgia, dyspnea, dysphonia, weight loss, focal pain, or mucosal bleeding. The pattern and extent of tobacco and alcohol use are pertinent as well, as is any history of prior head and neck tumors, including skin lesions. Information regarding recent treatment and diagnostic investigations is desirable, and any imaging studies should be reviewed first hand.

The head-and-neck examination is attuned to finding a primary carcinoma. Symptom complexes will sometimes indicate a likely anatomic site for the lesion; however, the entire mucosal surface of the upper aerodigestive tract should be assessed carefully by visual inspection (direct and indirect) and palpation. Adequate mucosal anesthesia is essential for a complete and comfortable evaluation. The use of flexible and rigid endoscopes permits the thorough inspection of the mucosa in a relatively painless fashion. The new fiberoptic endoscopes permit transnasal esophagoscopy as well. Digital palpation of the oral cavity and oropharynx should be done last, because this maneuver is uncomfortable even with good topical anesthesia.

Assessment of the neck provides for documentation of the location of enlarged lymph nodes, and for noting their size, location(s), and degree of mobility. Occipital nodes drain the posterior scalp behind an imaginary line connecting the tragal cartilages on each side. Postauricular nodes serve the posterior scalp, mastoid, and posterior ear. Parotid nodes are considered in extraglandular and intraglandular groups. The former drains the anterior scalp. The intraglandular lymph nodes are situated in the substance of the parotid; they serve as the basin for the anterior scalp and the parotid gland itself. Retropharyngeal nodes serve the posterior nasal cavity, sphenoid and ethmoid paranasal sinuses, hard and soft palate, nasopharynx, and posterior pharynx.

The cervical lymph nodes are arbitrarily but conventionally designated in anatomic "levels." Level Ia nodes are central and submental; they drain the anterior jaw, middle lower lip, anterior gingiva, and anterior tongue. The boundaries of the zone that define level Ia are the anterior bellies of the digastric muscle and the hyoid. Level Ib nodes are situated in the submandibular region, serving the lower and upper lip on the same side as well as the cheek, nose, medial canthus, and oral cavity in front of the anterior tonsillar pillar. Their compartment is defined by the mandibular body and the anterior and posterior bellies of the digastric muscle.

Levels IIa and IIb nodes are in the upper jugular region, along the superior one-third of the sternocleidomastoid (SCM) muscle. Their boundaries are the stylohyoid muscle, the posterior part of the SCM, and the inferior hyoid bone. Level IIa is separated from level IIb by the spinal accessory nerve (eleventh cranial nerve). Nodes located posterior to this nerve are designated as level IIb, whereas level IIa nodes are anterior. Level II is associated with lesions of the mouth, nose, naso-oropharynx, hypopharynx, larynx, and parotid.

Level III cervical nodes are in the middle jugular group, along the middle one-third of the SCM. They are bounded by a horizontal line through the inferior hyoid, a horizontal line through the inferior cricoid, the sternohyoid, and the posterior border of the SCM. Tumors in the mouth, oro-nasopharynx, base of tongue, and larynx tend to involve level III nodes.

Level IV nodes are the lower jugular groups, found along the inferior one-third of the SCM. Their anatomic compartment is defined by a horizontal line through the inferior cricoid, the clavicle, the sternohyoid, and the posterior border of the SCM. Nodes in level IV preferentially receive metastases from neoplasms in the hypopharynx, upper esophagus, thyroid gland, and larynx.

Levels Va and Vb nodes reside in the region bounded by the intersection of the SCM and the trapezius muscle, the clavicle, the posterior SCM, and the anterior trapezius. A horizontal line through the inferior cricoid divides Va (superior) from Vb nodes. Level Vb includes supraclavicular nodes. Lymph nodes in levels Va and Vb receive metastases from tumors in the naso-oropharynx, the skin of the posterior scalp and neck, and the upper aerodigestive tract.

Level VI nodes comprise pretracheal, paratracheal, perithyroidal, and precricoid (Delphian) nodes. This group is bounded by the hyoid, the suprasternal notch, and the common carotid arteries on each side. Neoplasms in the thyroid, larynx, pyriform sinus, and upper esophagus drain there.

When one knows the lymphatic drainage patterns of the head and neck, a more informed search for a primary lesion can be undertaken. If a neck mass is one-sided, the primary neoplasm will likely be found in an ipsilateral mucocutaneous site. Bilateral neck metastases suggest an origin from the midline (e.g., tongue base, nasopharynx, or epiglottis), or from a lateral lesion that extends past the anatomic midline. Precision in specifying the site of nodal involvement is also important. When isolated right supraclavicular lymphadenopathy is present, for example, the lung is an important potential site of tumor origin (1); if left supraclavicular (Virchow's) lymph nodes are involved, the stomach, retroperitoneum, and pelvic organs likewise must be considered as sources (2, 3).

Thyroid, salivary glandular, and soft-tissue abnormalities are also noted in the physical examination; careful inspection of the skin of the face, scalp, and neck completes the assessment. After completion of these procedures, biopsy may be recommended if a lesion has been localized. If radiographic imaging studies have not been obtained, they must be done to provide complete staging information. This step should be taken before manipulation or biopsy of the lesional area, to eliminate confusion regarding postoperative changes versus tumor growth. If no primary lesion is identified in the mucosal surfaces, FNA of the cervical mass(es) is typically performed to establish a histological diagnosis (Fig. 1).

Once a histological interpretation of metastatic carcinoma is available, the surgeon can then consult with radiologists and pathologists. This step facilitates further planning of additional investigations that may be necessary (4, 5). Close communication with other physicians not only enhances efficiency but also avoids unnecessary duplication of investigations and facilitates expedited scheduling. Patients for whom clinical examinations

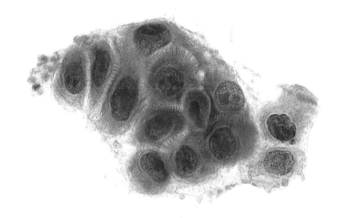

FIGURE 1 Fine-needle aspirate of an enlarged cervical lymph node, showing metastatic squamous cell carcinoma.

(including fiberoptic endoscopy) and adequate imaging studies fail to detect a primary lesion will require additional evaluations.

Current literature indicates that 5% to 10% of cervical metastases derive from unknown primary sources (4, 6–9). The location (4, 8–10) and morphologic details (4, 6, 11–19) of the metastatic tumor may provide useful clues regarding the possible location of an occult primary lesion. Level I to III nodal metastases most likely originate from tumors in the head and neck, predominantly squamous cell carcinomas (SCCs) of the upper aerodigestive tract 20–25). O'Brien et al. (26–30) have emphasized the importance of parotid and periparotid lymph-nodal metastasis from cutaneous malignancies. These potential primary tumors also must not be overlooked. Level IV and supraclavicular nodal metastases are almost related to primary disease below the level of the clavicles. Hence, the role of the otolaryngologist is limited in most of these cases, with the exception being examples of metastatic thyroid carcinoma (31–34).

Imaging examinations (including plain film radiographs and CT of the chest and abdomen in some cases) (35–36a) attempt to define and localize the presence of clinically occult tumors and to increase the yield of "speculative" biopsies. The staging and localization standard has been contrast-enhanced, thin-section, spiral CT (Fig. 2) (36–38). More recently, positron emission tomography (PET) (Fig. 3) and combined PET/CT studies

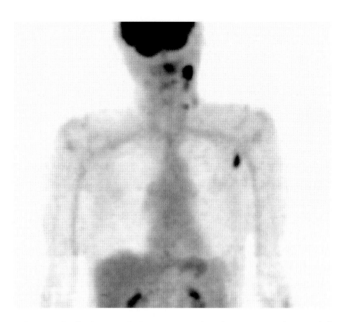

FIGURE 3 Positron emission tomography showing signals in a left cervical lymph node, a left axillary node, and the hard palate. Biopsy of the palatal lesion revealed squamous cell carcinoma, and the nodes were also involved by metastasis.

have been used increasingly, with encouraging results (6, 39, 40–45). Other authors have been less enthusiastic regarding the benefit of PET and PET/CT in this context, as compared with high-quality enhanced CT (40–45, 46).

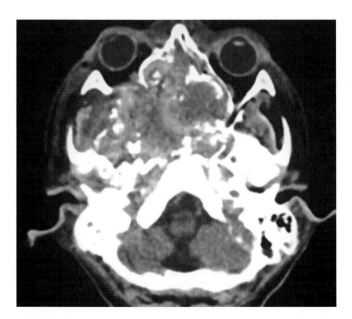

FIGURE 2 High-resolution CT of the head and neck in a patient who presented with right cervical lymphadenopathy. This study demonstrates a large destructive mass in the right nasal cavity and paranasal sinuses. The lesion proved to be a squamous cell carcinoma.

■ ENDOSCOPY AND "SPECULATIVE" BIOPSY

Although Dowell (4) and Hillen (10) have questioned the efficacy and cost efficiency of a concerted search for occult primary adenocarcinoma and undifferentiated carcinoma in the head and neck, the identification of occult primary SCC definitely influences treatment and long-term outcome (47, 48). Examination under anesthesia with esophagoscopy, direct laryngoscopy, and "speculative" biopsies of the nasopharynx, tongue base, and tonsil oropharynx are essential to detection of this tumor type (4, 6, 8, 9, 49–54). Patients who have undergone prior endoscopy without a diagnosis deserve consideration of a repeated examination under anesthesia (38, 39, 47, 55).

In each instance, careful inspection of the entire mucosal surface is done before any biopsy to avoid obstruction or distortion owing to postbiopsy bleeding. Any firm or friable areas are noted for later biopsy by palpation of the floor of the mouth, tongue, and tongue base. Suspicious areas should then be sampled generously, beginning with those that are most distally located. This provision avoids potential distortion owing to bleeding from the biopsy site(s). Large tissue samples are essential when performing "speculative" biopsies, especially from the tongue base and tonsil (53, 54). Specimens should be taken from both sides of the base of the tongue and another deeper biopsy is recommended from the base of each sampling site. If the patient has had a prior tonsillectomy, remnant tonsillar tissue should be biopsied in a similar fashion.

Many head-and-neck surgeons currently perform a bilateral tonsillectomy rather than doing simple punch biopsies of the tonsil (56–61). McQuone et al. (62) demonstrated that tonsillectomy identified an occult tonsillar tumor in several patients who had previously had negative results of "speculative" biopsies. That study also included one patient in whom an occult contralateral tonsillar SCC was found. Not all otolaryngological oncologists advocate bilateral tonsillectomy, but it is gaining increasing support in the evaluation of MCUO cases. An additional benefit of this procedure is the resulting symmetry of the oropharynx, with reduced subsequent confusion regarding the possible development of a new contralateral lesion (56, 62).

Mendenhall et al. (25) noted a relative increase in the identification of occult primary lesions in the tonsil and tongue base, and a decrease in those in the nasopharynx, hypopharynx, and supraglottis. These authors attribute such findings to improved clinical diagnosis of small primaries in the latter three locations with fiberoptic endoscopic examination. Such observations underscore the importance of careful and thorough preoperative assessment; they also support the importance of generous biopsy sampling.

■ TREATMENT AND PROGNOSIS

Depending on findings at endoscopy, primary lesions outside the nasopharynx are addressed surgically at the same time that a cervical lymphadenectomy is done. Alternatively, a neck dissection can be done separately (20, 22, 24, 63).

Patients with MCUO of the SCC type in the head and neck have a prognosis that is similar to others with metastatic nodal SCCs from known primary sites (64–66). With current modes of treatment, regional tumor control has improved but there has been no significant advance in overall disease-free survival. The respective three- and five-year disease-free survivals are 40% to 60% and 10% to 25% (23, 52, 66–70). Prognostic factors are focused on stage at presentation, the presence of extranodal spread by metastatic tumor, and the level of neoplastic differentiation (tumor grade) (71–73).

■ CONCLUSIONS

A comprehensive examination of the head and neck is indicated in the evaluation of all patients with cervical lymph nodal metastasis. The routine use of fiberoptic endoscopy in the clinic or office permits relatively painless inspection of the upper aerodigestive tract. When an occult primary SCC is suspected, evaluation under anesthesia, with endoscopy and "speculative" biopsies, is recommended. Any suspicious focus that is seen visually deserves tissue sampling. Occult primary neoplasms are most frequently found in the tonsils and tongue base. Thus, tonsillectomy, unilateral or bilateral, should be considered systematically in this setting, because it provides a generous sample of tissue and increases the diagnostic yield.

■ REFERENCES

1. Ellison E, LaPuerta P, Martin SE. Supraclavicular masses: results of a series of 309 cases biopsied by fine needle aspiration. *Head Neck* 1999; 21:239–46.

2. Negus D, Edwards JM, Kinmouth JB. Filling of cervical nodes from the thoracic duct and the physiology of Virchow's node: studies by lymphography. *Br J Surg* 1969; 56:699.

3. Mizutani M, Nawata S, Hirai I, Murakami G, Kimura W. Anatomy and histology of Virchow's node. *Anat Sci Int* 2005; 80: 193–8.

4. Dowell JE. Cancer from an unknown primary site. *Am J Med Sci* 2003; 326:35–46.

5. Pavlidis N, Briasoulis E, Hainsworth J, Greco FA. Diagnostic and therapeutic management of cancer of an unknown primary. *Eur J Cancer* 2003; 39:1990–2005.

6. Schmalbach CE, Miller FR. Occult primary head and neck carcinoma. *Curr Oncol Rep* 2007; 9:139–46.

7. Yakushiji S, Ando M, Yonemori K, et al. Cancer of unknown primary site: review of consecutive cases at the National Cancer Center Hospital of Japan. *Int J Clin Oncol* 2006; 11:421–5.

8. Guntinas-Lichius O, Peter-Klussmann J, Dinh S, et al. Diagnostic workup and outcome of cervical metastases from an unknown primary. *Acta Otolaryngol* 2006; 126:536–44.

9. Doty JM, Gossman D, Kudrimoti M, et al. Analysis of unknown primary carcinomas metastatic to the neck: diagnosis, treatment, and outcomes. *J Ky Med Assoc* 2006; 104:57–64.

10. Hillen HF. Unknown primary tumors. *Postgrad Med J* 2000; 76: 690–3.

11. Yalin Y, Pingzhang T, Smith GI, Ilankovan V. Management and outcome of cervical lymph node metastases of unknown primary sites: a retrospective study. *Br J Oral Maxillofac Surg* 2002; 40: 484–7.

12. Issing WJ, Taleban B, Tauber S. Diagnosis and management of carcinoma of unknown primary in the head and neck. *Eur Arch Otorhinolaryngol* 2003; 260:436–43.

13. Harwick RD. Cervical metastases from an occult primary site. *Semin Surg Oncol* 1991; 7:2–8.

14. Glynne-Jones RG, Anand AK, Young TE, Berry RJ. Metastatic adenocarcinoma in the cervical lymph nodes from an occult primary. *Clin Oncol* 1989; 1:19–21.

15. Hainsworth JD, Greco GA. Managing carcinoma of unknown primary site. *Oncology* 1988; 2:43–54.

16. Roh MS, Hong SH. Utility of thyroid transcription factor-1 and cytokeratin-20 in identifying the origin of metastatic carcinomas of cervical lymph nodes. *J Korean Med Sci* 2002; 17:512–7.

17. Tong CC, Luk MY, Chow SM, Ngan KC, Lau WH. Cervical nodal metastasies from occult primary: undifferentiated carcinoma versus squamous cell carcinoma. *Head Neck* 2002; 24:361–9.

18. Zuur CL, van Velthuysen ML, Schornagel JH, Hilgers FJ, Balm AJ. Diagnosis and treatment of isolated neck metastases of adenocarcinomas. *Eur J Surg Oncol* 2002; 28:147–52.

19. Wenig BM. Nasopharyngeal carcinoma. *Ann Diagn Pathol* 1999; 3:374–85.

20. Nieder C, Ang KK. Cervical lymph node metastases from occult squamous cell carcinoma. *Curr Treat Options Oncol* 2002; 3: 33–40.

21. Dutton JM, Graham SM, Hoffman HT. Metastatic cancer to the floor of the mouth: the lingual lymph nodes. *Head Neck* 2002; 24:401–5.

22. O'Mara W, Butler NN, Nemechek AJ. Carcinomas of unknown primary in the head and neck. *J La State Med Soc* 2001; 153:341–6.

23. Weber A, Schmoz S, Bootz F. CUP (carcinoma of unknown primary) syndrome in the head and neck: clinical features, diagnosis, and therapy. *Onkologie* 2001; 24:38–43.

24. Werner JA, Dunne AA. Value of neck dissection in patients with squamous cell carcinoma of unknown primary. *Onkologie* 2001; 24:16–20.

25. Mendenhall WM, Mancuso AA, Parsons JT, Stringer SP, Cassisi NJ. Diagnostic evaluation of squamous cell carcinoma metastatic to cervical lymph nodes from an unknown head and neck primary site. *Head Neck* 1998; 20:739–44.

26. O'Brien CJ. The parotid gland as a metastatic basin for cutaneous cancer. *Arch Otolaryngol Head Neck Surg* 2005; 131:551–5.

27. O'Brien CJ, McNeil EB, McMahon JD, Pathak I, Lauer CS. Incidence of cervical node involvement in metastatic cutaneous malignancy involving the parotid gland. *Head Neck* 2001; 23: 744–8.

28. O'Brien CJ, McNeil EB, McMahon JD, et al. Significance of clinical stage, extent of surgery, and pathologic findings in metastatic cutaneous squamous carcinoma of the parotid gland. *Head Neck* 2002; 24:417–22.

29. Bron LP, Traynor SJ, McNeil EB, O'Brien CJ. Primary and metastatic cancer of the parotid: comparison of clinical behavior in 232 cases. *Laryngoscope* 2003; 113:1070–5.

30. Vauterin TJ, Veness MJ, Morgan GJ, Poulsen MG, O'Brien CJ. Patterns of lymph node spread of cutaneous squamous carcinoma of the head and neck. *Head Neck* 2006; 28:785–91.

31. Verge J, Guixa J, Alejo M, et al. Cervical cystic lymph node metastasis as first manifestation of occult papillary thyroid carcinoma: report of seven cases. *Head Neck* 1999; 21:370–4.

32. Resta L, Piscitelli D, Fiore MG, et al. Incidental metastases of well-differentiated thyroid carcinoma in lymph nodes of patients with squamous cell head and neck cancer: eight cases with a review of the literature. *Eur Arch Otorhinolaryngol* 2004; 261: 473–8.

33. Mirallie E, Visset J, Sagan C, et al. Localization of cervical node metastasis of papillary thyroid carcinoma. *World J Surg* 1999; 23: 970–3.

34. Proye C, Gontier A, Quievreux JL, Carnaille B, et al. Decision-making for lymph node excision in surgery of thyroid cancer: extemporaneous examination of the external supraclavicular lymph nodes. *Chirurgie* 1990; 116:290–5.

35. Brouwer J, de Bree R, Hoekstra OS. Screening for distant metastases in patients with head and neck cancer: is chest computed tomography sufficient? *Laryngoscope* 2005; 115:1813–7.

36. Dillon WP, Harnsberger HR. The impact of radiologic imaging on staging of cancer of the head and neck. *Semin Oncol* 1991; 18: 64–79.

36a. Ong TK, Kerawala CJ, Martin IC, Stafford FW. The role of thorax imaging in staging head and neck squamous cell carcinoma. *J Craniomaxillofac Surg* 1999; 27:339–44.

37. Mevio E, Gorini E, Sbrocca M, et al. The role of positron emission tomography (PET) in the management of cervical lymph node metastases from an unknown primary tumor. *Acta Otorhinolaryngol Ital* 2004; 24:342–7.

38. Saleh EM, Mancuso AA, Stringer SP. Relative roles of computed tomography and endoscopy for determining the inferior extent of pyriform sinus carcinoma: correlative histopathologic study. *Head Neck* 1993; 15:44–52.

39. Miller FR, Hussey D, Beeram M, et al. Positron emission tomography in the management of unknown primary head and neck carcinoma. *Arch Otolaryngol Head Neck Surg* 2005; 131:626–9.

40. Gutzeit A, Antoch G, Kuhl H, et al. Unknown primary tumors: detection with dual-modality PET/CT-initial experience. *Radiology* 2005; 234:227–34.

41. Bohuslavvizki KH, Klutmann S, Kroger S, et al. FDG-PET detection of unknown primary tumors. *J Nucl Med* 2000; 41: 816–22.

42. Stokkel MP, Terhaard CH, Hordijk GJ, van Rijk PP. The detection of unknown primary tumors in patients with cervical metastases by dual-head positron emission tomography. *Oral Oncol* 1999; 35:390–4.

43. Aassar OS, Fischbein NJ, Caputo GR, et al. Metastatic head and neck cancer: role and usefulness of FDG-PET in locating occult primary tumors. *Radiology* 1999; 210:177–81.

44. Jungehulsing M, Scheidhauer K, Damm M, et al. 2[F]-fluoro-2-deoxy-D-glucose positron emission tomography is a sensitive tool for the detection of occult primary cancer (carcinoma of unknown primary syndrome) with head and neck lymph node manifestation. *Otolaryngol Head Neck Surg* 2000; 123:294–301.

45. Greven KM, Keyes JW Jr, Williams DW III, et al. Occult primary tumors of the head and neck: lack of benefit from positron emission tomography imaging with 2[F]-fluoro-2-deoxy-D-glucose. *Cancer* 1999; 86:114–8.

46. Jereczek-Fossa BA, Jassem J, Orecchia R. Cervical lymph node metastases of squamous cell carcinoma from an unknown primary. *Cancer Treat Rev* 2004; 30:153–64.

47. Mahoney EJ, Spiegel JH. Evaluation and management of malignant cervical lymphadenopathy with an unknown primary tumor. *Otolaryngol Clin North Am* 2005; 38:87–97.

48. Dhooge IJ, De Vos M, Albers FW, Van Cauwenberge PB. Panendoscopy as a screening procedure for simultaneous primary tumors in head and neck cancer. *Eur Arch Otorhinolaryngol* 1996; 253:319–24.

49. Birchall MA, Stafford ND, Walsh-Waring GP. Malignant neck lumps: a measured approach. *Ann R Coll Surg Engl* 1991; 73:91–5.

50. Jones AS, Cook JA, Phillips DE, Roland NR. Squamous carcinoma presenting as an enlarged cervical lymph node. *Cancer* 1993; 72:1756–61.

51. Haas I, Hoffmann TK, Engers R, Ganzer U. Diagnostic strategies in cervical carcinoma of an unknown primary (CUP). *Eur Arch Otorhinolaryngol* 2002; 259:325–33.

52. Charlton G, Singh B, Landers G. Metastatic carcinoma in the neck from an occult primary lesion. *S Afr J Surg* 1996; 34:37–9.

53. Gluckman JL, Robbins KT, Fried MP. Cervical metastatic squamous carcinoma of unknown or occult primary source. *Head Neck* 1990; 12:440–3.

54. Chang AR, Liang XM, Chan AT, et al. The use of brush cytology and directed biopsies for the detection of nasopharyngeal carcinoma and precursor lesions. *Head Neck* 2001; 23:637–45.

55. Nieder C, Gregoire V, Ang KK. Cervical lymph node metastases from occult squamous cell carcinoma: cut down a tree to get an apple? *Int J Radiat Oncol Biol Phys* 2001; 50:727–33.

56. Randall DA, Johnstone PA, Foss RD, Martin PJ. Tonsillectomy in diagnosis of the unknown primary tumor of the head and neck. *Otolaryngol Head Neck Surg* 2000; 122:52–5.

57. Koch WM, Bhatti N, Williams MF, Eisele DW. Oncologic rationale for bilateral tonsillectomy in head and neck squamous cell carcinoma of unknown primary source. *Otolaryngol Head Neck Surg* 2001; 124:331–3.

58. Kazak I, Haisch A, Jovanovic S. Bilateral synchronous tonsillar carcinoma in cervical cancer of unknown primary site (CUPS). *Eur Arch Otorhinolaryngol* 2003; 260:490–3.

59. Price T, Pickles J. Synchronous bilateral tonsillar carcinoma: role of fluoro-deoxyglucose positron emission tomography scanning in detecting occult primary tumors in metastatic nodal disease of the head and neck. *J Laryngol Otol* 2006; 120:334–7.

60. Lapeyre M, Malissard L, Peiffert D, et al. Cervical lymph node metastasis from an unknown primary: is a tonsillectomy necessary? *Int J Radiat Oncol Biol Phys* 1997; 39:291–6.

61. Reiter ER, Randolph GW, Pilch BZ. Microscopic detection of occult malignancy in the adult tonsil. *Otolaryngol Head Neck Surg* 1999; 120:190–4.

62. McQuone SJ, Eisele DW, Lee DJ, Westra WH, Koch WM. Occult tonsillar carcinoma in the unknown primary. *Laryngoscope* 1998; 108:1605–10.

63. Medini E, Medini AM, Lee CK, Gapany M, Levitt SH. The management of metastatic squamous cell carcinoma in cervical lymph nodes from an unknown primary. *Am J Clin Oncol* 1998; 21:121–5.

64. Fernandez JA, Suarez C, Martinez JA, et al. Metastatic squamous cell carcinoma in cervical lymph nodes from an unknown primary tumour: prognostic factors. *Clin Otolaryngol Allied Sci* 1998; 23:158–63.

65. Andruchow JL, Veness MJ, Morgan GJ, et al. Implications for clinical staging of metastatic cutaneous squamous carcinoma of the head and neck based on a multicenter study of treatment outcomes. *Cancer* 2006; 106:1078–83.

66. Grau C, Johansen LV, Jakobsen J, et al. Cervical lymph node metastases from unknown primary tumors: results from a national survey by the Danish Society for Head and Neck Oncology. *Radiother Oncol* 2000; 55:121–9.

67. Gabalski EC, Belles W. Management of the unknown primary in patients with metastatic cancer of the head and neck. *Ear Nose Throat J* 2000; 79:306–13.

68. Layland MK, Sessions DG, Lenox J. The influence of lymph node metastasis in the treatment of squamous cell carcinoma of the oral cavity, oropharynx, larynx, and hypopharynx: N0 versus N+. *Laryngoscope* 2005; 115:629–39.

69. Nguyen C, Shenouda G, Black MJ, et al. Metastatic squamous cell carcinoma to cervical lymph nodes from unknown primary mucosal sites. *Head Neck* 1994; 16:58–63.

70. McMahon J, Hruby G, O'Brien CJ, et al. Neck dissection and ipsilateral radiotherapy in the management of cervical metastatic carcinoma from an unknown primary. *Aust N Z J Surg* 2000; 70:263–8.

71. Christiansen H, Hermann RM, Martin A, et al. Neck lymph node metastasis from an unknown primary tumor: retrospective study and review of literature. *Strahlenther Onkol* 2005; 181:355–62.

72. Perez CA, Patel MM, Chao KS, et al. Carcinoma of the tonsillar fossa: prognostic factors and long-term therapy outcome. *Int J Radiat Oncol Biol Phys* 1998; 42:1077–84.

73. Wang RC, Goepfert H, Barber AE, Wolf P. Unknown primary squamous cell carcinoma metastatic to the neck. *Arch Otolaryngol Head Neck Surg* 1990; 116:1388–93.

9 Endoscopic Evaluation of the Gastrointestinal Tract

HENRY C. HO

MICHEL KAHALEH

VANESSA M. SHAMI

■ INTRODUCTION

Metastatic carcinoma of unknown primary site (CUP) is a common clinical entity. By some estimates, CUP constitutes about 3% to 5% of all malignancies (1, 2), although its true incidence is variable, depending upon the definition and the extent of clinical investigation that is applied. In general, CUP represents metastatic disease for which a primary site is undetectable at presentation. The initial evaluation of patients with presumed CUP need not be exhaustive. Instead, it is generally accepted that early evaluation should be geared toward the most likely primary sites, given the specifics of the clinical findings. One should generally obtain a thorough history and physical examination, complete blood count, urinalysis, blood chemistries, chest radiograph, and computed tomographic (CT) studies of the abdomen and pelvis in search of a primary lesion (3).

Although CUP implies the presence of advanced disease, almost by definition, a proportion of these patients will respond to therapy that may not necessarily be curative but may improve the quality of life and prolong survival (4, 5). Therefore, a principal goal in CUP cases is to identify those tumors that are likely to respond to treatment, while minimizing the use of costly or invasive tests, especially in reference to carcinomas that are known to resist therapy (6).

Approximately 80% of patients with metastases from an undiagnosed primary tumor will have an adenocarcinoma on pathological examination (7). In the majority of instances, this tumor type is known to originate in the pancreas, gastrointestinal (GI) tract, or lung. Unfortunately, some reports estimate that carcinomas of the esophagus, stomach, and colon account for nearly half of all cancer deaths in the United States and Europe (8). Clearly, then, examination of the alimentary system, including the liver, pancreas, intestines, and biliary tree, is important in CUP cases. This chapter describes traditional and novel approaches to the identification of GI malignancy in CUP cases, from an interventional endoscopist's perspective.

■ COLORECTAL NEOPLASMS

The majority of colorectal carcinomas are endoluminal tumors that arise from the mucosa. Colonoscopy is the single best diagnostic test for them, because it can visualize lesions throughout the entirety of the large bowel, allow for biopsy of mass lesions and detection of synchronous neoplasms, and enable the removal of polyps (9, 10). The air-contrast barium enema, as supplemented with flexible sigmoidoscopy, is also used, but the diagnostic yield of this procedural combination is less than that of colonoscopy for the evaluation of the lower GI tract. It is essential that the entire colon be examined for the presence of concurrent lesions. If the presence of luminal obstruction precludes a complete colonoscopy, a double-contrast barium enema or the use of newer modalities, such as CT-mediated virtual colonoscopy (CTVC) or MRI technology, may be applicable. CTVC has already been shown to outperform double-contrast barium enemas (which have traditionally been used if colonoscopy is impeded) at some institutions (11).

CTVC, represented by computer-enhanced spiral CT scanning after bowel preparation and air insufflation, allows for complete visualization of the colonic mucosa. The sensitivity of virtual colonoscopy, as compared to optical colonoscopy, ranges from 55% to 90% for detecting polyps larger than 10 mm, and 39% to 55% for smaller polypoid lesions (12–15). An enhanced method of CTVC uses three-dimensional image display and barium tagging of stool and retained fluids. This approach reduces the misidentification of the latter materials as lesional tissue, thus reducing false-positive results. One study compared the use of this technique for screening, and found it to perform comparably to optical colonoscopy (16). Nonetheless, there are no published reports that compare standard colonoscopy with CTVC for the diagnosis of CUPs in the lower GI tract. Currently, established indications for CTVC include evaluation of the colon after incomplete or unsuccessful colonoscopy, and visualization of the large bowel proximal to an obstructing neoplasm. Perhaps this procedure will be utilized along with colonoscopy in CUP cases in the future. CTVC can be performed on the same day that a conventional colonoscopy has been done, precluding the need for additional bowel preparation.

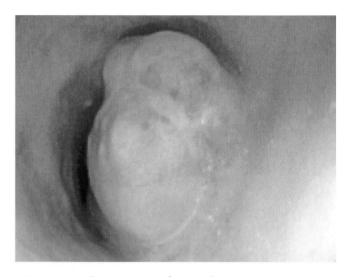

FIGURE 1   Endoscopic image of an esophageal mass.

■ TUMORS OF THE UPPER GI TRACT

If there is concern over the possibility of a neoplasm in the upper GI tract, a tissue diagnosis is best obtained via upper GI endoscopy. Even though it is more invasive and more costly, upper-tract endoscopy is more sensitive and more specific for the identification of gastroesophageal malignancies (Fig. 1) and duodenal lesions, as compared with alternative diagnostic strategies (17). The early use of upper GI endoscopy in patients with GI complaints has also been associated with increased detection of low-stage gastric carcinomas (18). The ability to do biopsies during endoscopy obviously adds to its clinical utility. Because up to 5% of malignant mucosal ulcers look benign grossly, it is imperative that all such lesions be evaluated by biopsy and histological assessment (19).

■ NEOPLASMS OF THE SMALL BOWEL

Primary small-intestinal tumors are rare. The most common among them are adenocarcinoma and carcinoid tumor (20). The small bowel may also be involved by

metastatic carcinomas originating in the breast, lung, stomach, colon, or kidney, by direct extension or hematogenous spread. Treatment of these lesions is generally palliative; limited resection or "intestinal bypass" will frequently relieve the symptoms they cause.

There is no single "best" method for imaging the small intestine in patients with suspected tumors in this location. The choices include radiographic procedures [CT scans, barium-swallow series, enteroclysis (Fig. 2)]

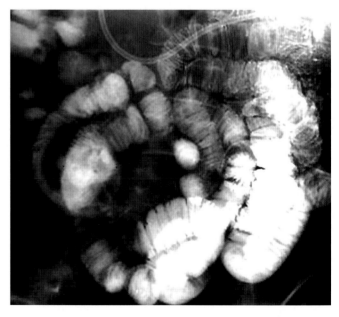

FIGURE 2   Enteroclysis involves the administration of barium and methyl-cellulose via an enterostomy tube placed in the small bowel. A double-contrast image is obtained of the mucosa.

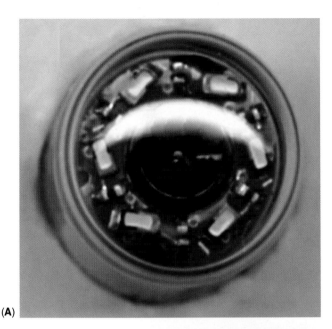

(A)

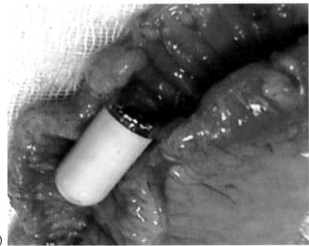

(B)

FIGURE 3 This wireless capsule endoscopy device (WCED) contains several light-emitting diodes and a central camera lens (**A**). The relationship of the device to the bowel lumen is shown in this resection specimen of small bowel, where the WCED was stopped by an area of stenosis (**B**).

and endoscopic methods [wireless capsule endoscopy (CE) (Fig. 3), "push" enteroscopy, double-balloon endoscopy (DBE)]. Unfortunately, differing examination techniques (frequency of fluoroscopy and compression radiography) limit small-bowel "follow-through" by barium-contrast study (21, 22), and patient discomfort and a relatively high radiation dose relate similarly to enteroclysis (23, 24). CE was designed primarily to provide diagnostic imaging of the small intestine, an anatomic site that has proved particularly difficult to visualize. Limited views of the esophagus, stomach, and cecum may also be acquired

via CE. The images that are acquired have excellent resolution and a magnification that is higher than that obtained by conventional endoscopy. Currently, CE is felt to be best indicated to investigate obscure GI bleeding. Its role is expanding, however, and may extend to the diagnosis of chronic diarrhea, malabsorption, and regional enteritis (25). Some studies that have compared CE with barium imaging and CT enteroclysis have shown a superior diagnostic yield of CE (26, 27). A possible place in the evaluation of CUP cases is yet to be defined for this modality.

Dedicated endoscopes that can pass through the entire small bowel are also available (28, 29). The main advantage of this direct or "push" enteroscopy, as compared with wireless CE, is an improved ability to obtain tissue samples and to perform therapeutic interventions. Nevertheless, the former procedure can be technically challenging. Most data comparing CE with push enteroscopy (PE) have been attuned to evaluations of GI bleeding. Early reports have suggested that CE delineates a definitive source for bleeding more frequently than does enteroscopy, with a higher diagnostic yield (30, 31). Some investigators have suggested that indirect studies do not permit detailed examination of the mucosa and have low sensitivity for flat, small, infiltrative, or inflammatory lesions (32). Although PE is effective for well-defined uses, it is best applied to lesions of the proximal small bowel (33).

Images recorded by CE can also be used in DBE. This new technique allows for examination of the entire small intestine, but it is time consuming and requires specialized training (34). One can envision that DBE could be complementary to CE by allowing for tissue sampling of lesions that are identified during wireless CE. Again, the relative roles of these methods in CUP cases must still be defined.

■ ENDOSCOPIC ULTRASONOGRAPHY

Endoscopic ultrasonography (EUS) combines a standard video endoscope with an ultrasound transducer to provide detailed images of the alimentary tract and surrounding structures (Fig. 4). It is a safe and accurate method for the diagnosis and staging of GI neoplasms (35). In addition, the development of "large-channel" endoscopes and new biopsy needles has enabled EUS-guided fine-needle aspiration (FNA) of the pancreas, liver, and mediastinum. The ability of EUS to guide a biopsy needle into lesions that are too small to be identified by CT or MRI, or too well sheathed by vascular structures to allow safe percutaneous sampling, has led to its use in several clinical settings. EUS-mediated FNA is most commonly employed to biopsy

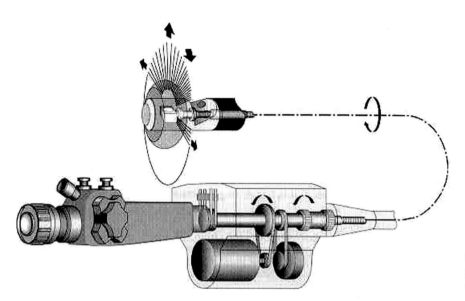

FIGURE 4 Endoscopy-mediated ultrasonography (EUS) utilizes a conventional endoscope to which a sonic transducer is attached.

peri-intestinal structures such as lymph nodes and masses in the pancreas, liver, adrenal glands, and bile ducts. It has also been used to aspirate peritoneal and pleural fluid. Applications for EUS in the assessment of CUP cases are definitely growing, because of its diagnostic power.

For example, EUS is considered to be superior to helical CT for detection of small pancreatic lesions (Fig. 5) (36, 37). Thus, in individuals with metastatic adenocarcinoma of unknown origin, especially in the setting of a high serum level of CA-19.9, EUS may be helpful in documenting the presence of a primary pancreatic cancer. At present, EUS is not routinely performed in all patients with CUP. However, Erickson and Garza reported that a greater number of pancreatic carcinomas were detected at a large referral center after the introduction of EUS. They suggested that this result might be attributable to the effects of the latter procedure (38).

Even in patients in whom a pancreatic mass is also identified by conventional cross-sectional imaging studies, EUS-FNA sampling can be helpful in distinguishing primary pancreatic tumors from metastatic extrapancreatic malignancies. Cytochemistry, immunohistochemistry, and the use of molecular tumor markers are potentially beneficial in this setting. In a study by Frischer-Ravens et al. 114 patients with pancreatic lesions underwent EUS-FNA sampling (39). In the 112 biopsies that were diagnostic, 56 showed primary pancreatic carcinoma, 12 demonstrated metastatic disease, and 44 had delineated benign lesions. In the patients who were found to have metastatic lesions, detection of the pancreatic metastases preceded diagnosis of the primary tumor in five of six patients with no prior history of malignancy.

EUS has also become a valuable tool in the localization of pancreatic endocrine tumors (PETs) of all types. Rosch et al. identified 32 of 39 such lesions (with a sensitivity of 82% and specificity of 95%) using EUS, even though they had not been detected with transabdominal ultrasound or CT (40). As another example, insulinomas (insulin-producing PETs) comprise the largest group of islet-cell tumors. They are usually biologically benign and solitary: 90% are intrapancreatic and 40% measure less than 1 cm. Detection rates of insulinomas with EUS are reported at approximately 80% and are highest with lesions in the pancreatic head (83–100%) (40–47). Thus, EUS is felt to be the preferred investigative modality in cases of suspected insulin-producing PET.

EUS is also helpful in cases of gastrinoma, both those that are sporadic and others that are associated with multiple endocrine neoplasia (MEN) type 1. Ninety percent of EUS-detected tumors of this type occur in the "gastrinoma triangle" (duodenum, head of pancreas, and peripancreatic soft tissue). In all, up to 50% originate outside the pancreas. EUS has the highest sensitivity (93%) for detection of intrapancreatic gastrinomas. Extrapancreatic tumors of this type are smaller and more difficult to image. Therefore, the sensitivity of EUS in finding them is much lower (approximately 50%) (42, 43, 48–50).

EUS may also have a role in screening asymptomatic patients with MEN1, a rare autosomal-dominant disorder that is caused by mutation and inactivation of the tumor-suppressor gene *MEN1*. About 40% to 60% of MEN1 patients develop pancreaticoduodenal tumors, and it is the most common cause of death in such individuals. The difficulty is that these islet cell tumors are often small and

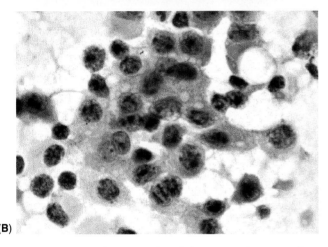

FIGURE 5 Linear endoscopy-mediated ultrasonographic image showing a pancreatic mass (**A**), fine-needle aspiration of which showed a pancreatic endocrine carcinoma (**B**).

mediastinum, and this compartment is easily accessible to EUS. Cytological samples of neoplasms that are obtained with EUS-FNA can be studied by special cytopathological techniques to help localize the site of tumor origin. EUS has been shown to have a 90% sensitivity in detecting lymph-node metastases in the superior mediastinum, AP window, subcarinal region, and periesophageal soft tissue. In combination with EUS, the specificity of FNA in this setting approximates 100% (52, 53). These procedures have definitely improved the diagnosis, staging, and treatment of lung carcinomas that are associated with mediastinal lymphadenopathy (54). Twenty-five percent of NSCLC patients lacking lymph node enlargement by CT are shown subsequently to have nodal metastasis by EUS-FNA (55).

EUS is also helpful in cases of mediastinal or intra-abdominal lymphadenopathy of unknown cause. In one analysis by Yasuda et al. 104 patients with enlarged mediastinal or intra-abdominal lymph nodes underwent EUS-FNA. The overall accuracy was 98%, yielding a diagnosis of lymphoma in 48 patients, metastatic solid tumors in 16, and benign conditions in 40 (56).

Like other imaging modalities discussed in this chapter, EUS is highly operator-dependent and has limited availability. Thus, it is generally limited to academic centers with a high case volume. Hence, the data cited in the aforementioned discussion should be viewed contextually as the products of experienced endoscopists practicing at large referral centers. New approaches to the evaluation of GI malignancy in CUP cases continue to improve and advancements in EUS-mediated imaging have occurred using such contrast-enhancing agents as "microbubbles." These developments may improve the identification of CUPs (57, 58) by delineating lesions that are not readily seen with conventional endosonography.

multiple. For example, in a retrospective study of 15 asymptomatic patients with MEN1, EUS demonstrated islet-cell tumors in 14 of them; 12 patients had multiple lesions (51). In that analysis, the number of tumors that were removed surgically exceeded the number predicted by EUS. Other data suggest that EUS, in combination with radionuclide-labeled somatostatin receptor scanning, may represent the best preoperative imaging strategy. One assessment showed that at least one of the latter two techniques identified all PETs (50).

As previously stated, the lungs are a common source for CUPs. Although pulmonary tumors are obviously not directly related to GI lesions, they are important contextually to illustrate the value of EUS in CUP cases. Roughly 85% of lung cancers are of the non–small cell type (NSCLC). In patients who lack extrathoracic metastases, the most common site of secondary involvement by NSCLC is the

CONCLUSIONS

CUP continues to be a difficult challenge for gastroenterologists. However, practitioners now have increased access to novel imaging systems such as CT colonography, MRI, and others. Moreover, there is ongoing development of endoscopic tools such as video CE, DBE, and EUS-enhanced imaging using microbubbles. Therefore, we expect that the detection of primary tumors in the setting of CUPs will dramatically improve in the future.

REFERENCES

1. Dowell JEM. Cancer from an unknown primary site. *Am J Med Sci* 2003; 326:35–46.

2. Abbruzzese JL, Lenzi R, Raber MN, Pathak S, Frost P. The biology of unknown primary tumors. *Semin Oncol* 1993; 20:238–43.

3. Souhami R, Tobias J. Cancer and Its Management. London, UK: Blackwell, 2005:364–8.

4. Hainsworth JD, Erland JB, Kalman LA, Schreeder MT, Greco FA. Carcinoma of unknown primary site: treatment with 1-hour paclitaxel, carboplatin, and extended-schedule etoposide. *J Clin Oncol* 1997; 15:2385–93.

5. Briasoulis E, Pavlidis N. Cancer of unknown primary origin. *Oncologist* 1997; 2:142–52.

6. Breslin NP, Wallace MB. EUS: a role in metastatic cancer with undiagnosed primary? *Gastrointest Endosc* 2001; 54:793–6.

7. Hainsworth JD, Greco FA. Management of patients with cancer of unknown primary site. *Oncology* 2000; 14:563–74.

8. Matthes K, Bounds BC, Collier K, Gutierrez A, Brugge WR. EUS staging of upper GI malignancies: results of a prospective randomized trial. *Gastrointest Endosc* 2006; 64:496–502.

9. Fong Y, Fortner J, Sun RL, Brennan MF, Blumgart LH. Clinical score for predicting recurrence after hepatic resection for metastatic colorectal cancer: analysis of 1001 consecutive cases. *Ann Surg* 1999; 230:309–18.

10. Saltz LB, Cox JV, Blanke C, et al. Irinotecan plus fluorouracil and leucovorin for metastatic colorectal cancer. Irinotecan Study Group. *N Engl J Med* 2000; 343:905–14.

11. Ferrucci JT. Double-contrast barium enema: use in practice and implications for CT colonography. *Am J Roentgenol* 2006; 187: 170–3.

12. Rockey DC, Paulson E, Niedzwiecki D, et al. Analysis of air contrast barium enema, computed tomographic colonography, and colonoscopy: prospective comparison. *Lancet* 2005; 365: 305–11.

13. Fenlon HM, Nunes DP, Schroy PC, et al. A comparison of virtual and conventional colonoscopy for the detection of colorectal polyps. *N Engl J Med* 1999; 341:1496–503.

14. Yee J, Akerkar GA, Hung RK, et al. Colorectal neoplasia: performance characteristics of CT colonography for detection in 300 patients. *Radiology* 2001; 219:685–92.

15. Cotton PB, Durkalski VL, Pineau BC, et al. Computed tomographic colonography (virtual colonoscopy): a multicenter comparison with standard colonoscopy for detection of colorectal neoplasia. *JAMA* 2004; 291:1713–9.

16. Pickhardt PJ, Choi JR, Hwang I, et al. Computed tomographic virtual colonoscopy to screen for colorectal neoplasia in asymptomatic adults. *N Engl J Med* 2003; 349:2191–200.

17. Van Dam JV, Brugge WR. Endoscopy of the upper gastrointestinal tract. *N Engl J Med* 1999; 341:1738–48.

18. Tan YK, Fielding JW. Early diagnosis of early gastric cancer. *Eur J Gastroenterol Hepatol* 2006; 18:821–9.

19. Graham DY, Schwartz JT, Cain GD, Gyorkey F. Prospective evaluation of biopsy number in the diagnosis of esophageal and gastric carcinoma. *Gastroenterology* 1982; 82:228–31.

20. Weiss N. Incidence of histologic types of cancer of the small intestine. *J Natl Cancer Inst* 1987; 78:653–6.

21. Maglinte DD, Burney BT, Miller RE. Lesions missed on small-bowel follow-through: analysis and recommendations. *Radiology* 1982; 144:737–9.

22. Gurian L, Jendrzejewski J, Katon R, et al. Small-bowel enema: an underutilized method of small-bowel examination. *Dig Dis Sci* 1982; 27:1101–8.

23. Thoeni RF, Gould RG. Enteroclysis and small-bowel series: comparison of radiation dose and examination time. *Radiology* 1991; 178:659–62.

24. Ott Dj, Chen YM, Gelfand DW, Van Swearingen F, Munitz HA. Detailed per-oral small bowel examination vs. enteroclysis. Part II. Radiographic accuracy. *Radiology* 1985; 155:31–4.

25. Magnano A, Privitera A, Calogero G, et al. The role of capsule endoscopy in the workup of obscure gastrointestinal bleeding. *Eur J Gastroenterol Hepatol* 2004; 16:403–6.

26. Eliakim R, Suissa A, Yassin K, Katz D, Fischer D. Wireless capsule video endoscopy compared to barium follow-through and computerized tomography in patients with suspected Crohn's disease—final report. *Dig Liver Dis* 2004; 36:519–22.

27. Hara AK, Leighton JA, Sharma VK, Fleischer DE. Small bowel: preliminary comparison of capsule endoscopy with barium study and CT. *Radiology* 2004; 230:260–5.

28. Monkemuller K, Weigt J, Treiber G, et al. Diagnostic and therapeutic impact of double-balloon enteroscopy. *Endoscopy* 2006; 38:67–72.

29. Ell C, May A, Nachbar L, et al. Push-and-pull enteroscopy in the small bowel using the double-balloon technique: results of a prospective European multicenter study. *Endoscopy* 2005; 37: 613–6.

30. Ell C, Remke S, May A, et al. The first prospective controlled trial comparing wireless capsule endoscopy with push enteroscopy in chronic gastrointestinal bleeding. *Endoscopy* 2002; 34:685–9.

31. Mylonaki M, Fritscher-Ravens A, Swain P. Wireless capsule endoscopy: a comparison with push enteroscopy in patients with gastroscopy and colonoscopy-negative gastrointestinal bleeding. *Gut* 2003; 52:1122–6.

32. Eliakim R. The impact of wireless capsule endoscopy on gastrointestinal diseases. *South Med J* 2007; 100:235–6.

33. Pennazio M, Arrigoni A, Risio M, Spandre M, Rossini FP. Clinical evaluation of push-type enteroscopy. *Endoscopy* 1995; 27:164–70.

34. Yamamoto H, Kita H. Double-balloon endoscopy: from concept to reality. *Gastrointest Endosc Clin N Am* 2006; 16:347–61.

35. Anandasabapathy S. Endoscopic ultrasound: indications and applications. *Mt Sinai J Med* 2006; 73:702–7.

36. Gloor B, Todd KE, Reber HA. Diagnostic workup of patients with suspected pancreatic carcinoma: the University of California-Los Angeles approach. *Cancer* 1997; 79:1780–6.

37. O'Malley ME, Boland GW, Wood BJ, et al. Adenocarcinoma of the head of the pancreas: determination of surgical unresectability with thin-section pancreatic-phase helical CT. *Am J Roentgenol* 1999; 173:1513–8.

38. Erickson RA, Garza AA. Impact of endoscopic ultrasound on othe management and outcome of pancreatic carcinoma. *Am J Gastroenterol* 2000; 95:2248–54.

39. Fritscher-Ravens A, Sriram PV, Krause C, et al. Detection of pancreatic metastases by EUS-guided fine needle aspiration. *Gastrointest Endosc* 2001; 53:65–70.

40. Rosch T, Lightdale CJ, Botet JF, et al. Localization of pancreatic endocrine tumors by endoscopic ultrasonography. *N Engl J Med* 1992; 326:1721–6.

41. Gouya H, Vignaux O, Augui J, et al. CT, endoscopic sonography, and a combined protocol for preoperative evaluation of pancreatic insulinomas. *Am J Roentgenol* 2003; 181:987–92.

42. Zimmer T, Scherubl H, Faiss S, et al. Endoscopic ultrasonography of neuroendocrine tumors. *Digestion* 2000; 62(Suppl. 1):45–50.

43. Anderson MA, Carpenter S, Thompson NW, et al. Endoscopic ultrasound is highly accurate and directs management in patients with neuroendocrine tumors of the pancreas. *Am J Gastroenterol* 2000; 95:2271–7.

44. Ardengh JC, Rosenbaum P, Ganc AJ, et al. Role of EUS in the preoperative localization of insulinomas compared with spiral CT. *Gastrointest Endosc* 2000; 51:552–5.

45. Glover JR, Shorvon PJ, Lees WR. Endoscopic ultrasound for localization of islet cell tumors. *Gut* 1992; 33:108–10.

46. Pitre J, Soubrane O, Palazzo L, Chapuis Y. Endoscopic ultrasonography for the preoperative localization of insulinomas. *Pancreas* 1996; 13:55–60.

47. Schumacher B, Lubke HJ, Frieling T, Strohmeyer G, Starke AA. Prospective study on the detection of insulinomas by endoscopic ultrasonography. *Endoscopy* 1996; 28:273–6.

48. Ruszniewski P, Amouyal P, Amouyal G, et al. Localization of gastrinomas by endoscopic ultrasonography in patients with Zollinger-Ellison syndrome. *Surgery* 1995; 117:629–35.

49. Wamsteker EJ, Gauger PG, Thompson NW, Scheiman JM. EUS detection of pancreatic endocrine tumors in asymptomatic patients with type 1 multiple endocrine neoplasia. *Gastrointest Endosc* 2003; 58:531–5.

50. Proye C, Malvaux P, Pattou F, et al. Noninvasive imaging of insulinomas and gastrinomas witih endoscopic ultrasonography and somatostain receptor scintigraphy. *Surgery* 1998; 124:1134–43.

51. Gauger PG, Scheiman JM, Wamsteker EJ, et al. Role of endoscopic ultrasonography in screening and treatment of pancreatic endocrine tumors in asymptomatic patients with multiple endocrine neoplasia type 1. *Br J Surg* 2003; 90:748–54.

52. Gress FG, Savides TJ, Sandler A, et al. Endoscopic ultrasonography, fine-needle aspiration biopsy guided by endoscopic ultrasonography, and computed tomography in the preoperative staging of non-small-cell lung cancer: a comparison study. *Ann Intern Med* 1997; 127:604–12.

53. Fritscher-Ravens A, Bohuslavizki KH, Brandt L, et al. Mediastinal lymph node involvement in potentially resectable lung cancer: comparison of CT, positron emission tomography, and endoscopic ultrasonography with and without fine needle aspiration. *Chest* 2003; 123:442–51.

54. Caddy GR, Chen RY. Current clinical applications of endoscopic ultrasound. *A NZ J Surg* 2007; 77:101–11.

55. Wallace MB, Ravenel J, Block MI, et al. Endoscopic ultrasound in lung cancer patients with a normal mediastinum on computed tomography. *Ann Thorac Surg* 2004; 77:1763–8.

56. Yasuda I, Tsurumi H, Omar S, et al. Endoscopic ultrasound-guided fine needle aspiration biopsy for lymphadenopathy of unknown origin. *Endoscopy* 2006; 38:919–24.

57. Bhutani MS, Hoffman BJ, Van Velse A, Hawes RH. Contrast-enhanced endoscopic ultrasonography with galactose microparticles: SHU508A (Levovist). *Endoscopy* 1997; 29:635–9.

58. Kasono K, Hyodo T, Suminaga Y, et al. Contrast-enhanced endoscopic ultrasonography improves the preoperative localization of insulinomas. *Endocr J* 2002; 49:517–22.

10 Radiological Assessments

ANDERS E. SUNDIN

ÅKE BERGLUND

■ DIAGNOSTIC CONSIDERATIONS IN CARCINOMA OF UNKNOWN PRIMARY SITE CASES

Detection Rates

When considering diagnostic imaging strategies for the localization of an occult tumor in a patient with carcinoma of unknown primary site (CUP), it is important to remember that even after extensive imaging studies, the primary neoplasm frequently escapes detection. Indeed, even at autopsy, it remains undetermined in roughly one-third of subjects. When the patient is still alive, a primary tumor is found in only 11% to 27% of cases (1–4), compared with 30% to 67% at postmortem examination (5–8). There is, however, considerable variation regarding these figures among different studies on the topic. A recent review (9) reported primary tumor-detection rates of 0% to 48% during life and 0% to 85% at autopsy.

The results of previous reports on radiological imaging of CUPs must also be interpreted with regard to the techniques available at the time the studies were performed, and their corresponding technical standards.

CT of the abdomen/thorax and pelvis is now routinely included in the radiological evaluation of patients with CUP, which was not the case before 1980. Accordingly, in earlier studies that lack CT data, a primary tumor was detected in only 11% to 26% of patients. More recently, with the inclusion of thoraco-abdominopelvic CT, a primary lesion has been detected in up to 33% of cases during life (10, 11). Current multidetector row–CT (MDCT) scanners now offer vastly superior spatial and temporal resolution, compared with the previous incremental CT technique. In addition to improving the delineation of anatomical details, MDCT scanners allow for the better use of intravenously administered contrast media. During the same examination, image acquisition may be performed in the arterial contrast enhancement phase for CT angiography; in the late arterial phase (or portal venous inflow phase) for depiction of well-vascularized visceral tumors; and in the venous phase for diagnosis of poorly vascularized organ-based lesions.

Moreover, acquisition of thin (mm to sub-mm) image sections allows for reformatting of transaxial images in coronal, sagittal, and oblique planes of visualization. Three-dimensional images may also be produced using the volume-rendering technique and maximum-intensity projections (MIP) to facilitate image interpretation and reproduction (e.g., at clinical hospital conferences). Almost by definition, current patients with CUP are subjected to several conventional radiological examinations, including MDCT. Criteria for CUP include a biopsy-proven carcinoma that is anatomically foreign to the site of tissue sampling, and the clinical absence of a definitive primary lesion despite a thorough physical examination, laboratory assessment, chest radiography, CT of the abdomen and pelvis, and mammography in women (12).

Histopathological Examination

A thorough histopathological assessment is fundamental to the evaluation of CUP cases; it should be done before considering a battery of imaging or endoscopic procedures. To ensure that the pathologist will have sufficient material to analyze, radiologists should generally eschew fine-needle aspiration in favor of a tru-cut biopsy. This permits immunohistochemistry (13–15), electron microscopy, cytogenetic analysis, and gene-chip microarray evaluation. In one recent study that used gene-expression profiling, a primary site could be confidently predicted for 11 of 13 CUPs (16). Close collaboration between radiologists, pathologists, and clinicians concerning the medical history, physical findings, and results of laboratory data optimizes the identification of a probable primary site in CUP cases.

Prognosis

The median survival of CUP patients has recently been reported to be in the range of six to nine months (5, 9). Nonetheless, other studies have documented a more favorable prognosis, with a median survival of 11 months (17, 18) or, conversely, a more adverse outcome with a median survival of two to three months (19–22). In view of the generally poor outlook for CUP patients, some of them, especially those with other significant comorbid conditions, will not benefit from extensive imaging studies. The latter evaluations may instead be more advantageous and justifiable for patients who are able to tolerate aggressive therapy.

A portion of CUP patients may be cured. Potential treatment-responsive patients include women with adenocarcinoma involving axillary lymph nodes only, women with isolated peritoneal carcinomatosis, men with blastic bone metastases and elevated serum levels of prostate-specific antigen, patients with squamous cell carcinoma in cervical lymph nodes only, patients with midline extragonadal germ cell tumors, and individuals with poorly differentiated adenocarcinomas or neuroendocrine carcinomas (NECs) (12, 18, 23).

The majority of CUP patients fall outside the subsets just listed. Nevertheless, other relatively favorable clinical findings include an age of more than 50 years (18–20), and topographic restriction of metastatic lesions to lymph nodes only (20, 23) or two or fewer metastatic sites (18). In contrast, unfavorable factors include liver metastases (18, 21, 22), adrenal involvement (18), poor overall clinical performance status (21, 22), other significant comorbid conditions (21), low serum albumin, lymphopenia (21), and high serum-alkaline phosphatase concentrations (17).

■ IMAGING STUDIES

Magnetic Resonance Imaging (MRI) of the Breasts

Metastatic patterns of spread are unpredictable in patients with CUP, and they often differ markedly from those seen in association with known primary tumor types (1, 3, 24).

In other words, carcinoma of the lung presenting as a CUP may demonstrate quite a different metastatic profile than a clinically obvious pulmonary cancer of the same histotype. However, in women with isolated axillary lymph node metastases of adenocarcinoma, an ipsilateral breast cancer is the most likely underlying lesion, even if the nodal tumor is a true CUP (ie, mammography fails to show the primary neoplasm). Further radiographic studies, such as MRI and ultrasonography (US), would have advantages for these patients and so any abnormalities that are seen should be biopsied (25–27). In pertinent publications on such cases, MRI has detected a primary breast carcinoma in 70% to 86% of cases (25, 26). Tumor localization was achieved in 40% of women who lacked a previous history of cancer and in 27% who had a prior or concurrent but contralateral breast carcinoma. Overall, MRI was effective in detecting an underlying tumor in 36% of cases (27). All of these lesions could also be localized by US and fine-needle aspiration. Interestingly, in 15 MRI-negative cases, no breast tumors were subsequently found during 12 to 53 months of follow-up surveillance (27).

Somatostatin-Receptor Scintigraphy

In the subset of patients with CUPs who have neuroendocrine differentiation, functional imaging by somatostatin-receptor scintigraphy (SRS) may be performed, employing ^{111}In-labeled octreotide (OctreoScan) (28). Positron emission tomography (PET) may also be performed with ^{68}Ga-labelled octreotide. In a recent study, it was shown to be superior to SRS for the detection of occult NECs (29). NECs with high proliferative activity and poor differentiation have also shown an increased uptake of [18F]-fluorodeoxy-glucose (FDG) (30, 31); one study demonstrated that FDG-PET imaging was effective in localizing 83% of high-grade NECs (31). Figure 1 shows the results of SRS in a patient who presented with liver metastases of an NEC.

Positron Emission Tomography

For oncological imaging, PET with FDG has evolved as a powerful functional modality. Generally, malignant tumors show an increased accumulation of FDG compared with most normal tissues, and FDG-PET therefore may be used advantageously to distinguish between these two substrates. It is an effective means of delineating the presence and size of malignant tumors. In addition, FDG-PET has utility in staging, therapeutic monitoring, and the detection of tumor recurrence. The clinical impact of FDG-PET and FDG-PET/CT has been reported in regard to different malignant neoplasms in a series of original publications and subject reviews (32–38). In one

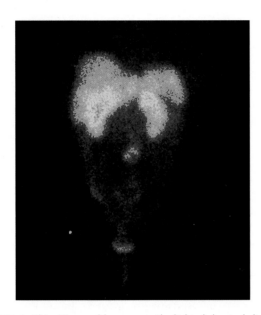

FIGURE 1 This 45-year-old woman with slight abdominal discomfort and other vague symptoms underwent CT of the abdomen, which showed multiple liver metastases; no primary tumor was detected. Biopsy of one liver lesion revealed metastatic carcinoma with neuroendocrine differentiation. Somatostatin-receptor scintigraphy (anterior view) showed high octreotide accumulation in the hepatic metastases and two small accumulations in the midline lower abdomen. The latter findings were consistent with mesenteric metastases from a midgut carcinoid; a review of the CT showed that they had been previously overlooked.

meta-analysis of the FDG-PET literature from 1993 to 2000, comprising 419 articles, the overall sensitivity and specificity of this method were estimated at 84% and 86%, respectively. Results of FDG-PET studies were said to have changed clinical management in approximately one-third of cases (32). Tumor types for which FDG-PET and PET/CT are regularly employed include non–small cell lung carcinomas (39–42); gastrointestinal carcinomas (43–45); lymphomas (46–48); carcinomas of the head and neck (49, 50); and melanomas (51, 52).

PET Technique

The PET tracer is generally administered as an intravenous bolus injection. In order to detect its accumulation in tumors and various normal tissues, the tracer must include a positron-emitting radionuclide. Such molecules are generally produced in a low-energy cyclotron and their half-lives are generally short (18F $t_{1/2} = 110$ min, 11C $t_{1/2} = 20$ min, 15O $t_{1/2} = 2$ min). The clinical use of 11C- and 15O-labelled PET tracers requires the availability of an in-house cyclotron and a radiochemistry laboratory. On the other hand, the relatively long half-life of 18F-labelled PET tracers permits their transportation over approximately two hours. Hence, PET centers may acquire FDG from nearby cyclotron facilities. FDG is usually

administered about one hour before the imaging procedure to allow the tracer to accumulate in tumor implants and diffuse from normal tissues. Nevertheless, some tumors are better visualized after three hours (53), and, for PET examination of patients with CUPs, where occult tumors are expected to be small, a longer accumulation time is desirable. By contrast, because of the 20-minute half-life of 11C, tracers based on this substance are administered about 20 minutes before PET examination.

A PET scanner includes a bed for the patient and a gantry that holds tens of thousands of detectors, arranged in rings. Axially, the detectors cover approximately 15 cm of the gantry. In order to perform a whole-body examination, the patient is moved in a stepwise fashion through the gantry. The bed typically stays in each "bed position" for a three-to-five-minute acquisition of image data. During a PET examination, the detection of tracer is made possible because positrons are emitted from nuclear protons. Within a few millimeters from the nucleus, positron collides with an electron. Upon this, both particles are annihilated and converted into high-energy (511 keV) photons that travel in opposite directions to simultaneously reach the detector ring. Lines of decay are registered by a computer in the PET camera. By using these data, transaxial images that represent regional radioactivity concentrations may be reconstructed to create emission scans.

A fraction of the photons do not reach the detector rings because of attenuation. In order to adjust for this, a compensatory measurement (transmission examination) is performed in each bed position, most often by rotating a gamma-emitting pin (rod source) around the patient for a few minutes. By using these attenuation data, emissions may be corrected and reconstructed into images that reflect accurate radioactivity concentrations (Bq/cm^3).

Examination times are considerably shorter with PET/CT scanners, because the CT scan is used for attenuation correction. Moreover, the CT examination provides an anatomical map for morphological correlation of functional image findings. The PET/CT examination is generally displayed in the form of transaxial, coronal, and sagittal PET and CT images. A software overlay is shown in which functional data in the PET images are fused with morphological information from CT images. The whole volume of PET data is typically displayed as an MIP that can be rotated to facilitate image reading. When needed, the CT examination may be modified regarding its acquisition parameters and the use of contrast media (54–58).

PET and PET/CT in CUP Cases

An established application for FDG-PET and FDG-PET/CT studies is the detection of occult primary tumors in CUP patients (32, 33, 38). Because FDG-PET and

FDG-PET/CT evaluations are performed as "whole-body" examinations, from the base of the skull to the proximal thighs, previously undiagnosed metastatic lesions may also be detected along with the primary tumors. In the literature on PET, a categorical distinction is usually made between patients who present with middle- or high-cervical lymph node metastases (usually associated with a carcinoma in the head and neck) and individuals with metastatic disease in other locations.

FDG-PET IN PATIENTS WITH CERVICAL LYMPH NODE METASTASES.

A review of 16 studies published between 1994 and 2003, including 302 patients with cervical lymph node metastases from CUP, showed that FDG-PET detected a primary tumor in 74 cases (25%) (59). Unrecognized metastases were diagnosed in 27% of the patients; regional in 16%, and distant in 11%. However, the overall incidence of false-positive FDG-PET studies was high (16%), especially in a subset of patients for whom a tonsillar carcinoma was favored (39%). False positivity also attended cases where tumors were suspected at the base of the tongue (21%) or the hypopharynx (8%). The definition of CUP, based on the diagnostic evaluation that had been done before FDG-PET examination, has differed among various studies. All patients had generally undergone imaging by CT and/or MRI, but in 10 of the 16 cases, they also had had panendoscopy. Only those with negative results of endoscopic evaluations were included in the assessment. A large variation in the detection rate of CUPs was found among papers included in this review. The least favorable result achieved was FDG-PET detection of a primary tumor in only 1 of 21 patients (5%). On the other hand, it detected previously unrecognized metastases in 9 of 21 (43%) patients (60). In contrast, another analysis of FDG-PET demonstrated better localization of primary lesions. It was successful in identifying a primary neoplasm in 11 of 15 patients (73%) (61). The details of the report, however, indicate that CT findings in four of the 15 patients were also suggestive of the primary cancers (61).

Additional studies have been published that report results of FDG-PET alone, but such publications principally address the impact of FDG-PET/CT in CUP patients. In one analysis of 26 patients with metastatic squamous cell carcinoma in cervical lymph nodes, FDG-PET detected the primary neoplasm in eight cases (31%) (62). In that series, FDG-PET was preceded by CT and/or MRI. Laryngoscopy/nasopharyngoscopy was performed after the PET examination. Out of 69 patients, 46 underwent FDG-PET, and the diagnostic capabilities of several different investigative methods were compared (63). A primary tumor was detected in 23 patients (33%). The best sensitivity was obtained with FDG-PET (69%), which was superior to panendoscopy (48%) and conventional (CT) imaging (32–50%). Nevertheless, the latter

modality had better specificity (87–95%) than FDG-PET (69%). Distant metastases were found in 6 of the 69 patients (9%), and they were all detected with FDG-PET. On the other hand, FDG-PET localized the primary lesion in only one patient among six who had occult tonsillar carcinoma (17%) (64). In another retrospective study on FDG-PET imaging of tumors in the head and neck, a subgroup of 18 CUP patients was analyzed; occult primary lesions were detected by FDG-PET in 7 of 18 cases (36%) (50).

FDG-PET/CT IN PATIENTS WITH CERVICAL LYMPH NODE METASTASES.

In a large cohort of 326 patients with CUP, a subgroup of 14 had exclusively nonsquamous metastatic cell carcinomas in cervical lymph nodes. The 14 individuals underwent FDG-PET or FDG-PET/CT studies, and a primary lesion was found in 50%. However, there was also one false-positive result (65). In another analysis of CUP patients with cervical lymph node metastases and extracervical metastases, the results of FDG-PET/CT studies and diagnostic CT were evaluated. A primary neoplasm was detected by FDG-PET/CT in 6 of 18 patients (33%) and a side-by-side evaluation of FDG-PET and CT revealed five tumors (28%). In each group, there was one false-positive result (66). Twenty-two percent of the patients had their occult primary lesions found with PET imaging alone. These differences in detection rate were not statistically significant if the study modalities used were taken into account. Figures 2 and 3 illustrate the value of FDG-PET-CT in two CUP patients presenting with cervical lymph node metastases.

Yet another publication on CUP with cervical lymph node involvement indicated that FDG-PET/CT results suggested a potential primary site in 26 of 38 patients (68%) (67). However, only 13 of those were histopathologically verified. One more study had a 36% detection rate by FDG-PET/CT among 85 patients with head and neck tumors (36%) (68).

FDG-PET AND FDG-PET/CT IN PATIENTS WITH EXTRACERVICAL METASTASES.

In a review of 10 studies that were published between 1998 and 2006, including 221 patients, the impact of FDG-PET (used in seven studies) and FDG-PET/CT (three studies) was evaluated in patients with extracervical metastases and negative conventional radiological assessments (e.g., plain film studies; CT; MRI) (69). Almost all patients (94%) were found to have one metastatic site only. FDG-PET and FDG-PET/CT detected a primary tumor in 41% of cases, and previously unseen metastases were found in 37%. Further analyses of these data showed that the primary tumor was found by FDG-PET/CT in 40% of cases and by FDG-PET in 39%.

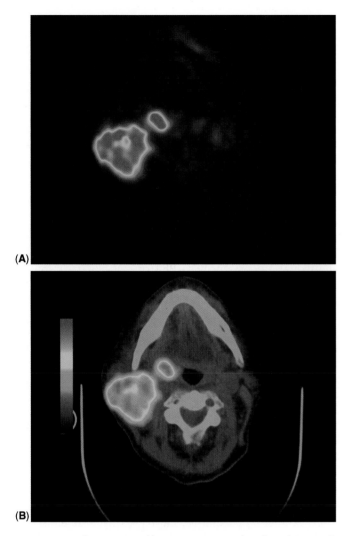

FIGURE 2 This 51-year-old woman presented with a large right cervical tumor, a biopsy of which revealed squamous cell carcinoma. Clinical examination and conventional radiological evaluations were negative. A transaxial [18F]-fluorodeoxy-glucose–positron emission tomography image shows the large cervical metastasis and demonstrates the primary tumor at the right tongue base (**A**). Anatomic localization of the lesion is better appreciated in the fusion of PET and CT (**B**).

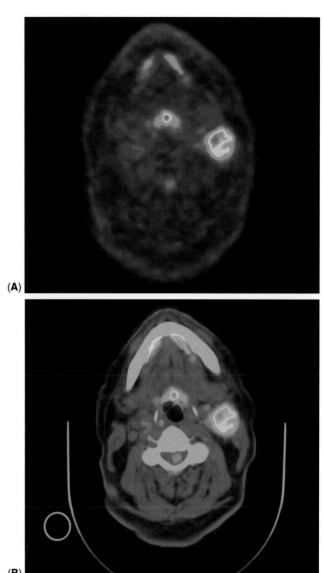

FIGURE 3 A 66-year-old man was found to have an enlarged left cervical lymph node; a biopsy showed metastatic small cell carcinoma. Conventional imaging by CT failed to demonstrate a primary tumor in the head, neck, or thorax. A transaxial [18F]-fluorodeoxy-glucose–positron emission tomography image shows the cervical lymph node metastasis and a primary neoplasm in the midline tongue base. Biopsy of the latter lesion and histological reevaluation of the lymph node specimen were consistent with one another, confirming that the tumor was of oropharyngeal origin (**A**). Its anatomic localization is better appreciated in the fusion of PET and CT (**B**).

There was considerable variation in reported detection rates of primary tumors among the publications included in this review (24–63%). In one report, FDG-PET detected primary lesions that were confirmed by tissue sampling in 24% of cases. The primary site was suggested by FDG-PET for an additional five patients, resulting in an overall detection rate of 44% (70). The best results were obtained by Mantaka et al. in which primary tumors that were seen with FDG-PET in 63% of cases were verified pathologically (71). Figure 4 illustrates the use of FDG-PET in a patient with cerebral metastasis of a CUP.

Another recent study (72), which was not included in the meta-analytic review, reported that FDG-PET/CT was 53% effective in delineating primary tumors in CUP patients with cervical and extracervical metastases. If only the latter subgroup (extracervical disease) was considered, the detection rate was 45%.

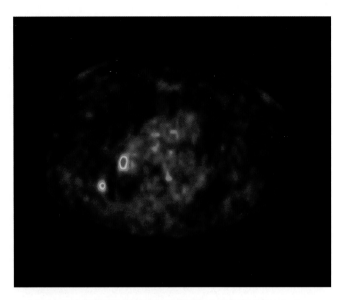

FIGURE 4 A 78-year-old woman underwent cranial exploration because of symptoms and signs of a brain tumor. Histopathologic examination revealed metastatic squamous cell carcinoma, and [18F]-fluorodeoxyglucose–positron emission tomography (FDG-PET)/CT was done subsequently to search for the primary tumor. A transaxial FDG-PET image shows the primary neoplasm in the lateral–posterior aspect of the right lung; a lymph node metastasis is also visible in the right pulmonary hilum.

Whole-Body MRI

No analysis has, to the best of our knowledge, yet been published on whole-body MRI (WB-MRI) in CUP patients. However, in a comparative study of FDG-PET/CT and WB-MRI, comprising 41 patients with a variety of tumor types, both methods were found to be equally unlikely to locate a primary tumor in four subjects with CUP (73). Comparable results were obtained in a more specific study of 21 head and neck carcinoma cases that were evaluated with WB-MRI (74).

A study by Schmidt et al. also demonstrated that among patients with a spectrum of malignancies, but not including CUPs, FDG-PET/CT and WB-MRI yielded consonant results regarding disease stage in 89% of cases. The accuracy of the individual imaging methods was 96% for FDG-PET/CT and 91% for WB-MRI (73). FDG-PET/CT detected more lymph nodal metastases than WB-MRI did. On the other hand, WB-MRI was superior at delineating distant metastases in bone and liver (73). Another such comparison—but not in CUP cases—showed that correct staging of the disease was achieved in 77% of patients by FDG-PET/CT and in 54% by WB-MRI (75). Statistically better substaging of T- and N-tumor parameters was achieved with FDG-PET/CT, but distant metastases were detected equally well by both methods. Other WB-MRI studies of oncology patients—but not including CUP cases—have compared imaging results with those obtained using conventional radiological and nuclear medicine techniques (76, 77). One publication indicated that it was feasible to perform WB-MRI in approximately 15 minutes; metastases were detected in 84% of cases, compared with 82% for conventional imaging techniques (76). Yet another study demonstrated metastases better with WB-MRI than with CT among a cross section of oncology patients. WB-MRI results produced a change in therapy in 10% of cases (77).

■ CONCLUSIONS

Patients with CUP are not uncommon, and they have a generally poor prognosis. Whether they should be imaged in an exhaustive manner depends on factors such as clinical performance status, comorbid conditions, age, the number of metastatic sites, liver or adrenal involvement, and specific histopathological diagnoses, among others. However, some subsets of CUP patients have a better outcome, and in these subjects the choice of specific diagnostic strategies has a definite impact on survival. To this end, close collaboration between radiologists, oncologists, pathologists, and other members of a multidisciplinary oncology team is essential. Between them, conclusions can be reached regarding the desirability and nature of additional imaging studies.

The purpose of radiographic evaluation in CUP cases is not only to detect the primary tumor but also to achieve reliable and objective staging of the disease. Similarly, the use of endoscopy is tailored to particular clinicopathologic CUP subsets. For example, laryngoscopy, bronchoscopy, and esophagoscopy would be appropriate for patients with cervical lymph node metastases of squamous cell or neuroendocrine carcinomas, whereas colonoscopy alone would likely be indicated in cases of CUP where metastases are restricted to the liver, and the tumor morphotype is adenocarcinoma.

The development of FDG-PET and FDG-PET/CT has clearly improved the detection rate of occult primary neoplasms in patients with CUP. Some authors have proposed that patients with cervical lymph node metastases should principally be studied with FDG-PET instead of CT and/or MRI. This is because it is highly unlikely that the latter two morphology-based methods will detect a primary tumor that could not be seen with PET (78, 79). Indeed, in some publications on CUP, FDG-PET/CT has been proposed as the initial imaging procedure that should be done, the results of which can then guide further diagnostic evaluations (80).

Published results on imaging techniques in CUP patients are sometimes difficult to compare, because the patient groups are often small, and specific diagnostic evaluations are variable in nature and with regard to the information they provide. Furthermore, PET results have been reported differently. Some authors have equated the primary-tumor detection rates with the proportion of patients with FDG-avid lesions; others have been more restrictive, requiring both FDG-avidity and surgical or histopathological confirmation.

In spite of continuing improvements in imaging technology, a considerable proportion of primary lesions in CUP cases still elude detection. This does not mean that technical advances have been fruitless in this context. As indicated, another important aspect to consider is the improved sensitivity of FDG-PET and FDG-PET/CT in diagnosing previously occult additional metastatic sites. In fact, some have even suggested that this factor may perhaps be the most important contribution of radiological evaluation to the current choice of treatment in CUP cases (79). Unfortunately, not all published FDG-PET and FDG-PET/CT studies of CUPs have reported such data, and this omission should be corrected in the future.

WB-MRI has definitely emerged as a new application for MRI in oncological imaging. WB-MRI examinations may be completed relatively rapidly, and comparative studies have shown roughly equal efficacy in staging liver and bone metastases vis-à-vis FDG-PET/CT. WB-MRI has been evaluated in a very limited number of CUP patients, and overall results have not shown it to have a clear benefit over other modalities. Additional studies in larger groups of patients will therefore be required to assess its contextual role.

■ REFERENCES

1. Nystrom JS, Weiner JM, Heffelfinger-Juttner J, Irwin LE, Bateman JR, Wolf RM. Metastatic and histologic presentations in unknown primary cancer. *Semin Oncol* 1977; 4:53–8.

2. Stewart JF, Tattersall MH, Woods RL, Fox RM. Unknown primary adenocarcinoma: incidence of overinvestigation and natural history. *Br Med J* 1979; 1:1530–3.

3. Le Chevalier T, Cvitkovic E, Caille P, et al. Early metastatic cancer of unknown primary origin at presentation. A clinical study of 302 consecutive autopsied patients. *Arch Intern Med* 1988; 148:2035–9.

4. Abbruzzese JL, Abbruzzese MC, Lenzi R, Hess KR, Raber MN. Analysis of a diagnostic strategy for patients with suspected tumors of unknown origin. *J Clin Oncol* 1995; 13:2094–10.

5. Didolkar MS, Fanous N, Elias EG, Moore RH. Metastatic carcinomas from occult primary tumors. A study of 254 patients. *Ann Surg* 1977; 186:625–30.

6. Maiche AG. Cancer of unknown primary. A retrospective study based on 109 patients. *Am J Clin Oncol* 1993; 16:26–9.

7. Blaszyk H, Hartmann A, Bjornsson J. Cancer of unknown primary: clinicopathologic correlations. *APMIS* 2003; 111: 1089–94.

8. Al-Brahim N, Ross C, Carter B, Chorneyko K. The value of postmortem examination in cases of metastasis of unknown origin-20-year retrospective data from a tertiary care center. *Ann Diagn Pathol* 2005; 9:77–80.

9. Pavlidis N, Briasoulis E, Hainsworth J, Greco FA. Diagnostic and therapeutic management of cancer of an unknown primary. *Eur J Cancer* 2003; 39:1990–2005.

10. Karsell PR, Sheedy PF 2nd, O'Connell MJ. Computed tomography in search of cancer of unknown origin. *JAMA* 1982; 248: 340–3.

11. McMillan JH, Levine E, Stephens RH. Computed tomography in the evaluation of metastatic adenocarcinoma from an unknown primary site. A retrospective study. *Radiology* 1982; 143:143–6.

12. Varadhachary GR, Abbruzzese JL, Lenzi R. Diagnostic strategies for unknown primary cancer. *Cancer* 2004; 100:1776–8.

13. Tot T. Cytokeratins 20 and 7 as biomarkers: usefulness in discriminating primary from metastatic adenocarcinoma. *Eur J Cancer* 2002; 38:758–63.

14. Milovic M, Popov I, Jelic S. Tumor markers in metastatic disease from cancer of unknown primary origin. *Med Sci Monit* 2002; 8(Suppl):MT25–MT30.

15. Pavlidis N, Kalef-Ezra J, Briassoulis E, et al. Evaluation of six tumor markers in patients with carcinoma of unknown primary. *Med Pediatr Oncol* 1994; 22:162–7.

16. Tothill RW, Kowalczyk A, Rischin D, et al. An expression-based site of origin diagnostic method designed for clinical application to cancer of unknown origin. *Cancer Res* 2005; 65:4031–40.

17. Abbruzzese JL, Abbruzzese MC, Hess KR, Raber MN, Lenzi R, Frost P. Unknown primary carcinoma: natural history and prognostic factors in 657 consecutive patients. *J Clin Oncol* 1994; 12:1272–80.

18. Hess KR, Abbruzzese MC, Lenzi R, Raber MN, Abbruzzese JL. Classification and regression tree analysis of 1000 consecutive patients with unknown primary carcinoma. *Clin Cancer Res* 1999; 5:3403–10.

19. Levi F, Te VC, Erler G, Randimbison L, La Vecchia C. Epidemiology of unknown primary tumors. *Eur J Cancer* 2002; 38: 1810–2.

20. van de Wouw AJ, Janssen-Heijnen ML, Coebergh JW, Hillen HF. Epidemiology of unknown primary tumors; incidence and population-based survival of 1285 patients in Southeast Netherlands, 1984–1992. *Eur J Cancer* 2002; 38:409–13.

21. Seve P, Sawyer M, Hanson J, Broussolle C, Dumontet C, Mackey JR. The influence of comorbidities, age, and performance status on the prognosis and treatment of patients with metastatic carcinomas of unknown primary site: a population-based study. *Cancer* 2006; 106:2058–66.

22. Shaw PH, Adams R, Jordan C, Crosby TD. A clinical review of the investigation and management of carcinoma of unknown primary in a single cancer network. *Clin Oncol (R Coll Radiol)* 2007; 19:87–95.

23. Chorost MI, Lee MC, Yeoh CB, Molina M, Ghosh BC. Unknown primary. *J Surg Oncol* 2004; 87:191–203.

24. Hillen HF. Unknown primary tumors. *Postgrad Med J* 2000; 76: 690–3.

25. Orel SG, Weinstein SP, Schnall MD, et al. Breast MR imaging in patients with axillary node metastases and unknown primary malignancy. *Radiology* 1999; 212:543–9.

26. Olson JA Jr, Morris EA, Van Zee KJ, Linehan DC, Borgen PI. Magnetic resonance imaging facilitates breast conservation for occult breast cancer. *Ann Surg Oncol* 2000; 7:411–5.

27. Obdeijn IM, Brouwers-Kuyper EM, Tilanus-Linthorst MM, Wiggers T, Oudkerk M. MR imaging-guided sonography followed by fine-needle aspiration cytology in occult carcinoma of the breast. *Am J Roentgenol* 2000; 174:1079–84.

28. Fuster D, Navasa M, Pons F, et al. In-111 octreotide scan in a case of a neuroendocrine tumor of unknown origin. *Clin Nucl Med* 1999; 24:955–8.

29. Gabriel M, Decristoforo C, Kendler D, et al. 68Ga-DOTA-Tyr3-octreotide PET in neuroendocrine tumors: comparison with somatostatin receptor scintigraphy and CT. *J Nucl Med* 2007; 48: 508–18.

30. Adams S, Baum R, Rink T, Schumm-Drager PM, Usadel KH, Hor G. Limited value of fluorine-18 fluorodeoxyglucose positron emission tomography for the imaging of neuroendocrine tumors. *Eur J Nucl Med* 1998; 25:79–83.

31. Pasquali C, Rubello D, Sperti C, et al. Neuroendocrine tumor imaging: can 18F-fluorodeoxyglucose positron emission tomography detect tumors with poor prognosis and aggressive behavior? *World J Surg* 1998; 22:588–92.

32. Gambhir SS, Czernin J, Schwimmer J, Silverman DH, Coleman RE, Phelps ME. A tabulated summary of the FDG PET literature. *J Nucl Med* 2001; 42(Suppl. 5):1S–93S.

33. Reske SN, Kotzerke J. FDG-PET for clinical use. Results of the 3rd German Interdisciplinary Consensus Conference, "Onko-PET III", 21 July and 19 September 2000. *Eur J Nucl Med* 2001; 28: 1707–23.

34. Kapoor V, McCook BM, Torok FS. An Introduction to PET-CT Imaging. *RadioGraphics* 2004; 24:523–43.

35. von Schulthess GK, Steinert HC, Hany TF. Integrated PET/CT: current applications and future directions. *Radiology* 2006; 238:405–22.

36. Ell PJ. The contribution of PET/CT to improved patient management. *Br J Radiol* 2006; 79:32–6.

37. Czernin J, Allen-Auerbach M, Schelbert HR. Improvements in cancer staging with PET/CT: literature-based evidence as of September 2006. *J Nucl Med* 2007; 48(Suppl. 1):78S–88S.

38. Blodgett TM, Meltzer CC, Townsend DW. PET/CT: form and function. *Radiology* 2007; 242:360–85.

39. Bunyaviroch T, Coleman RE. PET evaluation of lung cancer. *J Nucl Med* 2006; 47:451–69.

40. Kim BT, Lee KS, Shim SS, et al. Stage T1 non-small cell lung cancer: preoperative mediastinal nodal staging with integrated FDG PET/CT—a prospective study. *Radiology* 2006; 241:501–9.

41. Kim SK, Allen-Auerbach M, Goldin J, et al. Accuracy of PET/CT in characterization of solitary pulmonary lesions. *J Nucl Med* 2007; 48:214–20.

42. Nettelbladt OS, Sundin AE, Valind SO, et al. Combined fluorine-18-FDG and carbon-11-methionine PET for diagnosis of tumors in lung and mediastinum. *J Nucl Med* 1998; 39:640–7.

43. Chin BB, Wahl RL. 18F-fluoro-2-deoxyglucose positron emission tomography in the evaluation of gastrointestinal malignancies. *Gut* 2003; 52:23–9.

44. Kantorova I, Lipska L, Belohlavek O, Visokai V, Trubac M, Schneiderova M. Routine 18F-FDG PET preoperative staging of colorectal cancer: comparison with conventional staging and its impact on treatment decision making. *J Nucl Med* 2003; 44:1784–8.

45. Esteves FP, Schuster DM, Halkar RK. Gastrointestinal tract malignancies and positron emission tomography: an overview. *Semin Nucl Med* 2006; 36:169–81.

46. Juweid ME, Cheson BD. Role of positron emission tomography in lymphoma. *J Clin Oncol* 2005; 23:4577–80.

47. Rodriguez M, Ahlström H, Sundin A, et al. [18F] FDG PET in gastric non-Hodgkin's lymphoma. *Acta Oncol* 1997; 36:577–84.

48. Kasamon YL, Jones RJ, Wahl RL. Integrating PET and PET/CT into the risk-adapted therapy of lymphoma. *J Nucl Med* 2007; 48(Suppl. 1):19S–27S.

49. Kapoor V, Fukui MB, McCook BM. Role of [18F]FDG PET/CT in the treatment of head and neck cancers: principles, technique,

50. Ekberg T, Sorensen J, Engstrom M, Blomquist E, Sundin A, Anniko M. Clinical impact of positron emission tomography (PET) with (18F)fluorodeoxyglucose (FDG) in head and neck tumors. *Acta Otolaryngol* 2007; 127:186–93.

51. Belhocine TZ, Scott AM, Even-Sapir E, Urbain JL, Essner R. Role of nuclear medicine in the management of cutaneous malignant melanoma. *J Nucl Med* 2006; 47:957–67.

52. Bastiaannet E, Oyen WJ, Meijer S, et al. Impact of [18F]fluorodeoxyglucose positron emission tomography on surgical management of melanoma patients. *Br J Surg* 2006; 93:243–9.

53. Lin WY, Tsai SC, Hung GU. Value of delayed 18F-FDG-PET imaging in the detection of hepatocellular carcinoma. *Nucl Med Commun* 2005; 26:315–21.

54. Berthelsen AK, Holm S, Loft A, Klausen TL, Andersen F, Hojgaard L. PET/CT with intravenous contrast can be used for PET attenuation correction in cancer patients. *Eur J Nucl Med Mol Imaging* 2005; 32:1167–75.

55. Yau YY, Chan WS, Tam YM, et al. Application of intravenous contrast in PET/CT: does it really introduce significant attenuation correction error? *J Nucl Med* 2005; 46:283–91.

56. Brechtel K, Klein M, Vogel M, et al. Optimized contrast-enhanced CT protocols for diagnostic whole-body 18F-FDG PET/CT: technical aspects of single-phase versus multiphase CT imaging. *J Nucl Med* 2006; 47:470–6.

57. Kuehl H, Veit P, Rosenbaum SJ, Bockisch A, Antoch G. Can PET/CT replace separate diagnostic CT for cancer imaging? Optimizing CT protocols for imaging cancers of the chest and abdomen. *J Nucl Med* 2007; 48(Suppl. 1):45S–57S.

58. Pfannenberg AC, Aschoff P, Brechtel K, et al. Value of contrast-enhanced multi-phase CT in combined PET/CT protocols for oncological imaging. *Br J Radiol* 2007; 80:437–45.

59. Rusthoven KE, Koshy M, Paulino AC. The role of fluorodeoxyglucose positron emission tomography in cervical lymph node metastases from an unknown primary tumor. *Cancer* 2004; 101: 2641–9.

60. Fogarty GB, Peters LJ, Stewart J, Scott C, Rischin D, Hicks RJ. The usefulness of fluorine 18-labelled deoxyglucose positron emission tomography in the investigation of patients with cervical lymphadenopathy from an unknown primary tumor. *Head Neck* 2003; 25:138–45.

61. Kresnik E, Mikosch P, Gallowitsch HJ, et al. Evaluation of head and neck cancer with 18F-FDG PET: a comparison with conventional methods. *Eur J Nucl Med* 2001; 28:816–21.

62. Miller FR, Hussey D, Beeram M, Eng T, McGuff HS, Otto RA. Positron emission tomography in the management of unknown primary head and neck carcinoma. *Arch Otolaryngol Head Neck Surg* 2005; 131:626–9.

63. Guntinas-Lichius O, Peter Klussmann J, Dinh S, et al. Diagnostic work-up and outcome of cervical metastases from an unknown primary. *Acta Otolaryngol* 2006; 126:536–44.

64. Nabili V, Zaia B, Blackwell KE, Head CS, Grabski K, Sercarz JA. Positron emission tomography: poor sensitivity for occult tonsillar cancer. *Am J Otolaryngol* 2007; 28:153–7.

65. Paul SA, Stoeckli SJ, von Schulthess GK, Goerres GW. FDG PET and PET/CT for the detection of the primary tumor in patients with cervical non-squamous cell carcinoma metastasis of an unknown primary. *Eur Arch Otorhinolaryngol* 2007; 264:189–95.

66. Gutzeit A, Antoch G, Kuhl H, et al. Unknown primary tumors: detection with dual-modality PET/CT—initial experience. *Radiology* 2005; 234:227–34.

67. Wartski M, Le Stanc E, Gontier E, et al. In search of an unknown primary tumor presenting with cervical metastases: performance of hybrid FDG-PET-CT. *Nucl Med Commun* 2007; 28:365–7.

68. Fencl P, Belohlavek O, Skopalova M, Jaruskova M, Kantorova I, Simonova K. Prognostic and diagnostic accuracy of [(18)F]FDG-PET/CT in 190 patients with carcinoma of unknown primary. *Eur J Nucl Med Mol Imaging* 2007; 34(11):1783–92.

69. Seve P, Billotey C, Broussolle C, Dumontet C, Mackey JR. The role of 2-deoxy-2-[F-18]fluoro-D-glucose positron emission tomography in disseminated carcinoma of unknown primary site. *Cancer* 2007; 109:292–9.

70. Kolesnikov-Gauthier H, Levy E, Merlet P, et al. FDG PET in patients with cancer of an unknown primary. *Nucl Med Commun* 2005; 26:1059–66.

71. Mantaka P, Baum RP, Hertel A, et al. PET with 2-[F-18]-fluoro-2-deoxy-D-glucose (FDG) in patients with cancer of unknown primary (CUP): influence on patients' diagnostic and therapeutic management. *Cancer Biother Radiopharm* 2003; 18:47–58.

72. Ambrosini V, Nanni C, Rubello D, et al. 18F-FDG PET/CT in the assessment of carcinoma of unknown primary origin. *Radiol Med (Torino)* 2006; 111:1146–55.

73. Schmidt GP, Baur-Melnyk A, Herzog P, et al. High-resolution whole-body magnetic resonance image tumor staging with the use of parallel imaging versus dual-modality positron emission tomography-computed tomography: experience on a 32-channel system. *Invest Radiol* 2005; 40:743–53.

74. Herborn CU, Unkel C, Vogt FM, Massing S, Lauenstein TC, Neumann A. Whole-body MRI for staging patients with head and neck squamous cell carcinoma. *Acta Otolaryngol* 2005; 125: 1224–9.

75. Antoch G, Vogt FM, Freudenberg LS, et al. Whole-body dual-modality PET/CT and whole-body MRI for tumor staging in oncology. *JAMA* 2003; 290:3199–206.

76. Lauenstein TC, Goehde SC, Herborn CU, et al. Whole-body MR imaging: evaluation of patients for metastases. *Radiology* 2004; 233:139–48.

77. Schlemmer HP, Schafer J, Pfannenberg C, et al. Fast whole-body assessment of metastatic disease using a novel magnetic resonance imaging system: initial experiences. *Invest Radiol* 2005; 40: 64–71.

78. Schoder H, Yeung HW. Positron emission imaging of head and neck cancer, including thyroid carcinoma. *Semin Nucl Med* 2004; 34:180–97.

79. Basu S, Alavi A. FDG-PET in the clinical management of carcinoma of unknown primary with metastatic cervical lymphadenopathy: shifting gears from detecting the primary to planning therapeutic strategies. *Eur J Nucl Med Mol Imaging* 2007; 34: 427–8.

80. Jerusalem G, Rorive A, Ancion G, Hustinx R, Fillet G. Diagnostic and therapeutic management of carcinoma of unknown primary: radio-imaging investigations. *Ann Oncol* 2006; 17(Suppl. 10): x168–x176.

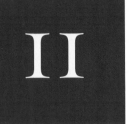

Chemotherapy

II

NICHOLAS PAVLIDIS

■ GENERAL ASPECTS

Carcinoma of unknown primary site (CUP) accounts for approximately 3% to 5% of all malignant tumors and is therefore one of the 10 most common cancer diagnoses in humans. The median age at presentation is approximately 60 years, with a marginally higher frequency in males (1, 2). CUP refers to patients who present with histologically confirmed metastatic carcinoma in whom a detailed medical history, complete physical examination, full blood count and biochemical evaluation, urinalysis and occult blood testing of stool, thorough pathological review of biopsy material, chest radiography, computed tomography (CT) of the abdomen and pelvis and, in certain cases, mammography, fail to identify a primary site for the lesion (3).

CUPs represent a heterogeneous group of malignancies that share a unique clinical behavior. In this set of tumors, most of which follow an aggressive biological and clinical course, there are no obvious etiological factors or known risks that contribute to the pathogenesis of the syndrome. Similarly, no specific genetic or phenotypic changes have been identified that might characterize this distinctive biological entity. It seems that the primary tumor in CUP cases may either have a slow growth rate, or it may possibly involute, resulting in the absence of clinical manifestations of a lesion at the primary site (4).

CUPs are categorized into four major subtypes by routine light microscopic criteria: (*i*) well-to-moderately differentiated adenocarcinoma, (*ii*) poorly differentiated adenocarcinomas, (*iii*) squamous cell carcinomas (SCCs), and (*iv*) undifferentiated neoplasms. The majority of patients have well- or moderately differentiated metastatic adenocarcinomas, 30% have poorly differentiated adenocarcinomas, 15% have SCCs, and the remaining 5% have undifferentiated neoplasms. The last group includes carcinomas not further specified, neuroendocrine carcinomas, malignant germ cell tumors, and embryonal malignancies (5).

The natural history of CUP patients differs considerably from that of individuals with known primary tumors. Early dissemination, a clinical absence of the primary tumor, unpredictability of metastatic patterns, and overall aggressiveness constitute the fundamental characteristics of CUP cases. The unpredictability of metastatic patterns refers to differences in the incidence of sites that are involved by metastases at diagnosis, when comparing CUP patients with those having known primary carcinomas (3, 4, 6, 7).

The diagnostic evaluation in such cases must include extensive pathological investigations and state-of-the-art imaging technology. Despite such assessments, the primary tumor usually remains undetected, even at autopsy. However, when they are discovered, tumors are most frequently found in the lungs or pancreas (3, 4).

■ CUPs: CLINICOPATHOLOGICAL ENTITIES

In order to provide appropriate therapeutic guidance, CUP entities should be classified as favorable or unfavorable subsets. Several clinicopathological entities in each category have been recognized based on their responses to treatment and outcome (Table 1).

Certain favorable subsets require specific treatment modalities and have a potential for a better-than-average outcome. Unfortunately, patients with tumors in unfavorable subsets are more common, and they have a generally dismal prognosis, with short survivals.

■ THERAPEUTIC MANAGEMENT OF CUP PATIENTS

History of Chemotherapy for CUP (1964–2007)

In the early 1960s and 1970s, systemic treatment for CUP was based mainly on fluorouracil- or adriamycin-containing regimens. Other cytostatics included in such regimens were cyclophosphamide, vinca alkaloids, and mitomycin-C. Treatment responses were seen in approximately 20% of cases, but with very few complete remissions. Median survival ranged between three and seven months (Table 2) (8–19).

Table 1 Favorable and unfavorable subsets of carcinoma of unknown primary site

Favorable Subsets	Unfavorable Subsets
Poorly differentiated carcinoma with midline nodal distribution	Adenocarcinoma metastatic to the liver or other organs
Women with papillary adenocarcinoma of peritoneal cavity	Malignant ascites from a nonpapillary adenocarcinoma
Poorly differentiated neuroendocrine carcinomas	Multiple cerebral metastases from an adenocarcinoma or squamous carcinoma
Women with adenocarcinoma involving only axillary lymph nodes	Multiple lung/pleural metastases from an adenocarcinoma
Squamous cell carcinoma involving cervical lymph nodes	Multiple metastatic bone disease from an adenocarcinoma
Men with blastic bone metastatic lesions from an adenocarcinoma with elevated serum prostate-specific antigen	
Isolated inguinal lymphadenopathy from squamous carcinoma	
Patients with a single small metastasis	

Table 2 Results from fluorouracil-anthracycline-based chemotherapy in patients with carcinoma of unknown primary site

Drug Combination	N	Response Rate (%)	Median Survival (Months)
FU vs. various (8)	103	6.2 vs. 2.6	9
FU vs. combinations vs. various (9)	213	16 vs. 9.5 vs. 8.5	3.5
CAF (10)	100	21	7+
FAM (11)	28	21.4	7.6
CAV (12)	20	50	8
AV (13)	38	13.2	7
FAM (14)	43	30.2	11
FU, DTIC, VCR, BCNU (15)	61	20	3.6
FAM (16)	29	10.3	3.5
AVM (17)	57	30	
PALA, MTX, FU (18)	21	5	
Etoposide (19)	25	8	

Abbreviations: AV, adriamycin, vindesine; AVM, adriamycin, vincristine, mitomycin; BCNU, carmustine; CAF, cyclophosphamide, adriamycin, fluorouracil; CAV, cyclophosphamide, adriamycin, vincristine; DTIC, decarbazine; FAM, fluorouracil, adriamycin, mitomycin; FU, fluorouracil; GCSF, granulocyte colony stimulating factor; MTX, methotrexate; PALA, N-phosphoacetyl-1-aspartate; VCR, vincristine.

Table 3 Phase II studies in carcinoma of unknown primary site patients using platinum-based regimens

Drug Combination	N	Response Rate (%)	Median Survival (Months)
FACP (20)	23	17	6
PVeB (21)	56	57	16
FAPH (22)	85	21	6
PEB (23)	34	79	8+
FEP (24)	36	22	11
PFL (25)	25	32	–
PE (26)	16	19	8
PVB ± Doxo (27)	68	56	–
P (28)	21	19	5
P-containing vs. Cb-containing (29)	48	29	4.3
PF (30)	15	53	–
P-based (31)	92	37.2	6.4
CbFL (32)	40	25	7.8
CbEpE (33)	62	37	10
PMiEp (34)	40	50	9.4
CbE (35)	26	23	5.6
PF (36)	44	27	–
ECF (37)	34	19	8.25
PE (38)	23	32	8
PAC (39)	22	50	10.7
ECF (40)	36	22	9
CA alternating with PE/GCSF (41)	82	39	10

(Continued)

Table 3 Phase II studies in carcinoma of unknown primary site patients using platinum-based regimens (*Continued*)

Drug Combination	N	Response Rate (%)	Median Survival (Months)
PMiF (42)	31	27	7.7
PEG (43)	30	36.6	7.2
CbEA (44)	102	26.5	9
CbG (45)	51	30.5	8.5

Abbreviations: A, adriamycin; B, bleomycin; C, cyclophosphamide; Cb, carboplatin; E, etoposide; Ep: epirubicin; F, fluorouracil; G, gemcitabine; H, hexamethymelamine; I, ifosfamide; L, leucovorin; Mi, mitomycin-C; P, cisplatin; Ve, vinblastine.

Platinum-based combination therapies appeared in the late 1980s. Other drugs that were used, beginning in that period, included etoposide, vinca alkaloids, anthracyclines, cyclophosphamide, bleomycin, and, more recently, other novel agents such as vinorelbine, gemcitabine, and irinotecan. From these studies, certain chemoresponsive entities emerged in relation to platinum-based chemotherapy, such as poorly differentiated carcinomas (PDCs) with a midline nodal-centered distribution, papillary peritoneal adenocarcinomatosis, and neuroendocrine carcinomas. Responses were improved to 40% to 50%, and several months were added to the median survival. In addition, long-term survivors in chemosensitive tumor subgroups were documented (Table 3) (20–45).

Since 2001, taxanes have been integrated with cisplatinum or carboplatinum-based regimens, but response rates and survivals have remained largely unchanged. Paclitaxel is the most commonly used taxane. Etoposide and gemcitabine have also been combined with paclitaxel or docetaxel (Table 4) (46–58). Table 5 presents a summary of results of chemotherapy for CUP patients during the last 40 years.

Treatment of Favorable Subsets

In Table 6, a review of the chemotherapy-related outcome of three chemoresponsive CUP subsets is outlined.

PDC with Midline Distribution

This subset behaves similarly to extragonadal malignant germ cell tumors and is seen mainly in men who are less than 50 years old. It usually affects midline lymph nodal chains (supraclavicular, mediastinal, or paraortic), but occasionally can be accompanied by concomitant parenchymal

■ **Table 4** Results from phase II studies in patients with carcinoma of unknown primary site using taxane-platinum-based regimens

Drug Combination	N	Response Rate (%)	Median Survival (Months)
P_LC_bE (46)	55	47	13.4
P_LCb (47)	77	38.7	13
P_LCbE (48)	71	48	11
PD_X (49)	22	33	8
D_X (50)	29	7	6
P_LPG (51)	29	50	–
P_LCbG (52)	120	25	9
$P_LCbE \rightarrow GI_R$ (53)	132	30	9.1
P_LP (54)	37	42	11
D_XG (55)	35	40	10
P_LCb (56)	22	23	6.5
P_LCbE (57)	78[a]	53	14.5
P_LCb(weekly) (58)	42	18	8.5

[a]Neuroendocrine CUP.

Abbreviations: Cb, carboplatin; D_x, docetaxel; E, etoposide; G, gemcitabine; I_R, irinotecan; P, cisplatin; P_L, paclitaxel.

■ **Table 5** Efficacy of chemotherapy in carcinoma of unknown primary site patients during the last 40 years

Drug-Based Chemotherapy	Response Rate (%)	Median Survival (Months)
5-Fluorouracil/ anthracyclines	13 (2–50)	7 (3.5–11)
Platinum	30 (17–79)	8 (4.3–72)
Taxanes/platinum	39 (7–50)	10 (6–48)

■ **Table 6** Results of platinum- and/or taxane-based chemotherapy in chemosensitive favorable carcinoma of unknown primary site subsets at a glance

CUP Subset	Response Rate/ Complete Responses	Median Survival (Months)
Poorly differentiated carcinoma with midline nodal distribution	30–50%/ 10–25%	13 (10–15%, long-term survivors)
Papillary adenocarcinoma of peritoneal cavity (women)	40–60%/ 25–35%	16 (10%, 5-yr survival)
Poorly differentiated neuroendocrine carcinoma	50–70%/ 15–30%	14.5 (24%, 3-yr survival)

Abbreviation: CUP, carcinoma of unknown primary site.

pulmonary lesions. Serum beta-human chorionic gonadotropin or alpha-fetoprotein levels are increased in around 20% of such cases. Midline PDC is characterized as a CUP subset that is sensitive to platinum-based chemotherapy, and it should be treated as would be poor prognosis germ cell malignancies. High rates of response, in up to 50% of cases, with 15% to 25% complete remission and 10% to 15% long-term disease-free survivors have been observed (23, 59).

Women with Papillary Adenocarcinoma of the Peritoneal Cavity

These patients should be managed as FIGO stage III ovarian carcinomas. Optimal surgical cytoreduction, followed by taxane and/or platinum-based systemic chemotherapy, is recommended. High response rates of up to 50%, including complete remissions in 30% to 35%, have been seen. The median survival in this group is 16 months, and five-year survivals of 10% have been realized. No data are available concerning the use of intraperitoneal chemotherapy in this subset of CUP patients (60, 61).

Poorly Differentiated Neuroendocrine Carcinoma

Poorly differentiated neuroendocrine carcinoma has been characterized as a highly chemoresponsive tumor with reference to cisplatin-based treatment. In 1988, Hainsworth et al. reported a response rate of 72% (with 24% complete responses) and 15% long-term disease-free survivors in this CUP subset. Recently, the same researchers, using a combination of paclitaxel, carboplatin, and etoposide, reported major tumor responses in 53% of cases, with 15% complete remissions. Median survival was 14.5 months, with 24% overall three-year survival (57, 62, 63).

Women with Adenocarcinoma Involving Only Axillary Lymph Nodes

In the CUP subgroup of female patients with only axillary lymph-nodal metastasis, locoregional treatment, with or without chemotherapy or hormonal therapy, is recommended. However, data from randomized large prospective studies are lacking. The management in this tumor subset is similar to that used for stage II or III breast carcinoma patients. Those with mobile lymph-node metastases (N1 disease) should undergo surgical axillary clearance followed by either simple mastectomy or radiation therapy to the breast. Adjuvant chemotherapy in premenopausal women, followed by tamoxifen administration in estrogen receptor (ER)–positive cases, is suggested. For postmenopausal patients with ER-positive neoplasms, tamoxifen is the treatment of choice. Patients with fixed lymph-node metastases (N2 disease) should be given preoperative neoadjuvant chemotherapy, following guidelines for stage III breast carcinoma. In nonresponding cases or in elderly patients, radical radiation therapy can be offered, and subsequent hormonal treatment can be given provided the tumor is ER positive (64–66).

SCC Involving Cervical Lymph Nodes

The management of patients with metastatic SCC in cervical lymph nodes should parallel established guidelines for locally advanced carcinomas of the head and neck. Locoregional treatment is most appropriate. The five-year survival in such cases ranges from 35% to 50%, depending on nodal status. Long-term disease-free survivors have been documented. Only cases showing pN1 neck disease without extranodal extension by metastasis should be managed surgically. All other patients require combined-modality treatment.

Radiation should be given to both sides of the neck and the mucosa of the entire pharyngeal axis and larynx. Locoregional failures occur more commonly if only ipsilateral cervical nodes are irradiated. Concurrent chemoradiotherapy is recommended for patients with N2 or N3 nodal disease (67, 68).

Men with Blastic Bone Metastases of Adenocarcinoma and Elevated Serum Levels of Prostate-Specific Antigen

This is a rare and relatively favorable prognosis CUP subgroup. It comprises men who should be managed as if they have metastatic prostatic carcinoma, usually including hormonal therapy (3, 69).

Isolated Inguinal Lymph Node Metastasis of SCC

In these rare cases, lymph nodal dissection with or without local radiation treatment is the recommended approach. Long-term disease-free survival has been documented. No systematic data on chemotherapy are available (3).

Patients with a Single Small Metastasis

Patients with a single small focus of metastatic carcinoma enjoy palliative benefit, or even long disease-free survival, after only local resection, with or without radiotherapy (3).

Treatment of Unfavorable CUP Subsets

Unfortunately, most CUP cases belong to prognostically unfavorable subgroups. The majority of patients have differentiated metastatic adenocarcinomas, and their clinical picture is characterized by disseminated metastases involving the liver, bones, lungs, or central nervous system.

Despite some response to chemotherapy in many cases, the ultimate prognosis is poor. In general, several platinum or taxane/platinum-based chemotherapy regimens have yielded better responses and relatively longer survivals compared with older treatment schemes.

One should always be cautious in regard to interpretation of these results, because of the heterogeneity of CUP populations, the retrospective nature of many studies, and biases concerning patient selection in reference to median age, performance status, and so on. Population-based data from European registries report a median age of 70 years and a survival of two to three months in an unselected CUP case population, whereas the median age was less than 60 years and median survival was six to seven months among patients who were enrolled in clinical protocols (2, 70). Based on three studies that were published between 1998 and 2005, with almost 400 CUP patients with liver metastases, more than 20% had responses to principally platinum-based chemotherapy regimens, and their median survival was less than seven months (71–73).

In conclusion, patients with unfavorable CUPs who are relatively young and have a good performance status should be offered platinum-based chemotherapy. Alternatively, optimal supportive care is recommended.

Randomized Prospective Studies of CUP

Prospective phase II randomized studies of treatment for CUP, with relatively small numbers of patients, are also available in the literature. Initially, nonplatinum combinations were compared, whereas more recent analyses have focused on platinum- and/or taxane-based combination regimens. None of the published randomized trials

Table 7 Prospective randomized studies in CUP site patients

Drug Combination	N	Response Rate (%)	Median Survival (Months)
MiA vs. CMF (74)	47	36 vs. 4.5	4.2 vs. 3
F vs. FAC (75)	36	0 vs. 0	3.5 vs. 3.0
MA vs. CVB (76)	95	42 vs. 32	4.1 vs. 5.8
MA vs. MAP (77)	55	7.1 vs. 18.5	5.5 vs. 4.6
EP/AC vs. high dose (78)	60	42 vs. 39	11 vs. 8
PD$_X$ vs. CbD$_X$ (79)	73	26 vs. 22	8 vs. 8
CbE vs. P$_L$F$_L$ (80)	34	19 vs. 19	8.3 vs. 6.4
PG vs. PI$_R$ (81)	80	42 vs. 25	22% vs. 23% (1 yr survival)
F vs. F + Mi (82)	88	11.6 vs. 20	6.6 vs. 4.7
PG vs. PI$_R$ (83)	80	55 vs. 38	8 vs. 6
P$_L$Cb vs. GV$_L$ (84)	90	21.5 vs. 21.5	10.7 vs. 6.9
PGbP$_L$ vs. PGbV$_L$ (85)	66	48.5 vs. 42.3	9.6 vs. 13.6

Abbreviations: F, fluorouracil; A, adriamycin; C, cyclophosphamide; Mi, mitomycin; M, methotrexate; Cb, carboplatin; E, etoposide; L, leucovorin; V, vincristine; B, bleomycin; G, gemcitabine; I$_R$, irinotecan; D$_X$, docetaxel; P$_L$, paclitaxel; V$_L$, vinorelbine; P, cisplatin.

Table 8 Second-line chemotherapy in CUP site patients

Drugs	N	Response Rate (%)	Median Survival (Months)
G (86)	39	8	–
FL (87)	25	0	9[a]
D$_X$G (88)	15	28	8[b]
GI$_R$ (89)	40	10	4.5

[a]From diagnosis.
[b]From start of second-line treatment.

Abbreviations: D$_x$, docetaxel; F, fluorouracil; G, gemcitabine; I$_R$, irinotecan; L, leucovorin.

were able to show any significant difference in clinical response or median survival (Table 7). Several other randomized phase III studies are still underway both in Europe and in the United States, comparing single versus combination chemotherapy, or platinum- versus non-platinum-based regimens. Both "good" and "poor" prognosis CUP patients have been included in such assessments (74–85).

"Second-Line" Chemotherapy

During the last six years, four phase II trials have been reported, including a total of 120 CUP patients who failed first-line treatment. Chemotherapeutic combinations with various cytostatics, such as fluorouracil, leucovorin, gemcitabine, irinotecan, or docetaxel, were administered. Most of them showed no substantially beneficial results. Nevertheless, in one small analysis using docetaxel and gemcitabine, a response rate of 28% and a median survival of eight months was observed, after initiating second-line treatment (Table 8) (86–89).

Targeted Treatments

There is anecdotal evidence of two CUP patients who were treated with thalidomide and steroids, and with the combination of trastuzumab and vinorelbine. Both individuals exhibited partial remissions lasting for 17 and 7 months, respectively (90, 91). In another phase II study, 51 patients were treated with bevacizumab and erlotinib as a second-line regimen. Four of them (8%) achieved a partial response, and 30 patients (59%) had stable disease with a median overall survival of eight to nine months (92).

■ PROGNOSTIC VARIABLES IN CUP CASES

Various independent prognostic factors have been identified in patients with CUPs. Several clinical, histopathological, serological, and biological analytes were found to be inversely correlated with survival. Among these, male sex, poor performance status, a high number of metastatic sites, unfavorable histopathologic subsets, the presence of hepatic metastases, elevated serum alkaline phosphatase levels, elevated serum lactate dehydrogenase levels, low serum albumin values, and lymphopenia were found to be the most important (93–97).

LATE SEQUELAE RELATED TO TREATMENT

Surgery-Related Sequelae

Clinically, long-term sequelae owing to surgical procedures in specific CUP subsets (such as women with adenocarcinoma in axillary lymph nodes, women with papillary adenocarcinoma of the peritoneal cavity, and patients with SCC in cervical lymph nodes) are no different than those seen in patients with known primary breast, ovarian, or head and neck carcinomas of similar clinical stages. Therefore, recommended surgical approaches for these groups of patients are comparable.

Radiotherapy-Related Sequelae

Sequelae related to radiotherapy, which is primarily employed in women with metastatic adenocarcinoma in axillary lymph nodes or cases with SCC in cervical lymph nodes, are likewise similar to those observed in cases of known primary breast and head and neck carcinoma.

Chemotherapy-Related Sequelae

In the majority of CUP patients, late sequelae of chemotherapy do not represent a serious clinical problem. This is principally true because median survival is typically no longer than one year. In a minority of patients with longer survivals, late toxicities are similar to those seen in patients who have been treated with platinum- and/or taxane-based chemotherapy for known primary carcinomas.

FOLLOW-UP

The short life expectancy of most CUP patients leaves little room for developing standarized recommendations for follow-up strategies. Generally speaking, after termination of therapy, patients with unfavorable subsets should visit outpatient clinics upon need, but patients with a favorable CUP subset diagnosis should be seen on a regular basis similar to that followed for the respective solid tumor, such as germ-line tumors for patients with middle-line distribution, ovarian cancer for carcinomatosis peritonei in women, and breast cancer for patients with axillary nodal metastases.

CUP GUIDELINE WEB SITES

Guideline recommendations for the treatment of CUPs are available on the following Web pages:

1. European Society for Medical Oncology (ESMO) Clinical Recommendations: www.esmo.org/reference/reference.guidelines.htm

2. National Cancer Institute's Physician Data Query (NCI/PDQ): http://www.cancer.gov/cancertopics/pdq/treatment/unknownprimary/healthprofessional

3. State of the Art Oncology in Europe (StART): www.startoncology.net

REFERENCES

1. Ries LAG, Eisner MP, Kosary CL, et al. SEER Cancer Statistics Review. Bethesda: National Cancer Institute, 1999.

2. Levi F, Te VC, Eler G, Randimbision L, La Vecchia C. Epidemiology of unknown primary tumors. *Eur J Cancer* 2002; 38:1810–2.

3. Pavlidis N, Briasoulis E, Hainsworth J, Greco FA. Diagnostic and therapeutic management of cancer of an unknown primary. *Eur J Cancer* 2003; 39:1990–2005.

4. Pavlidis N, Fizazi K. Cancer of unknown primary (CUP). *Crit Rev Oncol Hematol* 2005; 54(3):243–50.

5. Fritz A, Percy C, Jack A, et al., eds. *ICD-O. International Classification of Diseases for Oncology.* 3rd ed. Geneva: World Health Organization, 2000.

6. Nystrom JS, Weiner JM, Hellelfinger-Juttner J, Irwin LE, Bateman JR, Wolf RM. Metastatic and histologic presentation in unknown primary cancer. *Semin Oncol* 1977; 4:53–8.

7. Briasoulis E, Pavlidis N. Cancer of unknown primary origin. *Oncologist* 1997; 2:142–52.

8. Johnson R, Castro R, Ansfield F. Response of primary unknown cancers to treatment with 5-fluorouracil (NSC-19893). *Cancer Chemoth Reports* 1964; 38:63–4.

9. Moertel C, Reitemeier R, Schutt AJ, Hhn RG. Treatment of the patient with adenocarcinoma of unknown origin. *Cancer* 1972; 30:1469–72.

10. Valentine J, Rosenthal S, Arseneau J. Combination chemotherapy for adenocarcinoma of unknown primary origin. *Cancer Clin Trials* 1979; 2:265–8.

11. McKeen E, Smith F, Haidak D. Fluorouracil, adriamycin and mitomycin-C for adenocarcinoma of unknown origin (abstr). *Proc Am Assoc Cancer Res* 1980; 21:358.

12. Anderson H, Thatcher N, Rankin E, Wagstaff J, Scarffe JH, Crowther D. VAC (vincristine, adriamycin and cyclophosphamide) chemotherapy for metastasis carcinoma from an unknown primary site. *Eur J Cancer Clin Oncol* 1983; 19:49–52.

13. Fiore JJ, Kelsen DP, Gralla RJ, et al. Adenocarcinoma of unknown primary origin:treatment with vindesine and doxorubicin. *Cancer Treat Rep* 1984; 69:591–4.

14. Goldberg RM, Smith FP, Ueno W, Ahlgren JD, Schein PS. Fluorouracil, adriamycin and mitomycin in the treatment of unknown primary. *J Clin Oncol* 1986; 4:395–9.

15. Alberts AS, Falkson G, Falkson HC, van der Merwe MP. Treatment and prognosis of metastatic carcinoma of unknown primary: analysis of 100 patients. *Med Pediatr Oncol* 1989; 17 (3):188–92.

16. Al-Idrissi HY. Combined 5-fluorouracil, adriamycin and mitomycin–C in the management of adenocarcinoma metastasizing to the liver from an unknown primary site. *J Int Med Res* 1990; 18 (5):425–9.

17. Kambhu SA, Kelsen DP, Fiore J, et al. Metastatic adenocarcinomas of unknown primary site. Prognostic variables and treatment results. *Am J Clin Oncol* 1990; 13(1):55–60.

18. Kelsen D, Martin DS, Colofiore J, Sawyer R, Coit D. A phase II trial of biochemical modulation using N-phosphonacetyl–L-aspartate,

high-dose methotrexate, high-dose 5-fluorouracil, and leucovorin in patients with adenocarcinoma of unknown primary site. *Cancer* 1992; 70(7):1988–92.

19. van der Gaast A, Henzen-Logmans SC, Planting AS, Stoter G, Verweij J. Phase II study of oral administration of etoposide for patients with well—and moderately—differentiated adenocarcinomas of unknown primary site. *Ann Oncol* 1993; 4 (9):789–90.

20. Jadeja J, Legha S, Burgess M. Combination chemotherapy with 5-fluorouracil, adriamycin, cyclophosphamide, and cis-platinum in the treatment of adenocarcinoma of unknown primary and undifferentiated carcinomas. *Proc Am Soc Clin Oncol* 1983; 926 (abstr).

21. Greco FA, Vaughn WK, Hainsworth JD. Advanced poorly differentiated carcinoma of unknown primary site: recognition of a treatable syndrome. *Ann Intern Med* 1986; 142:547–53.

22. Becouarn Y, Brunet R, Barbe-Gaston C. Fluorouracil, doxorubicin, cisplatin and altretanine in the treatment of metastatic carcinoma of unknown primary. *Eur J Cancer Clin Oncol* 1989; 25:861–8.

23. van der Gaast, Verweij J, Henzen-Logmans SC, Rodenburg CJ, Stoter G. Carcinoma of unknown primary: identification of a treatable subset? *Ann Oncol* 1990; 1:119–22.

24. Raber MN, Faintuch J, Abbruzzese LJ, Sumrall C, Frost P. Continuous infusion 5-fluorouracil, etoposide and *cis*-diamminedichloroplatinum in patients with metastatic carcinoma of unknown primary origin. *Ann Oncol* 1991; 2:519–20.

25. Lenzi R, Abbruzzese J, Amato R. Cisplatin, 5-fluorouracil and follinic acid for the treatment of carcinoma of unknown primary: a phase II study. *Proc Am Soc Clin Oncol* 1991; 10:301(abstr).

26. Gill I, Guaglianone P, Grunberg SM, Scholz M, Muggia FM. High dose intensity of cisplatin and etoposide in adenocarcinoma of unknown primary. *Anticancer Res* 1991; 11:1231–5.

27. Hainsworth JD, Johnson DH, Greco FA. The role of etoposide in the treatment of poorly differentiated carcinoma of unknown primary site. *Cancer* 1991; 67(Suppl. 1):310–4.

28. Wagener DJ, de Mulder PH, Burghouts JT, Croles JJ. Phase II trial of cisplatin for adenocarcinoma of unknown primary site. IKZ/IKO Clinical Research Group. *Eur J Cancer* 1991; 27(6): 755–7.

29. Pavlidis N, Kosmidis P, Skarlos D, et al. Subsets of tumors responsive to cisplatin or carcboplatin combinations in patients with carcinoma of unknown primary site. *Ann Oncol* 1992; 3(8): 631–4.

30. Khansur T, Allred C, Little D, Anand V. Cisplatin and 5-fluorouracil for metastatic squamous cell carcinoma from unknown primary. *Cancer Invest* 1995; 13(3):263–6.

31. Farrugia DC, Norman AR, Nicolson MC, et al. Unknown primary carcinoma: randomized studies are needed to identify optimal treatments and their benefits. *Eur J Cancer* 1996; 32A(13):2256–61.

32. Rigg A, Cunningham D, Gore M, et al. A phase I/II study of leucovorin, carboplatin, and 5-fluorouracil (LCF) in patients with carcinoma of unknown primary site or advanced oesophagogastric/pancreatic adenocarcinomas. *Br J Cancer* 1997; 75(1):101–5.

33. Briasoulis E, Tsavaris N, Fountzilas G, et al. Combination regimen with carboplatin, epirubicin and etoposide in metastatic carcinomas of unknown primary site: a Hellenic Co-operative Oncology Group Phase II study. *Oncology* 1998; 55:426–30.

34. Falkson CI, Cohen GL. Mitomycin, epirubicin and cisplatin versus mitomycin-C alone as therapy for carcinoma of unknown primary origin. *Oncology* 1998; 55:116–21.

35. Warner E, Goel R, Chang J, et al. A multicenter phase II study of carboplatin and prolonged oral etoposide in the treatment of

cancer of unknown primary site (CUPS). *Br J Cancer* 1998; 77: 2376–80.

36. Lofts FJ, Gogas H, Mansi JL. Management of adenocarcinoma of unknown primary with a 5-fluorouracil-cisplatin chemotherapy regimen (CFT arm). *Ann Oncol* 1999; 10:1389–92.

37. Parnis FX, Olver IN, Kotasek D, et al. Phase II study of epirubicin, cisplatin and continuous infusion 5-fluorouracil (ECF) for carcinoma of unknown primary site. *Ann Oncol* 2000; 11(7): 883–4.

38. Voog E, Merrouche Y, Trillet-Lenoir V, et al. Multicentric phase II study of cisplatin and etoposide in patients with metastatic carcinoma of unknown primary. *Am J Clin Oncol* 2000; 23: 614–6.

39. Guardiola E, Pivot X, Tchicknavorian X, et al. Combination of cisplatin-doxorubicin-cyclophosphamide in adenocarcinoma of unknown primary site: a phase II trial. *Am J Clin Oncol* 2001; 24: 372–5.

40. Karapetis CS, Yip D, Virik K, et al. Epirubicin, cisplatin, and prolonged or brief infusional 5-fluorouracil in the treatment of carcinoma of unknown primary site. *Med Oncol* 2001; 18 (1):23–32.

41. Culine S, Fabbro M, Ychou M, Romieu G, Cupissol D, Pinguet F. Alternative bimonthly cycles of doxorubicin, cyclophosphamide, and etoposide, cisplatin with hematolopoietic growth factor support in patients with carcinoma of unknown primary site. *Cancer* 2002; 94(3):840–6.

42. Macdonald AG, Nicolson MC, Samuel LM, Hutcheon AW, Ahmed FY. A phase II study of mitomycin C, cisplatin and continuous infusion 5-fluorouracil (UCF) in the treatment of patients with carcinoma of unknown primary site. *Br J Cancer* 2002; 86:1238–42.

43. Balana C, Manzano JL, Moreno I, et al. A phase II study of cisplatin, etoposide and gemcitabine in an unfavourable group of patients with carcinoma of unknown primary site. *Ann Oncol* 2003; 14(9):1425–9.

44. Piga A, Gesuita R, Catalano V, et al. Identification of clinical prognostic factors in patients with unknown primary tumors treated with a platinum-based combination. *Oncology* 2005; 69 (2):135–44.

45. Pittman KB, Olver IN, Koczwara B, et al. Gemcitabine and carboplatin in carcinoma of unknown primary site: a phase 2 Adelaide Cancer Trials and Education Collaborative Study. *Br J Cancer* 2006; 95(10):1309–13.

46. Hainsworth JD, Erland JB, Kalman LA, Schreeder MT, Greco FA. Carcinoma of unknown primary site: treatment with 1-hour paclitaxel, carboplatin, and extended-schedule etoposide. *J Clin Oncol* 1997; 15(6):2385–93.

47. Briasoulis E, Kalofonos H, Bafaloukos D, et al. Carboplatin plus paclitaxel in unknown primary carcinoma: a phase II study. The Hellenic Cooperative Oncology Group study. *J Clin Oncol* 2000; 18:3101–17.

48. Greco FA, Burris HA 3rd, Erland EB, et al. Carcinoma of unknown primary site. *Cancer* 2000; 89:2655–60.

49. Bouleuc C, Saghatchian M, Di Tullio L, et al. A multicenter phase II study of docetaxel and cisplatin in the treatment of cancer of unknown primary site. *Proc Am Soc Clin Oncol* 2001; 137b:2298.

50. Darby AJ, Richardson L, Nokes L, Harvey M, Hassan A, Iveson T. Phase II study of single agent docetaxel in carcinoma of unknown primary site. *Proc Am Soc Clin Oncol* 2001; 100b: 2151.

51. Gothelf A, Daugaard G, Nelausen K. Paclitaxel, cisplatin and gemcitabine in the treatment of unknown primary tumors, a phase II study. *Proc ESMO* 2002; 25:88.

52. Greco FA, Burris HA 3rd, Litchy S, et al. Gemcitabine, carboplatin and paclitaxel for patients with carcinoma of unknown primary site: a Minnie Pearl Cancer Research Network study. *J Clin Oncol* 2002; 20:1651–6.

53. Greco FA, Rodriquez GI, Shaffer DW, et al. Carcinoma of unknown primary site: sequential treatment with paclitaxel/carboplatin/etoposide and gemcitabine/irinotecan: a Minnie Pearl Cancer Research Network phase II trial. *Oncologist* 2004; 9(6):644–52.

54. Park YH, Ryoo BY, Choi SJ, Yang SH, Kim HT. A phase II study of paclitaxel plus cisplatin chemotherapy in an unfavourable group of patients with cancer of unknown primary site. *Jpn J Clin Oncol* 2004; 34(11):681–5.

55. Pouessel D, Culine S, Becht C, et al. Gemcitabine and docetaxel as front-line chemotherapy in patients with carcinoma of an unknown primary site. *Cancer* 2004; 100(6):1257–61.

56. El-Rayes BF, Shields AF, Zalupski M, et al. A phase II study of carboplatin and paclitaxel in adenocarcinoma of unknown primary. *Am J Clin Oncol* 2005; 28(2):152–6.

57. Hainsworth JD, Spigel DR, Litchy S, Greco FA. Phase II trial of paclitaxel, carboplatin and etoposide in advanced poorly differentiated neuroendocrine carcinoma: a Minnie Pearl Cancer Research Network Study. *J Clin Oncol* 2006; 24(22):3548–54.

58. Berry W, Elkordy M, O'rourke M, Khan M, Asmaz L. Results of a Phase II study of weekly paclitaxel plus carboplatin in advanced carcinoma of unknown primary origin: a reasonable regimen for the community-based clinic? *Cancer Invest* 2007; 25(1):27–31.

59. van der Gaast A, Verweij J, Henzen-Logmans SC, Rodenburg CJ, Stoter G. Carcinoma of unknown primary: identification of a treatable subset. *Ann Oncol* 1990; 1:119–22.

60. Chen KT, Flam MS. Peritoneal papillary serous carcinoma with long-term survival. *Cancer* 1986; 58:1371–3.

61. Ransom DT, Patel SR, Keeney GL, Malkasian GD, Edmonson JH. Papillary serous carcinoma of the peritoneum. A review of 33 cases treated with platin-based chemotherapy. *Cancer* 1990; 66:1091–4.

62. Moertel CG, Kvols LK, O'Connell MJ, Rubin J. Treatment of neuroendocrine carcinomas with combined etoposide and cisplatin. Evidence of major therapeutic activity in the anaplastic variants of these neoplasms. *Cancer* 1991; 68:227–32.

63. Hainsworth JD, Johnson DH, Greco FA. Poorly differentiated neuroendocrine carcinoma of unknown primary site. A newly recognized clinicopathologic entity. *Ann Intern Med* 1988; 109:364–71.

64. Ellerbroek N, Holmes F, Singletary E, Evans H, Oswald M, McNeese M. Treatment of patients with isolated axillary nodal metastases from an occult primary carcinoma consistent with breast origin. *Cancer* 1990; 66:1461–7.

65. Jackson B, Scott-Conner C, Moulder J. Axillary metastasis from occult breast carcinoma: diagnosis and management. *Am Surg* 1995; 61:431–4.

66. Vlastos G, Jean ME, Mirza AN, et al. Feasibility of breast preservation in the treatment of occult primary carcinoma presenting with axillary metastases. *Ann Surg Oncol* 2001; 8:425–31.

67. Grau C, Johansen LV, Jakobsen J, Geertsen P, Andersen E, Jensen BB. Cervical lymph node metastases from unknown primary tumors. Results from a national survey by the Danish Society for Head and Neck Oncology. *Radiother Oncol* 2000; 55:121–9.

68. Nieder C, Gregoire V, Ang KK. Cervical lymph node metastases from occult squamous cell carcinoma: cut down a tree to get an apple? *Int J Radiat Oncol Biol Phys* 2001; 50:727–33.

69. Greco FA, Hainsworth JD. Cancer of unknown primary site. In: DeVita TV, Hellman S, Rosenberg SA, eds. *Cancer: Principles and Practice of Oncology*. 4th ed. Philadelphia: J.B. Lippincott Co., 1997:2423–43.

70. van de Wouw AJ, Janssen-Heijnen MLG, Coebergh JWW, Hillen HF. Epidemiology of unknown primary tumors; incidenceand population-based survival of 1285 patients in Southeast Netherlands, 1984–1992. *Eur J Cancer* 2002; 38:409–13.

71. Ayoub JP, Hesds KR, Abbruzzese MC, Lenzi R, Raber MN, Abbruzzese JL. Unknown primary tumors metastatic to liver. *J Clin Oncol* 1998; 16(6):2105–12.

72. Hogan BA, Thornton FJ, Brannigan M, et al. Hepatic metastases from an unknown primary neoplasm (UPN): survival, prognostic indicators and value of extensive investigations. *Clin Radiol* 2002; 57(12):1073–7.

73. Pouessel D, Thezenas S, Culine S, Becht C, Senesse P, Ychou M. Hepatic metastases from carcinomas of unknown primary site. *Gastroenterol Clin Biol* 2005; 29:1224–32.

74. Woods RL, Fox RM, Tattersall MH, Levi JA, Brodie GN. Metastatic adenocarcinomas of unknown primary site: a randomized study of two combination–chemotherapy regimens. *N Engl J Med* 1980; 303:87–9.

75. Shild RA, Kennedy PS, Chen TT, Athens JW, O'Bryan RM, Balcerzak SP. Management of patients with metastatic adenocarcinoma of unknown origin: a Southwest Oncology Group Study. *Cancer Treat Reports* 1983; 67:77–9.

76. Milliken ST, Tattershall MH, Woods RL, et al. Metastatic adenocarcinoma of unknown primary site. A randomized study of two combination chemotherapy regimens. *Eur J Cancer Clin Oncol* 1987; 23:1645–8.

77. Eagan RT, Therneau TM, Rubin J, Long HJ, Schutt AJ. Lack of value for cisplatin added to mitomycin/doxorubicin combination chemotherapy for carcinoma of unknown primary site. A randomized trial. *Am J Clin Oncol* 1987; 10(1):82–5.

78. Culine S, Fabbro M, Ychou M, Romieu G, Cupissol D, Rujol H. Chemotherapy in carcinomas of unknown primary site: a high-dose intensity policy. *Ann Oncol* 1999; 10:569–75.

79. Greco FA, Erland JB, Morrissey LH, et al. Carcinoma of unknown primary site: phase II trials with docetaxel plus cisplatin or carboplatin. *Ann Oncol* 2000; 11:211–5.

80. Dowell J, Garrett AM, Shyr Y, Johnson DH, Hande KR. A randomized phase II trial in patients with carcinoma of an unknown primary site. *Cancer* 2001; 91:592–7.

81. Lortholary A, Culine S, Bouzy J. Cisplatin in combination with either gemcitabine or irinotecan in carcinomas of unknown primary: results of a randomized phase II study. *Proc Am Soc Clin Oncol* 2002; 153a:609.

82. Assersohn L, Norman AR, Cunningham D, et al. A randomized study of protracted venous infusion of 5-fluorouracil (5-FU) with or without bolus mitomycin C (MMC) in patients with carcinoma of unknown primary. *Eur J Cancer* 2003; 39:1121–8.

83. Culine S, Lortholary A, Voigt JJ, et al. Cisplatin in combination with either gemcitabine or irinotecan in carcinomas of unknown primary site: results of a randomized phase II study-trial for the French Study Group on Carcinomas of Unknown Primary (GEFCAPI 01). *J Clin Oncol* 2003; 21(18):3479–82.

84. Huebner G, Steinbach S, Kohne CH, et al. Paclitaxel (P)/Carboplatin (C) versus gemcitabine (G)/vinorelbine (V) in patients with adeno- or undifferentiated carcinoma of unknown primary (CUP)—a randomized prospective phase-II trial. *Proc Am Soc Clin Oncol* 2005; 23:330s(abstr 4089).

85. Palmeri S, Lorusso V, Palmeri L, et al. Cisplatin and gemcitabine with either vinorelbine or paclitaxel in the treatment of carcinomas of unknown primary site: results of an Italian multicenter, randomized, phase II study. *Cancer* 2006; 107 (12):2898–905.

86. Hainsworth JD, Burris HA 3rd, Calvert SW, et al. Gemcitabine in the second-line therapy of patients with carcinoma of unknown primary site: a phase II trial of the Minnie Pearl Cancer Research Network. *Cancer Invest* 2001; 19:335–9.

87. Culine S, Ychou M, Fabbro M, Romieu G, Cupissol D. 5-Fluorouracil and leucovorin as second-line chemotherapy in carcinomas of unknown primary site. *Anticancer Res* 2001; 21: 1455–7.

88. Pouessel D, Culine S, Becht C, et al. Gemcitabine and docetaxel after failure of cisplatin-based chemotherapy in patients with carcinoma of unknown primary site. *Anticancer Res* 2003; 23 (3C):2801–4.

89. Hainsworth JD, Spigel DR, Raefsky EL, et al. Combination chemotherapy with gemcitabine and irinotecan in patients with previously treated carcinoma of an unknown primary site: a Minnie Pearl Cancer Research Network Phase II trial. *Cancer* 2005; 104(9):1992–7.

90. Frank RC, Kaplan F, Nair S. Response of carcinoma of unknown primary site affecting bone to thalidomide. *Lancet Oncol* 2005; 6: 534–5.

91. Asakura H, Takashima H, Mitani M, et al. Unknown primary carcinoma, diagnosed as inflammatory breast cancer, and successfully treated with trastuzumab and vinorelbine. *Int J Clin Oncol* 2005; 10:285–8.

92. Hainsworth JD, Spigel DR, Thompson DS, et al. Bevacizumab plus erlotinib in patients with carcinoma of unknown primary site: a phase II trial of the Minnie Pearl Cancer Research Network. *Proc Am Soc Clin Oncol* 2006; 24:129s(abstr 3033).

93. van der Gaast A, Verweij V, Planting AST, Hope WCJ, Stoter G. Simple prognostic model to predict survival in patients with undifferentiated carcinoma of unknown primary site. *J Clin Oncol* 1995; 13:1720–5.

94. Abbzuzzese J, Abbruzzese MC, Hess Kr, Raber MN, Lenzi R, Frost P. Unknown primary carcinoma: natural history and prognostic factors in 657 consecutive patients. *J Clin Oncol* 1994; 12:1272–80.

95. Culine S, Kramar A, Saghatchian M, et al. Development and validation of a prognostic model to predict the length of survival in patients with carcinomas of an unknown primary site. *J Clin Oncol* 2002; 20(24):4679–83.

96. Seve P, Sawyer M, Hanson J, Broussolle C, Dumontet C, Mackey JR. The influence of comorbidities, age and performance status on the prognosis and treatment of patients with metastatic carcinomas of unknown primary site: a population-based study. *Cancer* 2006; 106 (9):2058–66.

97. Seve P, Ray–Coquard I, Trillet–Lenoir V, et al. Low serum albumin levels and liver metastasis are powerful prognostic markers for survival in patients with carcinomas of unknown primary site. *Cancer* 2006; 107:2698–705.

12 Surgical Therapy for Metastatic Carcinomas of Unknown Origin

PERRY SHEN

LERON JACKSON

JEFFREY E. CARTER

EDWARD A. LEVINE

■ INTRODUCTION

Approximately 3% to 6% of patients presenting with metastatic disease from solid tumors can be classified as having metastatic carcinoma from an unknown primary site (CUP). CUP represents a heterogeneous group of metastatic tumors for which no primary site can be detected after a thorough medical evaluation. The primary lesion may either have a slow growth rate or possibly involute; therefore, it rarely becomes manifest during the clinical course (1, 2). CUP represents a unique entity in which it is presumed that a primary tumor is able to metastasize before the primary site becomes large enough to be identified. The natural history of these patients differs considerably. When grouped together, patients with metastases from an unknown primary site have a median survival of approximately six months (3).

CUP is a diagnosis of exclusion that is made only after an exhaustive clinical and pathological analysis has failed to identify a primary site (4, 5). Women should have a breast and pelvic exam and men should undergo complete prostate and testicular examination (6). The diagnosis of CUP applies to 5% to 10% of all cancer patients, making it the seventh most common malignancy (7). A primary tumor that has escaped clinical detection can be identified in 30% to 82% of cases at autopsy (8). Most large studies have shown that carcinomas of the lung and pancreas are the most common primary lesions that initially present as CUP. Other common malignancies, such as colorectal, breast, and prostate carcinoma, infrequently do so (9, 10, 11, 12).

The definition of CUP has varied over time according to inclusion criteria and the evolution of diagnostic tools. In the early 1970s, it was argued that the diagnosis of CUP could be made only if the primary tumor was not found at autopsy (13). A retrospective chart review by Stewart et al. in 1979 maintained that the most pertinent challenge for the clinician was to decide how aggressively to try to identify the primary site (14). In that analysis, there was no difference in median survival time between patients in whom the primary tumor site was found during life and others in whom it was not. Currently, it is felt that clinical investigations should be directed at finding *treatable* primary tumors.

The argument for pursuing the primary neoplasm aggressively in CUP patients is usually based on two beliefs—that finding it may allow for specific antitumor treatment and provide a better guide to prognosis. However, despite recent advances in molecular pathology, immunohistochemistry, and imaging technology, the diagnosis and therapy of patients with CUP remains a real dilemma. The majority of CUP patients are relatively resistant to systemic therapy and have short survivals, but certain clinicopathological subsets that are defined by

Table 1 Favorable and unfavorable subsets of CUP

Favorable Subsets	Unfavorable Subsets
1. Poorly differentiated carcinoma with midline distribution (extragonadal germ cell syndrome)	1. Adenocarcinoma metastatic to the liver or other organs
2. Women with papillary adenocarcinoma of peritoneal cavity	2. Nonpapillary malignant ascites (adenocarcinoma)
3. Women with adenocarcinoma involving only axillary lymph nodes	3. Multiple cerebral metastases (adeno- or squamous carcinoma)
4. Squamous cell carcinoma involving cervical lymph nodes	4. Multiple lung/pleural metastases (adenocarcinoma)
5. Isolated inguinal adenopathy (squamous carcinoma)	5. Multiple metastatic bone disease (adenocarcinoma)
6. Poorly differentiated neuroendocrine carcinomas	
7. Men with blastic bone metastases and elevated PSA (adenocarcinoma)	
8. Patients with a single, small, potentially resectable tumor	

Abbreviations: CUP, metastatic carcinoma from an unknown primary site; PSA, prostate specific antigen.

either clinical or pathological features do respond to treatment and have a better prognosis. These are listed in Table 1 (15).

The therapeutic strategy for CUP patients should be individualized according to the clinical subset. Oncologists must determine whether the patient belongs to any of the favorable or unfavorable subsets prior to recommending a specific intervention. Cases of CUP usually belong to two categories—metastatic involvement of lymph nodes only and those with visceral disease (16). The most common sites for secondary lesions are the lymph nodes, lungs, bone, and liver (17, 18). This is an important distinction, because patients with isolated nodal metastasis generally have a better prognosis after appropriate therapy (19).

Based on the clinical presentation and histology, the recommended treatment may be locoregional or systemic, and it may have curative or palliative intent. Historically, chemotherapy has been the cornerstone of management for patients with CUP (20). During the last 40 years, almost all cytotoxic drugs have been used in this context, either as single agents or in combinations.

During evaluation of the patient with CUP, communication between the surgeon and the pathologist is critical to ensure the appropriate collection and handling of tissue specimens and minimizing the need for repeated biopsies. Moreover, all available clinical information should be provided to the pathologist. In a review by Hainsworth and Greco (21), approximately 60% of patients with CUP were found to have well-differentiated or moderately well-differentiated adenocarcinomas, 5% had squamous carcinomas, and 35% had poorly differentiated and otherwise unclassifiable epithelial neoplasms (PDC-NOS). After histological confirmation, the next step in pathological assessment is usually immunostaining. This technique has revolutionized the ability to identify the origin of many metastases from unknown primary sources. In conjunction with the clinical history, histology and adjunctive staining procedures can delineate specific tumor lineages in 72% of cases (22). The results of immunostains are always correlated with light microscopic findings and the clinical picture to optimize diagnosis, because no single tumor marker is entirely specific.

Serum tumor products that are shed into the bloodstream represent other tests that can serve as adjuncts in defining the source of a metastatic tumor. Although most such markers lack a high level of specificity in determining the site of the primary, their use, together with morphological, pathological, and clinical information, may be helpful. Table 2 (6) lists the most commonly used markers and corresponding tumors. It is worthwhile to note that an isolated elevation of any one marker is not diagnostic and does not predict response to therapy. Elevations in these analytes must be interpreted in the clinical context, and they should only be used in specific situations where clinicopathologic data support their application.

Table 2 Serum tumor markers

Tumor Marker	Differential Diagnosis
α-Fetoprotein	Hepatocellular, germ cell
β-HCG	Trophoblastic, germ cell
CA15-3	Breast>ovary, lung, gastrointestinal
CA19-9	Pancreas, gastrointestinal
CA-125	Ovary, uterine>breast, lung
CEA	Carcinoma versus mesothelioma

Abbreviations: CEA, carcinoembryonic antigen; HCG, human chorionic gonadotropin; CA, carbohydrate antigen.

This chapter analyzes the subsets of patients with CUP who have been shown to derive benefit from surgical intervention. Generally, they have either lymph node metastases—in the cervical, axillary, or inguinal regions—or isolated visceral secondary lesions or solitary metastases in the bone or peritoneum. In these sites, certain histological tumor types will be discussed, such as occult breast carcinoma. Indications for surgery, the role of adjunctive therapies, clinical outcomes, and prognostic factors will be presented. Clinical treatment algorithms have been formulated for selected sections based on information in the pertinent literature.

CERVICAL NODAL METASTASES

Incidence and Evaluation

Approximately 2% to 8% of patients presenting with malignant cervical lymphadenopathy have a primary tumor that is not readily diagnosed by standard evaluation (23). Classically, the individual who presents with cervical nodal metastases is a middle-aged or elderly person with a history of chronic tobacco or alcohol use. Common tumor types in such cases include squamous cell carcinoma (SCC), adenocarcinoma, PDC-NOS, and melanoma. The primary site for most cervical metastatic SCCs is usually the oral cavity, larynx, or cervical esophagus. Possible sites of origin for metastatic cervical adenocarcinomas include the thyroid, stomach, breasts, and prostate. The most likely primary site for PDC-NOS in the head and neck region is the nasopharynx. The recommended pathway of diagnostic inquiry in patients with cervical lymph node metastases is outlined in Table 3 (24). This

approach was 87% successful in identifying a primary lesion in patients with metastatic cervical nodal SCC in a study of 267 patients (25).

Fine-needle aspiration (FNA) of the affected cervical nodes is the method of choice for histological diagnosis. FNA is 90% to 98% accurate in recognizing metastatic SCC (24, 26). A complete examination of the oral cavity, pharynx, and larynx is also warranted; indirect and direct laryngoscopy with mucosal biopsy is strongly recommended as well. Incisional biopsy of enlarged cervical nodes is somewhat controversial and may lead to higher rates of local recurrence and decreased survival after definitive treatment (27). Positron emission tomography (PET) is a potentially useful option if the primary site remains unidentified after direct and indirect endoscopy. In one study of 42 patients with metastatic cervical SCC and negative endoscopy, PET showed localized increased metabolic uptake in 20 of them (48%). Further investigation revealed a primary lesion in 10 of these, and previously unrecognized metastatic sites were also found in nearly one-third of the cases (28). Bronchoscopy is not generally performed when metastases are found in upper and mid-cervical lymph nodes, if thoracic computed tomography (CT) is normal and no pulmonary symptoms exist. CT is useful for characterizing the extent of disease. Other methods used to improve diagnosis are screening tonsillectomy, chromosomal analysis, and Epstein–Barr virus (EBV) detection in tumor tissue. Surveillance biopsies from the upper aerodigestive tract may also confirm the presence of genetic aberrations that are found in the metastatic tumor. EBV detection points to a nasopharyngeal site of origin, especially in young patients whose tumors show a PDC-NOS histology (29).

Role of Screening Tonsillectomy

Screening tonsillectomy is recommended in the diagnosis of patients with subdigastric, mid-jugulocarotid, or submandibular nodal metastases from an occult primary tumor. A recent study examined results for 87 patients who underwent screening tonsillectomy in that setting. Twenty-six percent of them had a tonsillar primary lesion, with involved lymph nodes in the subdigastric, submandibular, and mid-jugulodigastric groups in 38%, 28%, and 23% of cases respectively (30). In another series reported by Randall et al. (23), 6 of 14 T1 tonsillar carcinomas were occult, requiring tonsillectomy for diagnosis. Among the patients without identifiable primary sites after endoscopic evaluation, 6 of 34 (18%) had a diagnosis after tonsillectomy. Koch et al. (31) recommended bilateral tonsillectomy in patients who present with metastatic SCC in cervical nodes with an unknown anatomic source. The proposed rationale for bilateral tonsillectomy is to create a symmetric faucial arch to avoid

Table 3 Recommended diagnostic workup for cervical nodal metastases

History
Physical exam
Examination of oral cavity, pharynx, and larynx
Indirect laryngoscopy
Chest radiograph
CT and/or MRI of head and neck; PET
Laboratory studies (complete blood count, complete metabolic panel)
Direct endoscopy
Biopsy of nasopharynx, tonsils, base of tongue, pyriform sinuses, suspicious mucosal areas
Tonsillectomy (unilateral or bilateral)
Fine-needle aspirate of cervical node

Source: From Ref. 24.

confusion during posttreatment surveillance regarding recurrence and the presence of second primary tumors. Moreover, complete tonsillectomy can also capture rare cases of bilateral disease (32). In a series of 41 patients, four (10%) had bilateral tonsillar primary lesions.

Surgical Treatment

Several institutions have published their experiences in the treatment of cervical lymph node metastases from unknown primary sites (31, 33–35). Treatment of patients with SCC of unknown origin in the upper or mid-cervical lymph nodes should be predicated on guidelines for locally advanced SCC of the head and neck. Therapeutic options for *all* histological subtypes include radiation to the pharynx and both sides of the neck, radical neck dissection, or a combination of those interventions.

Surgery as Definitive Therapy

Patients who have a solitary positive cervical node containing SCC may be treated with neck dissection alone if there has been no prior open biopsy and if there is no extracapsular extension (ECE) by metastatic tumor (36). However, radiation therapy should be added when there are multiple positive nodes and/or ECE, to reduce the likelihood of local recurrence in the neck (37). In a study by Iganej et al. of 106 patients with metastatic SCC of unknown source, 41 had N1 or N2a disease without ECE. Surgery alone as the initial treatment yielded 81% tumor control above the clavicle (33).

Adjuvant Radiotherapy

Radiation as Definitive Therapy

Radiation treatment (RT) is generally not recommended as definitive therapy for CUP, except in patients with extremely advanced, bulky, or otherwise inoperable disease. The local failure rate in such patients is estimated at >50%, and the overall survival is poorer than that of patients treated with surgery alone. However, it must be acknowledged that the majority of patients given RT alone have more advanced disease and a poor prognosis, independent of the treatment modality used (33).

Postoperative RT

Postoperative RT is recommended for patients who have radical neck dissections and ECE by metastatic tumor or multiple positive nodes. RT can also target potential primary sites in the head and neck besides treating the affected nodal basins. Weir et al. published a retrospective analysis of 144 patients with cervical lymph node metastases from unknown primary tumors (38).

Eighty-five of them were given RT to the affected nodes alone, whereas 59 received radiation to the nodes as well as to potential primary sites in the head and neck (38). No survival difference was reported between the patient subgroups; the overall five-year survival for the entire cohort was 41%. However, the primary lesions were more likely to manifest themselves eventually in those patients who only had nodal irradiation. Among seven patients who subsequently developed a detectable primary tumor, only one (15%) had received radiation to affected cervical nodes and potential primary sites (37).

Some authors do not recommend routine postoperative RT for CUPs. Iganej et al. (33) published a retrospective analysis of 106 patients with N1, N2, and N3 disease. Initial treatment included excisional biopsy alone in 12 cases, radical neck dissection alone in 29, radiotherapy alone in 12, excisional biopsy followed by radiotherapy in 15, and radical neck dissection together with postoperative RT in 26. No significant difference was found in survival based on these treatment modalities. However, disease-free survival and overall outcome was worse for patients with advanced (N2b, N2c, and N3) disease. Tumor-free survival at five years was slightly higher (80%) for patients with N1 and N2a metastases, compared with approximately 50% for others who had more advanced disease. Overall survival at 10 years was slightly above 50% for patients with N1 and N2a disease and approximately 35% for patients with higher-stage tumors. The latter study suggests that, in the absence of advanced cervical metastatic disease, RT can be reserved for salvage therapy.

Outcomes and Survival

Recent analyses provide insight into an important clinical question; that is, whether bilateral cervical RT results in better prevention of local recurrence than unilateral RT. McMahon et al. assessed a prospectively compiled computerized database in which 38 patients had metastatic cervical SCC from an occult primary site (34). Radiotherapy was directed at the ipsilateral neck alone in 24 patients, whereas 10 were given comprehensive bilateral RT to cervical nodes and potential primary sites. Patients in the latter group had either bilateral metastases or a suspected nasopharyngeal carcinoma. The rate of disease control in the ipsilateral neck was 91%. Contralateral neck recurrence occurred in six cases (16%), none of which had received contralateral radiotherapy as part of the initial treatment. Of the six individuals who developed contralateral recurrences in the neck, all of them had had a radical neck dissection; five of the six also received RT directed at the ipsilateral neck. Two of the six showed evidence of distant metastases as well, precluding curative treatment.

A recent evaluation by Boscolo-Rizzo et al. (39) describes the clinical outcome of 90 patients with CUPs who presented with metastases to cervical lymph nodes. They were treated with radical or modified radical neck dissection and mucosal irradiation. Thirteen patients (14.4%) developed distant metastases 9 to 38 months after treatment, and the five-year actuarial incidence of distant disease was 19.1%. Nodal involvement of cervical levels IV and V ($p < 0.001$), the presence of nodal ECE ($p = 0.007$), and histological tumor grades of 3 and 4 ($p = 0.002$) significantly affected the risk of metastasis outside the head and neck. In multivariate analysis, distant failure was associated with involvement of cervical nodal levels IV and V ($p = 0.01$) and ECE ($p = 0.013$). The dose of RT was not significantly related to distant tumor recurrence.

Despite definitive treatment, 10% to 15% of patients with metastatic SCC of unknown origin will develop a clinically manifest lesion in the mucosa of the head or neck within five years and another 10% to 15% show distant metastases (40). The subsequent appearance of a primary tumor may potentially affect treatment, but little data is available on that point. In a recent assessment by McMahon et al. 5 of 38 patients with cervical metastases from CUPs developed obvious mucosal primary lesions after their initial presentation. Three of them then had salvage surgery and adjuvant radiotherapy. Two of those individuals were alive and disease free at one and three years of follow-up (34). However, another analysis suggested that the appearance of a primary tumor did not alter survival significantly (33).

Long-term disease-free survival with CUP of the head and neck approximates to 40% to 67% after definitive treatment. Data generated by Boscolo-Rizzo et al. demonstrated an actuarial overall survival of 71.7% and 59.9%, respectively, at two and five years of follow-up; actuarial disease-specific survival (DSS) rates at these time points were 73.6% and 62.8%, respectively. The level of cervical nodal involvement, the presence of ECE, and the N stage significantly affect the DSS. As is true of distant metastases, nodal involvement of levels IV and V ($p = 0.001$) and the presence of ECE ($p = 0.001$) negatively influenced actuarial DSS; the irradiation dose did not do so (39).

PDC-NOS may be sensitive to radiotherapy alone, or combination treatment of RT and chemotherapy (36). The five-year survival for the patients treated only with RT is 38% (15/40), whereas five-year survivals of others given chemotherapy alone were significantly lower. RT and chemotherapy together improved the outcome. Surgery alone also is not considered a viable option for CUPs of the head and neck that are poorly differentiated SCCs (36). Yang et al. reported on results of RT in 113 cases of cervical nodal metastasis from unknown primary tumors, with a five-year survival of 37%. The dose of radiotherapy was the main factor that affected survival, and those patients who were given >50 Gy enjoyed twice the survival rate as others who received less irradiation (41). In a study by Yalin et al. focusing on metastatic cervical nodal SCC, patients were given preoperative RT at a dose of <50 Gy, followed by radical neck dissection within six weeks. With this approach, a five-year survival rate of 53% was achieved (36). Preoperative irradiation may reduce the size of the tumor and possibly affect micrometastases as well. However, RT may make subsequent surgical dissection more difficult and negatively affect wound healing. The five-year survival rate of patients in the latter study who were given radiotherapy alone was 33% ($N = 3$). Four patients who were given chemotherapy, either alone or with RT, had supraclavicular nodal disease and a poorer prognosis (36).

Improved survival was reported in a group of eight patients with metastatic papillary adenocarcinoma that presented in cervical nodes. They underwent radical thyroidectomy and neck dissection (36), yielding a five-year survival of 62%. That group was compared with another eight patients with nonpapillary metastatic adenocarcinoma, of whom only one patient survived for more than five years. Six had metastatic disease in supraclavicular nodes, for which the primary site was most likely in the abdomen or thorax. The prognosis for such patients is poor, and treatment is often palliative. The presence of clinical N3 disease, ECE, poor tumor differentiation on histological studies, and positive surgical margins predict a poor survival in this cohort by univariate statistical analysis (34, 36).

Lower Cervical and Supraclavicular Sites

A biopsy showing metastatic SCC in the supraclavicular lymph nodes (especially right-sided ones) suggests a primary lung cancer; hence, fiberoptic bronchoscopy should be performed (even if the chest radiograph is negative) after a head and neck examination has failed to provide evidence of a primary tumor above the clavicles. Patients in this scenario should receive standard treatment for a lung carcinoma of advanced stage. Those who lack detectable disease below the clavicles should be treated using the same approach employed for those with a detectable thoracic tumor (41).

■ AXILLARY LYMPH NODE METASTASES— OCCULT BREAST CARCINOMA

Incidence and Diagnostic Workup

Women presenting with a unilateral axillary mass and a normal breast examination should be evaluated with mammography and/or MRI of the breasts, chest radiography, and FNA of the axillary lesion. If metastatic carcinoma is seen in the biopsy specimen, it should be evaluated for estrogen and progesterone receptor status and Her-2/*neu* gene amplification (42). Providing that a breast lesion is found, further diagnostic evaluation should follow standard guidelines for suspected mammary carcinoma. If no breast mass is apparent, patients with this clinical presentation should still be considered to have occult primary breast cancer if the histological image of the metastatic tumor is that of adenocarcinoma. The overall incidence of occult breast carcinoma with axillary metastasis is <1% of all breast cancer cases (43).

A retrospective study done by Muttarak et al. examined mammograms from 43 patients with palpable unilateral axillary masses and normal breasts on physical examination (44). Ninety-three percent of them had true lymph nodal enlargement, but other diagnoses included lipoma, fibroadenoma in the mammary axillary tail, and hematoma. Forty-one percent of the patients had benign lymphadenopathy with reactive lymphoid hyperplasia or acute infectious lymphadenitis, whereas 59% had intra-nodal malignancies. Metastases of nonmammary primary tumors, occult ipsilateral breast carcinomas, and previous contralateral breast carcinomas were all represented (45). No significant discrepancy in size was observed between malignant and benign lymph nodes. In this series, 80% of patients with breast carcinoma were subsequently found to show mammographic evidence of malignancy (45).

In another series reported by Obdeijn et al. 31 women with metastatic adenocarcinoma in axillary nodes and no known primary tumor had an MRI of the breasts taken, after mammography and physical examination revealed nothing (45). Two-thirds had no prior history of malignancy, but the remaining patients had had previous contralateral breast cancers. Sonography and FNA were performed on any contrast-enhancing lesion seen on MRI, and a primary intramammary tumor was identified in 40% of the 20 patients without a history of malignancy. A second primary neoplasm was found in 27% of the women with a history of breast cancer (46).

Definitive Local Treatment

Treatment should include modified radical mastectomy, or axillary lymphadenectomy and upper outer quadrantectomy, or RT to the breast. Occult breast cancer is identified in 33% to 82% of patients when mastectomy is performed when all clinical studies are negative (46–49). Once found, the primary tumor is usually <2 cm in diameter, and, in some cases, only ductal carcinoma in situ is identified. Upper outer quadrantectomy has been suggested as a breast-conserving surgical option. It is based on the premise that there is an increased density of

glandular tissue in that quadrant; (50); however, this approach is controversial and may miss up to 50% of tumors (51). Nevertheless, some form of definitive local therapy, whether represented by surgery or irradiation, should be implemented, because many patients with axillary CUP eventually develop a clinically manifest breast tumor. Administration of adjuvant therapy is based on the hormonal status of the tumor, its Her-2/*neu* gene expression, and selected clinical features, including menopausal status. If other sites besides the axilla are involved, the working diagnosis still may be metastatic breast carcinoma. A trial of empirical chemotherapy or hormonal therapy may offer at least palliative benefit in such cases.

Axillary Lymph Node Dissection

To achieve maximum locoregional tumor control as well as proper staging and prognostic information, a level I and II axillary lymph node dissection (ALND) is the current treatment standard for all patients with axillary nodal metastases from breast cancer; this is true regardless of whether the lesion is an occult or known primary. Vlastos et al. (52) found a trend toward improved survival in patients who underwent ALND, as compared with others who only had axillary nodal biopsy. However, the difference between the groups was not statistically significant. In patients with nonoccult breast carcinoma, the prognostic importance of the absolute number of involved lymph nodes is well known (53, 54). Survival in cases of occult breast carcinoma is also associated with the extent of nodal involvement. Patients with one to three positive nodes have a statistically significant survival benefit as compared with others with four or more positive involved nodes (87% vs. 42%; $p < 0.0001$) (54).

Surgical Management of the Breast

Several options exist for management of the breast in cases of axillary nodal CUP. They include mastectomy or observation alone, with or without RT. Even in instances where a carcinoma is found in the mastectomy specimen, the lesion is often either noninvasive or very small. Meterissian et al. found that 35 of 71 (49%) primary breast cancers that were undetectable by clinical examination were noninvasive; 27 of the 36 invasive tumors (75%) measured <1 cm (55). A nonsurgical option for occult primary breast cancer is observation, with or without irradiation. In patients who have undergone axillary biopsy/dissection and observation alone, the reported incidence of subsequently obvious breast carcinoma is 14% to 53% (49, 55). These figures contrast with others pertaining to women who have axillary nodal dissection and RT to the breast. In this group, the incidence of subsequent clinically manifest breast carcinoma is 12% to 33% (56–58). In patients who do not undergo mastectomy, the addition of RT has a significant impact on survival as compared with women who are only observed (83% vs. 50%, respectively; $p = 0.001$) (52).

Prognosis and Survival

No significant survival difference is appreciated in comparisons of axillary nodal CUP patients who undergo mastectomy versus those who have breast preservation and RT (75% vs. 79%, respectively) at five years. The second treatment option is therefore a reasonable alternative for these patients (53).

■ CUP METASTASES IN INGUINAL LYMPH NODES

Incidence and Workup

Metastatic carcinoma presenting in inguinal lymph nodes from an unknown primary source accounts for 1% to 3.5% of patients with CUP (59). Patients in this group are epidemiologically similar to others with inguinal metastases from clinically *obvious* primary lesions, with a median age of 50 to 59 years. The most frequent presenting symptom is a painful inguinal mass. The diagnostic approach includes a thorough historical survey, physical examination, chest radiography, and serum biochemistry (60). Further diagnostic modalities include an upper gastrointestinal (GI) barium series, barium enema, proctosigmoidoscopy or colonoscopy, cervical and endometrial biopsies, and intravenous pyelography (60). Other useful studies include endoscopic gastroduodenoscopy and cystoscopy (57). Common tumor types that are identified in inguinal nodal biopsy specimens include PDC-NOS, SCC, and adenocarcinoma (60). A more detailed list of possible neoplasms is provided in Table 4 (60).

Zaren and Copeland reported an M.D. Anderson experience of 2232 patients with inguinal node metastases. Primary sites of malignancy were clinically apparent in 2210 patients (99%) and were, in order of frequency, the skin of the lower extremities, uterine cervix, vulva, skin of the trunk, rectum and anus, ovary, and penis (60). The three-year survival rate for the remaining 22 patients—with inguinal CUP—was 50%. A primary source was identified subsequently in only 1 of the 22 cases.

Curative therapy is available for carcinomas of the vulva, vagina, cervix, and anus, even with regional lymph-node involvement. If no primary tumor is identified, lymphadenectomy with or without postoperative RT to the inguinal nodal basin may result in long-term survival (61).

Table 4 Primary histologies identified in patients with carcinoma metastatic to inguinal nodes	
Melanoma	27.4%
Squamous carcinoma	23.9%
Adenocarcinoma	9.8%
Unclassified carcinoma	4.5%
Papillary serous carcinoma	4.2%
Transitional cell carcinoma	2.8%
Bronchogenic carcinoma	2.2%
Unclassified sarcoma	<1%
Unclassified malignant neoplasms and 41 other rare malignancies account for the remainder of primary sites identified	

Note: Percentages based on histological examination of 2210 patients with inguinal node metastases.
Source: From Ref. 60.

Overall Survival and Locoregional Recurrence

A review of 56 patients with inguinal nodal metastases from an unknown primary neoplasm was published by Guarischi et al. (59). Five-year survival for cases with inguinal disease alone was statistically comparable to those with unilateral inguinal and iliac-obturator nodal metastases. Both patient groups had better survival than patients with systemic disease. Zaren and Copeland reported that 7 of 22 patients with inguinal nodal CUP had superficial inguinal node dissections but no adjuvant therapy (60). The disease-free interval in these patients ranged from 2 to 18 years, with an average of 7.7 years. No patients in the subgroup treated by superficial groin dissection died of their tumors, but those treated by local excision alone showed a 40% two-year overall survival.

■ PERITONEAL CARCINOMATOSIS FROM CUP

Peritoneal Papillary Serous Carcinoma

In women, adenocarcinoma showing diffuse peritoneal involvement usually originates in the ovary. Occasionally, primary mammary or GI tumors can present with in the same way, but that is distinctly less common. In some women with abdominal carcinomatosis, however, an organ-based site of origin cannot be identified (12, 62, 63).

The metastases in such cases often have the histological features of papillary serous ovarian tumors, including psammoma bodies. Disease is usually limited to the peritoneal cavity, and the CA-125 level is commonly elevated (>1000 U/mL) (6). This presentation has therefore been termed *primary peritoneal papillary serous carcinoma* (PPPSC) or "multifocal extraovarian serous carcinoma." The patients have a median age of 60 years, with no visible ovarian lesions. Some have had prior oophorectomies.

Initial reports documented excellent responses in small numbers of PPPSC cases that were treated with exploratory laparotomy and surgical cytoreduction to disease <1 cm, followed by cisplatin-based chemotherapy as used for advanced ovarian cancer (64, 65). Those results were subsequently confirmed in larger series (Table 5) (11, 12, 21, 66). Rates of response ranged from 32% to 39%, and some patients had complete remissions lasting for more than two years. Lele et al. (67) reported on a group of 23 patients with PPPSC. Applying the strategy of aggressive cytoreduction and cisplatin-based chemotherapy, they observed 22% complete clinical response with a median survival of 19 months and 26% long-term survival. The response and survival statistics are similar to those seen in cases of stage IIIB ovarian serous carcinoma. Patients with PPPSC should therefore be treated according to current guidelines for advanced stage ovarian cancer.

Intraperitoneal Hyperthermic Chemotherapy

Sebbag et al. (68) reported on 15 cases of peritoneal carcinomatosis from an unknown primary source, with nonserous histological profiles. Diagnostic tests included radiological studies and endoscopy of the upper and lower GI tract, scintigraphy, mammography, ultrasonography, and CT and MRI studies of the thorax, abdomen, and

pelvis. All patients were treated with cytoreductive surgery (CS) and intraperitoneal hyperthermic chemotherapy. One patient received intraperitoneal chemotherapy with cisplatin prior to the administration of CS. The latter procedure involved one or more of four peritoneotomy approaches—greater omentectomy plus splenectomy; lesser omentectomy with cholecystectomy; right and left subphrenic peritoneotomy; and complete pelvic peritoneotomy. Often, visceral resection of the gastric antrum, right colon, or rectosigmoid colon was required to achieve complete cytoreduction. The intraoperative intraperitoneal chemotherapy was given at a temperature of 41°C. The drug regimens included mitomycin-C (Mutamycin, Bristol-Myers Squibb, Oncology Division, Syracuse, NY) at 12/5 mg/m (2) or cisplatin at 50 mg/m (2). Patients with a significant amount of tumor remaining after surgery were treated postoperatively with additional cycles of intraperitoneal chemotherapy using 5-fluorouracil (Adrucil, Pharmacia and Upjohn Company, Kalamazoo, MI) at 650 mg/m (2). The first cycle was given in the first five postoperative days.

There were four women and 11 men in the study, with a median age of 49 years (range, 31–75 years). Five individuals presented with acute or subacute abdominal pain, whereas the other 10 had more indolent disease manifestations, with hernias or increasing abdominal girth. There was no difference in survival according to the mode of clinical presentation. Four patients (27%) had a second-look laparotomy after initial CS. The average operating time was seven hours (range, 1.5–15 hours). Ten patients (67%) received perioperative chemotherapy. Nine received postoperative chemotherapy later on, which was intraperitoneal (n = 1), systemic (n = 7), or both (n = 1). Four cases with an original diagnosis of peritoneal mesothelioma were reviewed, and the pathological diagnosis was revised to that of peritoneal carcinomatosis from an unknown primary source after immunohistochemical

■ Table 5 Treatment of women with peritoneal adenocarcinomatosis of an unknown primary site (peritoneal papillary serous carcinoma)

Study	No. of Patients	Treatment	Overall Rate of Response	Complete Response (%)	Disease-Free Survival >24 mo	Median Survival (mo)
Strnad et al. (11)	18	Surgical cytoreduction and cisplatin-based chemotherapy	39	39	17	23
Dalrymple et al. (12)	31	Surgical cytoreduction and chemotherapy	32	10	6	11
Ransom et al. (66)	33	Surgical cytoreduction and cisplatin-based chemotherapy		13	9	17

studies. Six patients had poorly differentiated peritoneal adenocarcinomas and nine had mucin-producing adeno-carcinomas. Six of the 15 tumors contained signet-ring tumor cells. Three patients had serious complications, represented by sepsis, significant neutropenia, and pulmonary embolism. One individual required reoperation for bowel ischemia. The overall morbidity was 27%. One postoperative death occurred in a debilitated patient with sepsis and long-standing intestinal obstruction. Mean follow-up after CS was 14.4 months (range, 1–60 months). Two patients developed distant metastases. At the end of the surveillance period, 11 were dead of disease (73%) and 4 (27%) were alive, one with persistent disease. The overall median survival was seven months after CS.

Peritoneal carcinomatosis with an unknown primary tumor is a rare malignancy that is included in the CUP category clinically. However, it is likely that this malignancy has its origin in the peritoneal surface, like peritoneal mesothelioma and Mullerian-type PPPSC. The interrelationship between different primary peritoneal malignancies is a puzzling issue. Peritoneal mesothelioma has a spectrum of histological subtypes ranging from sarcoma-like to epithelial (carcinoma-like) (Fig. 1) (68). Figure 2 presents a clinical algorithm that can be followed for the treatment of peritoneal carcinomatosis from an unknown primary source.

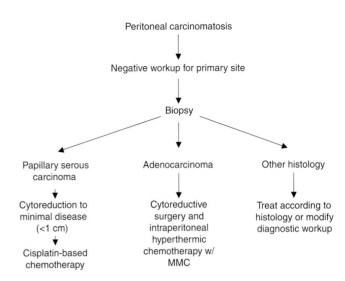

FIGURE 2 Clinical algorithm for management of peritoneal carcinomatosis from unknown primary. *Abbreviation*: MMC, mitomycin-C.

■ SINGLE-SITE METASTASES

Hepatic Metastases

Patients with CUP present with liver metastases in 30% of cases (69). The evaluation of these patients is as described earlier in this chapter. Additional information, such as a

history of cirrhosis or chronic infection with hepatitis B or C virus, may assist in determining whether primary hepatocellular carcinoma is also a consideration. Moreover, a fluorodeoxyglucose PET (FDG-PET) scan can also be helpful in evaluating extrahepatic disease. A previous study on head-and-neck disease noted that FDG-PET scans identified primary lesions in one-third of all cases concerning CUPs. They also assisted in choosing biopsy techniques, further diagnostic tests, and treatment (70).

Adenocarcinoma is the most frequent tumor type seen in hepatic metastases in CUP cases (72). This diagnosis is associated with a median survival of 5.9 months, according to a study of 58 patients at the Sloan-Kettering Cancer Center (72). A more recent review of 157 cases of hepatic metastasis included seven of adenocarcinoma-type CUP (76). Five of the seven patients underwent neoadjuvant and/or adjuvant chemotherapy in addition to radio-frequency ablation (RFA) or hepatic resection. Nine lesions in all were treated, six with RFA and three with hepatic surgery. The median diameter of the lesions was 5.4 cm (range, 1.3–15 cm). At nine months of follow-up, one patient was alive with no evidence of disease, four were alive with persistent tumor, and two had died. The median disease-free survival was 6.5 months, with a median overall survival of 9 months. The latter study suggests that surgical intervention, either with RFA or chemotherapy, might produce a survival benefit. More highly powered studies will be needed in the future to better clarify the role of local treatment.

Other publications have reviewed the role of hepatic resection for noncolorectal nonneuroendocrine (NCNNE) liver metastases in cases where the primary tumor was treated and the liver metastases were excised. Many of

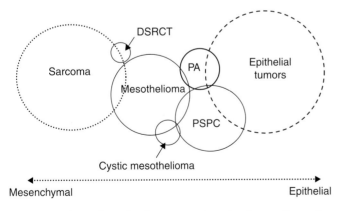

FIGURE 1 Interrelationship between peritoneal surface malignancies, sarcoma, and epithelial malignancies. *Abbreviations*: DSRCT, desmoplastic small round cell tumors; PA, peritoneal adenocarcinomatosis from an unknown primary site; PSPC, papillary serous peritoneal carcinoma.

these studies suggest that hepatic resection may offer as many as one-third of patients an opportunity for long-term survival. The largest analysis was a retrospective assessment of 1452 patients at 41 participating centers (73). The study divided cases into three categories based on five-year survival—favorable, intermediate, and poor. Individuals in the first category generally comprised patients with mammary, urological, and gynecological primary carcinomas and they showed five-year survivals of 41%, 48%, and 42%, respectively. There were 29 patients with hepatic CUPs, demonstrating a five-year overall survival of 38%. Those with GI primary lesions were placed in the intermediate category and had 15% to 30% survival at five years. Lastly, patients with lung or head and neck primary lesions were assigned to the poor-outcome category, with less than 15% five-year survival. The potential additional benefit of chemotherapy was not specifically addressed, but it was suggested that neo-adjuvant treatment increased overall five-year survival for all NCNNE liver metastases from 20% to 37%. This information provides additional support for multidisciplinary treatment by surgeons, medical oncologists, radiation oncologists, and diagnostic radiologists, in this cohort of CUP cases.

Management of hepatic lesions from CUPs has varied. Hogan et al. published a review of 88 patients with biopsy-proven hepatic metastases, accrued over a 10- year period (74). The primary neoplasm was identified in 18% of cases and was predominantly represented by adeno-carcinoma (79.5%), as seen in the previous literature (69). Among 16 patients who underwent surgical intervention, chemotherapy, and/or radiotherapy, the median survival was 49 days, compared with 52 days for other individuals who had no such treatment. This difference is not statistically significant (74).

Hemming et al. (75) studied 37 patients with NCNNE-type hepatic metastases. They were stratified into tumors of GI origin (pancreas, duodenum, gastric, esophagus, and small bowel) and non-GI neoplasms (renal, adrenal, testicular, ovarian, thyroid, breast, and unknown origins). Hepatic resection produced a median survival of 22 months and a five-year actuarial survival of 60% in the non-GI primary group and 0% in the GI group. This was a significant difference in both univariate and multivariate analyses. Unfortunately, only three patients with CUP were included in the non-GI group and their survival was not separately calculated.

There are no prospective randomized trials that have compared different modalities of therapy for hepatic metastases from CUPs, and published reports reflect small numbers of cases. Currently, recommended management includes a multidisciplinary review of therapeutic options by surgical oncologists, medical oncologists, and radiation oncologists. Hepatic metastases of CUPs are generally

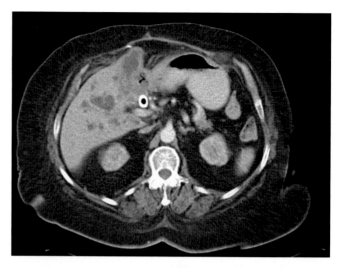

FIGURE 3 This CT of peripheral intrahepatic cholangiocarcinoma demonstrates multiple tumor nodules, simulating a metastatic tumor.

considered to reflect the presence of generalized rather than locoregional (e.g., portal venous-mediated) disease. Local intervention mainly is represented by hepatic resection when the clinical context allows it. RFA has been used for patients with lesions in unfavorable anatomic locations or others who are unable to tolerate hepatic resection. Most individuals are given adjuvant chemotherapy as well. Neoadjuvant chemotherapy may be used in patients with potentially resectable lesions to determine the biology of the disease prior to surgical intervention. Multifocal intrahepatic cholangiocarcinoma may be difficult to distinguish clinically from hepatic metastases of CUPs (Fig. 3), and resection should be

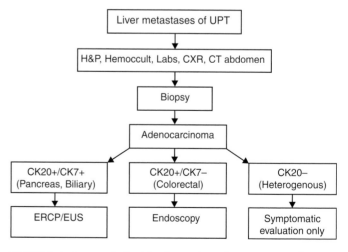

FIGURE 4 Proposed algorithm for workup of primary tumor for liver metastases from UPT. *Abbreviations*: UPT, unknown primary tumor; CXR, chest X-ray; ERCP, endoscopic retrograde pancreatography; EUS, endoscopic ultrasound.

considered when the former is included in the differential diagnosis. Further analyses will be necessary to clarify the role of neoadjuvant versus adjuvant chemotherapy, as well as RFA and resection in patients with isolated hepatic metastases of CUPs. A proposed algorithm is presented in Figure 4 to identify the primary tumor in liver metastases from CUP (76).

BRAIN METASTASES. The number of brain metastases is estimated to be 170,000 cases per year in the United States. It is thought to be increasing because of improved systemic therapy for carcinomas, which generates longer survivals. In addition, an improved sensitivity for detecting cerebral metastases has been obtained with MRI (Fig. 5). Brain metastases of carcinomas most commonly originate in the lung, breast, colon, and kidney (77).

Intracranial CUPs account for 10% to 15% of new cases of malignant brain tumors (78). A retrospective study of 47 patients with such lesions demonstrated a median overall survival of 3.4 to 4.8 months, and it included patients with extracranial disease as well (57% of patients). Those with single brain lesions had an overall survival of 7.3 months, in contrast with 3.9 months for individuals with multiple secondary tumors. Surgical

resection was performed in 15 cases (11 with single lesions and 4 with multiple). Of the remaining patients, 12 underwent stereotactic biopsy and 20 had a sampling of extracranial sites for diagnosis. The tumor type was adenocarcinoma in 31%, SCC in 9%, large cell undifferentiated carcinoma in 9%, small cell carcinoma in 9%, and other histological categories in 42%. Patients who had surgical resection of their brain implants with postoperative whole brain irradiation (WBRT) had a median overall survival of 9.5 months, as opposed to 3.6 months for others who had WBRT alone ($p = 0.0022$) (79). Additional retrospective studies also have reported that overall survival is improved by surgical resection in cases of solitary brain metastasis of CUPs (80).

The distribution of intracranial metastases generally reflects blood flow; hence, 80% are located in the cerebral hemispheres, most commonly in "watershed" areas at the interface of the gray and white matter (81). Symptoms of brain metastases are highly variable. Thus, any patient with a history of malignancy and unexplained neurological changes should be examined thoroughly with possible metastasis in mind. Headaches are the presenting symptom in 40% to 50% of cases and are generally characterized as dull and nonthrobbing; they can be associated with papilledema. Seizures are the manifestation of metastasis in 10% to 20% of cases, and cerebrovascular accidents occur in another 5% to 10%. Clinical evaluation now generally includes contrast-enhanced MRI, because it is more sensitive than CT scans (82). In general, searches for the primary lesion should begin with radiological examinations of the lungs (Fig. 6).

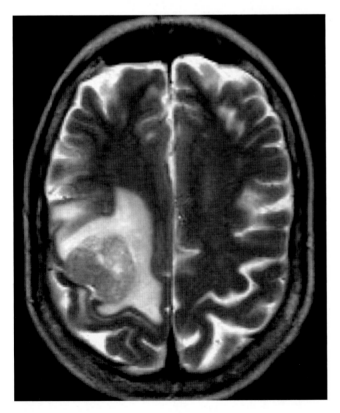

FIGURE 5 A large intracerebral metastasis is visible in this MRI of the brain.

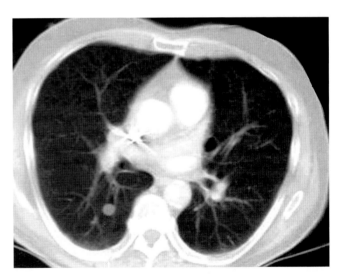

FIGURE 6 CT of the thorax shows a small nodule in the right lung field—representing bronchogenic carcinoma—in a case where the presenting clinical sign was metastasis to the brain.

Surgery for metastatic disease in the brain is performed to obtain local control of the lesions, to provide a histological diagnosis, and to treat neurological symptoms. Patients with biopsy-proven extracranial disease and high-quality imaging results showing probable brain metastases do not generally undergo surgical sampling of the latter. Otherwise, a stereotactic biopsy is usually done before initiating therapy. In cases of brain metastases of CUPs, external beam irradiation can extend survival by 12 to 20 weeks and the use of oral steroids can prolong it by 8 weeks (77). Definitive surgical therapy is generally offered only if systemic disease is felt to be adequately controlled.

In 1993, a retrospective review was reported of 56 patients seen at the M.D. Anderson Cancer Center, who had presented with multiple brain metastases. They were divided into two groups—those with multiple lesions that were all resected, and others with one or more metastases that were not surgically removed (83). An additional group of individuals with single-site metastases were matched for analysis of survival, recurrence, and improvement in symptoms. Statistical analysis showed that patients with multiple brain lesions that were completely excised had a median survival of 14 months; those with one or more unresected lesions had a median survival of six months ($p = 0.003$). Subjects with only one resected metastasis had a median survival of 14 months. Recurrence rates in these groups were not significantly different. Symptoms improved in 65% of patients with multiple incompletely resected lesions, 83% of those with multiple completely excised lesions, and 84% with single resected metastases.

The study concluded that patients with multiple completely excised brain lesions had similar survival times and symptomatic improvement as others with solitary resected metastases. Moreover, individuals in the second group who had postoperative WBRT showed improved survival, better quality of life, and decreased rates of recurrence (84). In a multicenter randomized study, Patchell et al. demonstrated a recurrence rate of 70% in cases where resection was done alone after 43 weeks. Only 18% of patients who had incomplete excisions and WBRT were alive at 48 weeks. The study concluded that subjects with single brain metastases who were treated with WBRT and surgical resection were less likely to develop intracranial recurrence than others managed with resection alone (78).

Additional therapeutic options now include stereotactic radiosurgery. This treatment modality has been used to extirpate lesions up to 4 cm in diameter, but it is most effective at treating metastases measuring <3 cm. The treatment is delivered through multiple cobalt sources or a linear accelerator. Radiosurgery can be employed for unresectable lesions, in patients unable to tolerate a craniotomy, and for tumors that are resistant to traditional radiotherapy. A retrospective study of 135 patients treated with linear accelerator–based radiosurgery demonstrated improved survival at one and two years for subjects with lesions <1 cm, compared with others who had larger metastases (85).

Bone Metastases

Metastatic lesions in bone are the initial presentation of CUP in 23% to 30% of patients (86). Osseous adenocarcinomatous metastases of unknown origin are third in frequency for CUPs, behind metastatic adenocarcinomas in the liver and lungs. Breast, lung, and prostate cancers most commonly spread to the bones and constitute up to 96% of such cases (87). Survival varies in this cohort based on the primary site, because some tumors are sensitive to hormonal modulation. The most common bony locations for metastases are the axial skeleton and long tubular bones. Pain is the leading symptom, ranging from dull aching to the severe lancinating pain associated with pathological fractures.

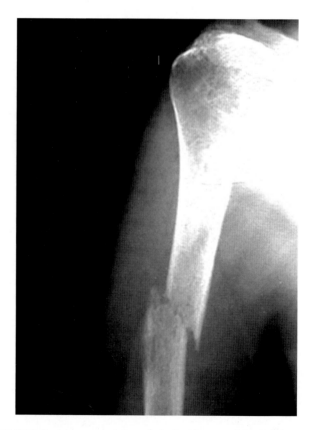

FIGURE 7   A transmetastatic pathological fracture of the right humerus is seen in this plain film, taken from a patient who later proved to have adenocarcinoma of the lung.

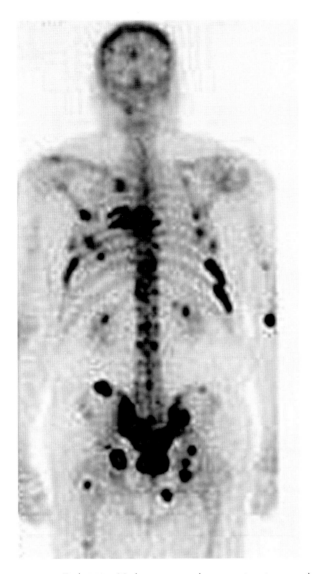

FIGURE 8 Technicium-99 bone scan, demonstrating innumerable bony metastases in a patient with renal cell carcinoma.

For the latter symptom, plain-film imaging of the bone in question should be performed, and thoracic anteroposterior radiographs and standard biochemical blood tests obtained as well. Plain bone films generally require lesions to measure at least 1 cm to be definitively detected (Fig. 7). Radionuclide scanning with technetium-99m methylene diphosphonate is reportedly more sensitive, and it can visualize lesions as small as 2 mm (Fig. 8). In recent years, FDG-PET imaging has been used as an alternative (88). This modality may alter treatment protocols in up to one-third of cases with osseous CUPs (70). After identifying a skeletal lesion, a tissue diagnosis is usually pursued. The most favored technique is core-needle biopsy of a readily accessible lesion. During biopsy, cultures for mycobacteria and fungi are recommended,

because osteomyelitis can simulate bone tumors radiographically. In regard to tumor markers, one study concluded that prostate-specific antigen is the only useful analyte in this context (87). Despite all investigative measures, primary sites for metastatic carcinomas presenting in bone are elusive in 21% of cases (87).

The management of osseous metastases generally takes the form of systemic treatment with hormonal agents or chemotherapy, or local treatment with irradiation and/or surgery. Generally, excision is reserved for patients who require palliative relief of symptoms, others who have lost the ability to ambulate, or individuals with limited disease who have progressive symptoms and signs despite chemotherapy and/or RT. Surgery is not indicated in patients with a life expectancy of less than four weeks. Moreover, individuals with prognoses of less than six months are less likely to heal fractures after stabilization (89). Restoration of the ability to ambulate has been shown to prolong survival (90).

Nonoperative interventions generally include braces, splints, or hard collar devices to stabilize the affected bones. Operative procedures comprise fixation or prosthetic replacement (Fig. 9). Patient selection for surgery should include careful assessment of additional comorbidities,

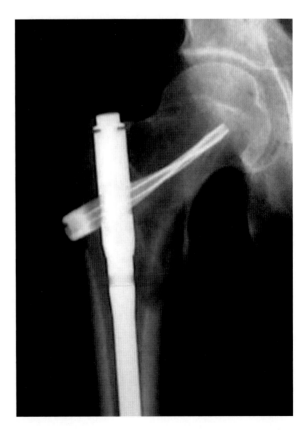

FIGURE 9 Pin-fixation of an intraosseous metastasis of breast carcinoma.

overall life expectancy, and the anatomic region of intervention. In a small series from Hong Kong, surgical spine stabilization resulted in an improvement on a visual analog pain scale from 9.3 to 1.9, and produced a mean survival of 13.1 months; one patient was alive after two years (90). Other studies concerning bone metastases from known primaries have demonstrated successful implantation of prosthetic joints; patients in these analyses sometimes survived for two or more years and had lessening of pain (91). In conclusion, subjects with osseous metastases from CUPs should undergo a thorough evaluation, biopsy of the lesions, and individualized care devised by a multidisciplinary team. Surgical intervention is appropriate for palliation of symptoms and to enable continued ambulation. Amputation has been reserved for distal lesions below the knee or elbow in patients without evidence of systemic disease (92).

■ CONCLUSIONS

The overall prognosis for patients with metastatic CUP is poor, but there are certain subsets that can be treated successfully. Those cohorts can be further refined with regard to those for whom surgical intervention has a therapeutic role. Resection of metastatic lymph-nodal disease from CUP is well described, and node dissection can be part of a multimodality treatment approach including RT and chemotherapy. Peritoneal carcinomatosis from CUP has a biological profile that is similar to that of metastatic ovarian cancer. In this setting, the application of aggressive CS, followed by systemic or intraperitoneal chemotherapy appears to be effective. The resection of single metastases from CUPs in various organs is mainly based on limited retrospective case series. Outcomes have been variable and the benefit of a localized approach needs to be judged on a case-by-case basis after review by a multidisciplinary oncology team.

■ REFERENCES

1. Jordan III WE, Shildt RA. Adenocarcinoma of unknown primary site. The Brooks Army Medical Center Experience. *Cancer* 1985; 55:857–60.
2. Galifano J, Westra WH, Koch W, et al. Unknown primary head and neck squamous cell carcinoma: molecular identification of the site of origin. *J Natl Cancer Inst* 1999; 91:599–604.
3. Greco FA, Vaughn WK, Hainsworth JD. Advanced poorly differentiated carcinoma of unknown primary site: recognition of a treatable syndrome. *Ann Intern Med* 1986; 104:547–53.
4. Frost P, Raber MN, Abbruzzese JL. Unknown primary tumors as a unique clinical and biologic entity: a hypothesis. *Cancer Bull* 1989; 41:139–41.
5. Abbruzzese JL, Abbruzzese MC, Lenzi R, Hess KR, Raber MN. Analysis of a diagnostic strategy for patients with suspected tumors of unknown origin. *J Clin Oncol* 1995; 13:2094–103.
6. Chorost MI, McKinley B, Tschoi M, Ghosh BC. The management of the unknown primary. *J Am Coll Surg* 2001; 193:666–77.
7. Greenlee RT, Murray T, Bolden S, et al. Cancer Statistics, 2000. *CA Cancer J Clin* 2000; 50:7–33.
8. Didolker MS, Fanous N, Elias EG, et al. Metastatic carcinomas from occult primary tumors. A study of 254 patients. *Ann Surg* 1997; 186:625–30.
9. Greco FA, Burris HA 3rd, Erland JB, et al. Carcinoma of unknown primary site. *Cancer* 2000; 89:2655–60.
10. Garrow GC, Greco FA, Hainsworth JD. Poorly differentiated neuroendocrine carcinoma of unknown primary tumor site. *Semin Oncol* 1993; 20:287–91.
11. Strnad CM, Grosh WW, Baxter J, et al. Peritoneal carcinomatosis of unknown primary site in women. A distinctive subset of adenocarcinoma. *Ann Intern Med* 1989; 111:213–7.
12. Dalrymple JC, Bannatyne P, Russell P, et al. Extraovarian peritoneal serous papillary carcinoma. A clinicopathologic study of 31 cases. *Cancer* 1989; 64:110–5.
13. Holmes FF, Fouts TL. Metastatic cancer of unknown primary site. *Cancer* 1970; 26:816–20.
14. Stewart JF, Tattersall MH, Woods RL, Fox RM. Unknown primary adenocarcinoma: incidence of overinvestigation and natural history. *Br Med J.* 1979 Jun 9; 1(6177):1530–3.
15. Pavlidis N, Briasoulis E, Hainsworth J, Greco FA. Diagnostic and therapeutic management of cancer of an unknown primary. *Euro J Cancer* 2003; 39:1990–2005.
16. Haskell CM, Cochran AJ, Barsky SH, et al. Metastasis of unknown origin. *Curr Probl Cancer* 1988; 12:5–58.
17. Kirsten F, Chi HE, Leary JA, et al. Metastatic adeno- or undifferentiated carcinoma from an unknown primary site: natural history and guidelines for identification of treatable subsets. *QJM* 1987; 62:143–61.
18. Le Chevalier T, Cvitkovic E, Caille P, et al. Early metastatic cancer of unknown primary origin at presentation: a clinical study of 302 consecutive autopsied patients. *Arch Intern Med* 1988; 148:2035–9.
19. Nystrom JS, Weiner JM, Heffelfinger-Juttner J, et al. Metastatic and histologic presentations in unknown primary cancer. *Semin Oncol* 1977; 4:53–8.
20. Ayoub JP, Hess KR, Abbruzzese MC, Lenzi R, Raber MN, Abbruzzese JL. Unknown primary tumors metastatic to the liver. *J Clin Oncol* 1998; 16:2105–12.
21. Hainsworth JD, Greco FA. Treatment of patients with cancer of an unknown primary site. *N Engl J Med* 1993; 329:257–63.
22. van der Gaast A, Verwij J, Planting AS, et al. The value of immunohistochemistry in patients with poorly differentiated adenocarcinomas and undifferentiated carcinomas of unknown primary. *J Cancer Res Clin Oncol* 1996; 122:181–5.
23. Randall DA, Johnstone P, Foss RD, et al. Tonsillectomy in diagnosis of the unknown primary tumor of the head and neck. *Otolaryngol Head Neck Surg* 2000; 122:52–5.
24. Mendenhall WM, Parsons JT, Mancuso AA, et al. Head and neck: management of the neck. In: Perez CA, Brady LW, eds. *Principles and Practice of Radiation Oncology.* 3rd edn. Philadelphia, PA: Lippincott Raven, 1998:1135–56.
25. Jones AS, Cook JA, Phillips DE, Roland NR. Squamous carcinoma presenting as an enlarged cervical lymph node. *Cancer* 1993; 72:1756.
26. Mui S, Li T, Rasgon M, et al. Efficacy and cost effectiveness of multihole fine-needle aspiration of squamous cell carcinoma of head and neck masses. *Laryngoscope* 1997; 107(6):759–64.

27. Pisharodi LR. False negative diagnosis in fine needle aspiration of squamous cell carcinoma of head and neck. *Diagn Cytopathol* 1997; 17:70.

28. McGuirt WF, McCabe BF. Significance of node biopsy before definitive treatment of cervical metastatic carcinoma. *Laryngoscope* 1978; 88:594.

29. Johansen J, Eigtved A, Buchwald C, et al. Implication of 18F-fluoro-2 deoxy-D-glucose positron emission tomography on management of carcinoma of unknown primary in the head and neck: a Danish cohort study. *Laryngoscope* 2002; 112:2009.

30. Nakao K, Yuge T, Mochiki M, et al. Detection of Epstein Barr virus in metastatic lymph nodes of patients with nasopharyngeal carcinoma and a primary unknown carcinoma. *Arch Otolarygol Head Neck Surg* 2003; 129:338.

31. Koch WM, Bhatti N, Williams MF, et al. Oncologic rationale for bilateral tonsillectomy in head and neck squamous cell carcinoma of unknown primary source. *Otolaryngol Head Neck Surg* 2001; 124:331–3.

32. Lapeyre M, Malissard L, Peiffert D, et al. Cervical lymph node metastasis from an unknown primary: is a tonsillectomy necessary? *Int J Radiat Oncol Biol Phys* 1997; 39:291–6.

33. Iganej S, Kagan R, Anderson P, et al. Metastatic squamous cell carcinoma of the neck from and unknown primary: management options and patterns of relapse. *Head and Neck* 2002; 24: 236–46.

34. McMahon J, Hruby G, O'Brien CJ, et al. Neck dissection and ipsilateral radiotherapy in the management of cervical metastatic carcinoma from an unknown primary. *Aust NZ J Surg* 2000; 70: 263–8.

35. Zuur CL, van Velthuysen MLF, Schornagel JH, Hilgers FJM, Balm AJM. Diagnosis and treatment of isolated neck metastases of adenocarcinomas. *EJSO* 2002; 28:147–52.

36. Yalin Y, Pingzhang T, Smith GI, Ilankovan V, et al. Management and outcome of cervical lymph node metastases of unknown primary sites: a retrospective study. *Br J Oral Maxillofac Surg* 2002; 40:484–7.

37. Mendenhall WM, Mancuso A, Amdur RJ, et al. Squamous cell carcinoma metastatic to the neck from an unknown head and neck primary site. *Am J Otolaryngol* 2001; 22:261–7.

38. Weir L, Keane T, Cummings B, et al. Radiation treatment of cervical lymph node metastases from an unknown primary: an analysis of outcome by treatment volume and other prognostic factors. *Radiother Oncol* 1995; 35:206.

39. Boscolo-Rizzo P, Gava A, Da Mosto MC. Carcinoma metastatic to cervical lymph nodes from an occult primary tumor: the outcome after combined-modality therapy. *Ann Surg Oncol* 2007; 14 (5):1575–82.

40. Erkal HS, Mendenhall WM, Amdur RJ, et al. Squamous cell carcinomas metastatic to cervical lymph nodes from an unknown head and neck mucosal site treated with radiation therapy alone or in combination with neck dissection. *Int J Radiat Oncol Biol Phys* 2001; 50(1) 55–63.

41. Yang ZH, Hu YH, Yan JH, et al. Lymph node metastases in the neck from an unknown primary. *Acta Radiol Oncol* 1983; 22: 17–22.

42. Bhatia SK, Saclarides TJ, Witt TR, et al. Hormone receptor studies in axillary metastases from occult breast cancers. *Cancer* 1987; 59:1170.

43. Jackson B, Scott-Conner C, Moulder J. Axillary metastases from occult breast carcinoma: diagnosis and management. *Am Surg* 1995; 61:431–4.

44. Muttarak M, Chaiwun B, Peh WCG. Role of mammography in diagnosis of axillary abnormalities in women with normal breast examination. *Australas Radiol* 2004; 48:306–10.

45. Obdeijn IMA, Brouwers-Kuyper EMJ, Tilanus-Linthorst MMA, et al. MR imaging guided sonography followed by FNA cytology in occult carcinoma of the Breast. *AJR* 2000; 174:1079–84.

46. Buchanan CL, Morris EA, Dorn PL, et al. Utility of breast MRI in patients with occult primary breast cancers. *Ann Surg Oncol* 2005; 12:1045.

47. Ashikari R, Rosen PP, Urban JA, Senoo T. Breast cancer presenting as an axillary mass. *Ann Surg* 1976; 183:415.

48. Merson M, Andreola S, Galimberti V, et al. Breast carcinoma presenting as axillary metastases without evidence of a primary tumor. *Cancer* 1992; 70:504.

49. Patel J, Nemoto T, Rosner D, et al. Axillary lymph node metastasis from an occult breast cancer. *Cancer* 1981; 47:2923.

50. Feigenberg Z, Zer M, Dintsman M. Axillary metastases from an unknown primary source: a diagnostic and therapeutic approach. *Isr J Med Sci* 1976; 12:1151–8.

51. Tench DW, Page DL. The unknown primary presenting with axillary lymphadenopathy. In: Bland KI, Copeland EM, eds. *The Breast: Comprehensive Management of Benign and Malignant Diseases*. Vol 2, 2nd edn. Philadelphia: WB Saunders, 1998: 1447–52.

52. Vlastos G, Jean ME, Mirza AN, et al. Feasibility of breast preservation in the treatment of occult primary carcinoma presenting with axillary metastases. *Ann Surg Oncol* 2001; 8(5).

53. Nemoto T, Vana J, Bedwani RN, Baker HW, McGregor FH, Murphy GP. Management and survival of female breast cancer: results of a national survey by the American College of Surgeons. *Cancer* 1980; 45:2917–24.

54. Carter CL, Allen C, Henson DE. Relation of tumor size, lymph node status, and survival in 24,740 breast cancer cases. *Cancer* 1989; 63:181–7.

55. Meterissian S, Fornage BD, Singletary SE. Clinically occult breast carcinoma: diagnostic approaches and role of axillary node dissection. *Ann Surg Oncol* 1995; 2:314–8.

56. van Ooijen B, Bontenbal M, Henzen-Logmans SC. Axillary nodal metastases from an occult primary consistent with breast carcinomas. *Br J Surg* 1993; 80:1299–300.

57. Campana F, Fourquet A, Ashby MA, et al. Presentation of axillary lymphadenopathy without detectable primary (T0N1b breast cancer): Experience at Institut Curie. *Radiother Oncol* 1989; 15: 321–5.

58. Fourquet A, De la Rochefordiere A, Campana F. Occult primary cancer with axillary metastases. In: Harris JR, Lippman ME, Morrow M, Hellman S, eds. *Diseases of the Breast*. 2nd edn. Philadelphia: Lippincott Williams & Wilkins, 1999:703–7.

59. Guarischi A, Keane TJ, Elhakim T. Metastatic inguinal nodes from and unknown primary neoplasm. *Cancer* 1987; 572–7.

60. Zaren HA, Copeland EM. Inguinal node metastases. *Cancer* 1978; 41(3):919–23.

61. Vilcoq JR, Calle R, Ferme F, Veith F. Conservative treatment of axillary adenopathy due to probable subclinical breast cancer. *Arch Surg* 1982; 117:1136–8.

62. Gooneratne S, Sassone M, Blaustein A, Talerman A. Serous surface papillary carcinoma of the ovary: a clinicopathologic study of 16 cases. *Int J Gynecol Pathol* 1982; 1:258–69.

63. August CZ, Murad TM, Newton M. Multiple focal extraovarian serous carcinoma. *Int J Gynecol Pathol* 1985; 4:11–23.

64. Hochster H, Wernz JC, Muggia FM. Intra-abdominal carcinomatosis with histologically normal ovaries. *Cancer Treat Rep* 1984; 68:931–2.

65. Chen KT, Flam MS. Peritoneal papillary serous carcinoma with long-term survival. *Cancer* 1986; 58:1371–3.

66. Ransom DT, Patel SR, Keeney GL, Malkasian GD, Edmonson JH. Papillary serous carcinoma of the peritoneum: a review of

33 cases treated with platin-based chemotherapy. *Cancer* 1990; 66:1091–4.

67. Lele SB, Piver MS, Matharu J, et al. Peritoneal papillary carcinoma. *Gynecol Oncol* 1988; 31:315–20.

68. Sebbag G, Shmookler BM, Chang D, Sugarbaker PH. Peritoneal carcinomatosis from an unknown primary site. Management of 15 patients. *Tumori* 2001; 87:67–73.

69. Mousseau M, Schaerer R, Lutz JM, Ménégoz F, Faure H, Swiercz P. Métastases hépatiques de site primitif inconnu. *Bull Cancer* 1991; 78:725–36.

70. Bohuslavizki KH, Klutmann S, Kroger S, et al. FDG PET detection of unknown primary tumors. *J Nucl Med* 2000; 41(5): 816–22.

71. Le Cesne A, Le Chevalier T, Caille T, et al. Metastases from cancers of unknown primary site: data from 302 autopsies. *Presse Med* 1991; 20:1369–73.

72. Kambhu, SA, Kelsen DP, Fiore J, et al. Metastatic adenocarcinoma of unknown primary site. prognostic variables and treatment results. *Am J Clin Oncol* 1990; 13:55–60.

73. Adam R, et al. Hepatic resection for noncolorectal nonendocrine liver metastases. *Ann Surg* 2006; 244(4):534–5.

74. Hogan BA, Thornton J, Brannigan M, et al. Hepatic metastases from an unknown primary neoplasm: survival, prognostic indicators and values of extensive investigations. *Clin Radiol* 2002; 57:1073–7.

75. Hemming AW, Sielaff TD, Gallinger S, et al. Hepatic resection of noncolorectal nonneuroendocrine metastases. *Liver Transplant* 2000; 6:97–101.

76. Hawksworth J, Geisinger K, Zagoria R, et al. Surgical and ablative treatment for metastatic adenocarcinoma to the liver from unknown primary tumor. *Am Surg* 2004; 70:512–7.

77. Nathoo N, Toms S, Barnett G. Metastases to the brain: current management perspectives. *Expert Rev Neurotherapeut* 2004; 4: 633–40.

78. Patchell R. Brain Metastases. *Handbook of Neurology* 1997; 25: 135–49.

79. Bartelt S, Lutterback J. Brain metastases in patients with cancer of unknown primary. *J Neuro-Onc* 2003; 64:249–53.

80. Nguyen L, Mayor M, Oswald M. Brain metastases as the only manifestation of an undetected primary tumor. *Cancer* 1998; 83: 2181–4.

81. Delattre JY, Krol G, Thaler HT, Posner JB. Distribution of brain metastases. *Arch Neurol* 1988; 45:741–4.

82. Wen P, Loeffler J. Management of brain metastases. *Oncology* 1999; 13:941–61.

83. Bindal RK, Sawaya R, Leavens ME, Lee JJ. Surgical treatment of multiple brain metastases. *J Neurosurg* 1993; 79:210–6.

84. Patchell RA, Tibbs PA, Regine WF. Postoperative radiotherapy in the treatment of single metastases to the brain: a randomized trail. *JAMA* 1998; 280:1485–9.

85. Chang E, Hassenbrusch SJ, Shiu AS, et al. The role of tumor size in the radiosurgical management of patients with ambiguous brain metastases. *Neurosurgery* 2003; 53:272–81.

86. Conroy T, et al. Histoire naturelle et evolution des metastases osseuses. Appropos des 429 observations. *Bull Cancer (Paris)* 1988; 1:296–7.

87. Destombe C, et al. Investigations for bone metastasis from an unknown primary. *Joint Bone Spine* 2007; 74:85–9.

88. Glasko C. The detection of skeletal metastases from mammary cancer by gamma camera scintigraphy. *Br J Surg* 1969; 50:3–28.

89. Gainor BJ, Buchert P. Fracture healing in metastatic bone disease. *Clin Orthop* 1983; 178:297–302.

90. Fung KY, Law SW. Management of malignant atlanto-axial tumors. *J Orth Surg* 2005; 13:232–9.

91. Harrington KD. Orthopaedic management of extremity and pelvic lesions. *Clin Orthop* 1995; 312:136–47.

92. Kawakita M, Kawamura J, Hida S, et al. *Hinyokika Kiyo* 1985; 31:463–73.

13

Postmortem Validation Studies of Carcinomas of Unknown Origin

KATHERINE CHORNEYKO

■ GENERAL CONSIDERATIONS

Metastasis of unknown origin (MUO) is typified by secondary tumor deposits due to an unknown primary site, despite a comprehensive diagnostic work-up. It is an umbrella term that encompasses any metastatic neoplasm for which the anatomic site of origin is unidentified. In the most common scenario, the tumor type is epithelial, and the syndrome is therefore termed *carcinoma of unknown primary* (CUP); however, other examples of MUO may represent melanomas, sarcomas, or other malignancies that are so poorly differentiated as to be truly unclassifiable. The overall incidence of CUPs among all malignancies varies from 4% to 10% (1). In 2003, the incidence in Canada was 19.5/100,000 in males and 14.0/100,000 in females. The overall incidence was 3% of all malignancies, a figure that has been stable over a 10-year timespan from 1993 to 2003 (2). The U.S. National Cancer Institute also quotes a similar figure for CUPs (3). Survival rates for patients with such lesions are generally extremely poor, and many individuals succumb very quickly.

An autopsy may well be requested in such cases in an attempt to identify the site of origin. On an individual basis, identification of the primary tumor can provide closure for family members, but it also supplies important information to physicians who were involved in the care of the patient. Correlation of autopsy findings with antemortem investigations and results of radiologic studies are important quality-assurance measures. Depending on the primary tumor site—if it is determinable—and other clinical findings, there may be genetic implications for other family members, and a discussion of risk factors such as smoking, diet, and sun exposure may be appropriate. On a larger scale, autopsy series have provided valuable and wide-ranging epidemiological information on this group of tumors.

The autopsy has been an important tool in the evolution of our understanding of disease in general. Anatomical dissections were carried out in ancient civilizations, but the significance of the findings that were uncovered was not understood, and they were usually interpreted in the context of the prevailing religious beliefs of the time (4). In the 1700s, Giovanni Batista Morgagni (1682–1771) performed over 700 autopsies and correlated clinical symptoms with pathologic findings. This led to a better understanding of conditions such as coronary artery disease, lobar pneumonia, and various malignancies. Subsequent physicians such as Baille (1761–1823), Rokitansky (1804–1878), Virchow (1821–1902), and Le Tulle (1853–1929) continued to correlate pathological conditions with clinical findings, and they more firmly established the value of autopsy technique as we know it today (4). A great deal of cumulative medical knowledge has been acquired since then, and much of it can be attributed to discoveries and observations made at autopsy. Despite this important and auspicious past, the medical autopsy rate has plummeted from 50% in the 1950s to 5% or less in most centers today (5).

The reasons generally cited to explain the low hospital autopsy rate include advances in medical diagnostic technology, a lack of education and experience regarding the value of the autopsy, concern regarding the transmission of infectious diseases, worries about litigation, and the objections of family members (5). A recent study examining physicians' attitudes toward the autopsy as a medical tool, however, found that most physicians are not particularly concerned about possible litigation stemming from unexpected findings at autopsy. In that survey, doctors who had been in practice for several years were more likely to have a strong belief in the relevance of autopsies than were younger physicians (5). That fact is likely related to a lack of exposure of young practitioners to necropsies. This is unfortunately a self-perpetuating problem, because low autopsy rates further diminish such familiarity. In spite of the global decrease in hospital autopsy rates, recent studies have ironically reaffirmed the value of autopsy in medical practice today (6, 7). The problem-oriented autopsy is especially encouraged, wherein attending physicians provide a clinical summary to the pathologist and raise specific questions to be answered at postmortem examination. In this scenario, the autopsy has been shown to be capable of answering 88% to 93% of the clinical questions that are posed (8).

Unfortunately, in most current health care settings, little time is provided for postmortem examinations. Shortages of professional and technical staff in pathology, the increasing volume and complexity of clinical practice, and fiscal constraints are all factors that conspire to make it difficult to perform autopsies. This is true even when complicated and puzzling clinical scenarios are encountered and a problem-oriented autopsy would be educationally beneficial.

One of the most challenging problems in clinical medicine is the scenario of a malignant tumor for which there is no identifiable primary site. Therapeutic decisions are typically made with the origin of a malignancy in mind; thus, in the absence of such knowledge, treatment choices are made more difficult. Postmortem investigations collectively have produced important contributions to our understanding of CUPs. They hopefully will continue to do so in the future, in order to improve therapy and ultimately enhance survival rates of patients with this peculiar set of tumors.

■ POSTMORTEM STUDIES

Limitations of Postmortem Data

In order to better understand the scenario of CUP, large studies that can document trends and patterns are necessary. Ideally, prospective standardized assessments would provide the most solid information; however, in any one center, these are difficult to undertake because of small volumes of cases and the subsequent length of time required to accrue sufficient data. Therefore, all of the data from autopsy studies pertaining to CUPs is principally retrospective.

Selection bias is one of the most important limitations in these types of investigations. Although one might anticipate that an autopsy would frequently be requested in cases of CUP, the actual percentage of patients who die of CUP and are necropsied is probably low. In one study where this figure was reported, 11.5% of patients dying of CUP had an autopsy performed (9). Patients with CUP who are not autopsied may have similar demographics and characteristics as those who are, but there has been no specific analysis to compare the two groups. In addition, the true incidence of patients with CUP could be under-represented in cancer registries, because primary sites of tumor are often assigned to patients based on the clinical scenario and "best available evidence," but without definite proof (9).

In light of the low incidence rate of CUP in general, any one study investigating this problem must span a number of years in order to collect sufficient numbers of cases. The time periods included in major retrospective studies in the English literature have ranged from 7 to 21 years; collectively, they span the years 1959 to 2000 (Table 1). During this period, however, significant changes in the field of immunohistochemistry (IHC) have occurred; thus, findings documented in autopsies that were done 20 or 30 years ago may not be completely relevant to current cases. Furthermore, in the past seven years, additional IHC markers have become available and are in widespread use. For example, the use of thyroid transcription factor-1 (TTF-1) (Fig. 1), an immunohistochemical marker for malignancies of lung and thyroid origin, was reported in 1996. This determinant entered general clinical use by the early 2000s (10). Therefore, by the very nature of the time periods they encompass, many studies on CUP are outdated in regard to current standards of pathology practice for assessing tumors of unknown origin.

Moreover, as a result of the retrospective nature of the investigations, there is an inherent lack of standardization. Even though autopsy techniques are, in general, universally similar, variable practices exist from center to center or pathologist to pathologist. For example, there may be variations in the amount of tissue sampled from organs that macroscopically show no abnormality. Although there *are* some limitations on this point, more generous sampling is obviously more likely to detect microscopic lesions that are not apparent macroscopically.

Retrospective Postmortem Studies

Despite the limitations of retrospective studies, a large amount of data has still been obtained from postmortem investigations of large groups of patients over time. In the English literature, six retrospective autopsy studies on

	Table 1 General information: retrospective autopsy studies				
Study	**Year of Publication and Time Span of Study**	**Number of Autopsy Cases Studied**	**Mean Age**	**Male:Female (%)**	**Primary Tumor Identified (%)**
Jordan and Shildt (11)	1985 (1971–1981)	18	58	59:41 (1.4:1)	72
Le Chevalier et al. (12)	1988 (1959–1980)	302[a]	53	75:25 (3:1)	79
Maiche (13)	1993 (1981–1988)	64	62	57:43 (1.3:1)	67
Mayordomo et al. (14)	1993 (1974–1990)	43	62	55:44 (1.3:1)	79
Blaszyk et al. (9)	2003 (1984–1999)	64	64	53:47 (1.1:1)	55
Al-Brahim et al. (1)	2005 (1980–2000)	53	66	59:41 (1.4:1)	51

[a]In 82 of these patients, the primary site was identified antemortem and confirmed at autopsy. The number of cases that came to autopsy with no known primary at the time of death was 220.

CUP of this type were published from 1980 to 2007 (Table 1). The number of cases in each series ranged from 18 to 302. In some of these analyses, examples of "CUP" were included in which the primary tumor had been identified during life and subsequently confirmed at autopsy; however, the majority of cases were true CUPs in which the anatomic origin of the neoplasm was unknown at the time of death. The mean age of the patients studied was 61 years, but there may very well be a selection bias pertaining to this figure; experientially, it is more likely that autopsies will be requested for younger patients. The male-to-female ratio ranged from 1.1–1.4:1 although in one study (from France), it was 3:1 (12). Apart from this latter statistic, these data generally correspond to population-based statistics on cancer, showing that males are slightly more likely than females to have CUP (2, 3). Such information suggests that, in at least one aspect, the demographics of the patients studied at autopsy are similar to cases in which a necropsy is not performed.

The autopsy was successful in identifying a primary site for CUP in 51% to 79% of cases. The most common anatomic origins were the lungs, pancreas, and gastro-intestinal and biliary tracts, followed, in smaller numbers, by the kidneys and liver (Table 2). These organs accounted for >50% of all primary sites for CUPs (Figs. 2–4). Pancreatic carcinoma, which has a relatively low incidence rate (approximately 3%) (2), was, in contrast, one of the most common forms of CUP. The pancreas and biliary tract are still difficult areas to image and sample during life; therefore, small tumors there may escape detection. Lung carcinoma, the second most common malignancy in both men and women (2), was also one of the most frequently detected primary tumors at autopsy in CUP cases. With the use of TTF-1 on premortem biopsy samples, it will be interesting to see if this fact is altered in future autopsy studies on CUP (because TTF-1-positive tumors would no longer be regarded as "CUPs"). Other less common primary sites, representing 5% or less of identified tumors at autopsy included the adrenals, thyroid, breasts, ovaries, oropharynx, liver, testes, and mediastinum (Fig. 5).

It is difficult to make comparisons between autopsy studies of CUP because they all spanned a considerable period of time and were, in large part, overlapping. There were, however, slight differences between them. For example, in some earlier studies, there was a tendency toward a higher percentage of primary tumors in the prostate or mesothelium, but these were not frequently seen in later series. This may again be related to improvements in the specificity of serum cancer markers [e.g., prostate-specific antigen (PSA)] as well as immunostains [PSA, various markers for mesothelioma (calretinin, WT-1, and podoplanin)].

It is worth considering that even the most recent autopsy study on CUP only includes cases accessioned up to the year 2000. In the past seven years, pathologists have seen a variety of new tissue markers besides TTF-1 and others just mentioned, for the identification of tumor origins. Some of these include Hep-Par1 for tumors of hepatic origin, renal cell carcinoma-antigen (RCC-Ag) for renal neoplasms, CDX2 for tumors of gastrointestinal origin, and monoclonal antibodies against various mucins to distinguish between mucin-producing adeno-carcinomas of various anatomic sites (15, 16). It is likely that the availability of these markers has increased

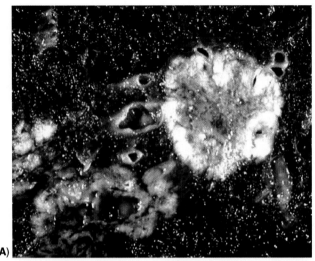

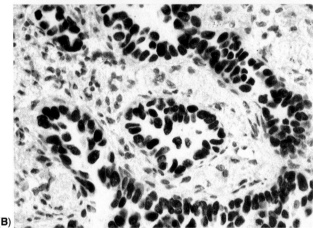

FIGURE 1 (**A**) Gross photograph of small peripheral adenocarcinoma of the lung, found at autopsy. (**B**) Immunoreactivity is seen in the tumor cells for thyroid-transcription factor-1, a marker of thyroid and pulmonary epithelial differentiation.

our ability to identify and subtype CUPs during life, but it may take additional years of study to see if this fact has an effect on cancer statistics and trends. One series assessed the percentage of CUP cases studied at autopsy in which histochemical or immunohistochemical studies were instrumental in pinpointing a primary site (1). It found that 85% of cases were amenable to determination of the tumor's anatomic origin simply by macroscopic and routine microscopic examination. This observation emphasizes the fact that, even in the *absence* of special investigations, necropsy is a successful tool in the identification of primary sites for CUPs. There have been no analyses to date that have assessed whether the growing repertoire of immunostains will alter such statistics.

Other tumor types besides carcinoma have been less commonly encountered in autopsy series on MUO (Table 2). Lymphoma accounted for up to 7% of cases in one study (14). This percentage represented three cases in which a premortem diagnosis of "undifferentiated neoplasm" was revised to one of non-Hodgkin's lymphoma at autopsy. In each of the cases, biopsy specimens had been suboptimal or were taken from an unusual site (for example, the pleura). This finding underscores the need for good tissue samples for accurate surgical pathological diagnosis. In general, with the current availability of flow cytometry and specific immunostains for hematopoietic neoplasms (Fig. 6), the diagnosis of lymphoma is virtually always possible during life. Hence, the scenario described above would be unusual indeed in modern practice. In regard to other noncarcinomatous tumor types in MUO cases, melanomas were found in four of six studies, ranging from 2% to 4% of cases; mesotheliomas were seen in three of the six studies, accounting for 2% to 5% of cases; and sarcomas were identified in three of six studies, representing 2% to 3% of cases.

Investigation of the clinical presentations of CUPs has failed to yield distinctive patterns that correlate with the anatomic sites of subsequently identified primary tumors. Clinical signs and symptoms are often related to the presence of *metastases*, rather than being indicators of tumor at the primary site (1). General deterioration (e.g., cachexia, malaise) was a common part of the presentation of CUPs, as well as respiratory or digestive-tract symptoms. Solitary lymph node enlargement was seen in a smaller number of cases (14). The causes of death in most CUP patients are similar to those of other individuals who die of disseminated malignancy with a *known* primary source. Respiratory insufficiency, gastrointestinal bleeding, cachexia, thromboembolism, and myocardial infarction are commonly seen terminal events (14).

Information concerning risk factors for malignancy in CUP cases is limited. In one study, 64% of the patients had a history of smoking (9), reaffirming that it is an important carcinogenic addiction.

Serum markers are frequently obtained premortem in many CUP cases, and they may sometimes be helpful as indicators of the likely primary site (see Chapter 6). Tumor-selective molecules such as PSA, thyroglobulin, chromogranin-A, and others may be useful if their levels in serum are elevated. However, not all neoplasms secrete or release the proteins they synthesize into the bloodstream. Furthermore, it is possible for tumors to secrete ectopic proteins that are not usually made in a particular primary site. As an example, synthesis of PSA by a nonprostatic small cell neuroendocrine carcinoma has been reported (17). This phenomenon may well result in erroneous classification of tumors if there is no histologic correlation. Prostatic acid

Table 2 Most common primary sites and pathology of CUP		
Study	**Most Common Primary Sites**	**Most Common Pathology**
Jordan and Shildt (11)	Lung, 28% Pancreas, 17% Gastric, 11% Biliary tract, 11% Mesothelium, 5%	All cases were adenocarcinomas (except for one case of mesothelioma)
Le Chevalier et al. (12)	Pancreas, 35% Gastrointestinal tract, 7% Lung, 6% Prostate, 5%	Adenocarcinoma, 45%[a] Undifferentiated carcinoma, 28% Squamous cell carcinoma, 15% Embryonal carcinoma, 4% Sarcoma, 3% Melanoma, 2% Other (not specified), 3%
Maiche (13)	Lung, 20% Kidney, 9% Gastrointestinal tract, 8% Pancreas, 6% Liver, 5%	Adenocarcinoma, 34%[b] Squamous cell carcinoma, 31% Anaplastic carcinoma, 28% Melanoma, 4% Sarcoma, 2% Clear cell carcinoma, <1% Mucocellular carcinoma, <1%
Mayordomo et al. (14)	Biliary tract, 16% Pancreas, 14% Lung, 12% Liver, 7% Lymph nodes (lymphoma), 7%	Adenocarcinoma, 53% Undifferentiated carcinoma, 11% Squamous cell carcinoma, 7% Lymphoma, 7% Hepatocellular carcinoma, 7% Neuroendocrine carcinoma, 7% Mesothelioma, 5% Melanoma, 2%
Blaszyk et al. (9)	Pancreaticobiliary, 20% Gastrointestinal tract, 14% Lung, 13%	Adenocarcinoma, 77%[c] Undifferentiated carcinoma, 12% Squamous cell carcinoma, 5% Neuroendocrine carcinomas, 4% Sarcoma, 1%
Al-Brahim et al. (1)	Lung, 30% Large bowel, 22% Pancreas, 15% Stomach, 11% Gallbladder, 7%	Adenocarcinoma, 70% Small cell carcinoma, 11% Undifferentiated carcinoma, 6% Anaplastic carcinoma, 6% Squamous cell carcinoma, 2% Melanoma, 2% Mesothelioma, 2% Neuroendocrine carcinoma, 2%

[a]These percentages include 82 cases where the primary site was identified antemortem.
[b]This percentage includes 45 cases in which there was no autopsy, but in which there was tissue available for histological examination.
[c]These percentages are based on 57 cases in which the diagnosis was made antemortem. Autopsy agreed with the antemortem diagnosis is 98% of cases.

phosphatase is not commonly used as a serum marker today, but in one early study, it was found to be elevated in some patients who did not have prostatic carcinoma at postmortem examination (12). Other serum markers such as carcinoembryonic antigen, β-human chorionic gonadotrophin, and α-fetoprotein are not specific for any given

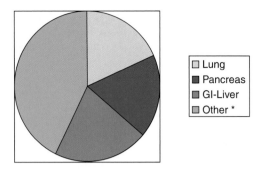

GI = Gastrointestinal tract
Other = Adenocarcinomas of kidney, prostate, and breast,
+ neuroendocrine carcinomas of nonpulmonary/pancreatic/
gastrointestinal origins

FIGURE 2 Summary of the most common primary sites for carcinoma with unknown primary, as identified at autopsy.

primary site. Hence, elevations of such determinants have correlated only very variably with the locations of primary tumors found at autopsy. This has led some authors to conclude that these proteins are not useful in delineating the origin of CUPs (12, 13).

There is an inherent expectation that the increasing sensitivity of diagnostic imaging, in conjunction with newer radiographic modalities, will improve the identification of primary tumors in CUP cases. Several reasons exist, however, to invalidate this assumption. No matter how sophisticated they are, diagnostic imaging methods cannot find all small tumors or those in locations that are inherently difficult to visualize. Tumors of the pancreas and biliary tract consistently represent relatively common primary neoplasms in CUP cases, as first discovered at autopsy. Yet, ultrasonography and computerized tomography (CT) have failed to identify them during life (14). The role of endoscopic retrograde cholangiopancreatography has not been specifically addressed in most studies on CUPs. It is an invasive procedure and would not likely be undertaken if the patient did not have specific symptoms related to the pancreas or biliary system.

Moreover, although radiological studies may demonstrate imaging abnormalities, biopsy tissue obtained from the areas in question may not be able to determine whether a tumor seen therein represents the primary lesion or a metastatic deposit. One study found that only 30% of lung nodules that were felt to be primary on the basis of radiologic studies were ultimately proven to be of pulmonary origin (12). In other words, the majority of those tumors were metastases from extrathoracic sites. Nevertheless, that study was undertaken before the availability of TTF-1 and other markers that help in defining a carcinoma as pulmonary in nature, and if it were repeated today, different results might be obtained.

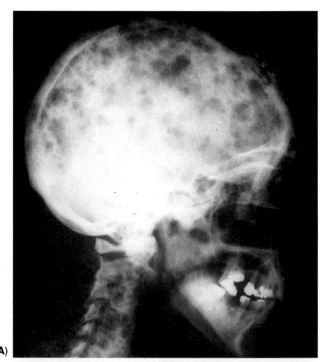

(A)

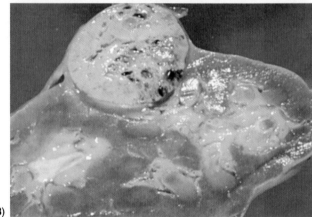

(B)

FIGURE 3 (**A**) Radiograph of bone-predominant metastatic carcinomatosis, extensively involving the skull. (**B**) A primary tumor was found in the kidney at autopsy.

Radiologically identified abnormalities must be confirmed by biopsy procedures to obtain tissue samples. If the specimens that are obtained prove to represent a benign neoplasm or a nonneoplastic process, further investigations are necessary. Patients with CUP generally have a short survival and may be medically unstable. Thus, there is often no time for extensive radiological or endoscopic procedures intended to detect a primary site.

All autopsy series to date have shown that adenocarcinomas are the most common histologic type of CUP, followed by squamous cell carcinoma and undifferentiated or anaplastic carcinoma in most studies (Table 2).

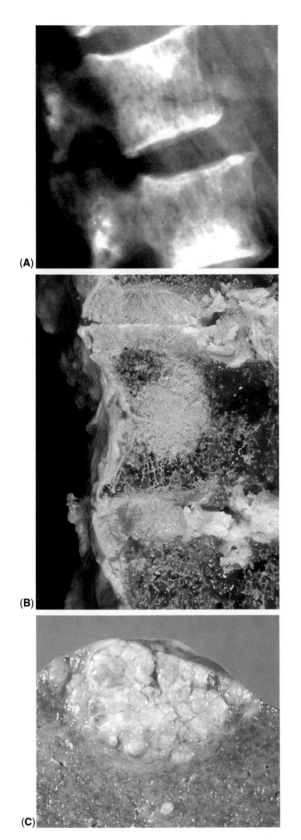

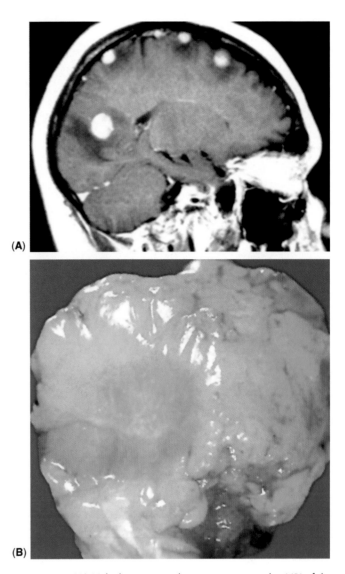

FIGURE 5 (**A**) Multiple metastatic lesions are seen in this MRI of the brain, taken from a middle-aged woman who presented with headaches. At autopsy, an invasive ductal adenocarcinoma of the left breast was found (**B**), measuring 7 mm in greatest dimension, which had eluded detection by mammography.

FIGURE 4 (**A**) Metastatic carcinoma is seen in the vertebrae in this radiograph, from an elderly man with back pain. At autopsy, the osseous lesions were confirmed (**B**), and a primary hepatocellular carcinoma was discovered (**C**).

Neuroendocrine carcinoma was identified in three of six studies and represented between 2% and 7% of cases (Fig. 7) (1, 9, 14). Other carcinoma histotypes, such as clear cell, mucoepidermoid, and germ cell, were occasionally seen (see Chapter 3). Where a premortem histological diagnosis has been available in CUP cases, correlation with autopsy findings has been variable. One study found a 98% concordance (9); however, in another series, it was only 65% (1). In some instances, disagreements in diagnosis were due to inadequate or suboptimal biopsies, but in others, significant interpretative revisions occurred even when premortem tissue samples were satisfactory. No specific

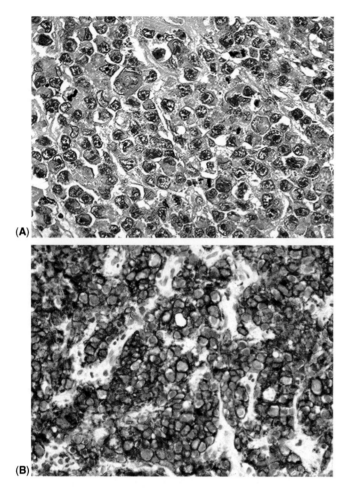

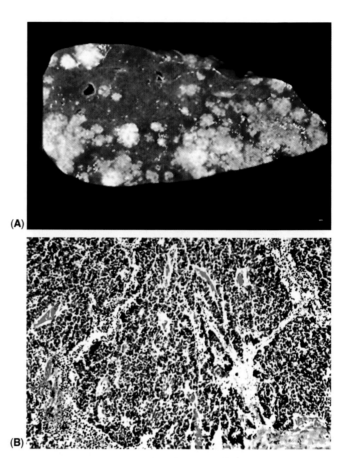

FIGURE 6 (**A**) The image of large cell non-Hodgkin's lymphoma may closely simulate that of undifferentiated carcinoma, melanoma, or selected sarcomas. However, immunostaining for CD45 (**B**) is capable of defining the hematopoietic nature of this tumor.

FIGURE 7 (**A**) Numerous metastatic lesions are present in this liver, as seen at autopsy, from an elderly man who presented with general malaise and weight loss. A small (6 mm) primary parahilar pulmonary high-grade neuroendocrine carcinoma (**B**) was found at necropsy. It had not been detected radiographically.

pattern was seen in such discrepancies; in one study, 12 of 17 diagnoses of undifferentiated carcinoma were revised at autopsy to others including non-Hodgkin's lymphoma, neuroendocrine carcinoma, hepatocellular carcinoma, mesothelioma, and melanoma (14). In another series, varying degrees of diagnostic change occurred, such as altering an interpretation of undifferentiated carcinoma to one of melanoma or mesothelioma, anaplastic carcinoma to adenocarcinoma, and poorly differentiated carcinoma (not further specified) to neuroendocrine carcinoma (1). This information once again affirms the value of necropsies in corroborating the tumor types in CUP cases.

The clinical outcome in patients with CUP is unpredictable, as it depends on a variety of factors, but in general, it is poor, as mentioned earlier. In the postmortem studies done to date, median survival after presentation has ranged from 1 to 15 months (Table 3). However, those patients who received some form of

treatment, irradiation or chemotherapy or both, did have longer survivals than those who were untreated. Some data have suggested that outcome is influenced by tumor histology. Although the numbers of cases are small, combined treatment (radiation and chemotherapy) of adenocarcinomas has shown some tendency toward longer survival as compared with similarly managed poorly differentiated carcinomas of other types (9, 11). The tissue burden of metastatic disease also correlates with survival. In one study, five-year survival rates for treated patients with metastases that were limited to cervical lymph nodes was 47%; in others who also had metastatic deposits in nodes outside the neck, it was 36% (13). In contrast, for patients who have metastases in many organ sites, the median survival is only nine months (13). The *pattern* of secondary disease may also impact survival. In one series, patients with liver or brain metastases had a worse outcome than others with lymph

Table 3 Survival rates in patients with CUP

Study	Median Survival Rates
Jordan and Shildt (11)	4 mo (treatment), <3 mo (no treatment)
Le Chevalier et al. (12)	5 mo (treatment and no treatment)
Maiche (13)	15 mo (combined chemo and radiation), 11 mo (radiotherapy alone), 3 mo (no treatment)
Mayordomo et al. (14)	1.4 mo (42 days, no treatment)
Blaszyk et al. (9)	7.5 mo (225 days, treatment); 2 mo (57 days, no treatment)
Al-Brahim et al. (1)	1 mo (treatment and no treatment)

Table 4 Common sites of metastases

Study	Most Common Primary Site	Main Sites of Metastases (%)
Jordan and Shildt (11)	Lung, 28% Pancreas, 17% Gastric, 11% Biliary tract, 11% Mesothelioma, 5%	NS
Le Chevalier et al. (12)	Pancreas, 35% Gastrointestinal tract, 7% Lung, 6% Prostate, 5%	Lymph nodes (37) Lung (19) Bone (13) Brain (10) Skin (9) Liver (5) Other (9)
Maiche (13)	Lung, 20% Kidney, 9% Gastrointestinal tract, 8% Pancreas, 6% Liver, 5%	Numerous sites (36) Bone (23) Cervical lymph nodes alone (16) Lymph nodes (10) Brain (7) Liver (5) Lung (4)
Mayordomo et al. (14)	Biliary tract, 16% Pancreas, 14% Lung, 12% Liver, 7% Lymphoma, 7%	Lymph nodes (77) Lung (70) Liver (58)
Blaszyk et al. (9)	Pancreaticobiliary, 20% Gastrointestinal tract, 14% Lung, 13%	NS
Al-Brahim et al. (1)	Lung, 30% Large bowel, 22% Pancreas, 15% Stomach, 11% Gallbladder, 7%	Lymph nodes (64) Liver (60) Lung (38) Adrenals (32) Gastrointestinal tract (25) Bone (19) Peritoneum (17) Brain (17)

Abbreviation: NS, not stated.

nodal or cutaneous metastases (12). Therefore, although the median survival of CUP patients is generally short, there are subgroups in which a better outcome is achievable. Regardless of where the primary site of a CUP may subsequently be found, the histologic type of the tumor, the degree of its differentiation, the burden of metastatic disease, and the distribution of metastases all seem to be important parameters that affect the survival of treated patients to some extent.

Autopsy studies have provided valuable information on the tissue distribution of metastases in CUP cases (Table 4). In retrospective investigations, the lymph nodes, liver, and lungs were the main sites of secondary disease. Nonetheless, many cases showed widespread metastases that were present in multiple sites (13). The pattern of metastasis in relation to the primary tumor site was frequently atypical, compared with cases where a primary neoplasm had been identified during life. For example, when they presented as CUPs, pancreatic and hepatic carcinomas tended to show a higher incidence of bone and lung involvement, as compared with "ordinary" malignancies of the pancreas and liver (11, 12). CUPs identified as originating in the gastrointestinal tract manifested more bone and brain involvement than alimentary tract carcinomas typically exhibit (12). Similarly, in cases where prostatic carcinoma was the source of a CUP, lung and liver metastases were more frequent than would otherwise be expected (Fig. 8) (12, 14). Up to 50% of pulmonary carcinomas may involve the bones, but in some series where CUPs were found to be of lung origin, osseous metastasis was much less prominent (9, 11). Therefore, it

would appear that although CUPs may be small and evade clinical detection, they have the ability to metastasize widely and in atypical patterns.

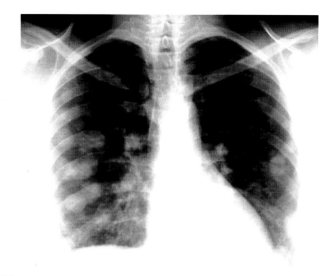

(A)

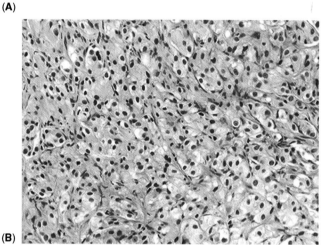

(B)

FIGURE 8 **(A)** Multiple nodular metastases are seen in both lung fields, in a chest radiograph taken from an elderly man who presented with cough. Percutaneous core biopsy of a pleural lesion **(B)**; the tumor cells were immunoreactive for prostate-specific antigen, establishing a prostatic origin for the tumor.

In light of this information, patterns of metastatic disease may be misleading in directing a search for the primary site (18). Furthermore, these findings add weight to the idea that CUP may represent a distinct clinical syndrome in which biological behavior differs from that of "ordinary" carcinomas (ie, those that are detected during life) that take origin in the same tissues or organs.

In all of the published autopsy studies on CUPs, a subset of cases continued to elude detection of a primary tumor, even after thorough postmortem examination. The percentage of such cases varied from 21% to 49%. Some authors noted that the detection rate of a primary tumor was lowest for poorly differentiated carcinomas, not further specified (9). The reasons for this fact may include the existence of very small primary lesions that evade

visualization (perhaps even with complete involution); a large burden of metastatic disease, which makes autopsy identification of a primary site very difficult; and autolysis of tissue after death, a change that degrades antigens and markedly limits immunohistochemical investigations.

Postmortem Studies Focusing on a Specific Metastatic Site of CUP

Cases of CUP have also been evaluated based on their dominant metastatic sites at presentation. The contribution of autopsy findings in those studies has been variable. Many reviews have documented cases in which primary tumors were diagnosed during life, but they included comparatively fewer cases in which the tumor origin had been undetermined after clinical investigation (ie, true cases of CUP) and before autopsy. In one series that evaluated CUPs presenting with bone involvement, the primary tumor was recognized premortem in 30% of cases and at necropsy in 35%; in the remainder, the site of origin was undetermined (19). In the latter group, approximately 70% of the patients died but no autopsy was performed; the others were either alive with disease or lost to follow-up at the time the study was done. In autopsied cases, the lung was found to be the most common site for the primary tumor. This observation contrasts with data pertaining to patients who presented with osseous metastases but had an identified primary carcinoma during life. In this cohort, the breast was the most common site for the primary tumors (19).

Such findings underscore the premise that tumors presenting as CUPs have a different biology than others that are histologically similar but obvious during life. In a separate study that also focused on skeletal metastases, the majority of cases (88%) involved a primary tumor that was identified premortem (20). In patients in whom a primary neoplasm was *not* identified during life (12%), an autopsy was performed in four of six cases, and a primary tumor was identified in three: one lung carcinoma, one hepatocellular carcinoma, and one bile duct carcinoma (20).

With regard to other predominant sites of metastatic disease, another study assessed CUPs that presented as intracerebral tumors. Among these, 27% of cases had no primary lesion identified after clinical investigations (21). Of the patients who died, autopsy was performed in 64% of cases (9 of 14), but no primary site was identified in any of them. A further study examined CUPs that manifested as malignant ascites of unknown origin; the majority of cases (80%) had an identifiable premortem primary tumor, but in those that did not, autopsy was helpful in defining the site of origin in 14% (22). In that series, the most common primary tumor locations in women were the ovaries, endometrium, and uterine cervix, whereas men tended to have lesions of the colon, rectum, and stomach (Fig. 9) (22).

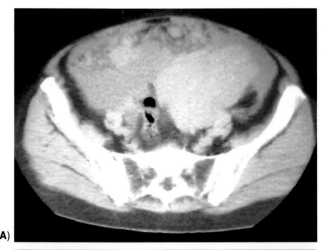

(A)

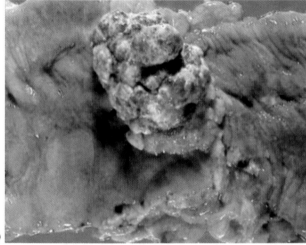

(B)

FIGURE 9 (**A**) This CT of the abdomen was obtained from a 48-year-old man who had vague abdominal discomfort, increasing girth, and evidence of ascites on physical examination. It was interpreted as showing diffuse peritoneal thickening, consistent with carcinomatosis. Paracentesis and cytological examination confirmed the presence of intraperitoneal adenocarcinoma. Although no source for the tumor was discovered during life, a primary carcinoma of the hepatic flexure (**B**) was found at autopsy.

Assessment of Case Reports

There is very little generalizable information that can be derived from published case reports, but they can provide a spectrum of information concerning unusual clinical presentations and evolutions. Individual cases are published for a variety of reasons, including atypical clinical findings or unusual tumor types, and therefore, they have a very high selection bias. A Boolean Medline search using the key words "autopsy/tumor/unknown primary," and spanning the years 1972 to 2007, yielded 171 articles from the English and non-English literature; 15% of them were case reports (Table 5). Almost half of these publications

were from the year 2000, and they therefore provide some information about the role of autopsy during the specified time period, albeit limited.

It is interesting to note that the most common sites of identifiable primary tumor at autopsy were the pancreas, biliary tract (including gallbladder), and gastrointestinal tract, representing data that are not dissimilar from those obtained in retrospective series. Furthermore, in some of the case reports, an atypical pattern of metastasis was noted. For example, a case of primary pancreatic adenocarcinoma that was found at autopsy presented clinically with neurological symptoms and intracerebral metastases (41), and a primary cholangiocarcinoma manifested as a metastatic deposit in a cervical lymph node (44). In their "usual" clinical forms, pancreatic and biliary tract tumors uncommonly involve either the brain or lymph nodes outside the abdomen (18). Only two examples of lung carcinomas that presented as CUPs were documented in case-report formats (34, 40). In one of them, premortem chest X-rays and CT scans showed atypical features in the area of the thorax where the primary tumor was ultimately identified, but these foci were considered by the radiologist to be inflammatory rather than neoplastic (40).

In approximately 30% of case reports on CUP, no primary tumor was identified, even at autopsy (26, 39). Disorders that altered normal anatomy (e.g., dysplasia or cystic disease of the kidneys) (24, 42) also figured in explanations of failure to recognize a primary tumor during life in some reports. Uncommon sites of supposed origin for CUPs (e.g., brain, adrenal) (28, 31) were also reported, emphasizing the need to consider many unusual anatomic locations in this context.

Consideration must also be given to the notion that unusual tumors may be *misidentified* as CUPs. A recently reported case of follicular dendritic cell tumor was determined to be the primary neoplasm, rather than a form of metastatic carcinoma, but that conclusion was reached only after an autopsy excluded other possibilities using extensive immunohistological and molecular investigations (46).

■ SUMMARY AND FUTURE DIRECTIONS

CUP continues to be a diagnostic and therapeutic challenge. Retrospective postmortem studies, as well as case reports, have provided important information about these tumors as a group and have confirmed the value of autopsy examination in such cases (Table 6). In individual instances, clinicians can direct their diagnostic efforts to the statistically most common anatomical sites of origin for particular tumor types, as identified in these studies.

■ Table 5 CUP autopsy case reports

Study	Clinical Scenario	Autopsy Findings
Nagelberg et al. 1985 (23)	39 yr female, 7 mo postpartum, pleural effusion, positive free beta subunit of chorionic gonadotropin	Widely disseminated poorly differentiated epidermoid carcinoma, no primary site identified
Shirai et al. 1986 (24)	33 yr female with bone metastases; antemortem biopsy showed adenocarcinoma	Widespread carcinoma with origin in dysplastic left kidney
Sunada et al. 1986 (25)	55 yr male, brain tumor and inguinal lymph nodes, antemortem histology strongly suggestive of amelanotic melanoma	No primary found
Bjornsson et al. 1986 (26)	10 yr female, no diagnosis antemortem	Primary intracranial choriocarcinoma
Bak et al. 1987 (27)	Multiple liver metastases	Adenocarcinoid tumor of the appendix
Freeman et al. 1991 (17)	Small cell carcinoma with unknown primary and elevated PSA and PAP	No definite primary identified, prostate free of tumor
Davila et al. 1993 (28)	38 yr patient with cranial nerve palsy and seizures, diagnosis of leptomeningeal carcinomatosis made on CSF exam	Leptomeningeal gliomatosis from astrocytoma of the hippocampus
Weber et al. 1993 (29)	71 yr male, *Salmonella enteritidis* septicemia	Bone marrow carcinomatosis, no primary site identified
Sakamoto et al. 1994 (30)	Not available (article in Japanese)	Autopsy confirmed gallbladder primary in 2 cases of CUP
Sakai et al. 1994 (31)	63 yr female, bone marrow positive for malignant cells	Malignant pheochromocytoma with metastases to lungs, liver, and lymph nodes
Torne et al. 1995 (32)	Widespread metastases to bone marrow and liver in third trimester of pregnancy	Infiltrating lobular carcinoma from 1.5 cm breast primary
Freidrich et al. 1997 (33)	66 yr female diagnosed with bone metastases from presumed breast primary	Primary signet-ring gastric carcinoma
Ise et al. 1998 (34)	60 yr female with metastatic tumor to bone marrow	Small focus of adenocarcinoma in the lung with widespread metastases
Pospiech et al. 2000 (35)	59 yr female with carcinomatous meningitis	No primary identified
Darvishian et al. 2002 (36)	35 yr male with familial visceral myopathy and generalized signet-ring cell carcinomatosis	No primary identified
Nakatsuji et al. 2001 (37)	Leptomeningeal carcinomatosis	No primary identified
Kloos et al. 2002 (38)	75 yr female with erythrodermia and skin biopsy showing pityriasis rubra pilaris, pleural effusion positive for malignant cells	Suspected breast primary

(Continued)

Table 5 CUP autopsy case reports (*Continued*)

Study	Clinical Scenario	Autopsy Findings
Ishihara et al. 2002 (39)	73 yr male with metastatic pulmonary tumors of unknown origin	Esophageal squamous cell carcinoma in situ with invasion and combined with choriocarcinoma and mucoepidermoid carcinoma
Sougawa et al. 2002 (40)	74 yr male, vertebral metastases of unknown origin	Primary pulmonary adenocarcinoma
Yamada et al. 2002 (41)	62 yr male, brain biopsy showing mucinous adenocarcinoma, no symptoms related to pancreatic disease	Papillary adenocarcinoma in the pancreatic head
Aita et al. 2003 (42)	71 yr female on long-term hemodialysis, peritoneal metastatic carcinoma	Sarcomatoid collecting duct carcinoma of the kidney with multicyst formation
Nabeshima et al. 2003 (43)	49 yr male with DIC, bone marrow metastases of adenocarcinoma with signet-ring cells	Poorly differentiated adenocarcinoma with signet-ring cells of the ampulla of Vater
Imamura et al. 2004 (44)	56 yr female with metastases to cervical lymph node	Undifferentiated cholangiocarcinoma
Braeuninger et al. 2005 (45)	68 yr male, leptomeningeal carcinomatosis	Gastric adenocarcinoma
Yakushijin et al. 2007 (46)	70 yr male with fatigue, anorexia, and abnormal cells of unknown origin in bone marrow	Follicular dendritic cell tumor with involvement of lymph nodes, liver, and spleen

Abbreviations: CSF, cerebrospinal fluid; CUP; carcinoma with unknown primary.

They often include the lungs, pancreas, biliary tree, and gastrointestinal tract. The intensity of a search for the primary site, however, must be balanced against the overall clinical status of the patient and the relative value of such information in future management. Without treatment, the survival of CUP patients is generally poor, emphasizing a need for quick and accurate evaluation of biopsies obtained from metastatic deposits. Pathologists who evaluate such samples should bear in mind the relative likelihood of various primary sites, vis-à-vis the clinical and histologic features of the lesions, and perform appropriate immunohistochemical and molecular studies as indicated.

Necropsy studies have confirmed that even if the primary site of a CUP cannot be determined, information concerning the type of tumor (i.e., adenocarcinoma, squamous cell carcinoma, undifferentiated carcinoma, etc.) is significant in terms of survival and treatment. From a cost-effectiveness perspective, thorough pathologic testing of biopsy samples is probably preferable to extensive radiological investigation, which is time consuming and expensive.

Table 6 Summary of information obtained from postmortem studies in cases of carcinoma with unknown primary sites

Autopsy can identify site of primary tumor in 51–79% of cases

Most common primary sites identified are lung, pancreas, gastrointestinal tract, and biliary tract

Pattern of metastases is atypical compared to known primaries of the same site

Correlation of antemortem and postmortem diagnoses ranges from 65% to 98%

Most common histological type of primary tumor is adenocarcinoma followed by squamous cell and undifferentiated carcinoma

Survival appears to be influenced by histological type of tumor and burden of metastatic disease

Improved median survival seen in patients who receive treatment (either combined chemotherapy/radiotherapy or radiation alone), while untreated patients have an extremely short survival (1–3 mo)

In this era of low hospital autopsy rates, and in light of data already available from published studies, one may question whether further postmortem assessments of CUP are necessary. Nevertheless, in individual cases, identification of a primary site will provide family members with an element of finality, concerning the reasons underlying the death of a loved one. Moreover, discussion of risk factors, and possibly genetic counseling, where appropriate, may follow.

Autopsy data improve the accrual of cancer statistics by identifying the primary sites of CUPs and also revising antemortem diagnosis in some instances. Pathologists who perform autopsies in specific CUP cases should sample judiciously from high-yield anatomic sites, even when no macroscopic lesion is identified.

Necropsy studies have strengthened the idea that the biology of tumors in CUP cases may be different from that of other tumors that originate from the same sites but are clinically detectable. The relative patterns of metastases are also often different. This information suggests that CUPs can be viewed as distinct tumor subsets, or perhaps as completely different tumor types, as compared with their histological counterparts. Thus, in the future, they may warrant very different therapeutic interventions.

Additional studies should focus not only on the identification of primary sites for CUPs but also on the biological characteristics of such tumors that confer an ability to metastasize early to atypical sites, with aggressive behavior. If immunohistochemical or molecular features can be found that identify specific subsets of CUPs, it is possible that treatment strategies can be targeted specifically to them. Molecular profiling of CUPs has already been reported (see Chapter 7), and it promises to be an important tool in the coming years (47, 48).

There are a number of other reasons supporting the continued use of the autopsy in cases of CUP (Table 7). For one, they should be able to determine whether improvements are realized in detection rates of primary sites, using new immunohistologic and molecular markers. As risk factors evolve and therapeutic strategies develop, necropsy studies can document changing trends in the biology of such neoplasms. A central national or international registry of CUP patients, including demographic data, selected risk factors, performance indicators, results of laboratory and radiological investigations, treatment details, survival, and postmortem findings, would be useful. Furthermore, a consolidated tissue bank of these tumors would greatly facilitate future investigations in molecular and genetic realms. The ever-increasing emphasis on cancer diagnosis and therapy will hopefully make these possibilities tenable in the future.

■ REFERENCES

1. Al-Brahim N, Ross C, Carter B, Chorneyko K. The value of postmortem examination in cases of metastasis of unknown origin—20 year retrospective data from a tertiary care center. *Ann Diag Pathol* 2005; 9:77–80.
2. Public Health Agency of Canada. Cancer Surveillance On-Line. http://dsol-smed.phac-aspc.gc.ca (accessed 4/17/07).
3. National Cancer Institute U.S. National Institutes of Health. http://www.cancer.gov/cancertopics/pdq/treatment/unknownprimary (accessed 4/17/07).
4. Finkbeiner WE, Ursell PD, Davis RL. *Autopsy Pathology. A Manual and Atlas.* 1st edn. Philadelphia: Churchill Livingstone, 2004:1–11.
5. Hooper JE, Geller SA. Relevance of autopsy as a medical tool. A large database of physician attitudes. *Arch Pathol Lab Med* 2007; 131:268–74.
6. Combes A, Mokhtari M, Couvelard A, et al. Clinical and autopsy diagnoses in the intensive care unit: a prospective study. *Arch Intern Med* 2004; 164:389–92.
7. Hwang DM, Chamberlain DW, Poutanen SM, Low DE, Asa SL, Butany J. Pulmonary pathology of severe acute respiratory syndrome in Toronto. *Mod Pathol* 2005; 18(1):1–10.
8. Bayer-Garner I, Fink L, Lamps L. Pathologists in a teaching institution assess the value of the autopsy. *Arch Pathol Lab Med* 2002; 126:442–7.
9. Blaszyk H, Hartmann A, Björnsson J. Cancer of unknown primary: clinicopathological correlations. *APMIS* 2003; 111(12):1089–94.
10. Holzinger A, Dingle S, Bejarano PA, et al. Monoclonal antibody to thyroid transcription factor-1: production, characterization and usefulness in tumor diagnosis. *Hybridoma* 1996; 15(1):49–53.
11. Jordan WE, Shildt RA. Adenocarcinoma of unknown primary site. The Brooke Army Medical Center experience. *Cancer* 1985; 55:857–60.
12. Le Chevalier T, Cvitkovic E, Caille P, et al. Early metastatic cancer of unknown primary origin at presentation. A clinical study of 302 consecutive studied patients. *Arch Intern Med* 1988; 148(9):2035–9.
13. Maiche AG. Cancer of unknown primary. A retrospective study based on 109 patients. *Am J Clin Oncol* 1993; 16(1):26–9.
14. Mayordomo JI, Guerra JM, Guijarro C, et al. Neoplasms of unknown primary site: a clinicopathological study of autopsied patients. *Tumori* 1993; 79:321–4.

■ **Table 7** Future role of autopsy studies in cases of CUP
Confirm antemortem findings
Determine influence of IHC and new diagnostic tests on identification of CUP
Document changing patterns of disease and the influence of new therapeutic strategies
Study molecular and genetic profiles
Collect samples for tissue banks
Further advance the understanding of the biology of these tumors

Abbreviations: CUP, carcinoma with unknown primary; IHC, immunohistochemistry.

15. Dennis JL, Hvidsten TR, Wit EC, et al. Markers of adenocarcinoma characteristic of the site of origin: development of a diagnostic algorithm. *Clin Cancer Res* 2005; 11(10):3766–72.

16. Nguyen MD, Plasil B, Wen P, Frankel WL. Mucin profiles in signet-ring carcinoma. *Arch Pathol Lab Med* 2006; 130(6):799–804.

17. Freeman NJ, Doolittle C. Elevated prostate markers in metastatic small cell carcinoma of unknown primary. *Cancer* 1991; 86(5): 1118–20.

18. Hess KR, Varadhachary GR, Taylor SH, et al. Metastatic patterns in adenocarcinoma. *Cancer* 2006; 106:1624–33.

19. Nottebaert M, Exner GU, von Hochstetter AR, Schreiber A. Metastatic bone disease from occult carcinoma: a profile. *Int Ortho* 1989; 13:119–23.

20. Katagiri H, Takahashi M, Inagaki J, et al. Determining the site of the primary cancer in patients with skeletal metastasis of unknown origin: a retrospective study. *Cancer* 1999; 86(3):533–7.

21. Giordana MT, Cordera S, Boghi A. Cerebral metastases as first symptom of cancer: a clinicopathologic study. *J Neurooncol* 2000; 50(3):265–73.

22. Ringenberg QS, Doll DC, Loy TS, Yarbro JW. Malignant ascites of unknown origin. *Cancer* 1989; 64(3):753–5.

23. Nagelberg SB, Marmorstein B, Khazaeli MB, Rosen SW. Isolated ectopic production of the free beta subunit of chorionic gonadotrophin by an epidermoid carcinoma of unknown primary site. *Cancer* 1985; 55(9):1924–30.

24. Shirai M, Ketagawa T, Nakata H, Urano Y. Renal cell carcioma originating from dysplastic kidney. *Acta Pathol Jpn* 1986; 36(8): 1263–9.

25. Sunada S, Date H, Satoh M, Iwasa H. A case of intracranial a melanotic melanoma [article in Japanese]. *No To Shinkei* 1986; 38(2):201–5.

26. Bjornsson J, Scheithauer BW, Leech RW. Primary intracranial choriocarcinoma: a case report. *Clin Neuropathol* 1986; 5(6): 242–5.

27. Bak M, Jorgensen LJ. Adenocarcinoid of the appendix presenting with metastases to the liver. *Dis Colon Rectum* 1987; 30(2):112–5.

28. Davila G, Duyckaerts C, Lasareth JP, et al. Diffuse primary leptomeningeal gliomatosis. *J Neurooncol* 1993; 15(1):45–9.

29. Weber J, Mettang T, Fritz. Lethal salmonella enteritidis meningoencephalitis in an adult with a carcinoma of an unknown primary site [article in German]. *Dtsch Med Wochenschr* 1993; 118 (3):53–6.

30. Sakamoto M, Serizawa H, Hibi T, et al. Two cases of metastases of unknown origin syndrome: confirmed gallbladder origin by autopsy [article in Japanese]. *Nippon Shokakibyo Gakkai Zasshi* 1994; 91(4):938–43.

31. Sakai C, Takagi T, Oguro M, et al. Malignant pheochromocytoma accompanied by microangiopathic hemolytic anemia: a case report. *Jpn J Clin Oncol* 1994; 24(3):171–4.

32. Torne A, Martinez-Roman S, Pahisa J, et al. Massive metastases from a lobular breast carcinoma from an unknown primary during pregnancy: a case report. *J Reprod Med* 1995; 40(9):676–80.

33. Freidrich T, Kellerman S, Leinung S. Atypical metastases of stomach carcinoma [article in German]. *Zentralbl Chir* 1997; 122(2):117–21.

34. Ise Y, Yanagawa H, Hirose T, et al. An autopsy case of cytokeratin 7-positive minute adenocarcinoma of the lung with systemic metastases. *Intern Med* 1998: 37(9):766–9.

35. Pospiech L, Orendorz-Fraczkowska K, Gawron W. A rare case of metastatic meningitis with unknown primary focus and atypical symptoms [article in Polish]. *Otolaryngol Pol* 2000; 54(Suppl. 31): 115–7.

36. Darvishian F, Bashan K. Familial visceral myopathy with carcinoma of unknown primary. *Ann Clin Lab Sci* 2002; 32(1): 93–7.

37. Nakatsuji Y, Sadahiro S, Watanabe S, et al. Leptomeningeal signet ring cell carcinomatosis presenting with ophthalmoplegia, areflexia and ataxia. *Clin Neuropathol* 2001; 20(6):272–5.

38. Kloos C, Muller UA, Hoffken K, et al. Paraneoplastic pityriasis rubra pilaris in metastatic adenocarcinoma without diagnosable primary [article in German]. *Dtsch Med Wochenschr* 2002; 127 (9):437–40.

39. Ishihara A, Mori T, Koono M. Diffuse pagetoid squamous cell carcinoma of the esophagus combined with choriocarcinoma and mucoepidermoid carcinoma: an autopsy report. *Pathol Int* 2002; 52(2):147–52.

40. Sougawa M, Ishihara H, Nagata K, et al. A case of metastatic bone tumor of missed lung cancer showing unusual manifestations on chest radiogram. *Radiat Med* 2002; 20(3):155–8.

41. Yamada K, Miura M, Miyayama H, et al. Brain metastases from asymptomatic adenocarcinoma of the pancreas: an autopsy report. *Surg Neurol* 2002; 58(5):332–6.

42. Aita K, Tanimoto A, Fujimoto Y, et al. Sarcomatoid collecting duct carcinoma arising in the hemodialysis associated acquired cystic kidney: an autopsy report. *Pathol Int* 2003; 53(7):463–7.

43. Nabeshima S, Kishihara Y, Nabeshima A, et al. Poorly differentiated adenocarcinoma with signet-ring cells of the Vater's ampulla without jaundice but with disseminated carcinomatosis. *Fukuoka Igaku Zasshi* 2003; 94(7):234–40.

44. Imamura S, Suzuki H. Head and neck metastases from occult abdominal primary site: a case report and literature review. *Acta Otolaryngol* 2004; 124(1):107–12.

45. Braeuninger S, Mawrin C, Malfertheiner P, et al. Gastric adenocarcinoma with leptomeningeal carcinomatosis as the presenting manifestation: an autopsy report. *Eur J Gastroenterol Hepatol* 2005; 17(5):577–9.

46. Yakushijin Y, Shikata H, Kito K, et al. Follicular dendritic cell tumor as an unknown primary tumor. *Int J Clin Oncol* 2007; 12 (1):56–8.

47. Buckhaults P, Zhang Z, Chen YC, et al. Identifying tumor origin using a gene expression-based classification map. *Cancer Res* 2003; 63(14):4144–9.

48. Ismael G, de Azambuja E, Awada A. Molecular profiling of a tumor of unknown origin. *NEJM* 2006; 355(10):1071–2.

Index

---

f indicate figures.
t indicate tables.